Find procedural videos for *Minimally Invasive and Office-Based Procedures in Facial Plastic Surgery* online at MediaCenter.thieme.com!

Simply visit MediaCenter.thieme.com and, when prompted during the registration process, enter the scratch-off code below to get started today.

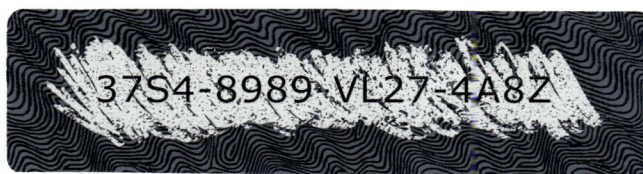

37S4-8989-VL27-4A8Z

This book cannot be returned once this panel has been scratched off.

Watch expert surgeons perform minimally invasive cosmetic facial plastic surgery procedures from the book in over 3 hours of video footage!

	WINDOWS	MAC	TABLET
Recommended Browser(s) **	Microsoft Internet Explorer 8.0 or later. Firefox 3.x	Firefox 3.x, Safari 4.x	HTML5 mobile browser. iPad — Safari. Opera Mobile — Tablet PCs preferred.
	** all browsers should have JavaScript enabled		
Flash Player Plug-in	Flash Player 9 or Higher* *Mac users: ATI Rage 128 GPU does not support full-screen mode with hardware scaling		Tablet PCs with Android OS support Flash 10.1
Minimum Hardware Configurations	Intel® Pentium® II 450 MHz, AMD Athlon™ 600 MHz or faster processor (or equivalent) 512 MB of RAM	PowerPC® G3 500 MHz or faster processor Intel Core™ Duo 1.33 GHz or faster processor 512MB of RAM	Minimum CPU powered at 800MHz 256MB DDR2 of RAM
Recommended for optimal usage experience	Monitor resolutions: • Normal (4:3) 1024×768 or Higher • Widescreen (16:9) 1280×720 or Higher • Widescreen (16:10) 1440×900 or Higher DSL/Cable internet connection at a minimum speed of 384.0 Kbps or faster WiFi 802.11 b/g preferred.		7-inch and 10-inch tablets on maximum resolution. WiFi connection is required.

Minimally Invasive and Office-Based Procedures in Facial Plastic Surgery

Thieme

Minimally Invasive and Office-Based Procedures in Facial Plastic Surgery

Fred G. Fedok, MD, FACS
Professor and Chief
Facial Plastic and Reconstructive Surgery
Otolaryngology–Head and Neck Surgery
Department of Surgery
The Hershey Medical Center
The Pennsylvania State University
Hershey, Pennsylvania

Paul J. Carniol, MD, FACS
Clinical Professor
Department of Otolaryngology–Head and Neck Surgery
Rutgers University Medical School
Newark, New Jersey

2014

Thieme
New York · Stuttgart

Thieme Medical Publishers, Inc.
333 Seventh Ave.
New York, NY 10001

Executive Editor: Tim Hiscock
Managing Editor: J. Owen Zurhellen
Editorial Assistant: Elizabeth Berg
Senior Vice President, Editorial and E-Product Development: Cornelia Schulze
Production Editor: Kenneth L. Chumbley
Medical Illustrator: Birck Cox
International Production Director: Andreas Schabert
Vice President, Finance and Accounts: Sarah Vanderbilt
President: Brian D. Scanlan
Compositor: Prairie Papers Inc.
Cover Illustration: Taken from *The Birth of Venus* (1486) by Sandro Botticelli. Image courtesy of the Uffizi Gallery, Florence, Italy, whose collection includes this painting.
Printer: Everbest Printing Co.

Library of Congress Cataloging-in-Publication Data

Minimally invasive and office-based procedures in facial plastic surgery / [edited by] Fred G. Fedok, Paul J. Carniol.
　　p. ; cm.
　Includes bibliographical references.
　ISBN 978-1-60406-567-1 (alk. paper)—ISBN 978-1-60406-568-8 (eISBN)
　I. Fedok, Fred G. II. Carniol, Paul J.
　[DNLM: 1. Cosmetic Techniques. 2. Face—surgery. 3. Ambulatory Surgical Procedures—methods. 4. Reconstructive Surgical Procedures—methods. 5. Surgical Procedures, Minimally Invasive—methods. WE 705]

　617.5′20592—dc23

2012044731

Important note: Medical knowledge is ever-changing. As new research and clinical experience broaden our knowledge, changes in treatment and drug therapy may be required. The authors and editors of the material herein have consulted sources believed to be reliable in their efforts to provide information that is complete and in accord with the standards accepted at the time of publication. However, in view of the possibility of human error by the authors, editors, or publisher of the work herein or changes in medical knowledge, neither the authors, editors, nor publisher, nor any other party who has been involved in the preparation of this work, warrants that the information contained herein is in every respect accurate or complete, and they are not responsible for any errors or omissions or for the results obtained from use of such information. Readers are encouraged to confirm the information contained herein with other sources. For example, readers are advised to check the product information sheet included in the package of each drug they plan to administer to be certain that the information contained in this publication is accurate and that changes have not been made in the recommended dose or in the contraindications for administration. This recommendation is of particular importance in connection with new or infrequently used drugs.

Some of the product names, patents, and registered designs referred to in this book are in fact registered trademarks or proprietary names even though specific reference to this fact is not always made in the text. Therefore, the appearance of a name without designation as proprietary is not to be construed as a representation by the publisher that it is in the public domain.

Printed in China

5 4 3 2 1

ISBN 978-1-60406-567-1

Also available as an e-book:
eISBN 978-1-60406-568-8

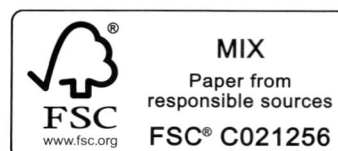

MIX
Paper from
responsible sources
FSC® C021256
www.fsc.org

To Adrienne Zoe and Eric Marshall, my children, who as infants and young children spent many hours sitting on my lap or next to me on the couch as I studied descriptions of procedures and surgical-technique videos during my years in training. They, in countless ways, made all the hours much more memorable.

Fred G. Fedok

To my sons, Michael, Alan, and Eric, and my wife, Renie. Thank you all for your thoughtful input and ongoing support in the completion of this book and my other endeavors. Your confident encouragements have made all things attainable and possible.

Paul J. Carniol

Contents

Video Contents...ix

Foreword xii

Preface..xiii

Contributors xv

1 Facial Aging, Cosmetic Concerns, and Facial Cosmetic Procedures 1
   Fred G. Fedok and Paul J. Carniol

2 Basic and Advanced Skin Care 8
   Lisa D. Grunebaum, Ilanit S. Samuels, and Leslie Baumann

3 Anesthesia and Analgesia for Facial Cosmetic Procedures..20
   Sadeq A. Quraishi

4 Techniques for Office Anesthesia: Local Anesthesia and Regional Block Techniques...............28
   David A. F. Ellis and YuShan Lisa Wilson

5 Superficial Chemical Peels 42
   Phillip R. Langsdon, David W. Rodwell III, Parker A. Velargo, Carol H. Langsdon, and Amanda Guydon

6 Medium-Depth Chemical Peels 47
   Fred G. Fedok and Dhave Setabutr

7 Hetter Chemical Peels 57
   Devinder S. Mangat

8 Deep Chemical Peels...68
   E. Gaylon McCollough

9 Skin Rejuvenation for Patients with Fitzpatrick Skin Types IV, V, and VI.......................................80
   Jennifer Parker Porter

10 Intense Pulsed Light (with and without Photodynamic Therapy) 91
    J. Randall Jordan

11 Laser Resurfacing with an Emphasis on Fractionated Technologies..98
    Louis M. DeJoseph and Paul J. Carniol

12 Treatment of Vascular Lesions...107
    William Russell Ries and Joseph E. Hall

13 Hair Removal 117
    Mark Hamilton and Jaimie DeRosa

14 Laser Treatment of Facial Scars 124
    Arden Edwards, Jennifer L. MacGregor, and Tina S. Alster

15 Surgical Treatment of Facial Scars 138
    Maurice Khosh

16 Treatment of Facial Imperfections with Dermal Fillers 147
    Georgann A. Poulos and Suzan Obagi

17 Treatment of Nasal Defects and Acne Scars with Microdroplet Silicone 158
    Jay G. Barnett and Channing R. Barnett

18 Soft Tissue Fillers for Facial Augmentation 166
    Thomas L. Tzikas

19 Facial Liposculpture and Fat Transfer 175
    Stephen E. Metzinger, James N. Parrish Jr., and Aldo B. Guerra

20 Neuromodulators 189
    Kartik Nettar, Jason P. Champagne, and Corey S. Maas

21 Endonasal Rhinoplasty 197
    Paul J. Carniol, Dhave Setabutr, and Fred G. Fedok

22 Office Rhinoplasty Techniques 209
    Ira D. Papel and Theda C. Kontis

23 Brow Rejuvenation 216
    Donn R. Chatham

24 Upper Eyelid Blepharoplasty 233
    Fred G. Fedok and Paul J. Carniol

25 Lower Blepharoplasty and Midface Rejuvenation 247
    Christina K. Magill and Jonathan M. Sykes

26 Avoidance and Management of Complications Following Lower Eyelid Surgery 257
    Farzad R. Nahai

27 Lip Rejuvenation 267
    Brian P. Maloney

28 Otoplasty and Earlobe Rejuvenation 277
    Edward H. Farrior

29 Short-Incision Facelift and Necklift 285
    Gregory J. Vipond and Harry Mittelman

30 Liposuction and Minimally Invasive Fat Reduction 300
    T. Gerald O'Daniel and Ron Hazani

31 Hair Transplantation 314
    Agata K. Brys and Daniel E. Rousso

Index 331

Video Contents

2.1 Advanced Skin Care: Superficial Chemical Peel, by Lisa D. Grunebaum
Dr. Grunebaum demonstrates a superficial chemical peel. This particular superficial peel may be used on a variety of skin types (it is very superficial). It contains hydroquinone, lactic acid, salicylic acid, and Kojic acid.

4.1 Supraorbital, Lacrimal, and Supratrochlear Nerve Blocks, by David A. F. Ellis
Dr. Ellis demonstrates nerve blocks of the supraorbital, lacrimal, and supratrochlear nerves.

4.2 Mental, Infratrochlear, and External Nasal Nerve Blocks, by David A. F. Ellis
Dr. Ellis demonstrates nerve blocks of the mental, infratrochlear, and external nasal nerves.

4.3 Infraorbital, Zygomatic-Facial, and Buccal Nerve Blocks, by David A. F. Ellis
Dr. Ellis demonstrates nerve blocks of the infraorbital, zygomatic-facial, and buccal nerves.

4.4 Zygomatic-Temporal Nerve Block, by David A. F. Ellis
Dr. Ellis demonstrates a nerve block of the zygomatic-temporal nerve.

4.5 Auriculo-Temporal Nerve Blocks, by David A. F. Ellis
Dr. Ellis demonstrates a nerve block of the auriculo-temporal nerve.

5.1 Enhanced Superficial Chemical Peel, by Dr. Phillip R. Langsdon and Carol H. Langsdon
Dr. Philip Langsdon and Carol Langsdon demonstrate the technique for a series of three progressive TCA peels. They use these progressive peels to optimize the results.

6.1 The 35% TCA/Jessner's Peel, by Fred G. Fedok
In this video, Dr. Fedok presents the science, technique, and the results of the 35% TCA peel/Jessner's.

7.1 Full-Face Hetter Peel, by Devinder S. Mangat
In this video, Dr. Mangat presents a detailed demonstration of the technique for the Hetter peel. This is an important for review prior to performing a Hetter peel.

8.1 The Baker-Gordon Peel, by E. Gaylon McCollough
Dr. McCollough demonstrates a Baker-Gordon Formula chemical peel of the upper eyelids and immediately adjacent regions.

10.1 Intense Pulsed Light with and without Photodynamic Therapy, by J. Randall Jordan
Dr. Jordan demonstrates the techniques for IPL and IPL with photodynamic therapy.

11.1 Fractionated CO2 Laser Resurfacing, by Louis M. DeJoseph
Dr. DeJoseph demonstrates fractionated CO2 laser resurfacing.

12.1   Laser Treatment of a Facial Port Wine Stain, by William Russell Ries
Dr. Ries demonstrates flashlamp pumped dye laser treatment of a port wine stain involving the left side of the face and lower eyelid region, as well as eye safety precautions for treating a lesion involving the eyelid.

13.1   Laser Hair Removal–Upper Lip, by Michele Gillen
Michelle Gillen of Hamilton Facial Plastic Surgery demonstrates laser hair removal of the upper lip with a 755 nm laser.

14.1   Laser Treatment of Scars, by Tina S. Alster
Dr. Alster demonstrates laser treatment of acne scars using a fractionated CO_2 laser and laser treatment of traumatic scars using a pulsed dye laser.

16.1   Filler Injection Techniques, by Suzan Obagi
At the start of this video, Dr. Obagi shows how she marks areas that will be treated with fillers. She then demonstrates her techniques for injecting three different facial fillers.

18.1   Tear Trough Correction with Diluted Restylane, by Thomas L. Tzikas
Dr. Tzikas demonstrates the injection of adiluted hyaluronic acid filler into a tear trough deformity.

18.2   Temporal Augmentation with CaHA, by Thomas L. Tzikas
Dr. Tzikas demonstrates the injection of calcium hydroxylapatite into the temporal region.

18.3   Intraoral Midface Augmentation with CaHA, by Thomas L. Tzikas
Dr. Tzikas demonstrates calcium hydroxylapatite injection of the midface using an intraoral approach.

18.4   Submalar PLLA, by Thomas L. Tzikas
Dr. Tzikas demonstrates the injection of poly-L-lactic acid filler into the submalar region.

18.5   Silikon 1000 Injection in the Perioral Region, by Thomas L. Tzikas
Dr. Tzikas demonstrates the injection of Silikon 1000 into the perioral region.

19.1   Facial Fat Grafting, by Drs. Metzinger, Guerra, and Parrish
Dr. Guerra gives a detailed demonstration of facial fat grafting. This includes harvesting of the fat as well as injection into several areas of the face.

20.1   Botulinum and Hyaluronic Acid Filler Enhancement of the Periorbital Area, by Corey S. Maas
Dr. Maas demonstrates the injection of botulinum toxin into the glabella and crow's feet regions. He also demonstrates the injection of a hyaluronic into the tear trough region.

21.1   Fundamental Aspects of the Endonasal Approach, by Fred G. Fedok
Dr. Fedok demonstrates various incisions and techniques used in endonasal rhinoplasty.

22.1   Needle Shave of a Nasal Dorsal Irregularity, by Ira D. Papel
Dr. Papel demonstrates the needle shave of a nasal dorsal irregularity. In this video, using this minimally invasive technique, Dr Papel reduces a limited dorsal imperfection.

23.1   Concepts in Brow Rejuvenation, by Donn R. Chatham
Dr. Chatham demonstrates several concepts in brow rejuvenation, which can be used on men or women.

24.1   Upper Blepharoplasty, by Fred G. Fedok
Dr. Fedok demonstrates upper blepharoplasty.

25.1   Midface Lift (Lower Eyelid Approach), by Jonathan M. Sykes
Dr. Sykes demonstrates a midface lift through a lower eyelid approach. This includes a detailed demonstration of the procedure.

26.1   Ectropion Repair: Lower Lid Reconstruction with Enduragen, by Farzad R. Nahai
Dr. Nahai demonstrates lower eyelid ectropion repair using a dermal collagen implant. This is one of the techniques that can be used for treatment of ectropion.

27.1 Hyaluronic Acid Injection for Lip Augmentation, by Brian P. Maloney
Dr. Maloney demonstrates lip augmentation with hyaluronic acid filler and the details of his technique.

27.2 Dermal Matrix Lip Augmentation and Vermillion Advancement, by Brian P. Maloney
Dr. Maloney demonstrates dermal matrix lip augmentation and vermillion advancement.

27.3 Upper Lip Enhancement with Nasal Base Resection, Hyaluronic Acid Filler, and Botulinum Toxin, by Brian P. Maloney
Dr. Maloney demonstrates upper lip enhancement with nasal base resection, hyaluronic acid filler, and botulinum toxin.

28.1 Otoplasty, by Edward H. Farrior
Dr. Farrior gives a precise demonstration of his technique for correcting prominent ears.

29.1 Short Incision Facelift: Multi-Vector SMAS Plication, by Harry Mittelman
Dr. Mittelman demonstrates the use of a multi-vector SMAS plication in conjunction with a short incision rhytidectomy.

30.1 Laser-Assisted Lipolysis, by T. Gerald O'Daniel
Dr. O'Daniel starts this with a demonstration of the issues being considered in one patient for whom he is planning facial rejuvenation surgery. As part of this rejuvenation procedure, he demonstrates laser-assisted lipolysis.

31.1 Follicular Unit Transplantation Surgery, by Daniel E. Rousso
Dr. Rousso gives a comprehensive presentation of his technique for hair transplantation. This starts with a presentation of the technique for harvesting the grafts and then preparing the grafts. It continues with a demonstration of follicular unit transplantation surgery.

Foreword

The most striking initial impression on picking up *Minimally Invasive and Office-Based Procedures in Facial Plastic Surgery* is its elegant simplicity. It immediately reflects the beauty and value of a superbly written book.

Dr. Fedok and Dr. Carniol, both experienced and respected practitioners and educators in facial plastic surgery, highlight the expanding role of minimally invasive procedures in aesthetic facial surgery. They have collected a coterie of leading experts who have reflected on their experience and relate their wisdom in a text that is both extensive and incisive at the same time. It paints the broad strokes and fills in the details.

Minimally Invasive and Office-Based Procedures in Facial Plastic Surgery begins with chapters on the aging process, skin care, and anaesthesia. It then discusses the various chemical peels and lasers for skin resurfacing before reviewing their application, along with surgical techniques, for treatment of scars. Subsequent chapters emphasize the importance of tissue volume management through various fillers, fat, and liposuction techniques. Neuromodulators are reviewed before the final chapters outline the extensive scope of more minimally invasive surgical procedures. These include the full gamut of techniques available today, beginning with endonasal and office rhinoplasty procedures. A variety of brow, blepharoplasty, mid face, and lower face rejuvenation procedures are detailed. Final specialty chapters describe lip rejuvenation, otoplasty, fat reduction, and hair transplantation procedures.

This book will be a highly treasured and very functional reference for the novice and experienced facial plastic surgeon, plastic surgeon, or dermatologist. Each chapter begins with key concepts that highlight the essence of the topic. An introduction, followed by relevant basic science or anatomical information and patient selection, provide valuable background prior to the concise description of technical components of the procedure. Chapters conclude with postoperative care, expected results, and complications.

For the nascent practitioner, this consistent organization provides a simple, memorable, and useful paradigm to grasp the topic. For the experienced practitioner, the experience and wisdom of the authors is apparent, the state of the art is defined, and its application to one's own specific patients can be ascertained. The chapters are all beautifully illustrated and have a large number of excellent tables that engage the reader and enhance the textual message. Postoperative photographs confirm the efficacy of the techniques described. References, often extensive, provide the immediate opportunity to obtain more specific or broader information if so desired. A number of chapters have supplementary video clips to enhance the educational experience.

Minimally Invasive and Office-Based Procedures in Facial Plastic Surgery is a collaborative, comprehensive, and concise presentation of important innovations and the state of the art as it is practiced today. Its information provides the basis for essential understanding and reflective contemplation of technical advances yet to be discovered. It is a convenient text that will prove to be a valuable and definitive resource for those seeking superior results in aesthetic facial surgery.

Peter A. Adamson, MD, FRCSC, FACS
Professor and Head
Division of Facial Plastic and Reconstructive Surgery
Department of Otolaryngology–Head and Neck Surgery
University of Toronto
Toronto, Ontario, Canada

Preface

Facial cosmetic surgery arose from many beginnings, with many practitioners and disciplines contributing to surgical techniques that aim to correct congenital and acquired facial imperfections and the unrelenting deleterious impact of aging. Over relatively few decades, the biology of many of these maladies has become better understood, surgical techniques have evolved, and technologies have been created. Along with the rapid expanse of general information and knowledge that characterizes our modern era, there has been a similar explosion in the knowledge surrounding cosmetic concerns. This collection of knowledge is at once a science, a discipline, and a craft.

In recognizing this rapidly advancing collection of knowledge and the accompanying desire to create a credible teaching vehicle, we conceptualized this book. Our first goal was to have experts from a variety of specialties and practice settings teach areas important to the practice of cosmetic surgery. Thus, all of the authors assembled are recognized experts in the practice of facial cosmetic procedures. Our second goal was to provide a "how-to" orientation within the book to propel the less experienced surgeon, as well as the more experienced surgeon, to new skill levels through the presentation of these expert methods. Finally, while this book does not cover all facial plastic procedures, it does address the ones that are most commonly performed. Specifically, the focus is on procedures that are generally of relatively short duration and that can be performed in an office or outpatient surgery center setting.

We invite you to read on, enjoying the graphics, the well-structured text, and the technique-laden videos. It has been a great privilege to work with all our contributors and to further our own knowledge as we reviewed their submitted chapters. We are confident you will find the information within to be valuable to your practice and to enhance your concepts of cosmetic surgery. In keeping with the essence of medical training and practice: we teach, we learn, and patients benefit. Enjoy!

Acknowledgments

Drs. Fedok and Carniol would like to give special thanks to the following individuals:

A most special thanks to Kim Gordon who had the nearly impossible task of keeping us moving ahead in this project, guiding the contributing authors, and using a finely sharpened editing scalpel to form the chapters into a consistent presentation for the editors at Thieme. We are indebted to her work in the creation of this book. (I, of course, am personally indebted to her also for all of her loving support and partnership in our life together. FGF)

To Beth Shultz who tirelessly worked to coordinate the communications and numerous electronic files between Drs. Fedok and Carniol, the numerous authors, and Thieme.

To Tim Hiscock, Owen Zurhellen, Elizabeth Berg, and the Thieme staff who stood by prodding, waiting, and doing everything else that superb editors and publishers do in the production of this new and innovative book.

To Birck Cox who artistically interpreted the concepts and images presented by the authors to create the exceedingly lucid artwork for this book.

Fred G. Fedok
Paul J. Carniol

Contributors

Tina S. Alster, MD
Director
Washington Institute of Dermatologic Laser Surgery
Clinical Professor of Dermatology
Georgetown University
Washington, DC

Channing R. Barnett, MD
Private Practice
Barnett Dermatology
Assistant Clinical Professor
Department of Dermatology
Columbia Presbyterian Medical Center
New York, New York
Attending Physician
James J. Peters VA Medical Center
Bronx, New York

Jay G. Barnett, MD
Private Practice
Barnett Dermatology
New York, New York

Leslie Baumann, MD
CEO
Baumann Cosmetic and Research Institute
Miami, Florida

Agata K. Brys, MD
Center for Facial Plastic and Hair Restoration Surgery
Hawthorn Medical
North Dartmouth, Massachusetts

Paul J. Carniol, MD, FACS
Clinical Professor
Department of Otolaryngology–Head and Neck
   Surgery
Rutgers University Medical School
Newark, New Jersey

Jason P. Champagne, MD
Director
The Champagne Center
Baton Rouge, Louisiana

Donn R. Chatham, MD
Chatham Facial Plastic Surgery
Louisville, Kentucky

Louis M. DeJoseph, MD
Facial Plastic Surgeon
Premier Image Cosmetic and Laser Surgery
Clinical Instructor
Department of Otolaryngology–Head and Neck
   Surgery
Emory University School of Medicine
Atlanta, Georgia

Jaimie DeRosa, MD, MS
Assistant Professor
Harvard Medical School
Department of Otolaryngology–Head and Neck
   Surgery
Massachusetts Eye and Ear Infirmary
Boston, Massachusetts

Arden Edwards, MD
PGY-5 Internal Medicine/Dermatology Resident
Georgetown University–Washington Hospital Center
Department of Dermatology
Washington, DC

David A. F. Ellis, MD, FRCSC
Professor, Division of Facial Plastic Surgery
Department of Otolaryngology–Head and Neck
   Surgery
University of Toronto
Toronto, Canada

Edward H. Farrior, MD
Medical Director
Farrior Facial Plastic Surgery Center
Associate Clinical Professor of Otolaryngology
University of South Florida
Tampa, Florida
Visiting Associate Professor of Otolaryngology
University of Virginia
Charlottesville, Virginia

Fred G. Fedok, MD, FACS
Professor and Chief
Facial Plastic and Reconstructive Surgery
Otolaryngology–Head and Neck Surgery
Department of Surgery
The Hershey Medical Center
The Pennsylvania State University
Hershey, Pennsylvania

Lisa D. Grunebaum, MD
Assistant Professor of Facial Plastics and
    Reconstructive Surgery and Clinical Dermatology
Departments of Otolaryngology and Dermatology
University of Miami Miller School of Medicine
Miami, Florida

Aldo B. Guerra, MD, FACS
Guerra Plastic Surgery Center
Scottsdale, Arizona

Amanda Guydon, BA
Aesthetician
The Langsdon Clinic
Germantown, Tennessee

Joseph E. Hall, MD
Resident Physician
Department of Otolaryngology–Head and Neck
    Surgery
Vanderbilt University Medical Center
Nashville, Tennessee

Mark Hamilton, MD
Clinical Assistant Professor
Department of Otolaryngology–Head and Neck
    Surgery
Indiana University School of Medicine
Indianapolis, Indiana

Ron Hazani, MD, FACS
Craniofacial Fellow
Division of Plastic and Reconstructive Surgery
Harvard Medical School
Massachusetts General Hospital
Boston, Massachusetts

J. Randall Jordan, MD, FACS
Professor and Vice Chair
Department of Otolaryngology–Head and Neck
    Surgery and Communicative Sciences
University of Mississippi Medical Center
Jackson, Mississippi

Maurice Khosh, MD, FACS
Assistant Clinical Professor
Department of Otolaryngology–Head and Neck
    Surgery
Columbia University
New York, New York

Theda C. Kontis, MD, FACS
Assistant Professor
Department of Otolaryngology–Head and Neck
    Surgery
Johns Hopkins Hospital
Facial Plastic Surgicenter, Ltd.
Baltimore, Maryland

Carol H. Langsdon, RNP, BSN
The Langsdon Clinic
Germantown, Tennessee

Phillip R. Langsdon, MD, FACS
Professor
Chief, Division of Facial Plastic Surgery
Department of Otolaryngology–Head and Neck
    Surgery
University of Tennessee Health Science Center
Memphis, Tennessee
Director
The Langsdon Clinic
Germantown, Tennessee

Jennifer L. MacGregor, MD
Columbia University Medical Center
Union Square Laser Dermatology
New York, New York

Corey S. Maas, MD, FACS
The Maas Clinics for Aesthetic and Facial Plastic
    Surgery
Associate Clinical Professor
University of California–San Francisco
San Francisco, California

Christina K. Magill, MD
Clinical Fellow, Facial Plastic and Reconstructive
    Surgery
Department of Otolaryngology–Head and Neck
    Surgery
University of California–Davis
Davis, California

Brian P. Maloney, MD, FACS
President
The Maloney Center PC
Atlanta, Georgia

Devinder S. Mangat, MD, FACS
Professor for Facial Plastic Surgery
Department of Otolaryngology–Head and Neck
    Surgery
University of Cincinnati
Cincinnati, Ohio
Private Practice
Cincinnati, Ohio
Vail, Colorado

E. Gaylon McCollough, MD, FACS
McCollough Plastic Surgery Clinic
Professor, Facial Plastic Surgery
Department of Surgery
University of South Alabama
Gulf Shores, Alabama

Stephen E. Metzinger, MD, MSPH, FACS
Aesthetic Surgical Associates
Clinical Associate Professor
Department of Surgery
Division of Plastic and Reconstructive Surgery
Tulane University Health Sciences Center
New Orleans, Louisiana

Harry Mittelman, MD
Fellowship Director
American Academy of Facial Plastic and
    Reconstructive Surgery
Los Altos, California

Farzad R. Nahai, MD
Rhinoplasty by Nahai
Atlanta, Georgia

Kartik Nettar, MD
Department of Head and Neck Surgery–Facial
    Plastic and Reconstructive Surgery
Kaiser Permanente
Woodland Hills Medical Center
Woodland Hills, California

Suzan Obagi, MD
Associate Professor of Dermatology
Associate Professor of Plastic Surgery
University of Pittsburgh Medical Center
Director
The Cosmetic Surgery and Skin Health Center
Pittsburgh, Pennsylvania

T. Gerald O'Daniel, MD, FACS
Private Practice
Clinical Assistant Professor, Surgery
University of Louisville Department of Plastic Surgery
Louisville, Kentucky

Ira D. Papel, MD, FACS
Associate Professor
Department of Otolaryngology–Head and Neck
    Surgery
Johns Hopkins University
Facial Plastic Surgicenter
Baltimore, Maryland

James N. Parrish Jr., MD, FACS
Mid-Louisiana Surgical Specialists
Alexandria, Louisiana

Jennifer Parker Porter, MD, FACS
Owner
Chevy Chase Facial Plastic Surgery, LLC
Chevy Chase, Maryland
Clinical Associate Professor
Department of Otolaryngology–Head and Neck
    Surgery
Georgetown University Medical Center
Washington, DC

Georgann A. Poulos, MD
Cosmetic Dermatology Fellow
The Cosmetic Surgery and Skin Health Center
Department of Dermatology
University of Pittsburgh Medical Center
Pittsburgh, Pennsylvania

Sadeq A. Quraishi, MD, MHA
Assistant Professor
Department of Anesthesia, Critical Care and Pain
    Medicine
Harvard Medical School
Massachusetts General Hospital
Boston, Massachusetts

William Russell Ries
Associate Professor
Department of Otolaryngology–Head and Neck
    Surgery
Vanderbilt University Bill Wilkerson Center
Nashville, Tennessee

David W. Rodwell III, MD
Resident
Department of Otolaryngology–Head and Neck
    Surgery
University of Tennessee Health Science Center
Memphis, Tennessee

Daniel E. Rousso, MD, FACS
Private Practice
Rousso Facial Plastic Surgery Clinic
Birmingham, Alabama

Ilanit S. Samuels, PA-C, MCMS
Cosmetic Dermatology
Baumann Cosmetic and Research Institute
Miami, Florida

Dhave Setabutr, MD
Resident
Division of Otolaryngology
The Hershey Medical Center
Pennsylvania State University
Hershey, Pennsylvania

Jonathan M. Sykes, MD, FACS
Professor
Department of Otolaryngology–Head and Neck
  Surgery
Director, Facial Plastic and Reconstructive Surgery
University of California–Davis Medical Center
Sacramento, California

Thomas L. Tzikas, MD
Private Practice
Facial Plastic Surgery
Delray Beach, Florida

Parker A. Velargo, MD
Chief Resident
Department of Otorhinolaryngology–Head and Neck
  Surgery
University of Tennessee Health Science Center
Memphis, Tennessee

Gregory J. Vipond, MD, FRCSC
Gregory J. Vipond, MD, Inc.
Otolaryngology Section
Methodist Hospital of Southern California
Arcadia, California

YuShan Lisa Wilson, MD
Associates in Otolaryngology–Head and Neck
  Surgery
Division of Facial Plastics
Worcester, Massachusetts

1 Facial Aging, Cosmetic Concerns, and Facial Cosmetic Procedures

Fred G. Fedok and Paul J. Carniol

Key Concepts

- Facial aging results from both intrinsic and extrinsic factors.

- Sunlight is the most significant external influence for aging of the skin.

- Volume loss occurs at both the skeletal and soft tissue levels of the face.

- Reversal of many of the signs of facial aging can be accomplished with the selection of appropriate techniques and technologies.

■ Introduction

This book presents and graphically illustrates frequently used surgical and minimally invasive techniques to correct many common facial cosmetic concerns. Cosmetic problems arise from aging, trauma, hereditary conditions, and exposure to powerful extrinsic factors, such as cigarette smoking and ultraviolet radiation. Changes occur superficially in both the epidermal and dermal skin components, as well as in the deeper aspects of the facial anatomy. Numerous methods and technologies are available to treat facial cosmetic problems. These "tools" can be categorized in many ways; however, most fall within the bounds of surgical procedures, light and laser technologies, chemical peels, and the use of injectable implants and fillers. A description of the aging process will help set the stage for discussion of the various technologies.

■ Facial Aging-Related Problems

Facial aging can result from a variety of causes. Some factors are intrinsic and uncontrollable; others are extrinsic and controllable to a certain degree. All human beings appear to age along a common progression; however, differences related to lifestyle, gender, and ethnicity can be seen. For example, it is noted that the Asian face ages with certain characteristics that are different from the Caucasian face.[1] Similar comparisons can be noted among other ethnic groups. Furthermore, different ethnic groups may express cultural differences in their goals for aesthetic facial surgery, and these should be considered when planning procedures.

The apparent rate of biological aging varies among individuals. Intrinsic aspects of aging appear to be highly controlled by heredity and are not largely influenced by the individual. In contrast, extrinsic factors are heavily determined by a person's habits, nutrition, and exposure to deleterious factors, such as ultraviolet light and cigarette smoking. Facial aging, for the individual, occurs with various accelerations and decelerations and does not appear to proceed at an even rate. What is apparent, however, is the commonality of progression across various ethnicities that enables certain generalities to be observed (**Fig. 1.1**).

People either consciously or unconsciously assign an apparent age to themselves and others based on facial appearance. A person's facial appearance is the visible declaration of the biological changes in the individual's basic facial structures. Aging leads to sagging, alterations in texture, and changes in facial volume and the underlying skeleton, which affect the perception of age. Once these age-related chang-

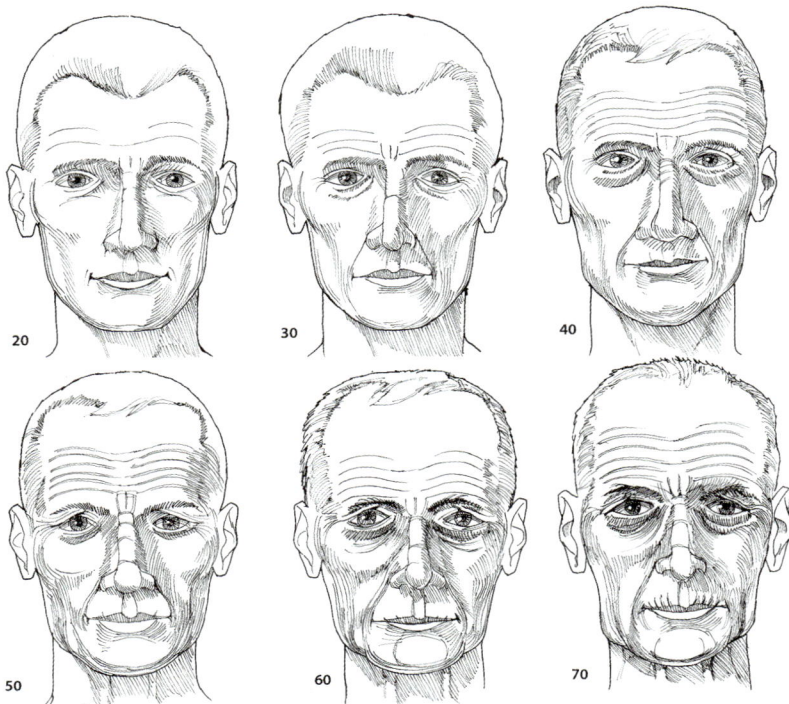

Fig. 1.1 Artist's representation of the progression of facial aging as depicted at consecutive decades during adulthood.

es have occurred, very few are reversible. However, they can be improved through makeup, cosmetic skin care, and cosmetic rejuvenative surgical and minimally invasive techniques.[2]

Changes in the Skin

The facial skin is continually exposed to a variety of external conditions, such as wind, cold, heat, and ultraviolet radiation. The last factor is the principal agent causing extrinsic aging of the skin, with effects that are significant enough to warrant the term "photoaging." This exposure extends throughout an individual's life, although it is postulated that the ultraviolet exposure occurring early in one's life is responsible for most of the changes in the skin decades later. Some authors have speculated that ~50 to 75% of a person's total lifetime ultraviolet radiation exposure occurs before 20 years of age.[3] People with fairer complexions are most susceptible to the harmful effects of ultraviolet radiation.

Sun-damaged epidermis is histologically disorganized and thickened compared with nonexposed skin. Keratinocytes lose their distinctive alignment, and a progressive flattening of the cellular architecture occurs. Dyskaryotic changes are seen in the superficial layers of the epidermis. In response to long-term exposure to sunlight, epidermal melanocytes enlarge, proliferate, and migrate to higher levels of the epidermis. This chronic stimulation of melanocytes leads to dyschromias, spotty hyperpigmentation, and the proliferation of pigmented keratoses. These changes are reflected in the dull uneven texture and pigmentation of adult sun-exposed skin.

In the deeper layers of the skin, ultraviolet radiation causes different long-term changes in addition to those seen in the epidermis. In sun-damaged skin, the region immediately beneath the epidermis develops a band of densely packed collagen with little or no elastic content.[3] Beneath this region is a broad zone of electron-dense, elastotic material. Here, curled entangled masses of the elastin-staining material are found among degenerated collagen fibrils. Elastotic degeneration of dermal architecture is a consistent histologic feature of cutaneous photodamage. These occurrences are responsible for many of the changes seen as wrinkling.[4]

Part of the aging of the skin is an inevitable degenerative process with changes that are superimposed on the external aging factors in each individual, thus producing the endless variety of problems that present. As part of the intrinsic skin-aging process, the skin varies in thickness. Skin thickness in women reaches a maximum at ~ 35 years of age and decreases gradually thereafter. In men, the curve is different, with the peak thickness occurring at 45 years of age.[5] There is a diversity of cell size and shape. The dermatoepithelial abutment is flattened with the loss of rete ridges, rendering skin fragile and susceptible to injury from shearing forces. The dermis of senescent skin is characterized by marked cellular atrophy and a corresponding reduction in metabolic activity. The percentage of newly synthesized collagen in the dermis decreases.[6] As a result, the skin is less distensible, poorly resilient, and prone to fine wrinkling.[7] As the dermis thins, there is a decrease in collagen content, degeneration of elastic fibrils, decreased water content, and the gradual addition of stable cross-links between collagen fibrils.[8]

Changes in Fat and Volume

Changes in the deeper soft tissue structures of the face complete the picture of the aging face. The face loses volume through several mechanisms. There appears to be actual fat atrophy, as well as a redistribution of fat. These alterations in the fat distribution are secondary to changes in the suspensory apparatus of the facial tissue. Principal among these suspensory mechanisms are the facial ligaments (**Fig. 1.2**): (1) zygomatic ligament, (2) mandibular ligament, (3) masseteric-cutaneous ligament, and (4) platysma-auricular ligament.[9]

In addition to the exaggeration of age-related changes from subcutaneous fat atrophy, further malposition of fibrofatty tissues and muscles and atrophy of the facial skeleton create a relative excess of skin. Absorption of the skull and facial bones occurs with advancing age. This is most prominent in the areas of the maxilla, the mandible, and the anterior nasal spine, for example, in the widening of the width of the orbital aperture.

Changes in the Brow

The procerus muscle creates transverse wrinkles at the nasal root. Descent of the lateral portion of the eyebrows may produce characteristic "hooding" of the eyes. Also, during the thirties, deeper wrinkles across the forehead begin to develop because of the action of the frontalis muscle. There is a gradual ptosis of the forehead soft tissue caused by gravity. Frequently, patients unconsciously maintain a continuously contracted frontalis to overcome this, producing deep and permanent forehead furrows.

Changes in the Periorbital Region

The changes around the eyes are closely linked to those in the forehead. Excess skin of the upper eyelids frequently appears in the late thirties because of the ptosis of the brows, as well as the developing laxity of the skin of the upper eyelid. Characteristic age-related "bags" of the lower eyelid are caused by loss of midface volume and descent of the midface, as well as weakening of the orbital septum. Photodamage, with resultant dermatochalasis, further accentuates the undesirable changes in the lower eyelid, thus producing rhytids and skin redundancy.

Fine wrinkles generally begin to appear in individuals during their twenties, deepening as they approach their thirties. "Crow's feet" may occur around the eyes in the late twenties, or earlier in persons prone to squinting. These are secondary to the contraction of the orbital portion of the orbicularis oculi muscle

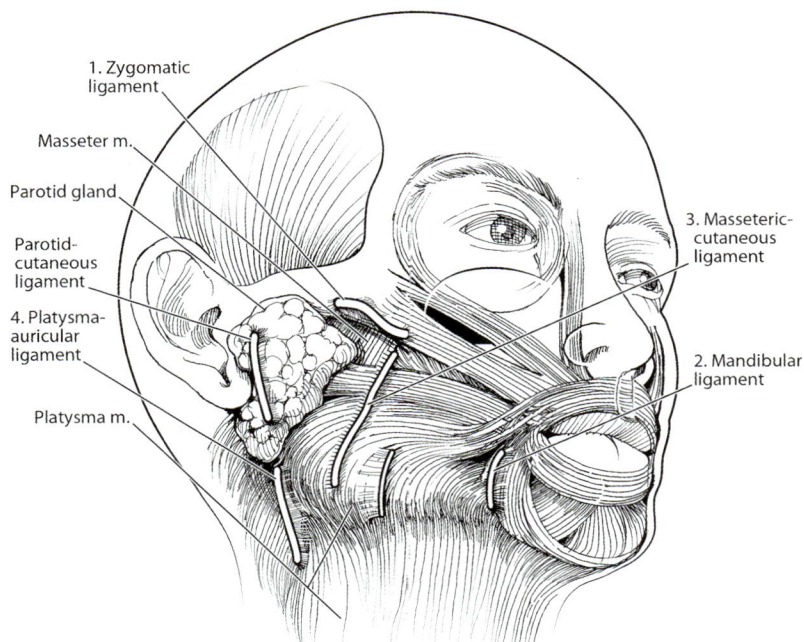

Fig. 1.2 Graphic depiction of the approximate anatomic locations of the facial ligaments: *(1)* zygomatic ligament, *(2)* mandibular ligament, *(3)* masseteric-cutaneous ligament, and *(4)* platysma-auricular ligament.

and are accentuated by elevation of the upper cheek by the zygomatic head of the quadratus labii superioris muscles. Vertical glabellar lines resulting from the contraction of the bilateral corrugator supercilii muscles frequently develop during the thirties.

Changes in the Nasolabial Region

With the attenuation of the suspensory structures in aging, several developments occur. In the lower face, many of these changes are seen to create deepening of the nasolabial fold. The nasolabial fold represents the point at which the fibers of the quadratus labii superioris, zygomaticus, and risorius muscles interdigitate and insert into the dermis.[10] Beyond the age 20 group, the groove created by these attachments grows longer and apparently deeper, eventually becoming a prominent feature of the face.

This apparent deepening in the nasolabial fold is largely caused by the more anteromedial and inferior projection of the cheek mass in older individuals and is not secondary to retrusion of the nasolabial fold itself. Sagging of the cheek soft tissue mass may form a prominence over relatively deeply creased nasolabial grooves, producing a more pronounced deformity. The descent of the midfacial structures is reflected not only in changes in the nasolabial fold, but also in more superiorly age-related changes. As the cheek mass descends, its superior projection becomes significantly lower in the older individual, leaving a paucity of soft tissues in its place.[11-13] This creates the obvious hollowing over the inferior orbital rim causing the characteristic biconvexity of midfacial aging. In all, these midface changes are multifactorial, with the common denominator of volume loss.

Changes in the Superficial Muscular Aponeurotic System (SMAS)

There is a gradual ptosis of the superficial muscular aponeurotic system (SMAS) with its overlying soft tissues in the lateral cheek and parotid region. SMAS

ptosis plays a role in the development of jowling, which disturbs the smooth, youthful contours of the mandibular line. Sagging of the SMAS and platysma extends to the neck platysma, with relaxation and lengthening of the suspensory ligaments. This gradually opens the cervicomental angle, eliminating its youthful contour. Diastasis and hypertrophy of the leading edge of the platysma muscles bilaterally produce vertical bands that bowstring across the cervicomental angle, during the fifties and later (**Fig. 1.3**).

Changes in the Nose

The most significant alterations associated with nasal aging occur in the suspension of the cartilages. The relationship between the upper and lower lateral cartilages slowly dehisces, and the support mechanisms of the tip and interdomal ligaments gradually weaken.[11] There are also changes in the medial crura. There is a downward rotation of the lobule and absorption of the fat pad in front of the anterior nasal spine, causing the feet of the medial crura to diverge and move posteriorly to produce a shortening and retraction of the columella and further downward rotation of lobule (**Fig. 1.4**). As a result, the nose is actually longer. It also appears relatively longer secondary to the vertical shortening of the lower third of the face from absorption of components of the maxilla and the mandible.

Changes in the Lips

The lips are a key feature of the central lower face. Along with the eyes and the nose, the lips and their intricate contours comprise some the integral details of the face. Fine vertical and radial wrinkling begins to appear and to increase over time during the forties. This is secondary to the underlying action of the orbicularis oris muscle. Fine vertical wrinkles perpendicular to the fibers of the orbicularis oris muscle appear on the upper lip during the late forties or early fifties. These wrinkles will appear earlier in in-

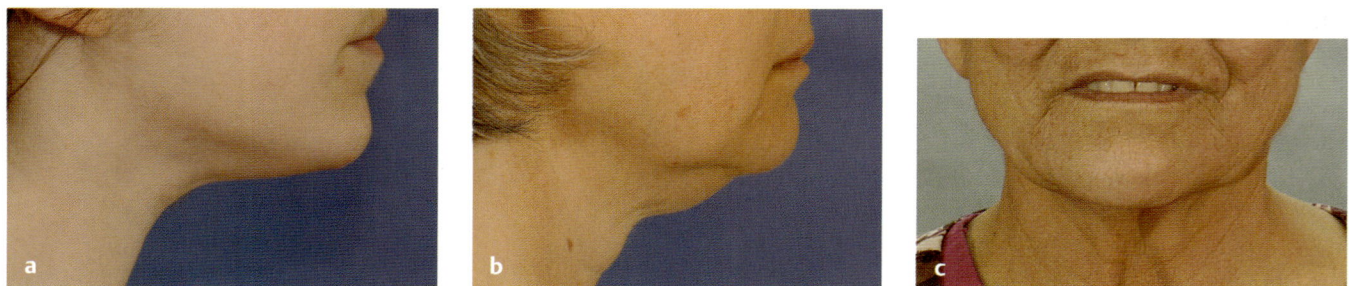

Fig. 1.3 **(a)** This patient illustrates many desirable features of the youthful neck and jaw line. **(b)** Changes associated with aging, with the relaxation and attenuation of the support of the superficial muscular aponeurotic system (SMAS)/platysma and obliteration of the cervicomental angle. **(c)** Jowling and platysmal bands secondary to the relaxation of the SMAS and platysma.

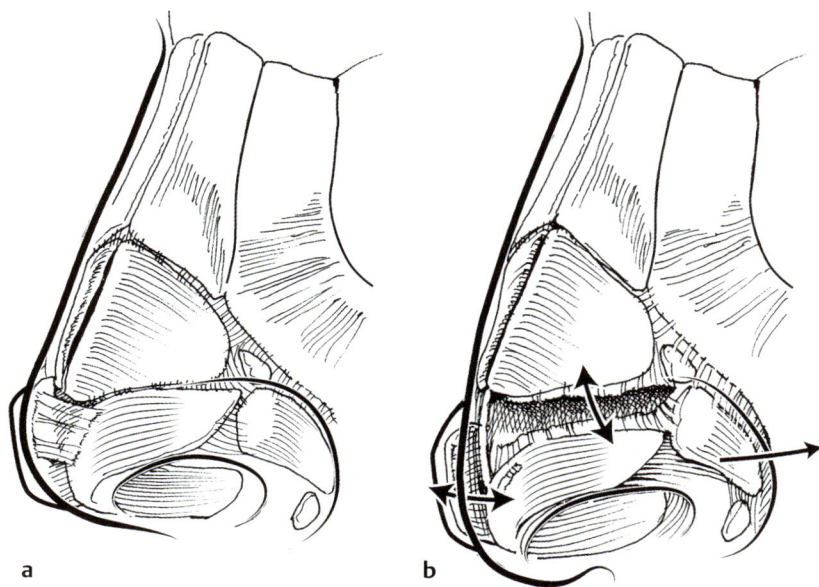

Fig. 1.4 Artist's depiction of the aging-associated changes of the nose with progressive loss of tip support, tip ptosis, and elongation. **(a)** A youthful nose, and **(b)** an aging nose.

dividuals who use tobacco. A horizontal mentolabial crease occurs after age 40, secondary to contraction of the underlying mentalis muscle. In youth, the lips are round and full with sharply detailed anatomy in the "Cupid's bow" and a sharp demarcation of the vermilion. With aging, the upper lip lengthens and descends vertically. There is a loss of the underlying tone and bulk of the orbicularis oris muscle. The projection of the vermilion slowly loses its firm support and descends, causing a loss of fullness in the exposed red lip (**Fig. 1.5**).

■ Facial Rejuvenation

Over time, various technologies and techniques have evolved to reverse, camouflage, and correct the multitude of cosmetic problems and blemishes. Many of these technologies and techniques are highly reliable, safe, and aimed at specific targets, given advances in science and anatomy. This book addresses these cosmetic issues, focusing on the following areas.

Methods to correct sagging and laxity of the skin have been largely surgical in nature, to date. These techniques remain "tried-and-true"; and although they are among the more invasive of cosmetic procedures, they generally produce the most dramatic results. For the purposes of this presentation—whereas there are promising, less-invasive skin-tightening technologies on the horizon—the surgical approaches appear to be the most reliable.

Improving the character of the skin by correcting dyschromias, fine wrinkling, and skin laxity through resurfacing continues to evolve. Traditionally, chemi-

cal peeling provided the mechanism to create a semi-controlled injury to the skin. The skin can be injured to several different levels, depending on the agent and how it is utilized. This selective variability allows for variation in patient selection as to skin type, the degree of cosmetic problem, the length of time to obtain healing, and the minimization of complications. Similar to dermabrasion, the deeper the injury, the more dramatic the result. However, the deeper the injury, the greater the likelihood of an undesirable result. In all cases, the final benefit to the patient's skin is largely secondary to the natural healing properties of the skin, not the depth of injury. This healing involves the reepithelialization of the skin, with improvement in texture and pigmentation. Tightening of the skin and the effacement of wrinkles are the result of the synthesis of new collagen bundles and the deposition of elastin.

Various chromophores are targeted with the application of laser technologies of different wavelengths. These technologies more selectively target undesirable aspects of the skin anatomy, including vascular lesions, dyschromias, unwanted hair, and water. A variety of ablative and nonablative laser technologies have allowed resurfacing to be applied to an even greater cross-section of patient skin types. Improved safety has allowed resurfacing to be performed by a greater selection of facial plastic, plastic surgical, ocular plastic, and dermatologic colleagues.

In the late 1970s and early 1980s, liposuction was popularized as a method to recontour the soft tissue in the facial area and the neck. Suction-assisted lipectomy can be performed independently or as an adjunctive procedure with facelifting, and it can involve laser-assistive technologies. In the 1980s,

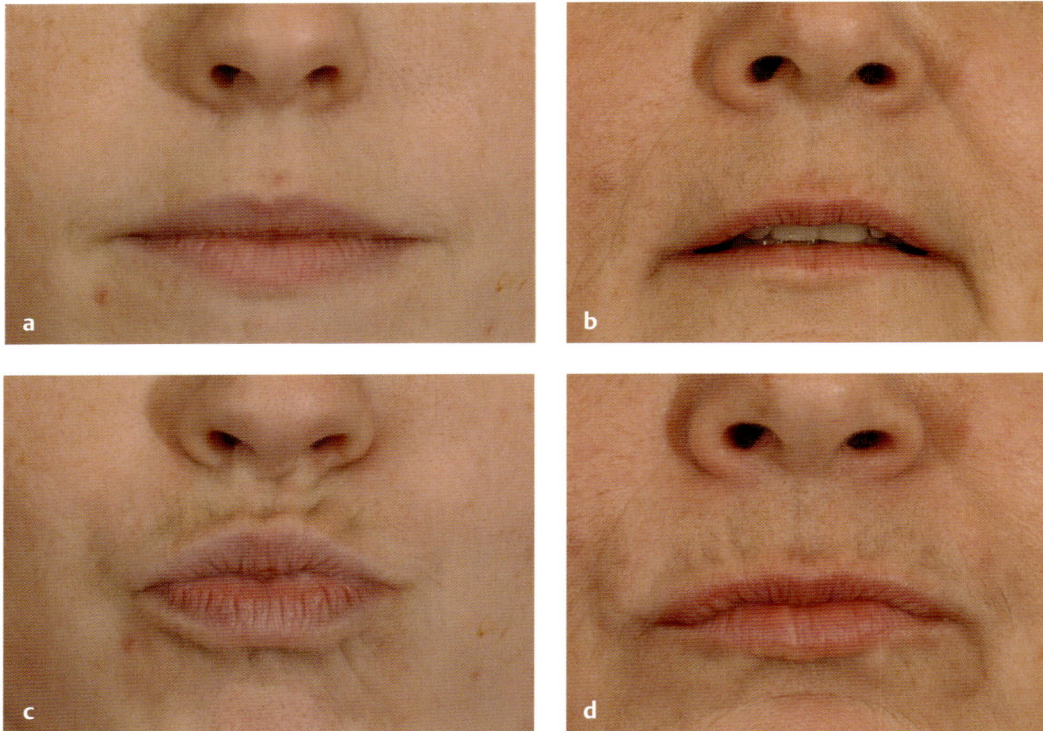

Fig. 1.5 **(a,c)** A patient in her twenties, and **(b,d)** another patient in her forties. With aging there is a draping or lengthening of the upper lip, thinning of the bulk of the red lip, and the appearance of radial rhytids that are accentuated with muscle activity.

the transfer of fat became more popular and has achieved a present peak of popularity as a means to use the patient's own fat to correct other contour deformities (i.e., volume depletion and depressions). The management of volume in the face now has bimodal attention. In areas of excess, fat removal is performed; in areas of volume depletion, fat is injected. Over all, this has allowed the practitioner to improve the areas of the face that were never adequately addressed with either resurfacing or facelifting alone.

There is a wealth of nonautogenous fillers becoming available. It is outside the scope of this particular chapter to elaborate on them. These fillers are commercially obtainable with several different underlying chemistries and physical characteristics. The duration of effect is also variable. At this time, they are safe and popular.

Finally, onabotulinum's popularity is based on its sizable safety margin, its availability, and its efficacy

for the treatment of some of the more vexing cosmetic facial problems. The use of onabotulinum toxin affords a very safe, reliable, and reproducible method to temporarily correct rhytids and hyperfunctioning lines, and to actually stabilize or lift the brows.

■ Conclusion

Over the past several decades, detailed study of the face has increased our knowledge of the cellular and structural changes that occur with aging. Additionally, there have been significant advancements in the development of new technologies, products, and surgical techniques. This current understanding of aging, coupled with these tools, has improved the ability of surgeons to reverse many of the cosmetic problems associated with aging and acquired and inherited deformities.

References

1. Shirakabe Y. The Oriental aging face: an evaluation of a decade of experience with the triangular SMAS flap technique in facelifting. Aesthetic Plast Surg 1988;12(1): 25–32

2. Fedok FG. The aging face. Facial Plast Surg 1996;12(2): 107–115

3. Consensus Development Panel. National Institutes of Health summary of the Consensus Development Conference on Sunlight, Ultraviolet Radiation, and the Skin. Bethesda, Maryland, May 8-10, 1989. [Review] J Am Acad Dermatol 1991;24(4):608–612

4. Kligman AM, Baker TJ, Gordon HL. Long-term histologic follow-up of phenol face peels. Plast Reconstr Surg 1985; 75(5):652–659

5. Leveque JL, Corcuff P, de Rigal J, Agache P. In vivo studies of the evolution of physical properties of the human skin with age. Int J Dermatol 1984;23(5):322–329

6. Bailey AJ, Robins SP, Balian G. Biological significance of the intermolecular crosslinks of collagen. Nature 1974; 251(5471):105–109

7. Daly CH, Odland GF. Age-related changes in the mechanical properties of human skin. J Invest Dermatol 1979; 73(1):84–87

8. Miyahara T, Murai A, Tanaka T, Shiozawa S, Kameyama M. Age-related differences in human skin collagen: solubility in solvent, susceptibility to pepsin digestion, and the spectrum of the solubilized polymeric collagen molecules. J Gerontol 1982;37(6):651–655

9. Furnas DW. The retaining ligaments of the cheek. Plast Reconstr Surg 1989;83(1):11–16

10. Ellis DA, Ward DK. The aging face. J Otolaryngol 1986; 15(4):217–223

11. Rubin LR, Mishriki Y, Lee G. Anatomy of the nasolabial fold: the keystone of the smiling mechanism. Plast Reconstr Surg 1989;83(1):1–10

12. Hamra ST. Repositioning the orbicularis oculi muscle in the composite rhytidectomy. Plast Reconstr Surg 1992; 90(1):14–22

13. Yousif NJ. Changes of the midface with age. Clin Plast Surg 1995;22(2):213–226

2 Basic and Advanced Skin Care

Lisa D. Grunebaum, Ilanit S. Samuels, and Leslie Baumann

Key Concepts

- Skin typing with the Baumann Skin Typing System (BSTS) allows for effective skin care by accounting for important variations in each individual patient.

- Specific cosmeceutical ingredients are useful for each skin type; practitioners and patients alike should be familiar with the myriad possibilities.

- Retinoids, antioxidants, and sunscreens are keystones to any good skin-care regimen.

- Minimally invasive procedures, such as superficial peels, microdermabrasion, and intense pulsed light (IPL), are helpful adjuncts for improving skin appearance—particularly unwanted pigment and redness.

■ Introduction

The traditional skin-type designations (i.e., dry, oily, combination, and sensitive) are insufficient in terms of directing physicians and consumers to proper product selection because these labels do not address various cutaneous characteristics, including the tendency to develop wrinkling or pigmentation. In the opinion of the authors, the BSTS is a better option for identifying skin type using a wider range of cutaneous factors based on four main skin parameters: oily versus dry; sensitive versus resistant; pigmented versus nonpigmented; and wrinkled versus tight (unwrinkled). Evaluating the skin using all four parameters results in 16 potential skin-type permutations, because these dichotomies are not mutually exclusive (**Table 2.1**). The BSTS can guide both physicians and patients/consumers in finding the most appropriate skin products. The Baumann Skin Type (BST) acts as a standardized forum in which to informatively discuss skin care. The BST is derived from a scientifically validated questionnaire, the Baumann Skin Type Indicator (BSTI), intended to ascertain baseline skin type.[1] The resulting data can be used to help identify the most suitable products and procedures for patients. This chapter briefly touches on skin-care science according to the format of the BSTS, before discussing selected minimally invasive techniques.

■ Background: Basic Science of Procedure

Dry skin is characterized by an impaired barrier, lack of natural moisturizing factor (NMF), or decreased sebum production; whereas oily skin is characterized by increased sebum production. A higher BSTI score indicates increased sebum production (oily skin); a lower score indicates reduced skin hydration (dry skin); and a score in the middle of this parameter indicates "normal" skin. Changes in climate, or traveling from one climate to another, can result in fluctuations between oily and dry skin.

Sensitive skin is characterized by inflammation and presents as acne, rosacea, burning and stinging sensations, or skin rashes. Individuals who receive a high score in the "S" portion of the BSTI are more likely to have more than one type of sensitive skin. Resistant skin is typified by a strong stratum corneum (SC) that confers cutaneous protection from allergens, other environmental factors, and water loss. Although resistant skin—as compared with sensitive skin—is less prone to acne, it is also less amenable to topical treatments, thus requiring stronger skin-care products and in-office procedures.

Pigmented skin within the BSTS framework refers not to skin color, but to the tendency to develop hyperpigmentation—particularly preventable or treat-

Table 2.1 Baumann Skin Type determined by the Baumann Skin Type Indicator

	Oily, pigmented	Oily, nonpigmented	Dry, pigmented	Dry, nonpigmented
Wrinkled, sensitive	OSPW	OSNW	DSPW	DSNW
Tight, sensitive	OSPT	OSNT	DSPT	DSNT
Wrinkled, resistant	ORPW	ORNW	DRPW	DRNW
Tight, resistant	ORPT	ORNT	DRPT	DRNT

Abbreviations: DRNT, dry, resistant, nonpigmented, tight; DRNW, dry, resistant, nonpigmented, wrinkled; DRPT, dry, resistant, pigmented, tight; DRPW, dry, resistant, pigmented, wrinkled; DSNT, dry, sensitive, nonpigmented, tight; DSNW, dry, sensitive, nonpigmented, wrinkled; DSPT, dry, sensitive, pigmented, tight; DSPW, dry, sensitive, pigmented, wrinkled; ORNT, oily, resistant, nonpigmented, tight; ORNW, oily, resistant, nonpigmented, wrinkled; ORPT, oily, resistant, pigmented, tight; ORPW, oily, resistant, pigmented, wrinkled; OSNT, oily, sensitive, nonpigmented, tight; OSNW, oily, sensitive, nonpigmented, wrinkled; OSPT, oily, sensitive, pigmented, tight; OSPW, oily, sensitive, pigmented, wrinkled.

able with skin-care products and/or procedures (i.e., ephelides, melasma, postinflammatory hyperpigmentation, and solar lentigines). Nonpigmented skin is often seen in people with light skin who do not tan easily. Knowing a patient's "P" score can guide practitioners in adjusting chemical-peel strengths and laser settings to prevent the development of postinflammatory hyperpigmentation.

The fourth parameter (wrinkled versus unwrinkled skin) is inextricably linked to aging. Cutaneous aging results from the complex intersection of intrinsic and extrinsic factors. Intrinsic aging derives from individual heredity and the natural effects of the passage of time. Extrinsic aging results from exogenous insults and manifests in premature skin aging, especially in the face. Rhytid formation, engendered by changes in the dermal layer of skin, is the primary manifestation of skin aging. Importantly, despite myriad false claims to the contrary, few skin care products are proven to adequately penetrate the dermis to improve deep wrinkles; therefore, preventing rhytids is the goal of dermatologic antiaging skin care.[2] Unwrinkled skin is skin that has been largely protected from exogenous aging factors. The remainder of this chapter focuses on specific aspects of the four BSTS parameters, as well as selected facial cosmetic procedures.

■ Technical Aspects of Procedure

Dry Skin

Basic Skin Care Formulations

Dry skin can be treated by augmenting SC hydration with occlusive or humectant ingredients and smoothing rough surfaces with an emollient. Occlu-

sives coat the SC and decelerate transepidermal water loss (TEWL); humectants attract water from the atmosphere and the epidermis; emollients soften and smooth the skin. Cleansing agents are used by people of all skin types. Surfactants are the primary active ingredients in cleansers. Cleansing products include bar surfactants, superfatted soaps, transparent soaps, combination bars, synthetic detergent bars, and liquid surfactants. Patients with dry skin should be advised to select nonfoaming agents, such as a cleansing milk, oil, or cream.

Moisturizers

Moisturizers raise water content in the SC by inhibiting TEWL through occlusive ingredients or by enhancing the integrity of the skin barrier. This is achieved via delivery of fatty acids, ceramides, and cholesterol to the skin, and controlling the calcium gradient. Moisturization is also achieved by augmenting NMF levels, glycerol (glycerin), and other humectants (e.g., hyaluronic acid). In addition, skin hydration is improved by fostering epidermal capacity to absorb important circulatory components, such as glycerol and water through aquaporin channels. Most moisturizers, which are designed to improve skin hydration, are oil-in-water emulsions (e.g., creams and lotions) or water-in-oil emulsions (e.g., hand creams).

Occlusives

Widely used in skin-care cosmetics, occlusives are oily substances that can dissolve fats and coat the SC to inhibit TEWL, resulting in an emollient effect. Petrolatum and mineral oil are among the most effective occlusives. A purified mixture of hydrocarbons derived from petroleum (crude oil) and used as a skin-care product since 1872, petrolatum, the gold standard of occlusives, displays a water vapor loss resistance 170 times that of olive oil.[3] The hydrocarbon molecules present in petrolatum prevent oxidation, giving it a long shelf life.[4] However, petrolatum has a greasy texture that many patients find unappealing. Cosmetic-grade mineral oil, a noncomedogenic agent derived from the distillation of petroleum in gasoline production, has been available for more than 100 years and is one of the more commonly used oils in skin products.[5] It is important to note that occlusives are effective only while on the skin; TEWL returns to prior levels upon removal of the agent. In moisturizers, occlusives are often combined with humectants. Lanolin, paraffin, squalene, dimethicone, propylene glycol, beeswax, soybean oil, grapeseed oil,[6] and other "natural" oils (e.g., sunflower seed, evening primrose, olive oil, and jojoba oils) are also among typically used occlusive ingredients.[7-11] Linoleic acid, an omega-6 fatty acid present in sunflower, safflower, and other oils, is an essential fatty acid, obtained from the diet or through topical application, necessary for the production of ceramide in the skin's barrier.

Humectants

Humectants are water-soluble substances with high water-absorption capacity. These compounds can attract water from the deeper epidermis and dermis in low-humidity conditions, which can aggravate dry skin.[8] Consequently, humectants are combined with occlusive ingredients to achieve the desired effect. In cosmetic moisturizers, humectant ingredients protect against evaporation and thickening of the product, thus extending the shelf life. Humectants can also change skin appearance by drawing water into the skin, causing mild SC swelling that makes the skin look smoother and less wrinkled. Manufacturers often capitalize on this phenomenon in touting some moisturizers as "antiwrinkle creams" even though no long-term antiwrinkling effects are imparted. Glycerin, urea, sorbitol, sodium hyaluronate, propylene glycol, alpha hydroxy acids (AHAs), and sugars are among the normally used humectant ingredients. Glycerin (glycerol) is a potent humectant with hygroscopic ability comparable to NMF,[9] paving the way for the SC to retain a significant amount of water even in a dry environment. Urea, included in hand creams since the 1940s,[10] is a constituent of the NMF and displays mild antipruritic activity.[11] Notably, the humectant hyaluronic acid does not penetrate into the dermis when applied topically.

Emollients

Emollients render a smooth appearance by filling the spaces between desquamating corneocytes and increasing cohesion, resulting in a flattening of the curled edges of the individual corneocytes. In addition, several emollients exhibit humectant and occlusive qualities. Occlusives that also confer an emollient effect include lanolin, mineral oil, and petrolatum. Several natural ingredients also impart such benefits. These include oatmeal, shea butter, vitamins C and E, coffeeberry, green tea, coenzyme Q10, niacinamide, soy, and glycyl-L-histidyl-L-lysine-Cu^{2+} (GHK-Cu), a copper tripeptide complex used for many years to enhance wound healing and more recently shown to augment collagen synthesis.[12,13]

Ideal moisturizers contain both humectant and occlusive ingredients. Glycerin is one of the better humectants because it can cross aquaporin channels and penetrate into the dermis. The best occlusive ingredients are oils that contain antioxidants and/or linoleic acid, including safflower, sunflower, olive, walnut, peanut, and grapeseed oils.

Sensitive Skin

Sensitive skin has defied easy characterization. Two classification systems have been proffered in the last 10 years, but a definitive typing system for sensitive skin remains elusive.[24,25] Nevertheless, sensitive skin is classified in the BSTS based on clinical manifestations: Type 1 (open and closed comedones and pimples; the acne or S1 type); Type 2 (facial flushing due to heat, spicy food, emotion, or vasodilation; the flushing rosacea or S2 type); Type 3 (burning, itching, or stinging; the S3 type); and Type 4 (developing contact dermatitis and irritant dermatitis and often associated with an impaired SC; the S4 type) (**Table 2.2**). Individuals can suffer from combinations of sensitive skin subtypes. The following discussion focuses on the primary topical treatments for sensitive skin.

Topical Treatments for Sensitive Skin

Corticosteroids

Corticosteroids block proinflammatory genes that encode cytokines, cell adhesion molecules, and other mediators, thus inhibiting the inflammatory process.[26] In particular, corticosteroids selectively induce anti-inflammatory proteins such as MAPK phospha-

Table 2.2 Types of sensitive skin

S1—Acne
S2—Rosacea
S3—Burning and stinging
S4—Susceptibility to contact and irritant dermatitis

tase and annexin I, which physically interact with and suppress cytosolic phospholipase A_2a ($cPLA_2a$).[27] Consequently, corticosteroids inhibit arachidonic acid release and a subsequent conversion to eicosanoids.[28] The use of topical corticosteroids is generally safe for short-term treatment of inflammatory skin diseases. However, long-term use can produce adverse cutaneous effects (e.g., acne, folliculitis, hirsutism, purpura, pigmentary changes, skin atrophy, striae, and telangiectasia).[29,30] Chronic topical corticosteroid use has also led to more serious systemic side effects, such as avascular osteonecrosis, glaucoma, hyperglycemia, hypothalamic-pituitary axis (HPA) suppression, and posterior subcapsular cataracts.[31–39] Although corticosteroids can effectively treat rosacea, they should be avoided for this indication because their use engenders compensatory redness upon discontinuation and their protracted use can thin the skin.

Cyclooxygenase Inhibitors

Several nonsteroidal anti-inflammatory drugs (NSAIDs) specifically target the bioactive lipids produced by arachidonic acid. For example, ibuprofen has shown success in treating acne because inflammatory acne lesions are infiltrated with neutrophils, and ibuprofen inhibits leukocyte chemotaxis.[32] Sunburn can also be treated with NSAIDs. In a randomized double-blind crossover study of 19 psoriatic patients receiving ultraviolet B (UVB) phototherapy conducted more than 30 years ago, researchers compared ibuprofen with placebo and evaluated signs and symptoms of UVB-induced inflammation. A statistically significant difference was found only in the technician's assessment of erythema; however, findings suggested that ibuprofen was more effective than placebo in delivering symptomatic relief of UVB-induced inflammation following high doses of UVB-phototherapy for psoriasis. Based on the observation that dermal prostaglandins are increased after UVB irradiation, it is thought that an NSAID that interrupts prostaglandin synthesis may attenuate UVB-induced inflammation.[33]

Salicylic Acid

Salicylates have demonstrated anti-inflammatory and antimicrobial activity in experimental as well as clinical settings.[34] Salicylic acid, a member of the aspirin family, interrupts the arachidonic acid cascade, thus exerting analgesic and anti-inflammatory effects. Salicylates control inflammation by inhibiting proinflammatory gene expression. Salicylic acid decreases the frequency and severity of acne eruptions by mitigating acne-related inflammation and delivering exfoliating activity to the pores. Because it is lipophilic, it is better able than glycolic acid to penetrate the sebum in skin pores, which accounts

for its popularity in OTC acne products. Salicylic acid 2% cleansers are effective treatment options for rosacea patients with oily skin.

Sulfur/Sulfacetamide

Sulfur, usually an adjuvant therapy, is used primarily to treat acne, seborrheic dermatitis, rosacea, scabies, and tinea versicolor.[35] Elemental sulfur and its various forms (e.g., sulfides, sulfites, and mercaptans) act as anti-inflammatory agents and reportedly display antifungal, antimicrobial, and antiparasitic activity.[36] Sulfur is often combined with sodium sulfacetamide, a sulfonamide agent with antibacterial properties, specifically acting as a competitive antagonist to para-aminobenzoic acid (PABA), an essential component for bacterial growth,[37] and *Propionibacterium acnes*.[38] The keratolytic and anti-inflammatory activity of sulfur and the antibacterial properties of sulfacetamide in a topical formulation render an effective treatment for acne vulgaris, rosacea, and seborrheic dermatitis.[39] Sulfur is often found with sodium sulfacetamide in cream, lotion, gel topical suspension, cleanser, and silica-based mask preparations. However, the odor of many of these products has been likened to rotten eggs, thus limiting their popularity.

Natural Ingredients

In the past 20 years, botanically derived products have gained widespread use and interest in the United States.[40] Indeed, several such ingredients, including aloe vera,[41,42] chamomile,[43,44] feverfew,[45,46] ginseng,[47,48] licorice extract,[49,50] mushrooms,[51,52] oatmeal,[53] selenium,[54,55] and turmeric, have been shown in recent years to impart anti-inflammatory activity.[56,57]

Pigmented Skin

Skin color is derived fundamentally from the incorporation of melanin-containing melanosomes, produced by the melanocytes, into epidermal keratinocytes and their subsequent degradation. The focus of the BSTS system regarding this skin parameter is on general treatments for hyperpigmentation.

Tyrosinase Inhibitors

Tyrosinase is the enzyme that controls melanin production, as it is the rate-limiting enzyme for the biosynthesis of melanin in epidermal melanocytes. Given what appears to be its pivotal role in melanogenesis, tyrosinase activity is targeted in various products designed to decrease melanin formation by suppressing tyrosinase.

Hydroquinone

The use of hydroquinone (HQ) leads to the reversible suppression of cellular metabolism by affecting both DNA and RNA synthesis. In addition, HQ efficiently inhibits tyrosinase, diminishing its activity by 90 %.[58] Although HQ is effective alone, it is usually combined with other agents (e.g., azelaic, glycolic, and kojic acids, and tretinoin).[59] For many years, HQ was the first-line therapy for postinflammatory hyperpigmentation and melasma.[60] Concerns about its safety, however, led to a ban for general cosmetic purposes in Europe in 2000. In Asia, HQ is legal but highly regulated. In the United States, the FDA has long been considering the status of HQ, but it has not yet decided whether to ban it in OTC products. HQ has never been etiologically linked with human cancer. Pigmentation of the eye and permanent corneal damage are the most serious adverse health effects seen in workers exposed to HQ.[61] Exogenous ochronosis is also associated with topically applied HQ,[62] although only 30 cases of ochronosis have been ascribed to HQ use in North America.[63] Skin rashes and nail discoloration have also been linked to HQ use. The safety debate within the FDA about this standard-bearing tyrosinase inhibitor has provided the impetus for manufacturers to research and develop newer, less problematic skin-lightening agents.

Aloesin

Derived from aloe vera, aloesin inhibits the hydroxylation of tyrosine to DOPA, as well as the oxidation of DOPA to DOPAchinone, and it suppresses melanin production in cultured normal melanocytes.[64] In a 2002 study on the inhibitory effect of aloesin and/or arbutin on pigmentation in human skin after UV radiation, investigators determined that pigmentation was inhibited compared with control: 34% by aloesin, 43.5% by arbutin, and 63.3% by the co-treatment with aloesin and arbutin.[65] A study published that same year indicated that aloesin and some chemically related chromones inhibit tyrosinase more effectively than arbutin and kojic acid.[66]

Arbutin

Arbutin, a naturally occurring B-D glucopyranoside composed of a molecule of HQ bound to glucose, is found in the leaves of pear trees and herbs such as wheat and bearberry. The depigmenting mechanism of arbutin involves a reversible inhibition of melanosomal tyrosinase activity, rather than blocking the expression and production of tyrosinase.[67] Traditionally used in Japan for depigmenting purposes, arbutin is now thought to be less effective than a synthetic derivative. Indeed, deoxyarbutin has shown, in vitro and in vivo, greater suppression of tyrosinase than arbutin.[68]

Kojic Acid

Kojic acid (5-hydroxy-2-hydroxymethyl-gamma-pyrone), a fungal metabolite of various species of *Aspergillus*, *Acetobacter*, and *Penicillium*,[69] inhibits tyrosinase activity, mainly by chelating copper, leading to a cutaneous whitening effect.[70] The combination of kojic and glycolic acids has been shown to be more effective than 10% glycolic acid and 4% HQ for the treatment of hyperpigmentation.[71,72] Kojic acid 1% products are usually suggested for twice-daily use for 1 to 2 months or until the desired cosmetic result is achieved; however, sensitization to 1% creams has been reported.[73] Kojic acid derivatives have been reported to exhibit enhanced efficiency by dint of greater skin penetration.[74] They have been extensively used in cosmetic products, especially in Japan.[75]

Licorice Extract

Glabridin (*Glycyrrhiza glabra*), a key active ingredient in licorice extract, suppresses tyrosinase activity in cell cultures without altering DNA synthesis. In guinea pig skin, topical applications of 0.5% glabridin have exhibited the capacity to suppress UVB-induced pigmentation and erythema.[76] In the clinical setting, glabridin has been used effectively to treat melasma[77] and has also displayed a depigmenting benefit greater than HQ.[78]

Emblicanin

Emblica, an extract of the *Phyllantus emblica* fruit, contains the tannins emblicanin A and emblicanin B. Emblica is photochemically and hydrolytically stable and is thought to be as effective as HQ and kojic acid, but it has not been associated with adverse side effects. It acts as an inhibitor of tyrosinase and/or tyrosinase-related proteins (TRP-1 & 2) and peroxidase/H_2O_2,[79] and as a broad-spectrum cascading antioxidant.

Melanosome-Transfer Inhibitors

Niacinamide

Niacinamide, also known as nicotinamide, is the biologically active amide of vitamin B_3. It has been demonstrated to suppress melanosome transfer to epidermal keratinocytes by up to 68% in an in vitro model and to render improvement in undesired facial pigmentation.[80] It is important to note that the effects of niacinamide on pigmentation have been shown to be reversible.[81] In a 2005 study, twice-daily application of a 5% niacinamide preparation for 8 weeks yielded significant improvement in hyperpigmentation, as did the use of 3.5% niacinamide combined with retinyl palmitate.[82]

Soy

Soymilk and the soymilk-derived proteins soybean trypsin inhibitor (STI) and the Bowmann-Birk inhibitor (BBI) can inhibit the activation of PAR-2, a G-protein-coupled receptor found to regulate the ingestion of melanosomes by keratinocytes in culture,[83] thus spurring skin depigmentation.[84] Significantly, topical soybean extract application has been shown in human trials to lighten hyperpigmentations.[85,86] Soy is likely both safe and effective, with negligible side effects, particularly since the suppressing of melanosome transfer is reversible. It is best to use soy that has been chemically altered to remove estrogenic properties. Formulation of soy is difficult, so brand names are more reliable than generic products. The authors have noted that Johnson & Johnson has one of the best formulations using "active soy," with estrogenic components removed and small soy proteins preserved.

Lignin Peroxidase

Lignin peroxidase is produced extracellularly during submerged fermentation of the fungus *Phanerochaete chrysosporium*[3] and then is purified from the fermented liquid medium.[87] Trademarked as Melanozyme (Lonza of Switzerland, Zurich), lignin peroxidase is a glycoprotein active at pH 2–4.5 that identifies eumelanin in the epidermis and breaks it down without impacting melanin biosynthesis or inhibiting tyrosinase. Melanozyme is proprietary and available only in the new skin-lightening product known as Elure (Syneron Medical Ltd., Ilit, Israel). The product includes an activator containing hydrogen peroxide (0.12%) that oxidizes, thereby activating the lignin peroxidase, which otherwise would be unable to lighten the skin.

Wrinkled Skin

Wrinkled skin is more readily prevented than successfully treated. Well-known effective behaviors to avert photoaging include the use of broad-spectrum sunscreen (blocking UVA and UVB) and sun avoidance during the peak hours of 10 am to 4 pm. A routine skin-care regimen that entails topical retinoid application may also aid in the prevention and treatment of cutaneous aging. Topical retinoids foster collagen synthesis and thwart the matrix metalloproteinases (MMPs) active in collagen and elastin degradation.[88,89] Also important in the dermatologic arsenal against wrinkling are antioxidants, which countervail the oxidative stress and free radicals created by UV irradiation.

Retinoids

For many years, retinoids, a family of compounds derived from vitamin A, have been used topically and systemically to treat dermatologic disorders, especially acne. Indeed, more than 25 years ago, female acne patients reported smoother skin and fewer wrinkles after treatment.[90] This led to a clinical trial showing that patients treated with tretinoin experienced improvement in sunlight-induced epidermal atrophy, dysplasia, keratosis, and dyspigmentation.[91] Additional findings from several clinical trials led to the FDA's approval of tretinoin (Renova [Ortho Dermatologics, Quebec, Canada]) to treat photodamage. Renova and Avage (Allergan, Courbevoie, France) are the only topical agents approved for this purpose.

Significantly, tretinoin may also play a role in the *prevention* of cutaneous aging. UVB exposure upregulates the development of multiple MMPs; and the activation of MMP genes promotes the production of collagenase, gelatinase, and stromelysin, which fully degrade skin collagen.[92] However, the induction of these MMPs has been demonstrated to be inhibited by the application of tretinoin.[93] Collagen synthesis has also been shown to be diminished by dint of UV exposure. Such a reduction in procollagen production has been demonstrated as a result of cutaneous pretreatment with tretinoin; therefore, consistently pretreating the skin with topical retinoids appears to have the potential to prevent as well as treat photodamage.[94] Collagen synthesis in photoaged human skin has also been promoted by the use of retinoids.[95] Specifically, levels of collagen type I have been partially restored by the topical application of tretinoin 0.1% to photodamaged skin. The metabolic precursor of tretinoin, retinol, is a key ingredient found in various OTC cosmetic products advertised as "anti-wrinkle" creams.[96]

Although they bear little structural resemblance to retinol, the newest retinoids impart biological action via the same nuclear receptors modulated by the active natural metabolite of vitamin A, retinoic acid. Third-generation retinoids, of which there are now more than 2,500 products,[97] are more photostable than the first- and second-generation formulations.[98] However, a recent report by the Environmental Working Group has stirred controversy about one retinoid—retinyl palmitate—suggesting that it may promote skin cancer development.[99] The American Academy of Dermatology has responded by denying that there is any such evidence.[100] What we do know is that retinyl palmitate delivers some sunscreen effects by absorbing UVB, but it may also absorb UVA and act as a photosensitizer. Whereas it is undetermined whether retinyl palmitate actually imparts a carcinogenic effect, it has been established that retinol penetrates human skin more effectively than retinyl palmitate.[100,101] In addition, several retinoids have been shown to exert anticarcinogenic effects. The authors recommend retinol or tretinoin products, not retinyl palmitate.

Antioxidants

Several antioxidants have demonstrated significant capacity to exert photoprotective effects. Although a suitable discussion of this subject is beyond the scope of this chapter, it is worth noting that the list of antioxidants or antioxidant-containing compounds associated with such effects includes, but is not limited to, vitamins C[102,103] and E,[104] coenzyme Q10,[105] grapeseed extract,[106,107] resveratrol,[108,109] green tea,[110,111] lycopene,[112] feverfew,[113] turmeric,[114] idebenone,[115] and coffeeberry.[111,112]

Sunscreens

Sun exposure deposits UV radiation into skin and is known to not only to cause skin cancer, but also to contribute to the appearance of aged skin, wrinkles, and uneven skin tone due to mottled pigmentation. UV radiation is made up of 96.5% UVA and 3.5% UVB on an average summer day. UVB is more likely to cause squamous cell carcinoma and can be blocked by glass, whereas UVA is believed to be a cause of melanoma and can penetrate glass. UVA can also penetrate deep into the skin and cause wrinkles. There are many different sunscreens available, all with varying Sun Protection Factor (SPF) displayed on the label. SPF numbers refer only to the amount of protection against UVB and not UVA, meaning that sunscreen SPF does not reveal how well the particular sunscreen guards against UVA absorption.

There are two types of sunscreens: physical blockers and chemical blockers. Physical blockers, otherwise known as "barrier sunscreens," reflect UV radiation. Because there is no systemic absorption, physical blockers (e.g., titanium dioxide, zinc oxide, and magnesium oxide) rarely cause an allergic reaction. Chemical blockers (e.g., avobenzone) are usually combined with physical blockers for periods of increased sun exposure. Chemical sunscreens absorb the UV radiation, and the chemicals in sunscreens are systemically absorbed. Therefore, there is a risk of allergic reactions with chemical blockers, and they are contraindicated in small children. The authors endorse a regimen that begins first with an antioxidant product layer followed by an antioxidant-containing sunscreen, or two different types of broad-spectrum sunscreens. The best products include avobenzone (now in a stable form known as Helioplex [Neutrogena, Los Angeles, CA]), Mexoryl (LaRoche Posay, Clichy, FR)-containing products, and the physical blockers zinc oxide and titanium dioxide.

Hydroxy Acids (Peels)

Alpha Hydroxy Acids

AHAs, a group of water-soluble, naturally occurring compounds with a hydroxy group in the α position, function as humectants and exfoliants. Lactic acid (derived from sour milk), glycolic acid (from sugarcane), citric acid (from citrus fruits), malic acid (from apples), tartaric acid (from grapes), and phytic acid (from rice) are members of this versatile family of compounds.[14] Lactic and glycolic acids were the first AHAs to reach the market and remain the most commonly used. For more than 35 years, topical formulations using AHAs have been known to affect epidermal keratinization.[15] Of note, the FDA requires preparations containing AHAs to include a label warning that sun protection should accompany product use.

Lactic Acid

First used in 1943 to treat ichthyosis,[16] lactic acid is a popular AHA present in several at-home products and prescription moisturizers. Lactic acid is the only AHA that is also a component of the NMF, which, as suggested above, plays an important role in skin hydration. Notably, the application of the L-isomer of lactic acid to keratinocytes increases the ratio of ceramide 1 linoleate to ceramide 1 oleate, which is significant insofar as a lower ceramide 1 linoleate to ceramide 1 oleate ratio is associated with atopic dermatitis and acne.[17,18] Lactic acid also confers anti-aging effects, as suggested by a double-blind vehicle-controlled study in which an 8% L-lactic acid formula performed better than vehicle in treating photoaged skin, with statistically significant amelioration of skin roughness, mottled hyperpigmentation, and sallowness.[19]

Glycolic Acid

Glycolic acid, known as "the lunchtime peel" because it can be completed effectively and discreetly within a lunch hour without conspicuous signs, is the AHA most often used in chemical peels in practitioners' offices. In 1996, the application of AHAs was shown through histological examination to increase skin thickness by 25%; augment acid mucopolysaccharides in the dermis; enhance elastic fiber quality; and increase collagen density.[20] Treatment with AHAs has also been demonstrated to spur collagen synthesis in vivo and in vitro using fibroblast cultures. Such results have been seen in vitro using glycolic acid, which has also increased fibroblast proliferation.[21] Glycolic acid, unlike several peels, must be neutralized after use to prevent burning. Consequently, glycolic acid should be used only on small areas of the body where it can be rapidly applied and neutralized.

Beta Hydroxy Acid

Salicylic acid is a chemical exfoliant derived from willow bark, wintergreen leaves, and sweet birch; however, it is also available in synthetic form.[22] Although labeled as the only beta hydroxy acid (BHA) because the aromatic carboxylic acid has a hydroxy group in the β position, the carbons of aromatic compounds are traditionally given Arabic numerals rather than Greek letter designations typical for the nonaromatic structures. The BHA label was bestowed for marketing purposes at the time the peels were introduced, and to benefit from the popularity of AHAs. Although the BHA peel is a newer category of chemical peels, salicylic acid has a long and varied history of utility in skin care.

As a chemical peel, salicylic acid is available in over-the-counter (OTC) home products, typically in 0.5 to 2% concentrations suitable for treating acne, rosacea, photoaging, and hyperpigmentation. It is also included in several in-office peels that combine ingredients, such as the Jessner's Peel, the PCA Peel (Physician's Choice, Inc., Chicago, IL), the Miami Peel (Quintessence, Miami, FL) ▶ Video 2.1, and the Pigment Plus Peel (Biomedic, IV Seasons Skin Care, Inc., Boulder, CO). Most cosmetic dermatologists use preparations of 20 or 30% salicylic acid for in-office peels, which—comparable to the effects of AHA peels—have shown success in fading pigment spots, ameliorating surface roughness, and diminishing fine lines.[23] Unlike AHAs, however, BHA impacts the arachidonic acid cascade, exhibiting anti-inflammatory activity and provoking less irritation than AHA peels. The lipophilic nature of salicylic acid also renders a stronger comedolytic effect than AHA peels, allowing BHA to penetrate the sebaceous material in the hair follicle and exfoliate the pores. BHA does not need to be neutralized, as do the AHAs, and the frost is apparent upon completion of the peel.

■ Postoperative Care

Very little, if any, information is published from an evidence-based standpoint regarding specific pre- and postfacial procedure skin care. However, the authors of this chapter suggest strongly that careful pre- and postprocedure skin care is paramount to maximal outcome. Consideration should be given to *three layers* of the face when studying optimal facial enhancement. Skin, volume, and skeletal structure correspond to the outer, middle, and deep layers of the face. Only optimization of all three layers will lead to the best results. A personalized day-to-day skin-care system is important for all-around "outer layer" maintenance, as discussed elsewhere in this chapter. Other aspects of the skin-care regimen may need to be added (or discontinued) for a period of time when preparing for a procedure. Most importantly, *all* patients must wear a daily sunscreen with SPF 30 or greater, whether or not a more invasive procedure is imminent.

Most patients who seek facial enhancement from peels and/or lasers hope to improve the appearance of photoaging—rhytids, pigment, texture and/or erythema/telangiectasias. The majority of individuals can tolerate and benefit from the use of a retinoid for rhytid improvement, as previously discussed. Given tretinoin's proven benefit in neocollagenesis,[88] the authors believe that the use of a retinoid product up to 5 days prior to a peel or laser procedure safely encourages increased laser or peel effectiveness and healing.[116,117] Patients who undergo superficial (epidermal only) peeling or nonablative laser treatments can return to retinoid use approximately 1 week after treatment; use can resume approximately 2 weeks after ablative laser treatments.

Pretreatment with HQ is a well-documented practice for patients at higher risk for postinflammatory hyperpigmentation. However, this exercise is limited by the fact that only epidermal melanocytes are susceptible to HQ and these cells are removed with ablative resurfacing, limiting utility of pretreatment HQ.[110] If instituted, pretreatment should begin 2 to 4 weeks prior to laser or peel. Posttreatment with HQ is usually reserved for unwanted hyperpigmentation. A concentration of at least 4% HQ combination therapy with added steroids and retinoid may be even more effective.[118,119] However, other ingredients may be used prophylactically and to maintain pigment improvement long term. Also, nonprescription topical agents that incorporate ingredients such as soy, kojic acid, or glycolic acid are documented to provide enhancement in pigment and overall skin brightness, and can be added to the daily skin-care regimen. An added advantage of nonprescription topical products is that their use may be continued to help maintain procedural results. Postlaser erythema is another potential cosmetic problem that can be treated with the addition of a targeted cosmeceutical. A well-stabilized vitamin C topical formulation has shown promise in this area.[120]

Many companies market postlaser/postprocedure "recovery" kits. Great care must be taken to avoid irritation and allergic dermatitis during the sensitive days following procedures. The simplest occlusive, such as petrolatum (Aquaphor [Eucerin, Wilton, CT]), should be used for 24 to 72 hours after ablative laser resurfacing. In one study at the University of Miami Miller School of Medicine (unpublished data), the use of one of two alternative marketed occlusive dressings on one side of the chest after ablative resurfacing versus Aquaphor led to unacceptably high rates of irritation, pruritus, and prolonged erythema in the non-Aquaphor side.

■ Expected Results

Microdermabrasion

Microdermabrasion is a painless resurfacing procedure requiring no anesthesia or recuperation time. Without provoking side effects, microdermabrasion diminishes fine wrinkles, enhances skin texture, treats comedones, and eliminates excess skin oil.[121] The microdermabrasion instrument drives sterile micronized aluminum oxide crystals at the skin, while using vacuum suction to remove these particles along with the desquamated skin. The force with which the particles are propelled and the speed at which the device is passed over the skin determine the depth of the treatment. Microdermabrasion is intended to remove the outer layer of the epidermis to foster natural exfoliation.[122] A concomitant benefit is that it seems to facilitate transdermal delivery of some medications.[123,124] Microdermabrasion devices are classified as cosmetic rather than medical and are therefore not regulated by the FDA, allowing manufacturers' marketing claims to go unchallenged or unproven. Acne, acne scarring, striae distensae, and photoaging are the common indications for microdermabrasion.[123] Consequently, this procedure is used for facial rejuvenation, treating other dyspigmented areas, facilitating transdermal delivery of medications, and selectively decreasing full-thickness SC without harming deeper tissues.[125]

Intense Pulsed Light

IPL devices emit noncoherent light with wavelengths between 500 and 1,200 nm. IPLs look and act like lasers, but technically are not lasers because they lack coherent, monochromatic light. The newer systems can pump true laser devices in a separate handpiece. Therefore, one system can be used for several indications. IPLs have been used to remove hair as well as to treat acne, erythema, keratosis pilaris, lentigines, nevus flammeus, photodamage, poikiloderma, spider veins, telangiectasias, and venous malformations.[126] No topical anesthesia is required for IPL procedures.

A patient's skin type and sun protection status should be determined before treatment. For example, treating a recently tanned patient can cause hypopigmentation due to the absorption of melanin by the device. Patients are cautioned to avoid solar exposure before and after treatments. Practitioners are advised to lengthen pulse widths and delays between pulses when using IPLs on patients with darker skin types (Fitzpatrick IV and V).[127,128] Pulses should be placed close together for patients with severe photodamage. Far spacing can cause striping, which can also occur when higher fluences are used and pulses are not placed closely together. This complication can be resolved by addressing the untreated areas. A full-face procedure typically takes 15 minutes. Photodamage usually requires three to five sessions at 1-month intervals.[129] IPLs allow for the management of vascular and pigmented lesions with one instrument. In addition, they offer rapid treatment times; therefore, patients can receive therapy during brief windows, such as a lunch period. Consistent, reproducible results, with few if any side effects (e.g., minimal if any downtime and perhaps mild darkening of treated lentigines, and erythema of treated areas) are also associated with IPL procedures.

■ Conclusion

To achieve optimal results for patients—whether they are having surgery or receiving dermal fillers, botulinum toxin injections, or laser treatments—the proper skin-care regimen, including topical products, must be recommended. Ascertaining the patient's Baumann Skin Type is the first step in ideal skin care. Armed with an understanding of a patient's BST, the physician can select a skin-care regimen best suited to the individual's skin type. To improve the likelihood of patient compliance, the skin-care regimen should be reviewed at each patient visit.

References

1. Baumann L. The Skin Type Solution. New York, NY: Bantam Dell; 2006
2. Baumann L. How to prevent photoaging? J Invest Dermatol 2005;125(4):xii–xiii
3. Spruit D. The interference of some substances with the water vapour loss of human skin. Dermatologica 1971;142(2):89–92
4. Morrison D. Petrolatum. In: Loden M, Maibach H, eds. Dry Skin and Moisturizers. Boca Raton, FL: CRC Press; 2000:251
5. DiNardo JC. Is mineral oil comedogenic? J Cosmet Dermatol 2005;4(1):2–3
6. Draelos Z. Moisturizers. In: Atlas of Cosmetic Dermatology. New York, NY: Churchill Livingstone; 2000:83
7. Darmstadt GL, Mao-Qiang M, Chi E, et al. Impact of topical oils on the skin barrier: possible implications for neonatal health in developing countries. Acta Paediatr 2002;91(5):546–554
8. Idson B. Dry skin: moisturizing and emolliency. Cosmetics and Toiletries 1992;(July)107:69–78
9. Chernosky ME. Clinical aspects of dry skin. J Soc Cosmet Chem 1976;27(8):365–376
10. Harding C, Bartolone J, Rawlings A. Effects of natural moisturizing factor and lactic acid isomers on skin function. In: Loden M, Maibach H, eds. Dry Skin and Moisturizers. Boca Raton, FL: CRC Press; 2000:236
11. Kligman AM. Dermatologic uses of urea. Acta Derm Venereol 1957;37(2):155–159

12. Maquart FX, Pickart L, Laurent M, Gillery P, Monboisse JC, Borel JP. Stimulation of collagen synthesis in fibroblast cultures by the tripeptide-copper complex glycyl-L-histidyl-L-lysine-Cu²⁺. FEBS Lett 1988;238(2):343–346

13. Maquart FX, Bellon G, Chaqour B, et al. In vivo stimulation of connective tissue accumulation by the tripeptide-copper complex glycyl-L-histidyl-L-lysine-Cu²⁺ in rat experimental wounds. J Clin Invest 1993;92(5):2368–2376

14. Lawrence N, Brody HJ, Alt TH. Chemical peeling. In: Coleman W, Hanke W, eds. Cosmetic Surgery of the Skin. 2nd ed. St. Louis, MO: CV Mosby; 1997:85–111

15. Van Scott EJ, Yu RJ. Control of keratinization with alpha-hydroxy acids and related compounds. I. Topical treatment of ichthyotic disorders. Arch Dermatol 1974;110(4):586–590

16. Stern EC. Topical application of lactic acid in the treatment and prevention of certain disorders of the skin. Urol Cutaneous Rev 1946;50:106

17. Yamamoto A, Serizawa S, Ito M, Sato Y. Stratum corneum lipid abnormalities in atopic dermatitis. Arch Dermatol Res 1991;283(4):219–223

18. Wertz PW, Miethke MC, Long SA, Strauss JS, Downing DT. The composition of the ceramides from human stratum corneum and from comedones. J Invest Dermatol 1985;84(5):410–412

19. Stiller MJ, Bartolone J, Stern R, et al. Topical 8% glycolic acid and 8% L-lactic acid creams for the treatment of photodamaged skin. A double-blind vehicle-controlled clinical trial. Arch Dermatol 1996;132(6):631–636

20. Ditre CM, Griffin TD, Murphy GF, et al. Effects of alpha-hydroxy acids on photoaged skin: a pilot clinical, histologic, and ultrastructural study. J Am Acad Dermatol 1996;34(2 Pt 1):187–195

21. Kim SJ, Park JH, Kim DH, Won YH, Maibach HI. Increased in vivo collagen synthesis and in vitro cell proliferative effect of glycolic acid. Dermatol Surg 1998;24(10):1054–1058

22. Draelos Z. Rediscovering the cutaneous benefits of salicylic acid. Cosm Derm Suppl 1997;10(Suppl. 4):4–5

23. Ahn HH, Kim IH. Whitening effect of salicylic acid peels in Asian patients. Dermatol Surg 2006;32(3):372–375, discussion 375

24. Yokota T, Matsumoto M, Sakamaki T, et al. Classification of sensitive skin and development of a treatment system appropriate for each group. IFSCC Mag 2003;6(4):303–307

25. Pons-Guiraud A. Sensitive skin: a complex and multifactorial syndrome. J Cosmet Dermatol 2004;3(3):145–148

26. Tuckermann JP, Kleiman A, McPherson KG, Reichardt HM. Molecular mechanisms of glucocorticoids in the control of inflammation and lymphocyte apoptosis. Crit Rev Clin Lab Sci 2005;42(1):71–104

27. Kim SW, Rhee HJ, Ko J, et al. Inhibition of cytosolic phospholipase A2 by annexin I. Specific interaction model and mapping of the interaction site. J Biol Chem 2001;276(19):15712–15719

28. Rhen T, Cidlowski JA. Antiinflammatory action of glucocorticoids—new mechanisms for old drugs. N Engl J Med 2005;353(16):1711–1723

29. Cohen DE, Heidary N. Treatment of irritant and allergic contact dermatitis. Dermatol Ther 2004;17(4):334–340

30. Marks R. Adverse side effects from the use of topical corticosteroids. In: Maibach HI, Surger C, eds. Topical Corticosteroids. Basel: Karger; 1992:170–183

31. Walsh P, Aeling JL, Huff L, Weston WL. Hypothalamus-pituitary-adrenal axis suppression by superpotent topical steroids. J Am Acad Dermatol 1993;29(3):501–503

32. Kaminsky A. Less common methods to treat acne. Dermatology 2003;206(1):68–73

33. Black AK, Fincham N, Greaves MW, Hensby CN. Time course changes in levels of arachidonic acid and prostaglandins D2, E2, F2 alpha in human skin following ultraviolet B irradiation. Br J Clin Pharmacol 1980;10(5):453–457

34. Wu KK. Salicylates and their spectrum of activity. Curr Med Chem Anti Inflamm Anti Allergy Agents. 2007;6(4):278–292

35. Lin AN, Reimer RJ, Carter DM. Sulfur revisited. J Am Acad Dermatol 1988;18(3):553–558

36. Konaklieva MI, Plotkin BJ. Anti-inflammatory sulfur-containing agents with additional modes of action. Curr Med Chem Anti Inflamm Anti Allergy Agents 2007;6:271

37. Plexion SCT.™ (sodium sulfacetamide 10% and sulfur 5%) [package insert]. Scottsdale, AZ: Medicis; The Dermatology Company; 2001

38. Tarimci N, Sener S, Kilinç T. Topical sodium sulfacetamide/sulfur lotion. J Clin Pharm Ther 1997;22(4):301

39. Gupta AK, Nicol K. The use of sulfur in dermatology. J Drugs Dermatol 2004;3(4):427–431

40. Baumann LS. Less-known botanical cosmeceuticals. Dermatol Ther 2007;20(5):330–342

41. Talmadge J, Chavez J, Jacobs L, et al. Fractionation of Aloe vera L. inner gel, purification and molecular profiling of activity. Int Immunopharmacol 2004;4(14):1757–1773

42. Lee JK, Lee MK, Yun YP, et al. Acemannan purified from *Aloe vera* induces phenotypic and functional maturation of immature dendritic cells. Int Immunopharmacol 2001;1(7):1275–1284

43. Safayhi H, Sabieraj J, Sailer ER, Ammon HP. Chamazulene: an antioxidant-type inhibitor of leukotriene B4 formation. Planta Med 1994;60(5):410–413

44. Safayhi H, Sabieraj J, Sailer ER, Ammon HP. Chamazulene: an antioxidant-type inhibitor of leukotriene B4 formation. Planta Med 1994;60(5):410–413

45. Kwok BH, Koh B, Ndubuisi MI, Elofsson M, Crews CM. The anti-inflammatory natural product parthenolide from the medicinal herb Feverfew directly binds to and inhibits IkappaB kinase. Chem Biol 2001;8(8):759–766

46. Martin K, Sur R, Liebel F, et al. Parthenolide-depleted Feverfew (*Tanacetum parthenium*) protects skin from UV irradiation and external aggression. Arch Dermatol Res 2008;300(2):69–80

47. Ahn JY, Choi IS, Shim JY, et al. The immunomodulator ginsan induces resistance to experimental sepsis by inhibiting Toll-like receptor-mediated inflammatory signals. Eur J Immunol 2006;36(1):37–45

48. Rhule A, Navarro S, Smith JR, Shepherd DM. *Panax notoginseng* attenuates LPS-induced pro-inflammatory mediators in RAW264.7 cells. J Ethnopharmacol 2006;106(1):121–128

49. Agarwal R, Wang ZY, Mukhtar H. Inhibition of mouse skin tumor-initiating activity of DMBA by chronic oral feeding of glycyrrhizin in drinking water. Nutr Cancer 1991;15(3-4):187–193

50. Barfod L, Kemp K, Hansen M, Kharazmi A. Chalcones from Chinese liquorice inhibit proliferation of T cells and production of cytokines. Int Immunopharmacol 2002;2(4):545–555

51. Sliva D. *Ganoderma lucidum* (Reishi) in cancer treatment. Integr Cancer Ther 2003;2(4):358–364

52. Xie JT, Wang CZ, Wicks S, et al. *Ganoderma lucidum* extract inhibits proliferation of SW 480 human colorectal cancer cells. Exp Oncol 2006;28(1):25–29

53. Dick LA. Colliodal emollient baths in pediatric dermatoses. Arch Pediatr 1958;75(12):506–508

54. Leverkus M, Yaar M, Eller MS, Tang EH, Gilchrest BA. Posttranscriptional regulation of UV induced TNF-alpha expression. J Invest Dermatol 1998;110(4):353–357

55. Stewart MS, Cameron GS, Pence BC. Antioxidant nutrients protect against UVB-induced oxidative damage to DNA of mouse keratinocytes in culture. J Invest Dermatol 1996;106(5):1086–1089

56. Rico MJ. Rising drug costs: the impact on dermatology. Skin Therapy Lett 2000;5(4):1–2, 5

57. Srimal RC, Dhawan BN. Pharmacology of diferuloyl methane (curcumin), a non-steroidal anti-inflammatory agent. J Pharm Pharmacol 1973;25(6):447–452

58. Nordlund JJ. Postinflammatory hyperpigmentation. Dermatol Clin 1988;6(2):185–192

59. Guevara IL, Pandya AG. Melasma treated with hydroquinone, tretinoin, and a fluorinated steroid. Int J Dermatol 2001;40(3):212–215

60. Penney KB, Smith CJ, Allen JC. Depigmenting action of hydroquinone depends on disruption of fundamental cell processes. J Invest Dermatol 1984;82(4):308–310

61. DeCaprio AP. The toxicology of hydroquinone—relevance to occupational and environmental exposure. Crit Rev Toxicol 1999;29(3):283–330

62. Lawrence N, Bligard CA, Reed R, Perret WJ. Exogenous ochronosis in the United States. J Am Acad Dermatol 1988;18(5 Pt 2):1207–1211

63. Nordlund JJ, Grimes PE, Ortonne JP. The safety of hydroquinone. J Eur Acad Dermatol Venereol 2006;20(7):781–787

64. Jones K, Hughes J, Hong M, Jia Q, Orndorff S. Modulation of melanogenesis by aloesin: a competitive inhibitor of tyrosinase. Pigment Cell Res 2002;15(5):335–340

65. Choi S, Lee SK, Kim JE, Chung MH, Park YI. Aloesin inhibits hyperpigmentation induced by UV radiation. Clin Exp Dermatol 2002;27(6):513–515

66. Piao LZ, Park HR, Park YK, Lee SK, Park JH, Park MK. Mushroom tyrosinase inhibition activity of some chromones. Chem Pharm Bull (Tokyo) 2002;50(3):309–311

67. Maeda K, Fukuda M. Arbutin: mechanism of its depigmenting action in human melanocyte culture. J Pharmacol Exp Ther 1996;276(2):765–769

68. Boissy RE, Visscher M, DeLong MA. DeoxyArbutin: a novel reversible tyrosinase inhibitor with effective in vivo skin lightening potency. Exp Dermatol 2005;14(8):601–608

69. Bhat R, Hadi SM. Photoinactivation of bacteriophage lambda by kojic acid and Fe(III): role of oxygen radical intermediates in the reaction. Biochem Mol Biol Int 1994;32(4):731–735

70. Hira Y, Hatae S, Inoue T, et al. Inhibitory effects of kojic acid on melanin formation. In vitro and in vivo studies in black goldfish. J Jpn Cosmet Sci Soc. 1982;6:193

71. Ellis DA, Tan AK, Ellis CS. Superficial micropeels: glycolic acid and alpha-hydroxy acid with kojic acid. Facial Plast Surg 1995;11(1):15–21

72. Garcia A, Fulton JE Jr. The combination of glycolic acid and hydroquinone or kojic acid for the treatment of melasma and related conditions. Dermatol Surg 1996;22(5):443–447

73. Nakagawa M, Kawai K, Kawai K. Contact allergy to kojic acid in skin care products. Contact Dermat 1995;32(1):9–13

74. Lee YS, Park JH, Kim MH, Seo SH, Kim HJ. Synthesis of tyrosinase inhibitory kojic acid derivative. Arch Pharm (Weinheim) 2006;339(3):111–114

75. Cabanes J, Chazarra S, Garcia-Carmona F. Kojic acid, a cosmetic skin whitening agent, is a slow-binding inhibitor of catecholase activity of tyrosinase. J Pharm Pharmacol 1994;46(12):982–985

76. Yokota T, Nishio H, Kubota Y, Mizoguchi M. The inhibitory effect of glabridin from licorice extracts on melanogenesis and inflammation. Pigment Cell Res 1998;11(6):355–361

77. Amer M, Metwalli M. Topical liquiritin improves melasma. Int J Dermatol 2000;39(4):299–301

78. Holloway VL. Ethnic cosmetic products. Dermatol Clin 2003;21(4):743–749

79. Chaudhuri RK. Emblica cascading antioxidant: a novel natural skin care ingredient. Skin Pharmacol Appl Skin Physiol 2002;15(5):374–380

80. Hakozaki T, Minwalla L, Zhuang J, et al. The effect of niacinamide on reducing cutaneous pigmentation and suppression of melanosome transfer. Br J Dermatol 2002;147(1):20–31

81. Greatens A, Hakozaki T, Koshoffer A, et al. Effective inhibition of melanosome transfer to keratinocytes by lectins and niacinamide is reversible. Exp Dermatol 2005;14(7):498–508

82. Otte N, Borelli C, Korting HC. Nicotinamide—biologic actions of an emerging cosmetic ingredient. Int J Cosmet Sci 2005;27(5):255–261

83. Seiberg M, Paine C, Sharlow E, et al. Inhibition of melanosome transfer results in skin lightening. J Invest Dermatol 2000;115(2):162–167

84. Paine C, Sharlow E, Liebel F, Eisinger M, Shapiro S, Seiberg M. An alternative approach to depigmentation by soybean extracts via inhibition of the PAR-2 pathway. J Invest Dermatol 2001;116(4):587–595

85. Hermanns JF, Petit L, Martalo O, Piérard-Franchimont C, Cauwenbergh G, Piérard GE. Unraveling the patterns of subclinical pheomelanin-enriched facial hyperpigmentation: effect of depigmenting agents. Dermatology 2000;201(2):118–122

86. Nazzaro-Porro M. The use of azelaic acid in hyperpigmentation. Rev Contemp Pharmacother 1993;4:415

87. Woo S, Cho J, Lee B, Kim E. Decolorization of melanin by lignin peroxidase from *Phanerochaete chrysosporium*. Biotechnol Bioeng 2004;9:256–260

88. Woodley DT, Zelickson AS, Briggaman RA, et al. Treatment of photoaged skin with topical tretinoin increases epidermal-dermal anchoring fibrils. A preliminary report. JAMA 1990;263(22):3057–3059

89. Fisher GJ, Datta SC, Talwar HS, et al. Molecular basis of sun-induced premature skin ageing and retinoid antagonism. Nature 1996;379(6563):335–339

90. Kligman L, Kligman AM. Photoaging—retinoids, alpha hydroxy acids, and antioxidants. In: Gabard B, Elsner P,

Surber C, Treffel P, eds. Dermatopharmacology of Topical Preparations. New York, NY: Springer; 2000:383

91. Kligman AM, Grove GL, Hirose R, Leyden JJ. Topical tretinoin for photoaged skin. J Am Acad Dermatol 1986;15(4 Pt 2):836–859

92. Fisher GJ, Wang ZQ, Datta SC, Varani J, Kang S, Voorhees JJ. Pathophysiology of premature skin aging induced by ultraviolet light. N Engl J Med 1997;337(20):1419–1428

93. Fisher GJ, Datta SC, Talwar HS, et al. Molecular basis of sun-induced premature skin ageing and retinoid antagonism. Nature 1996;379(6563):335–339

94. Fisher GJ, Talwar HS, Lin J, Voorhees JJ. Molecular mechanisms of photoaging in human skin in vivo and their prevention by all-trans retinoic acid. Photochem Photobiol 1999;69(2):154–157

95. Woodley DT, Zelickson AS, Briggaman RA, et al. Treatment of photoaged skin with topical tretinoin increases epidermal-dermal anchoring fibrils. A preliminary report. JAMA 1990;263(22):3057–3059

96. Kafi R, Kwak HS, Schumacher WE, et al. Improvement of naturally aged skin with vitamin A (retinol). Arch Dermatol 2007;143(5):606–612

97. Kligman AM. The growing importance of topical retinoids in clinical dermatology: a retrospective and prospective analysis. J Am Acad Dermatol 1998;39(2 Pt 3):S2–S7

98. Weiss JS. Current options for the topical treatment of acne vulgaris. Pediatr Dermatol 1997;14(6):480–488

99. Environmental Working Group, EWG. 2010 Sunscreen Report. http://www.ewg.org/2010sunscreen/full-report/new-fda-study-sunscreen-additive-may-speed-cancer-growth/. Accessed April 24, 2011

100. Wang SQ, Dusza SW, Lim HW. Safety of retinyl palmitate in sunscreens: a critical analysis. J Am Acad Dermatol 2010;63(5):903–906

101. Duell EA, Kang S, Voorhees JJ. Unoccluded retinol penetrates human skin in vivo more effectively than unoccluded retinyl palmitate or retinoic acid. J Invest Dermatol 1997;109(3):301–305

102. Darr D, Combs S, Dunston S, Manning T, Pinnell S. Topical vitamin C protects porcine skin from ultraviolet radiation-induced damage. Br J Dermatol 1992;127(3):247–253

103. Dunham WB, Zuckerkandl E, Reynolds R, et al. Effects of intake of L-ascorbic acid on the incidence of dermal neoplasms induced in mice by ultraviolet light. Proc Natl Acad Sci U S A 1982;79(23):7532–7536

104. Weber C, Podda M, Rallis M, Thiele JJ, Traber MG, Packer L. Efficacy of topically applied tocopherols and tocotrienols in protection of murine skin from oxidative damage induced by UV-irradiation. Free Radic Biol Med 1997;22(5):761–769

105. Hoppe U, Bergemann J, Diembeck W, et al. Coenzyme Q10, a cutaneous antioxidant and energizer. Biofactors 1999;9(2-4):371–378

106. Bagchi D, Bagchi M, Stohs SJ, et al. Free radicals and grape seed proanthocyanidin extract: importance in human health and disease prevention. Toxicology 2000;148(2-3):187–197

107. Bagchi D, Garg A, Krohn RL, Bagchi M, Tran MX, Stohs SJ. Oxygen free radical scavenging abilities of vitamins C and E, and a grape seed proanthocyanidin extract in vitro. Res Commun Mol Pathol Pharmacol 1997;95(2):179–189

108. Aziz MH, Reagan-Shaw S, Wu J, Longley BJ, Ahmad N. Chemoprevention of skin cancer by grape constituent resveratrol: relevance to human disease? FASEB J 2005;19(9):1193–1195

109. Adhami VM, Afaq F, Ahmad N. Suppression of ultraviolet B exposure-mediated activation of NF-kappaB in normal human keratinocytes by resveratrol. Neoplasia 2003;5(1):74–82

110. Katiyar SK, Ahmad N, Mukhtar H. Green tea and skin. Arch Dermatol 2000;136(8):989–994

111. Vayalil PK, Mittal A, Hara Y, Elmets CA, Katiyar SK. Green tea polyphenols prevent ultraviolet light-induced oxidative damage and matrix metalloproteinases expression in mouse skin. J Invest Dermatol 2004;122(6):1480–1487

112. Arab L, Steck S. Lycopene and cardiovascular disease. Am J Clin Nutr 2000; 71(6, Suppl)1691S–1695S, discussion 1696S–1697S

113. Baumann LS. Less-known botanical cosmeceuticals. Dermatol Ther 2007;20(5):330–342

114. Baumann L. Botanical ingredients in cosmeceuticals. J Drugs Dermatol 2007;6(11):1084–1088

115. Farris P. Idebenone, green tea, and coffeeberry extract: new and innovative antioxidants. Dermatol Ther 2007;20(5):322–329

116. Alt TH. Technical aids for dermabrasion. J Dermatol Surg Oncol 1987;13(6):638–648

117. Goldberg D. Complications in cutaneous laser surgery. New York: Taylor & Francis; 2004:30

118. Goldman MP. The use of hydroquinone with facial laser resurfacing. J Cutan Laser Ther 2000;2(2):73–77

119. West TB, Alster TS. Effect of pretreatment on the incidence of hyperpigmentation following cutaneous CO2 laser resurfacing. Dermatol Surg 1999;25(1):15–17

120. Alster TS, West TB. Effect of topical vitamin C on postoperative carbon dioxide laser resurfacing erythema. Dermatol Surg 1998;24(3):331–334

121. Lawrence N. New and emerging treatments for photoaging. Dermatol Clin 2000;18(1):99–112

122. Alkhawam L, Alam M. Dermabrasion and microdermabrasion. Facial Plast Surg 2009;25(5):301–310

123. Karimipour DJ, Karimipour G, Orringer JS. Microdermabrasion: an evidence-based review. Plast Reconstr Surg 2010 125(1):372–377

124. Prausnitz MR, Langer R. Transdermal drug delivery. Nat Biotechnol 2008;26(11):1261–1268

125. Gill HS, Andrews SN, Sakthivel SK, et al. Selective removal of stratum corneum by microdermabrasion to increase skin permeability. Eur J Pharm Sci 2009;38(2):95–103

126. Manstein D, Herron GS, Sink RK, Tanner H, Anderson RR. Fractional photothermolysis: a new concept for cutaneous remodeling using microscopic patterns of thermal injury. Lasers Surg Med 2004;34(5):426–438

127. Negishi K, Tezuka Y, Kushikata N, Wakamatsu S. Photorejuvenation for Asian skin by intense pulsed light. Dermatol Surg 2001;27(7):627–631, discussion 632

128. Kawada A, Shiraishi H, Asai M, et al. Clinical improvement of solar lentigines and ephelides with an intense pulsed light source. Dermatol Surg 2002;28(6):504–508

129. Bitter PH. Noninvasive rejuvenation of photodamaged skin using serial, full-face intense pulsed light treatments. Dermatol Surg 2000;26(9):835–842, discussion 843

3 Anesthesia and Analgesia for Facial Cosmetic Procedures

Sadeq A. Quraishi

Key Concepts

- Appropriate patient selection is fundamental to maintaining a safe and efficient office-based cosmetic practice.

- National, state, medical specialty–specific practice advisories, and local facility policies define minimum standards of care and monitoring.

- Short-acting intraoperative sedation, muscle relaxation, and analgesia combined with long-acting antiemesis are the fundamental goals of an ideal anesthetic.

- "Twilight" anesthesia often presents greater challenges than a plain local anesthetic or even general anesthesia.

■ Introduction

The safest anesthetic techniques are usually local and general anesthesia.[1] Many patients who undergo facial cosmetic procedures require more than just light sedation, and many receive deep intravenous sedation without an endotracheal tube. "Twilight" anesthesia or monitored anesthesia care, although it may sound serene and peaceful, is not without risks. The highest likelihood for complications lies in an anesthetic that is in between the local and general anesthetic levels—requiring the most skill and diligence to manage. Patients who are sedated but who do not have an endotracheal tube or laryngeal mask airway in place are more likely to have airway problems than patients who are either completely awake or asleep with an airway device in place.[2] Whereas this technique can work well in expert hands with appropriately selected patients, all members of the cosmetic surgery team should be familiar with the pre-, intra-, and postanesthetic challenges in office-based surgeries. As such, this chapter presents critical information that should be shared with all members of the operative team, but is primarily directed toward the surgeon and anesthesiologist or anesthetist.

■ Patient Selection

Many office-based procedure rooms are equipped to handle cases that require only local anesthesia with or without sedation; few are set up to deliver general anesthesia. Therefore, patient selection is of the utmost importance.[3] In essence, selection involves assessment of overall health status and the likelihood of a patient to safely tolerate the necessary anesthetics. The American Society of Anesthesiologists (ASA) has classified risk for anesthesia by preexisting illness of the patient and the surgery to be performed (**Table 3.1**). It is safest to limit office-based surgery under local anesthesia with/or without intravenous sedation to patients with an ASA I or ASA II classification.[4] An airway assessment should also be performed on all patients if deep sedation is to be given (**Fig. 3.1**). A Mallampati score of greater than II may be associated with a higher likelihood of airway complications if a patient becomes excessively sedated. In such cases, sedation directed by a trained anesthesia provider may offer an extra margin of safety. If the delivery of a general anesthetic is required, patient suitability in an office-based setting must be in line with the facility policies and in consultation with an appropriate anesthesia provider.

Table 3.1 American Society of Anesthesiologists (ASA) classifications

ASA category	Definition
I	Healthy patient in need of invasive procedure for localized disease
II	Patient with mild/moderate systemic disease (e.g., high blood pressure, well controlled by therapy)
III	Patient with severe systemic disease (e.g., complicated diabetes mellitus)
IV	Patient with life-threatening systemic disease (e.g., irregular angina, hepatic or renal failure)
V	Seriously ill patient with poor prognosis (e.g., heart attack with cardiogenic shock)
E	Patient requiring emergency surgery (this code is added to category V when the patient needs an urgent procedure)

Source: ASA Relative Value Guide 2002, American Society of Anesthesiologists, p. xii, Code 99140.

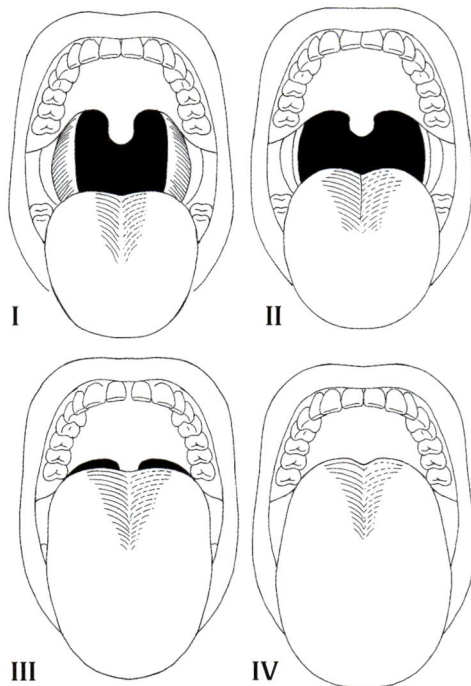

Fig. 3.1 Depiction of the modified Mallampati classification. (*Source:* Samsoon GL, Young JR. Difficult tracheal intubation: A retrospective study. Anaesthesia 42(5):487–490.)

■ Technical Aspects of Procedure

Monitoring

Requirements for the monitoring of patients during office-based procedures can vary by national mandates (e.g., the Joint Commission), state regulations (e.g., Department of Health), professional society practice advisories (e.g., ASA Guidelines for Office-Based Anesthesia), and local facility policies.[3,5] If intravenous sedation is to be administered, it is recommended that procedure rooms have the following basic equipment to accommodate these cases:

1. Oxygen
2. Suction
3. EKG (electrocardiogram)
4. Automatic blood pressure monitor
5. Pulse oximeter
6. Adequate ventilation
7. An operating table or reclining operating chair
8. Adequate space to transfer a patient to a gurney
9. Adequate lighting
10. Equipment to manage airway emergencies and a crash cart within the room may provide an extra margin of safety.

Although there is discussion on the inclusion of routine capnography (CO_2 monitoring) for moderate to deep sedation cases, it is generally not a requirement. The requirements for rooms that are set up to deliver general anesthesia with controlled ventilation are beyond the scope of this chapter. However, if gas anesthetics (except for nitrous oxide) and/or succinylcholine are to be used, a malignant hyperthermia cart must be readily obtainable in case of a crisis.

Patients who receive only local anesthetics or minimal sedation may be fast-tracked to Phase II recovery, depending on individual patient response to sedation. Patients who receive moderate to heavy sedation or general anesthesia must go to Phase I recovery, where frequent pulse oximetry, cardiac monitoring, and supplemental oxygen, as well as the equipment and personnel able to perform advanced cardiac life support in the event of an emergency must be available.

NPO Guidelines

Aspiration pneumonia is a serious risk when patients receive moderate or deep sedation. In general, patients who present for facial cosmetic procedures should adhere to the ASA guidelines for preoperative fasting (**Table 3.2**). NPO is from the Latin for "nothing by mouth."

Table 3.2 ASA NPO guidelines

Ingested material	Minimum fast (hours)[a]
Clear liquids[b]	2 h
Breast milk	4 h
Infant formula	6 h
Nonhuman milk	6 h
Light meal[c]	6 h

Abbreviations: h, hours; NPO, from Latin for "nothing by mouth."
Note: The guidelines recommend no routine use of gastrointestinal stimulants, gastric acid secretion blockers, or oral antacids.
[a]Fasting times apply to all ages.
[b]Examples: Water, fruit juice without pulp, carbonated beverages, clear tea, black coffee.
[c]Example: Dry toast and clear liquid. Fried or fatty foods may prolong gastric emptying time. Both amount and type of food must be considered.
Source: Practice guidelines for preoperative fasting and the use of pharmacologic agents to reduce the risk of pulmonary aspiration: application to healthy patients undergoing elective procedures. Anesthesiology 2011;114:495–511.

Local Anesthetics

Local anesthetics[6] work by reversibly blocking nerve conduction. They predominantly block the sensation of sharp pain. Therefore, it is important to share with patients that, in an area that has been adequately anesthetized, the patient will not feel the sharp needle stick during suture placement or incisions with a scalpel, but may feel a vague sensation of pressure.

The two most commonly used local anesthetics are lidocaine and bupivacaine (**Table 3.3**). Lidocaine (Xylocaine, AstraZeneca, LP, Wilmington, DE) is the most typically used and least expensive agent. The usual total dose that can safely be given is 3 to 5 mg/kg

body weight of plain solution or 5 to 7 mg/kg when epinephrine is used as part of the local anesthetic solution. The anesthesia becomes effective after 5 to 10 minutes and lasts, on average, from 45 minutes for a plain local anesthetic solution to ~ 90 minutes for an epinephrine-containing solution. It is important to note that lidocaine doses up to 35 mg/kg are often used during tumescent liposuction. Although such doses of lidocaine exceed the usual recommended maximum, plasma levels achieved through a tumescent technique are generally low and considered safe.

Bupivacaine (Marcaine, Hospira Inc., Lake Forest, IL; Sensorcaine, AstraZeneca Pharmaceuticals LLP, Wilmington, DE; Abbott Laboratories, Abbott Park, IL) is a longer-acting agent than lidocaine, but it is also more expensive and has the possibility of more severe toxicity. The usual total dose that can safely be administered at one time is 2 to 3 mg/kg. Although it takes 10 to 15 minutes to become effective, anesthesia lasts ~ 2 to 4 hours. The addition of epinephrine to bupivacaine does not appear to hasten the onset or prolong the duration of anesthesia. In addition, bupivacaine provides residual pain control after the procedure is completed.

If both lidocaine and bupivacaine are available, they can be mixed together in equal parts and administered with one syringe. This combination gives the advantages of a quicker onset of anesthesia from the lidocaine and a longer duration of action from the bupivacaine. The onset of action of this mixed solution is slower than lidocaine alone and does not last as long as bupivacaine alone.

Cocaine is a topical ester local anesthetic that is used for its rapid onset and excellent hemostatic effect. It is unique among the local anesthetic agents because of its vasoconstrictive properties and its ability to elicit a euphoric effect through stimulation of the central nervous system (CNS). However, excessive stimulation of the sympathetic nervous system can result in multiple untoward cardiovascular responses (tachycardia, hypertension, diaphoresis, and vasospasm). Cocaine is one of the more toxic anesthetics

Table 3.3 Local Anesthetics

Drug	Class	Onset	Duration (hours)	Dose
Cocaine	Ester	Rapid	1–2 h	3 mg/kg
Tetracaine	Ester	Delayed	2–3 h	1 mg/kg
Lidocaine	Amide	Rapid	1–2 h	3–5 mg/kg plain 5–7 mg/kg (epinephrine)
Bupivacaine	Amide	Delayed	2–4 h	3 mg/kg

Abbreviation: h, hours.

in use and, therefore, should be used with caution and in experienced hands. The recommended dosage is up to 3 mg/kg (up to 200 mg). Tetracaine (Pontocaine, Lippomix, Inc., Novato, CA) is another topical ester anesthetic used frequently in head and neck anesthesia. Maximum recommended dosage is 1 mg/kg.

Adverse reactions to local anesthetics (especially the esters) are not uncommon, but true allergy is very rare. Reported adverse reactions include delayed swelling, localized dermatitis, or mucosal inflammation at the site of administration due to delayed-type (type IV) hypersensitivity.[7] Allergic reactions to the esters are usually due to sensitivity to their metabolite, para-aminobenzoic acid, and do not result in cross-allergy to amides. Therefore, amides can be used as an alternative in such patients. General systemic adverse effects are due to the effects of local anesthetics on the conduction of electrical impulses in the CNS (causing tinnitus and seizures) and the heart (causing arrhythmias), which may be severe and potentially fatal. However, toxicity is typically associated with plasma levels that are rarely achieved if proper anesthetic techniques are adhered to (i.e., maximum dose calculation and aspiration prior to injection to minimize likelihood of intravascular injection). Twenty percent intravenous fat emulsion (Intralipid, Fresenius Kabi, Clayton, NC) rescue has recently been shown to be an effective treatment for cardiotoxicity from local anesthetic overdose. Therefore, offices that use large amounts of local anesthetic in a single patient should strongly consider stocking Intralipid in their crash carts.

It is often useful to add specific drugs to the local anesthetic solutions to optimize the anesthetic effect, minimize discomfort, and/or improve the surgical field. Epinephrine and sodium bicarbonate are the most commonly utilized adjuvants. Epinephrine is a potent vasoconstrictor, reducing bleeding at the operative site. It also decreases absorption of the anesthetic agent and is responsible for prolonging the duration of short-acting local anesthetics like lidocaine. Lidocaine and bupivacaine are available in premixed solutions with epinephrine, but these can also be prepared in the office by experienced personnel.

Both lidocaine and bupivacaine are acidic and, therefore, painful when injected. One way to lessen this pain is to add injectable sodium bicarbonate to the local anesthetic solution prior to infiltration. It is essential to use commercially prepared bicarbonate for injection. In general, 1 mL of bicarbonate to every 9 mL of lidocaine or to every 19 mL of bupivacaine works well. The addition of too much bicarbonate to the anesthetic solution can lead to the formation of crystals.

■ Sedatives

In general, there are four levels of sedation (**Table 3.4**). Minimal sedation is also known as anxiolysis. This entails a drug-induced state during which the patient responds normally to verbal commands. Cognitive function and coordination may be impaired, but ventilatory and cardiovascular functions are unaffected. Moderate sedation/analgesia (often referred to as conscious sedation) is a drug-induced depression of consciousness during which the patient responds purposefully to verbal command, either alone or accompanied by light tactile stimulation. No interventions are necessary to maintain a patent airway. Spontaneous ventilation is adequate, and cardiovascular function is usually maintained. Deep

Table 3.4 ASA definitions of general anesthesia and levels of sedation/analgesia

	Minimal sedation (anxiolysis)	Moderate sedation/analgesia (conscious sedation)	Deep sedation/analgesia	General anesthesia
Responsiveness	Normal response to verbal stimulation	Purposeful response to verbal or tactile stimulation	Purposeful response after repeated or painful stimulation	Unarousable, even w/ painful stimulus
Airway	Unaffected	No intervention required	Intervention may be required	Intervention often required
Spontaneous ventilation	Unaffected	Adequate	May be inadequate	Frequently inadequate
Cardiovascular function	Unaffected	Usually maintained	Usually maintained	May be impaired

Source: Used with permission from Continuum of Depth of Sedation: Definition of General Anesthesia and Levels of Sedation/Analgesia, 2009. American Society of Anesthesiologists. A copy of the full text can be obtained from ASA, 520 N. Northwest Hwy., Park Ridge, IL 60068–2573.

sedation/analgesia is a drug-induced depression of consciousness during which the patient cannot be easily aroused, but responds purposefully following repeated or painful stimulation. Spontaneous ventilatory function may be impaired, and the patient may require assistance to maintain a patent airway. Cardiovascular function is usually sustained. General anesthesia is a drug-induced loss of consciousness during which the patient is not arousable, even to painful stimuli. The ability to maintain independent ventilatory function is often impaired, and assistance is often required in preserving a patent airway. Positive pressure ventilation may be required due to depressed spontaneous ventilation or drug-induced depression of neuromuscular function (paralytics). Cardiovascular function may be impaired.

Oral and intramuscular administration of sedatives[6] is a perfectly acceptable method of providing minimal to moderate sedation. However, these routes of administration run the risk of unpredictability for time to onset, duration of action, and quality of maximal sedative effect. Consequently, injectable drugs are often chosen to reliably attain a desired level of sedation to facilitate the success of the surgical procedure and to speed the postoperative recovery. Benzodiazepines, alkylphenols, N-methyl-D aspartate (NMDA) receptor antagonists, and α_2-agonists are the most widely accepted drugs to provide anxiolysis, amnesia, modified consciousness, and skeletal muscle relaxation. Predominantly, sedatives do not provide analgesia and are typically used as an adjunct to local anesthesia or in measured concert with opioids. However, one must be aware of possible idiosyncratic reactions, such as increased anxiety, restlessness, and disinhibition—especially present in the very young or elderly. Dosing guidelines for IV sedation are presented in **Table 3.5**.

Lorazepam (Ativan, Biovail Pharmaceuticals, Inc., Bridgewater, NJ), diazepam (Valium, Roche Laboratories, Nutley, NJ), and midazolam (Versed, Roche Laboratories, Nutley, NJ) are the most customarily used benzodiazepines in clinical practice. Speed of onset, duration of action, and higher likelihood of paradoxical reactions make lorazepam a less-desired drug to use in an office-based or ambulatory care setting. Intravenous diazepam administered in doses of 2.5 to 5.0 mg increments (up to 0.3 mg/kg) can produce conscious sedation adequate for outpatient procedures. Intravenous midazolam is also an excellent sedative that is approximately four times more potent than diazepam. In doses of 1 to 2.5 mg (up to 0.1 mg/kg), midazolam can produce sedation appropriate for use in outpatient surgery and is often preferred over diazepam because of its shorter duration of action and lack of venous irritation on injection. Midazolam also causes more amnesia than diazepam, and this may occur even with relatively light levels of sedation. It may even induce retrograde amnesia, in that patients may be unable to recall presurgical events that occurred while they were fully conscious.

Suppression of the respiratory drive occurs with the use of benzodiazepines. Flumazenil (Romazicon, Epocrates, Inc., San Mateo, CA) is a competitive antagonist at the benzodiazepine receptor. Incremental intravenous doses of 0.2 to 1 mg are usually effective for reversal of all the effects of benzodiazepines; however, they should be used with caution in patients chronically dependent on benzodiazepines because abrupt withdrawal may induce seizures. The duration of action of flumazenil varies from 15 to 140 minutes, with re-sedation being a risk, especially if longer-acting benzodiazepines are used. This short duration of action typically correlates well with the reversal of midazolam.

Propofol (Diprivan, AstraZeneca, LP, Wilmington, DE) is an alkylphenol that has increased in popularity owing to its very rapid onset and short duration of action. The half-life is 30 to 60 minutes; however, a third compartment with slower elimination half-life is also present, indicating the possibility of accumulation after very long infusions. The recommended maintenance infusion rate of propofol var-

Table 3.5 Typical dosing for IV sedation

Drug	Bolus dose	Infusion dose
Propofol	0.25–1 mg/kg	10–75 µg/kg/min
Ketamine	0.3–0.6 mg/kg	300–600 µg/kg/h
Dexmedetomidine	Not recommended	0.2–0.7 µg/kg/h
Fentanyl	25–50 µg	Not recommended
Alfentanil	5–10 µg/kg	0.25–1 µg/kg/min
Remifentanil	0.1–0.3 µg/kg	0.025–1 µg/kg/min

Abbreviations: IV, intravenous; h, hour; m, minute.

ies between 100 and 200 mg/kg/min for hypnosis and 25 and 75 mg/kg/min for sedation. Amnesia is typically not profound with the use of propofol, and an excitatory phenomenon is observed in ~ 15% of cases. Propofol has antiemetic effects that are very advantageous, especially where opioids are used concomitantly. There is usually dose-related respiratory and cardiovascular depression, which may be exacerbated with accompanying use of potent opioids.

Ketamine (Ketalar, La Roche-Posay) is an NMDA receptor antagonist that causes dissociative anesthesia. Unlike most other sedatives, ketamine has a wide therapeutic range, possesses analgesic properties, and has a very low incidence of respiratory depression. However, laryngospasm (unknown cause) is potentially a dangerous complication but is rare and usually transient. Psychic side effects may be troublesome, but they can be minimized by the co-administration of a benzodiazepine or a similar hypnotic. Recovery may be delayed, especially if more than 2 mg/kg is given. Therefore, ketamine works best as part of a multimodal sedation/pain management strategy.

Until recently, α_2-agonists in ambulatory surgery were limited to oral clonidine (Catapres, Boehringer Ingelheim Pharmaceuticals, Ridgefield, CT) and clonidine solution for use in regional anesthesia—nerve blocks, spinal anesthesia, among others. Intravenous clonidine is not approved by the U.S. Food and Drug Administration despite worldwide use to provide preoperative sedation and anxiolysis, and to decrease intraoperative anesthetic requirements. However, dexmedetomidine (Precedex, Hospira, Lake Forest, IL) is approved for intravenous use in the United States and is a highly CNS-selective α_2-agonist. It has a half-life of ~ 2 hours. A unique type of sedation may be produced in which patients can be aroused readily and then return to a sleeplike state when left alone. Dexmedetomidine has minimal analgesic properties and, thus, works best with local anesthesia and/or sparing use of short-acting opioids. Higher infusion rates of dexmedetomidine may, however, lead to complete loss of responsiveness and amnesia. Because of its sympatholytic and vagomimetic actions, dexmedetomidine may be associated with hypotension and profound bradycardia, therefore requiring delivery in a monitored setting.

Opioids

Opioids[6] are primarily used to provide analgesia during procedural sedation. Although all opioids also cause varying degrees of sedation, the effect is inconsistent. Depending on the route of administration and the agent used, responses can vary greatly among in-dividual patients. As such, the effects of intravenous opioids are most predictable as long as they are used as analgesics to supplement other primarily sedating drugs or sub-optimal local anesthesia. The selection of opioids for outpatient surgeries should be limited to shorter-acting agents such as fentanyl (Sublimaze, Akorn, Inc., Buffalo Grove, IL), alfentanil (Alfenta, Jansson Pharmaceuticals, Johnson & Johnson Pharmaceutical Research Development, New Brunswick, NJ), or remifentanil (Ultiva, Mylan Pharmaceuticals, Morgantown, WV). All opioids have profound respiratory depressant effects, are associated with bradycardia, and can cause muscle rigidity. The risk of postoperative nausea and vomiting increases significantly when opioids are used to manage intra- and postoperative pain.

Fentanyl is the most commonly used opioid for outpatient anesthesia. It typically produces analgesia and euphoria when administered in 25 to 50 µg doses for a loading dose of 1 to 3 µg/kg. The onset of action is ~ 5 minutes, with peak activity at ~ 10 minutes and duration of action for 45 to 60 minutes. Fentanyl is highly lipophilic and accumulates in the body very quickly. As a result, fentanyl infusions should be used cautiously in office-based surgery.

Alfentanil is shorter acting than fentanyl. Whereas sedation and euphoria with alfentanil may be more profound than with fentanyl, respiratory depression occurs for a briefer period. An intravenous loading dose of 5 to 10 µg/kg typically produces effects within 1 to 2 minutes and lasts for ~ 20 minutes. For surgical cases of moderate length, an alfentanil infusion may be considered. Remifentanil is an ultra-short-acting opioid and is typically run as an infusion. It has a half-life of 8 to 10 minutes even after prolonged infusions.

Naloxone (Narcan, ENDO Pharmaceuticals, Newark, DE) is an opioid antagonist that can be used in cases of overdose. It has a half-life of ~ 30 to 60 minutes, making it effective for reversal of generous doses of all three intravenous opioids discussed above. Naloxone should be used with caution in opioid-dependent patients because it can induce acute withdrawal symptoms. It is typically given in doses of 0.1 to 0.2 mg every 1 to 2 minutes until the desired level of opioid reversal is achieved.

Antiemetics

Postoperative nausea and vomiting (PONV) is one of the most distressing complications after surgery. Indeed, many patients rank PONV over pain as their primary concern related to recovery from surgery. Risk factors for PONV include: female sex, history of nonsmoker, prior history of PONV or motion sickness, use of intra- and postoperative opioids, use of gas anesthetics, and duration of surgery. The routine use of antiemetic prophylaxis is highly encouraged in patients who will receive

Table 3.6 Common antiemetics with dosing and adverse effects

Drug	Dose	Timing	Adverse effects
Ondansetron (Zofran[a])	4–8 mg (IV)	At end of surgery	Headache, lightheadedness, elevated liver enzymes
Dolasetron (Anzemet[b])	12.5 mg (IV)	At end of surgery	Headache, lightheadedness, elevated liver enzymes
Granisetron (Kytril[c])	0.35–1 mg (IV)	At end of surgery	Headache, lightheadedness, elevated liver enzymes
Tropisetron (Navoban[d])	5 mg (IV)	At end of surgery	Headache, lightheadedness, elevated liver enzymes
Dexamethasone (Decadron[e])	5–10 mg (IV)	Before induction of anesthesia	Vaginal itching or anal irritation with IV bolus
Prochlorperazine (Compazine[f])	5–10 mg (IV)	At end of surgery	Sedation, hypotension, EPS
Promethazine (Phenergan[g])	6.25–12.5 mg (IV)	At end of surgery	Sedation, hypotension, EPS
Scopolamine (Transderm Scop[h])	Transdermal patch	Prior evening or 4 h before end of surgery	Sedation, dry mouth, visual disturbances
Aprepitant (Emend[i])	40 mg (PO)	1–3 h prior to induction of anesthesia	Headache, lightheadedness, elevated liver enzymes

Abbreviations: EPS, extrapyramidal symptoms; h, hours; IV, intravenous; PO, by mouth.
[a]GlaxoSmithKline Pharmaceuticals, Research Triangle Park, NC.
[b]Sanofi-Aventis US, Bridgewater, NJ.
[c]Roche Laboratories, Nutley, NJ.
[d]Novartis, East Hanover, NJ.
[e]Merck & Co., Inc., Whitehouse Station, NJ.
[f]GlaxoSmithKline, Philadelphia, PA.
[g]Baxter Healthcare Corp., Deerfield, IL.
[h]Novartis Consumer Health, East Hanover, NJ.
[i]Merck & Co., Inc., Whitehouse Station, NJ.

opioids.[6] Several therapeutic agents, from different classes, can be used to minimize the possibility of PONV in high-risk patients (**Table 3.6**). The use of intraoperative propofol appears to reduce the incidence of PONV.

■ Complications and Their Management

Despite a work environment dedicated to the safety of patients, unexpected and unwanted complications related to anesthetic management may occur. Therefore, it is critical that all perioperative staff understand the essential steps in managing these situations. Being prepared for emergencies is the most important step in managing them effectively.

Malignant Hyperthermia

If gas anesthetics (other than nitrous oxide) and/or succinylcholine are used in the practice setting, all perioperative staff should be prepared to manage a malignant hyperthermia (MH) crisis.[8] Upon clinical suspicion of MH, all available help should be solicited, the patient should be removed from any source of triggering agents, a secured airway should be established, and 100% oxygen should be delivered. Dantrolene (Dantrium, JHP Pharms, Rochester, MI) should be reconstituted as soon as possible and delivered intravenously at a dose of 2.5 mg/kg every 5 minutes until symptoms abate (i.e., hyperthermia, rigidity, hemodynamic instability). Large-bore intravenous access should also be established to provide aggressive fluid resuscitation. Packing the body with bags of ice and/or gastric lavage with cold fluid may be helpful while waiting for emergency medical services to transfer the patient to an intensive care unit or emergency department. For 24-hour assistance, the MH Hotline can be reached at: (U.S.) 1–800–644–9737 or (outside the U.S.) 00–1–303–389–1647.[9]

Local Anesthetic Overdose

When excessive amounts of local anesthetics reach the systemic circulation, signs and symptoms of toxicity may become apparent.[6] CNS symptoms are often subtle or absent; cardiovascular signs, particularly hypotension or bradycardia, are frequently the only manifestations of severe local anesthetic toxicity, and can occur 1 hour or more after local anesthetic administration. CNS excitation (agitation, confusion, twitching, seizure), depression (drowsiness, obtundation, coma, apnea), or nonspecific neurologic symptoms (metallic taste, circumoral paresthesias, diplopia, tinnitus, dizziness) are typical of local anesthetic toxicity. Progressive hypotension and bradycardia, leading to asystole, are commonly associated with severe cardiovascular toxicity. Ventricular ectopy, multiform ventricular tachycardia, and ventricular fibrillation are also often seen with severe overdose. Airway management is critical and will usually require 100% oxygen and a secured airway in settings of moderate to severe toxicity (i.e., more than just CNS excitation). Initiation of seizure suppression with benzodiazepines and, if needed, cardiopulmonary resuscitation should not be delayed. While transfer to the nearest facility with cardiopulmonary bypass capability is being arranged, 20% lipid emulsion (Intralipid) infusion should be initiated as follows: bolus 1.5 mL/kg intravenously over 1 minute followed by continuous infusion at 0.25 mL/kg/min.[10] Boluses may be repeated every 5 minutes for persistent cardiovascular collapse. The infusion rate may be doubled if blood pressure returns but remains low. An Intralipid infusion should be run for a minimum of 30 minutes.

Sedative/Opioid Overdose

The degree of sedation and respiratory depression determines the most effective intervention strategy.[2] In the setting of a maintained respiratory drive but mild or moderate airway obstruction, a jaw thrust, nasal trumpet, or oral airway with or without an increase in the rate of oxygen delivery may be sufficient. Apnea requires more aggressive management and usually requires careful reversal of benzodiazepines (with flumazenil) or opioids (with naloxone) with an increased rate of oxygen delivery.[6] Aggressive airway management, including a secured airway, during apnea is critical because not only are hypoxia and hypercarbia undesirable, but also the risk of as-

piration increases significantly. If a patient requires pharmacological reversal of sedatives or opioids during a procedure or in the recovery area, extended postoperative monitoring should be instituted.[3]

■ Conclusion

A rigorous patient selection process, an environment dedicated to safety, and a culture of open communication between members of the perioperative team are essential to a successful facial cosmetic practice. Whereas many minimally invasive procedures can be performed safely with preoperative oral sedatives and analgesics in addition to generous use of intraoperative local anesthetics, patient and/or surgeon preferences may dictate the use of intravenous agents. In all instances where intravenous sedatives and opioids are to be used, collaboration with a skilled anesthesia provider should be strongly considered to optimize perioperative outcomes.

References

1. Hausman LM, Dickstein EJ, Rosenblatt MA. Types of office-based anesthetics. Mt Sinai J Med 2012;79(1): 107–115
2. Perrott DH. Anesthesia outside the operating room in the office-based setting. Curr Opin Anaesthesiol 2008; 21(4):480–485
3. American Society of Anesthesiologists Clinical Standards, Guidelines, and Statements. http://www.asahq.org/For-Healthcare-Professionals/Standards-Guidelines-and-Statements.aspx. Accessed 12/04/2012
4. Kurrek MM, Twersky RS. Office-based anesthesia: how to start an office-based practice. Anesthesiol Clin 2010; 28(2):353–367
5. The Joint Commission section on Ambulatory Healthcare. http://www.jointcommission.org/accreditation/ambulatory_healthcare.aspx
6. Miller RD, Eriksson LI, Fleisher LA, Wiener-Kronish JP, Young WL. Anesthesia. 7th ed. Philadelphia: Elsevier/Churchill Livingstone; 2010
7. Melamed J, Beauchec WN. Delayed-type hypersensitivity (type IV) reactions in dental anesthesia. Allergy Asthma Proc 2007;28(4):477–479
8. Larach MG, Dirksen SJ, Belani KG, et al; Society for Ambulatory Anesthesiology; Malignant Hyperthermia Association of the United States; Ambulatory Surgery Foundation; Society for Academic Emergency Medicine; National Association of Emergency Medical Technicians. Special article. Creation of a guide for the transfer of care of the malignant hyperthermia patient from ambulatory surgery centers to receiving hospital facilities. Anesth Analg 2012;114(1):94–100
9. Malignant Hyperthermia Association US. http://www.mhaus.org/healthcare-professionals. Accessed 12/04/2012
10. Killoran PV, Cattanc D. From bedside to bench and back: perfecting lipid emulsion therapy for local anesthetic toxicity. Anesthesiology 2011;115(6):1151–1152

4 Techniques for Office Anesthesia: Local Anesthesia and Regional Block Techniques

David A. F. Ellis and YuShan Lisa Wilson

Key Concepts

- Local anesthetics in regional nerve blocks provide analgesia by blocking pain transmission along specific nerve fibers.

- The target of local anesthetics is the sodium channel.

- The degree of nerve blockage depends on the particular local anesthetic drug used and its concentration and volume.

- Knowledge of reliable anatomic bony and muscular landmarks is the key to precise local anesthetic placement.

- Detailed description of anatomy and techniques of regional blocks of the face, neck, and anterior chest are reviewed in this chapter.

- The secret to achieving full-face analgesia via local anesthetics is familiarity with the important but less universally known blocks of the external nasal, anterior ethmoid, lacrimal, buccal, zygomaticotemporal, and auriculotemporal nerves.

- Systemic toxicity from clinical dosages of local anesthetics is a potential but uncommon event.

- Cardiotoxicity is more frequent with high-potency, lipid-soluble agents such as bupivacaine and ropivacaine.

■ Introduction

A growing demand for cosmetic procedures outside the operating room has driven the need for physicians skilled in the practice of local anesthesia. The delivery of local anesthetic care is a blend of artistry and science. The ability to safely and effectively apply these techniques can make all the difference in creating good surgical results as well as pleased and satisfied patients. The use of local anesthetics in an office setting ranges from topical application, local infiltration, and field blocks to, importantly, regional blocks. The key to successful regional anesthesia relies heavily on detailed knowledge of local anatomy; and nowhere else is this as demanding as in the head and neck. Proper application of local anesthetics plays a critical role in procedures ranging from repair of lacerations to lesion-directed biopsies and full-face ablative laser resurfacing.

The advantages of local, compared with general, anesthesia are many. First, the airway is not compromised; therefore, the patient can control breathing, eliminating the risk of respiratory depression and all its untoward consequences. Second, a patient who is awake is also able to aid in positioning. This assists in surgical maneuvers like assessment of upper eyelid skin excision in blepharoplasty to ensure appropriate lagophthalmos. Third, the immediate postoperative recovery is smoother, without the coughing or bucking seen with extubation. Fourth, there is better postoperative pain control because the local anesthetic wears off slowly. Fifth, bleeding is less, due to the vasoconstrictive properties of concomitant epinephrine and lack of vasodilatory effects of inhalation agents. Sixth, early discharge is possible because patients do not experience a depressed level of consciousness. Last, costs are reduced because operating-room fees and hospital stays can be avoided.

The disadvantages of using only local anesthesia are many, as well. First, some patients are fearful of undergoing surgery while awake. Second, local anesthetics have systemic side effects that can reach toxic levels. Third, techniques for injecting local anesthetics are learned, thus poor injection skill may result in inadequate anesthesia and unnecessary pain. Fourth, the effects of local anesthesia are not immediate—particularly in the case of nerve blocks—so proper planning and time management need to be factored into the procedure to ensure optimal patient comfort. Fifth, if intraneural injection occurs, there is a very small risk of permanent nerve damage. Last, local anesthetics have decreased potency in an acidic environment such as an infected area.

Background: Basic Science of Procedure

Cocaine, an extract of the coca leaf, was the first successful local anesthetic.[1] Although Sigmund Freud published extensively on cocaine and its effects, the recognition for the discovery of local anesthesia belongs to Karl Köller, a friend and colleague of Freud. In 1884, with the application of cocaine to the conjunctiva and cornea of animals, Köller introduced the first use of local anesthetic in surgery.[2-4] By 1892, the use of cocaine in peripheral nerve blocks had been launched by W.S. Halsted, professor of surgery at Johns Hopkins University and later the creator of the residency system in surgery.[3]

Local anesthetics are classified biochemically into two groups: amides and esters. Structurally, each consists of an aromatic benzene ring joined to an amino group with either an ester or an amide linkage. Of note, the amide link is less heat-labile and therefore more stable in settings of pH or temperature fluctuations. Both groups are also categorized as weak bases, and thus can exist in one of two forms—a lipid-soluble neutral form or a charged hydrophilic form. The neutral form is understood to contribute to penetration of the drug into the neural cytoplasm; whereas the charged form is the active structure that interacts with the sodium channels.

Local anesthetic agents act by targeting the sodium channel. This sodium channel blockade results in an attenuation of neural action potential formation and propagation. Studies reveal that a 50% loss in action potential must be achieved before clinical loss of function is evident.[5] After application of local anesthetics to a peripheral nerve, the first sense to be blocked is temperature, followed by sharp pain, and then light touch.

Systemic absorption of local anesthetics is governed by several factors. The anesthetic's pharmacokinetic properties, dose, site of injection, and the addition of a vasoconstrictive agent all influence the rate of absorption. The rate of absorption differs among individual local anesthetics. More lipid-soluble anesthetics demonstrate slower rates of absorption. Local anesthetics are known to vasoconstrict vessels at low doses but in concentrations used for clinical practice actually vasodilate via direct action on smooth muscles of vessel walls. The only exception to this rule is cocaine, which consistently produces vasoconstriction.[4] In vessel-rich areas, higher peak plasma levels can be achieved in a short period of time unless concomitant vasoconstrictors are utilized. The greatest rate of systemic absorption is seen with intercostal nerve blocks, as compared with other sites in the body.[5] Use of vasoconstricting agents—the most popular, epinephrine—clinically results in longer duration of anesthesia, decreased risk of toxic side effects, and reduced bleeding in the surgical field. In a 70 kg healthy individual, the toxic dose of 1% lidocaine with 1:100,000 epinephrine is 50 mL or 7 mg/kg.

Clearance of local anesthetics is determined by their chemical linkage. Amino esters are hydrolyzed by plasma cholinesterases, whereas amino amides are degraded hepatically by carboxylesterases and cytochrome P450 enzymes. Therefore, cardiac and hepatic disease states may alter pharmacokinetics, and lower dosages of local anesthetics should be indicated. Renal disease, alternatively, has very little effect on the pharmacokinetics of local anesthetics.

The choice of local anesthetic depends on the length of procedure or surgery and preference for postoperative analgesia (**Table 4.1**). Esters include cocaine (Lannett Company Inc., Philadelphia, PA), procaine (Hospira, Inc., Lake Forest, IL), and tetracaine (Alcon Laboratories, Inc., Ft. Worth, TX). Commonly used amides are lidocaine (APP Pharmaceuticals, LLC, Schaumberg, IL), prilocaine (Dentsply Pharmaceuticals, York, PA), mepivacaine (Hospira, Inc., Lake Forest, IL), bupivacaine (Hospira, Inc., Lake Forest, IL), and ropivacaine (Naropin, APP Pharmaceuticals, Schaunberg, IL).

Patient Selection

A frank discussion needs to take place to reconcile both patient expectations and procedure-specific factors, when performing procedures under only local anesthetic. Patient factors such as psychological reserve, pain tolerance, anxiety, stamina, and tolerance must be thoroughly evaluated. Because the patient

Table 4.1 Common anesthetic agents

Agent	Onset (min)	Peak (min)	Duration (min, h)
Esters			
Cocaine	Immediate	–	45 min
Procaine	2–5	<15	60 min
Tetracaine	2–8	–	4–5 h
Amides			
Lidocaine	3–5	–	1–2 h
Bupivacaine	2–10	30	3–6 h
Ropivacaine	1–15	20–45	5–8 h

Abbreviations: min, minutes; h, hours.

will be awake throughout the procedure, the physician needs to be candid in terms of the intensity of stimulation anticipated and the duration of the operation. Often these procedure-specific factors depend considerably on the skill of the physician as well. The operative team also needs to be sensitive with respect to conversation, music, and sudden noises during the surgery. If any of these points pose a concern to either the patient or physician, further sedation options, ranging from light or "conscious" sedation to general anesthesia, can be explored (**Table 4.2**). In our clinical practice, for surgeries requiring full-face regional blocks, we routinely utilize "conscious" sedation (ASA [American Society of Anesthesiologists] category I and II patients) with Versed (Roche Laboratories, Nutley, NJ) and fentanyl titrated to help mitigate the discomfort of multiple regional blocks. This is not absolutely necessary; however, we find

Table 4.2 Levels of anesthesia

1	No sedation or analgesia
2	Light sedation and/or analgesia—"conscious" sedation
3	Moderate sedation and/or analgesia
4	Deep sedation
5	General anesthesia

that most patients prefer this combination to ensure a pleasant process.

True allergic reactions to local anesthetics are very rare. Antigenicity, mediated either through a type I (IgE) or type IV (cellular immunity) reaction toward local anesthetics, is often related to the presence of its ester or amide linkage. It is known that esters are more likely to cause an allergic reaction. Reports of true type I allergic reactions are purported to be a result of the ester's hydrolysis into its *para*-amino-benzoic acid constituent, which is a documented allergen.[5] Alternatively, allergic reactions may be a result of added preservatives, such as methylparaben or metabisulfite.

Frequently, clinical history points toward intolerance of the epinephrine within the local anesthetic, as opposed to a true allergic reaction. Epinephrine is a sympathomimetic amine and both an α- and β-adrenergic stimulant. It is an excellent vasoconstrictor with potential systemic side effects. Epinephrine has been shown to increase heart rate, stroke volume, cardiac output, and oxygen consumption in the cardiovascular system. Further, it may act as an irritant to the myocardium, predisposing to premature ventricular contractions and other dysrhythmias. Epinephrine should be limited to 0.04 mg in patients with a cardiac history. Most local anesthetics include 1:100,000 epinephrine, which is equivalent to 0.01 mg/mL (**Table 4.3**).[6] This agent is contraindicated in patients to whom β-adrenergic stimulation is harmful, and who present with unstable angina, malignant arrhythmias, and uncontrolled hypertension.[7] Anyone taking medications that alter the effects of catecholamines—such as tricyclic antidepressants or monoamine oxidase inhibitors (MAOIs)—should also avoid epinephrine.

Table 4.3 Lidocaine, epinephrine, and cocaine

Agent	Concentration	Dosage
Lidocaine	0.5%	5 mg/mL
	1%	10 mg/mL
	2%	20 mg/mL
Epinephrine	1:100,000	10 µg/mL
	1:200,000	5 µg/mL
	1:1,000	1,000 µg/mL
Cocaine	4%	40 mg/mL

■ Technical Aspects of Procedure

Topical Anesthetics

Local anesthetics are also commercially available in topical preparations for both the skin and mucous membranes. Although topical agents are not injected, one must still be mindful of potential systemic toxicity because a high degree of permeability is seen with topical application. For the oral mucosa, 10% aerosol lidocaine or 4% viscous lidocaine is an effective agent. For the conjunctiva and cornea of the eyes, 4% ophthalmic tetracaine is an ideal option. The vasoconstrictive properties of 4% cocaine make it a favorite among rhinologic surgeons. However, cocaine also acts as a mucosal irritant in chronic abuse, making it the culprit in septal perforations. Medical indications for cocaine use are scrutinized not only because of its history of addiction and abuse, but also because of its considerable central nervous system (CNS) and cardiovascular toxicity.[4] The result of cocaine in conjunction with epinephrine in local injection can be catastrophic—leading to malignant hypertension and cardiovascular insufficiency if it prevents significant re-uptake of norepinephrine at nerve endings.

Many preparations for topical cutaneous applications are marketed for intact skin. Several nonprescription-strength formulations of lidocaine 4 to 5% are also available. EMLA (AstraZeneca Pharmaceuticals, LP, Wilmington, DE) is an oil-in-water emulsion of 2.5% prilocaine and 2.5% lidocaine that was approved by the Food and Drug Administration (FDA) in 1992.[8] It works best when applied to the skin under an occlusive dressing for at least 45 to 60 minutes. LET (lidocaine 4%, epinephrine 0.1%, and tetracaine 0.5%), either as an aqueous solution or in a methylcellulose gel, is popular for laceration repairs. Standard dosage is 1 to 3 mL for ~ 20 to 30 minutes. The gel formulation may be applied directly onto the wound and surrounding skin without occlusion. Ultimately, we prefer to use our own topical preparation, which can be compounded as up to 30% lidocaine in Lipothene (LipoThene, Inc., Pacific Grove, CA). It provides quicker onset and is more effective than most other formulations.

Regional Blocks of the Face

The trigeminal nerve (cranial nerve V) supplies sensory innervations to the face (**Fig. 4.1**). Distributions of the trigeminal nerve can be further classified into three divisions: ophthalmic (V_1), maxillary (V_2), and mandibular (V_3). The ophthalmic, maxillary, and mandibular branches exit the skull through three separate foramina: the superior orbital fissure (**Fig. 4.2**), the foramen rotundum, and the foramen ovale, respectively. Within each division are several named

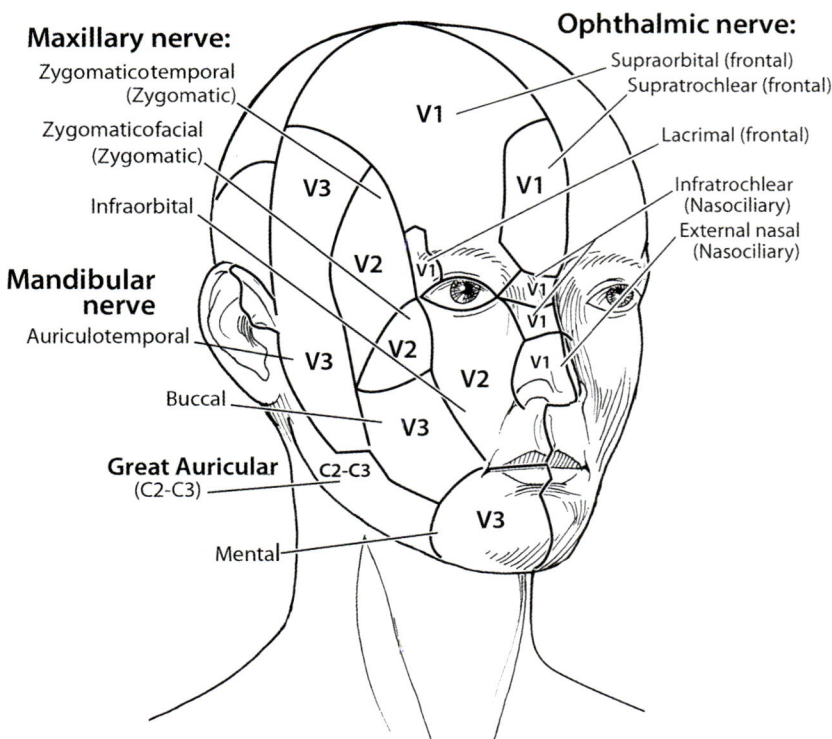

Fig. 4.1 Sensory distributions of trigeminal nerve—ophthalmic, maxillary, and mandibular divisions. Be aware that these distributions may be variable from patient to patient.

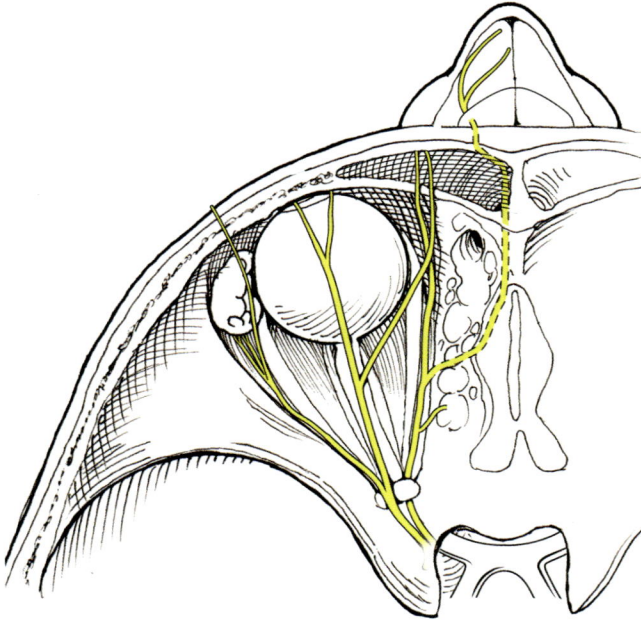

Fig. 4.2 Ophthalmic division of the trigeminal nerve. Axial view of ophthalmic division of the trigeminal nerve in relationship to orbit, optic nerve, optic chiasm, and skull base.

nerves. Only the ones that are pertinent to regional blocks are addressed here (**Fig. 4.3**).

Injection of local anesthetics does not have to be painful. There are several modifications that can be integrated to lessen the discomfort of injection. Cool solutions can be more painful than those at body temperature. Rapid infiltration also hurts more than slow injection. Addition of sodium bicarbonate will alter the pH of the anesthetic solution and help to attenuate the discomfort. Minimizing the number of injections

by performing an effective regional block first will improve patient comfort. Addition of hyaluronidase will further help to accelerate the spread of the anesthetic and increase diffusion. Our standard technique utilizes 9 mL of 2% Xylocaine with 1:100,000 epinephrine mixed with 1 mL (150 units) of hyaluronidase.

Ophthalmic Division V₁

Supraorbital Nerve—Pertinent Anatomy

This nerve is located by the supraorbital notch, which is palpable in the supraorbital rim of the frontal bone (**Fig. 4.4**). A vertical line can be drawn connecting this landmark with the infraorbital and mental foramen, which is a line drawn through the inner limbus of the eye. If measuring from the midline, this nerve reliably exits the skull between 2.5 and 2.7 cm. This measurement is important because the notch cannot always be palpated. In 60% of patients, the nerve is in the notch, whereas 32% of the time, it exits through a foramen. Supernumerary branches occur in 8% of all cases. After exiting, the nerve divides into two branches—a medial and a lateral. The medial branch runs on the surface of the frontalis; the lateral branch courses under the frontalis. There are instances where only the lateral branch exits from a separate foramen above the rim.[9]

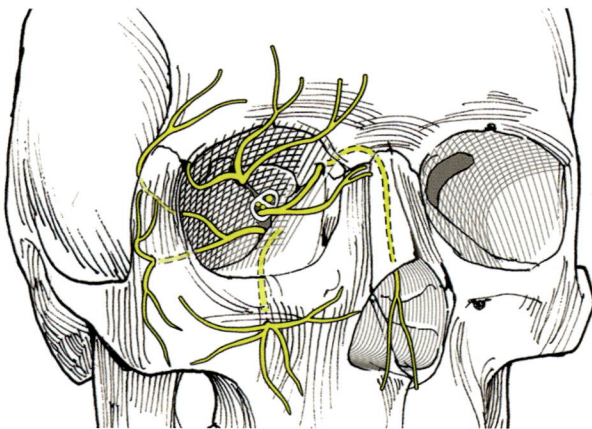

Fig. 4.3 Relationship of bony orbital rim to nerve exits. Nerve blocks associated with bony landmarks allow the practitioner to produce more reliable analgesia than those that depend solely on surface landmarks.

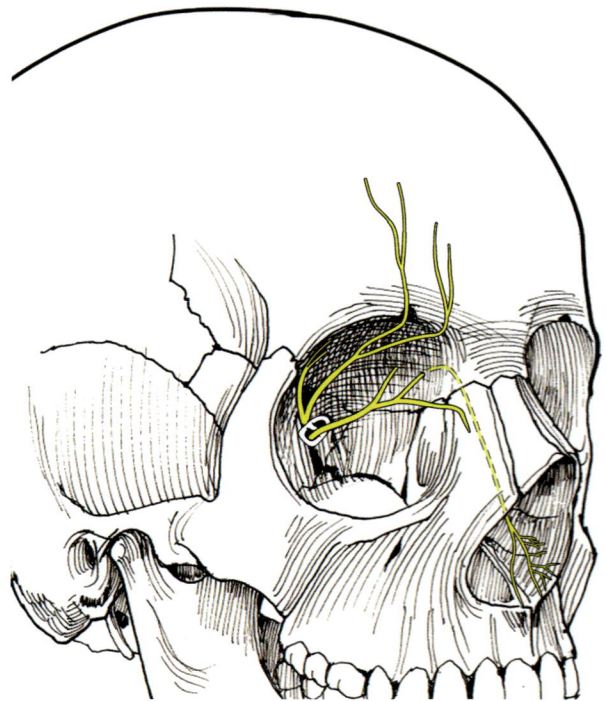

Fig. 4.4 Supraorbital nerve. The supraorbital nerve reliably exits via a notch (shown here) or foramen ~ 2.5 to 2.7 cm from midline.

Technical Aspects of Procedure

Inject 1 to 1.5 mL of local anesthetic under the edge of the superior orbital margin just lateral to the supraorbital notch ▶ **Video 4.1**.

Area of Anesthesia

The area of anesthesia is the medial and lateral forehead, back to the vertex of the head, and anterior scalp.

Supratrochlear Nerve—Pertinent Anatomy

This smaller nerve exits between the superior oblique muscle within the orbit and the supraorbital notch/foramen, eventually piercing through both the medial portion of the frontalis and corrugator supercilii muscles.

Technical Aspects of Procedure

Inject 1 mL of local anesthetic at the superior bony orbital margin, 1 cm superior to the caruncle of the eye ▶ **Video 4.1**.

Area of Anesthesia

The area of anesthesia is the central part of the forehead, inner canthal region, and glabella.

Infratrochlear Nerve—Pertinent Anatomy

This is a branch of the nasociliary nerve of the ophthalmic division of the trigeminal nerve. It courses forward along the medial wall of the orbit.

Technical Aspects of Procedure

Inject 1 mL of local anesthetic inferior to the medial aspect of the eyebrow at the level of the caruncle, just over the periosteum ▶ **Video 4.2**.

Area of Anesthesia

The area of anesthesia is the skin of the eyelids and side of the nose near the inner canthus.

Lacrimal Nerve—Pertinent Anatomy

The lacrimal nerve, also a branch of the ophthalmic division of the trigeminal nerve, runs along the upper border of the lateral rectus muscle and passes close to the periosteum of the orbital plate of the frontal bone. It branches off to the lacrimal gland, although some fibers pierce the orbital septum, exiting the orbit, to reach the skin and periosteum of the superolateral bony margin above the eyebrow.[10]

Technical Aspects of Procedure

Inject 1 mL of local anesthetic under the eyebrow just over the periosteum and in line with the lateral limbus ▶ **Video 4.1**.

Area of Anesthesia

The area of anesthesia is the infrabrow skin lateral to the pupil, and on occasion, forehead skin up to 2 cm above the brow.

Anterior Ethmoidal Nerve—Pertinent Anatomy

A branch of the nasociliary nerve of the ophthalmic division of the trigeminal nerve, this nerve supplies sensation to the mucosa of the lateral wall of the nose. Regional block of this nerve supplies sufficient anesthesia for even lateral osteotomies in rhinoplasty.

Technical Aspects of Procedure

Inject 0.5 mL of local anesthetic into the anterior border of the middle turbinate.

Area of Anesthesia

The area of anesthesia is the mucosa (internal lining) of the lateral wall of the nose.

External Nasal Nerve—Pertinent Anatomy

A part of the anterior ethmoidal branch of the nasociliary nerve, the external or dorsal nasal nerve first supplies the anterior septal mucosa and lateral nasal wall anteriorly before emerging from a small groove at the lower border of the nasal bones (**Fig. 4.5**). It passes 6 to 10 mm off the midline and runs under the transverse nasalis muscle. [1]

Technical Aspects of Procedure

Inject 0.5 mL of local anesthetic subcutaneously at the junction of the upper lateral cartilage and nasal bones ▶ **Video 4.2**.

Area of Anesthesia

The area of anesthesia is the nasal ala, nasal vestibule, and tip.

Maxillary Division V$_2$

Infraorbital Nerve—Pertinent Anatomy

The infraorbital nerve branches from the maxillary division and passes through the infraorbital foramen, exiting deep to the levator labii superioris muscle. The infraorbital foramen lies in a vertical line drawn from the inner limbus or ~ 2.7 cm from midline and ~ 1 cm inferior to the lower orbital margin (**Fig. 4.6**).

Technical Aspects of Procedure

The approach of the needle may be transcutaneous or transoral; however, the direction of the needle must be from below because there is often a signifi-

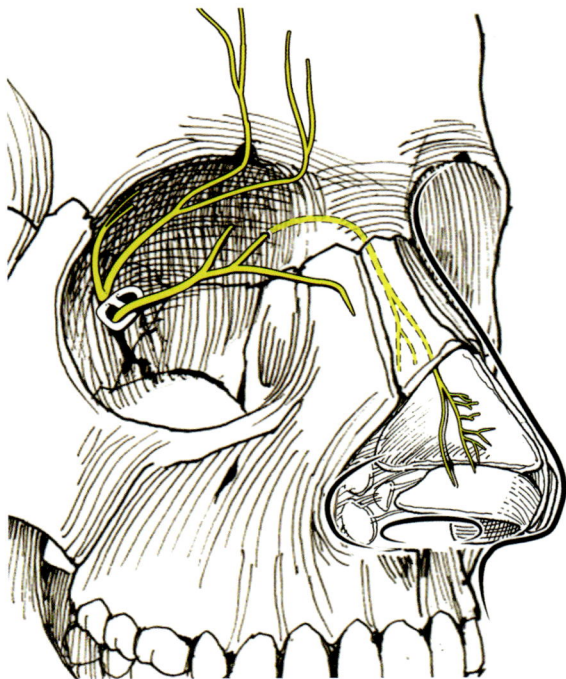

Fig. 4.5 External nasal nerve. The nasociliary nerve passes through the anterior ethmoidal foramen as the anterior ethmoidal nerve, supplying branches to the mucous membrane of the nasal cavity. Its terminal branch forms the external nasal nerve—emerging between the inferior border of the nasal bone and the upper lateral cartilages of the nasal dorsum.

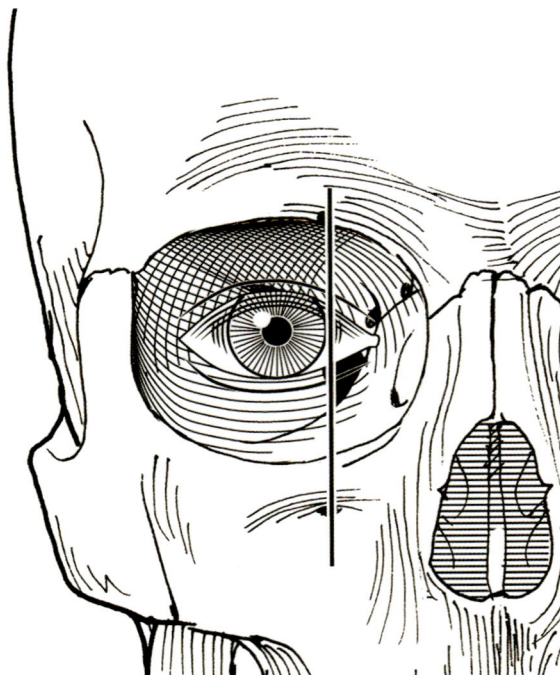

Fig. 4.6 Inner limbus line. A vertical line drawn through the inner limbus approximates the location of the supraorbital and infraorbital foramen.

cant bony ridge overlying the foramen (**Fig. 4.7**). Care should be taken to prevent injecting directly into the foramen because permanent numbness has been described. Inject 1 to 1.5 mL of local anesthetic after aspiration ▶ **Video 4.3**.

Area of Anesthesia

The area of anesthesia is the skin of the lower eyelid; lateral aspects of the nose, cheek, and upper lip; and mucous membranes of the cheek and upper lip.

Zygomaticotemporal Nerve—Pertinent Anatomy

This nerve runs along the lateral wall of the orbit to exit through the zygomaticotemporal foramen—a canal in the zygomatic bone behind the rim of the orbit (**Fig. 4.8**). It enters the temporal fossa and then resurfaces at the inferior aspect of the frontozygomatic suture (**Fig. 4.9**).

Technical Aspects of Procedure

After aspiration, inject 1 mL of local anesthetic posterior to the lateral orbital margin and 1 cm inferior to the frontozygomatic suture line ▶ **Video 4.4**.

Area of Anesthesia

The area of anesthesia is the anterior temple skin.

Zygomaticofacial Nerve—Pertinent Anatomy

This tiny nerve arises in the pterygopalatine fossa and runs along the inferior lateral border of the orbit, exiting from a foramen in the zygomatic bone (**Fig. 4.10**) piercing the orbicularis oculi muscle.

Technical Aspects of Procedure

Inject 0.5 mL of local anesthetic along the periosteum of the medial zygomatic arch (bony cheek prominence), ~ 1.5 cm lateral to the orbital rim at the level of the inferior orbital margin ▶ **Video 4.3**.

Area of Anesthesia

The area of anesthesia is the skin over the cheek prominence and the lateral lower eyelid.

Intramuscular Lip Block—Pertinent Anatomy

Sensory innervation of the upper lip is mainly derived from bilateral infraorbital nerves. In clinical practice, however, the midline of the lip (Cupid's bow) may not be adequately anesthetized with infraorbital nerve blocks. This area can be addressed by

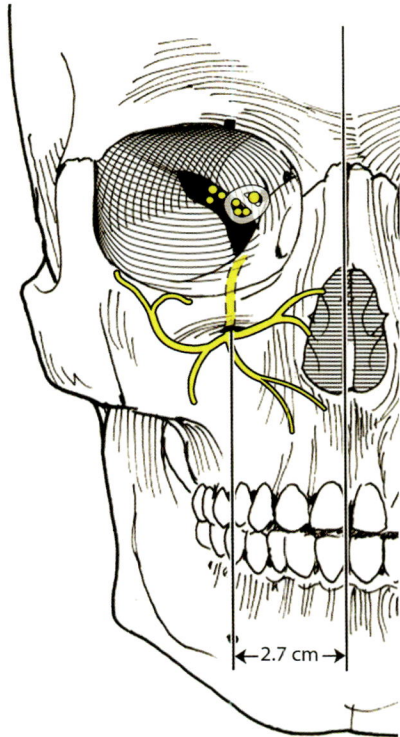

Fig. 4.7 Infraorbital nerve. The infraorbital nerve exiting through the infraorbital foramen can be found ~ 2.7 cm from midline and 1 cm inferior to the lower orbital margin. Note the bony ridge overlying the foramen.

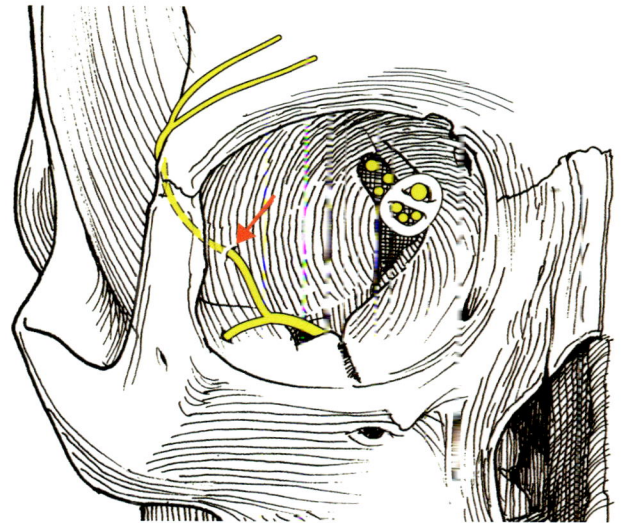

Fig. 4.8 Zygomaticotemporal foramen. The zygomaticotemporal nerve exits through the zygomatic bone behind the rim of the orbit via the zygomaticotemporal foramen (*arrow*).

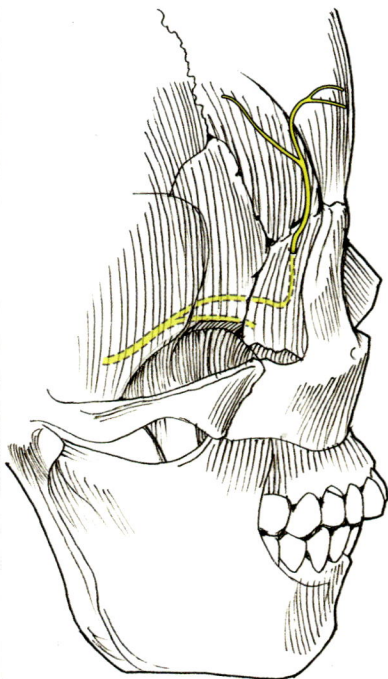

Fig. 4.9 Zygomaticotemporal nerve. This nerve resurfaces at the inferior aspect of the frontozygomatic suture line.

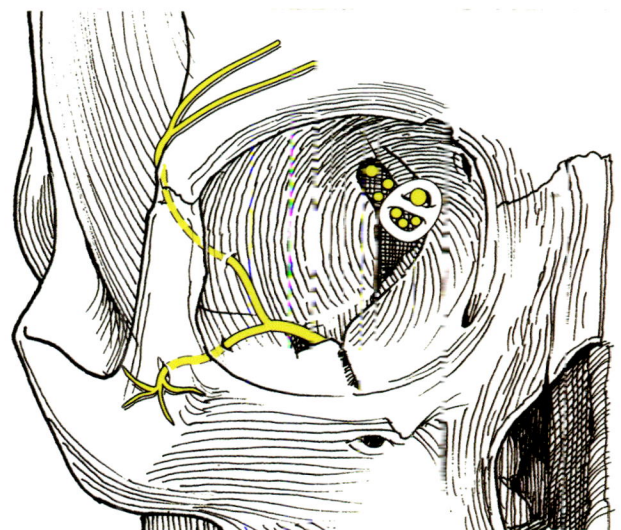

Fig. 4.10 Zygomaticofacial nerve. The zygomaticofacial nerve runs along the inferior lateral border of the orbit and exits via a foramen located on the convex malar surface of the zygomatic bone near its center.

anesthetizing the nasopalatine nerve (traditionally provides sensory innervation to the palate), which passes through the incisive foramen. Often an intramuscular nerve block is faster than an infraorbital block, without causing as much distortion as straight local infiltration of the lip.

Technical Aspects of Procedure

Administer five injections of 0.5 mL of local anesthetic across the mucosa—into the upper lip musculature (**Fig. 4.11**). Be sure to spread out the injections past the lip–cheek groove and include the nasal base.

Area of Anesthesia

The area of anesthesia is the upper lip.

Mandibular Division V₃

Auriculotemporal Nerve—Pertinent Anatomy

The auriculotemporal nerve passes posterior to the neck of the mandible (**Fig. 4.12**), carrying postganglionic parasympathetic fibers to the parotid gland before it turns superiorly and anteriorly between the temporomandibular joint and the external auditory canal to supply the auricle. It then crosses over the root of the zygomatic process of the temporal bone, deep to the superficial temporal artery, and follows the course of this artery to supply the skin of the temporal region and lateral scalp. Regional block of this nerve in conjunction with buccal and mental nerve blocks obviates the need for the riskier V₃ block at the foramen ovale.

Technical Aspects of Procedure

Inject 1 to 1.5 mL of local anesthetic deep and posterior to the neck of the mandibular condyle ▶ **Video 4.5**.

Area of Anesthesia

The area of anesthesia is the skin of the posterior temple and lateral cheek, and anterior surface of pinna.

Buccal Nerve—Pertinent Anatomy

This nerve runs between the two heads of the lateral pterygoid muscle before it courses underneath the tendon of the temporalis and masseter muscles. The nerve then continues on the surface of the buccinator muscle (**Fig. 4.13**).

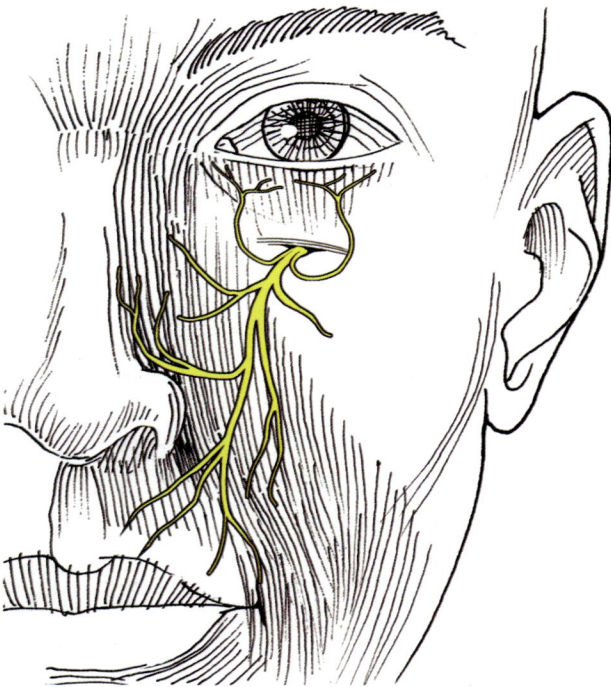

Fig. 4.11 Intramuscular lip branches. Intramuscular lip block is performed with local infiltration of five injections across the mucosa—into the upper lip musculature—targeting the lip branches.

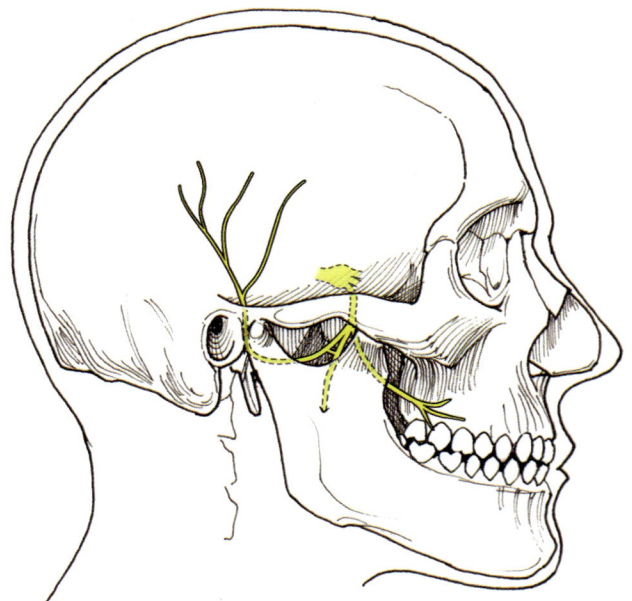

Fig. 4.12 Auriculotemporal nerve. The auriculotemporal nerve passes posterior to the neck of the mandible and then crosses over the root of the zygomatic process of the temporal bone to supply the skin of the anterior pinna, temporal region, and lateral scalp.

branches off the inferior alveolar nerve before the latter exits the mental foramen. Because both the mental and mylohyoid nerves are branches of the inferior alveolar nerve, an alternative is an inferior alveolar block at the lingula. This is a common block in dentistry but is rarely necessary for facial cosmetic procedures. However, due to moderate variability of the branching of the nerve to the mylohyoid off the inferior alveolar nerve, failure rates of 15 to 20% are reported in the dental literature.[14]

Technical Aspects of Procedure

To block the mental nerve, inject 1 mL of local anesthetic between the first and second premolars in the gingival labial sulcus approximately halfway between the gumline and the inferior border of the mandible. To block the terminal sensory branches of the nerve to the mylohyoid, use a 1.5-inch needle to inject 0.5 mL of local anesthetic into the vestibule directly in front of the anterior teeth; then advance the needle to inject another 0.5 mL beyond the lower border of the mandible in the supraperiosteal plane ▶ **Video 4.2**.[15]

Area of Anesthesia

The area of anesthesia is the skin of the chin and the lower lip, and the mucosa of the lower lip. The sensation of the skin at the mandibular line is variable.

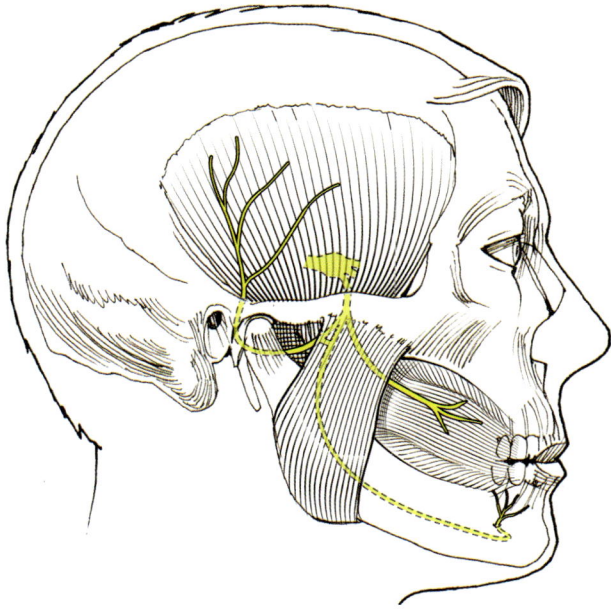

Fig. 4.13 Buccal nerve. The buccal nerve courses underneath the tendon of the temporalis and masseter muscles before continuing on the surface of the buccinator muscle.

Technical Aspects of Procedure

Inject 1 to 1.5 mL of local anesthetic at the middle third of the anterior border of the masseter muscle ▶ **Video 4.3**.

Area of Anesthesia

The area of anesthesia is the skin of the cheek over the buccinator muscle, buccal mucosa, and lateral oral commissure.

Mental Nerve—Pertinent Anatomy

The mental nerve is a branch of the inferior alveolar nerve. This nerve exits via the mental foramen, which is located between the apex of the first and second mandibular premolars (**Fig. 4.14**). The location of this foramen may vary from 6 to 10 mm anterior or posterior to this landmark.[12] The nerve is located between the gumline and the inferior border of the mandible. After exiting, it divides into three branches below the depressor anguli oris muscle. The three branches supply the red lower lip, the skin between the vermilion border to the labiomental crease, and the skin of the chin, respectively.

Although traditionally viewed as a motor nerve, the nerve to the mylohyoid also confers some sensation to the chin.[13] This nerve travels in a groove on the medial surface of the mandibular ramus and

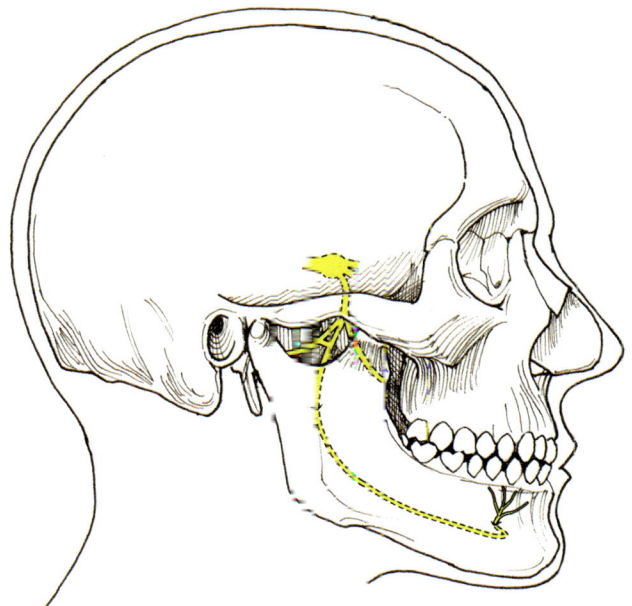

Fig. 4.14 Mental nerve. The mental nerve exits via the mental foramen, which is located between the apex of the first and second mandibular premolars.

Regional Blocks of the Neck

Cervical Plexus C$_2$, C$_3$

Pertinent Anatomy

The segmental spinal nerves of the upper cervical spine exit the vertebrae posterior to the vertebral arteries. The cervical plexus of C$_2$ and C$_3$ then divides into dorsal and ventral rami (**Fig. 4.15**). The greater and lesser occipital nerves make up the dorsal ramus. The ventral ramus includes the great auricular nerve, anterior cutaneous nerve of the neck, and the supraclavicular nerve. The dorsal ramus supplies sensory innervation to the posterior scalp, neck, and shoulders.

Technical Aspects of Procedure

To block the ventral ramus, inject 2 to 3 mL of local anesthetic at the posterior border of the sternocleidomastoid muscle approximately one third to one half of the distance inferior to the mastoid tip. A useful pearl is that the great auricular nerve is found ~ 6.5 cm below the lower border of the external auditory canal along the sternocleidomastoid muscle.[15]

Area of Anesthesia

The area of anesthesia includes the edges of this dermatome, which can be quite variable—anterior neck skin up to the lower jaw to just inferior of the clavicles.

Regional Blocks of the Chest

Anterior Cutaneous Nerves of Thorax

Pertinent Anatomy

The intercostal nerves of the thorax arise from the anterior division of the paravertebral nerves. An intercostal nerve typically has four branches: postganglionic gray communicantes, posterior cutaneous, lateral cutaneous, and anterior cutaneous branches (**Fig. 4.16**). The upper thoracic nerves run within their respective intercostal spaces at the inferior margin of the rib. The nerves travel along with the artery and vein in the costal groove. As they approach the midline, the nerves turn anteriorly and pierce the overlying external costal muscles and pectoralis major to terminate as the anterior cutaneous nerve near the lateral border of the sternum. The anterior cutaneous branches supply innervation to the midline of the chest with some contralateral crossover. There are notable variations in T1, especially. T1 and T2 send nerve fibers to the upper limbs and the upper thorax.

Technical Aspects of Procedure

Inject 1 mL of local anesthetic in the first and second intercostal groove just lateral to the sternum and immediately inferior to the rib (**Fig. 4.17**). To prevent pneumothorax, contact with the rib first is advised, followed by "walking" the needle off the inferior edge.[16] Prior to injection, aspiration should be per-

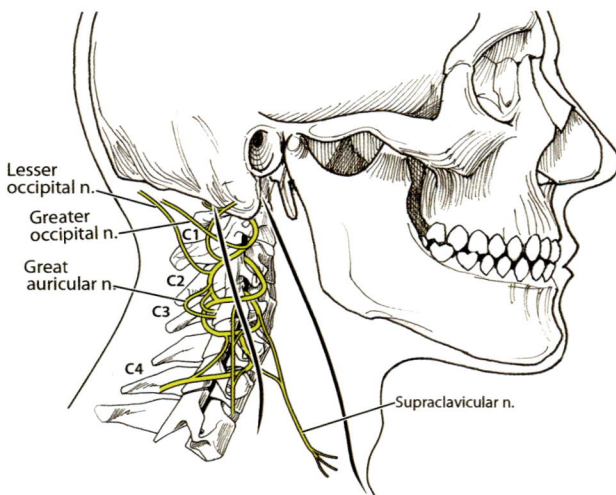

Fig. 4.15 Cervical plexus of C$_2$, C$_3$—dorsal and ventral rami. The greater and lesser occipital nerves make up the dorsal rami. The ventral ramus includes the great auricular nerve, anterior cutaneous nerve of the neck, and the supraclavicular nerve.

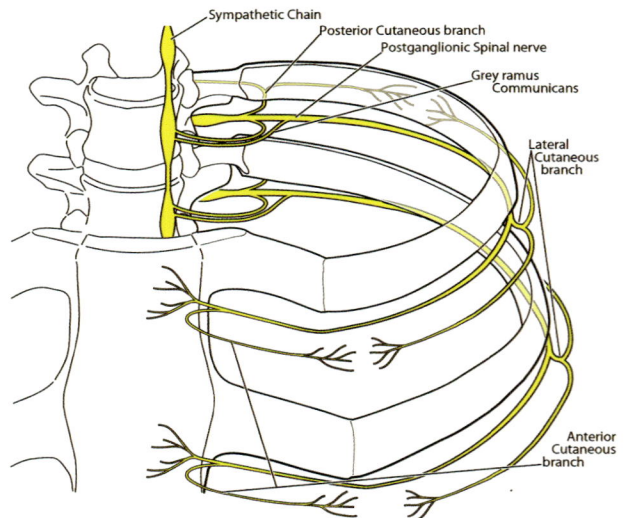

Fig. 4.16 Four branches of intercostal nerve anatomy. Postganglionic gray communicantes, posterior cutaneous, lateral cutaneous, and anterior cutaneous branches.

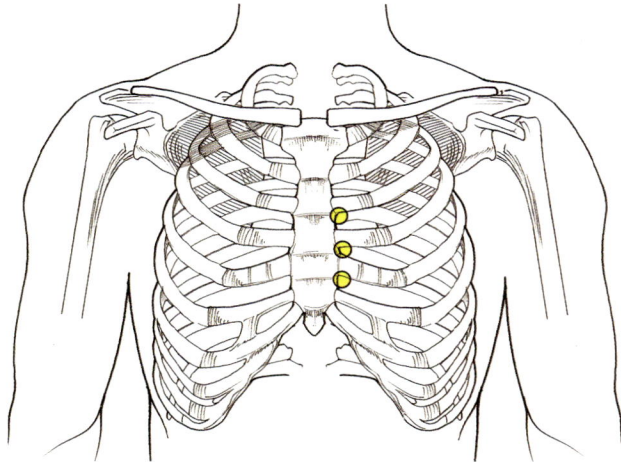

Fig. 4.17 Anterior thorax. Injection should be placed (yellow dot) just lateral to the sternum and immediately inferior to the rib. Care must be taken when performing these injections to avoid pneumothorax.

formed to check for air or blood so that intra-arterial or intrapleural injection is prevented.

Area of Anesthesia

The area of anesthesia is the skin of the front of the chest in the décolleté area based upon dermatomal distribution.

■ Complications and Their Management

Clearly, the best way to avoid systemic local anesthetic complications is prevention of excessive doses in highly vascular areas. Accepted maximal doses for healthy adults exist in the literature (**Table 4.4**); however, much controversy prevails because numerous studies have published safe plasma lidocaine levels despite administration of dosages above recommended levels. Subjective signs of toxicity are evident at 3 to 5 µg/mL, whereas cardiopulmonary arrest occurs at levels above 20 µg/mL.[17] Although the current recommended dose of lidocaine is 7 mg/kg or a total of 50 mL (or 500 mg) of 1% lidocaine with 1:100,000 epinephrine in healthy adults, doses up to 55 mg/kg have been used in tumescent liposuction.[18] High-dose diluted lidocaine with epinephrine has also been used successfully for facelifts at dosages of 21 mg/kg.[19,20] Toxic levels may result from inadvertent intravascular injection as well. A maneuver to minimize this risk is aspiration back into the syringe to check for blood before injection.

Table 4.4 Maximum dosage

Agent	Maximal Dosage
Lidocaine (Xylocaine[a])	4.5 mg/kg
Lidocaine (Xylocaine) 1 or 2% with epinephrine	7 mg/kg
Cocaine 4% topical	2 mg/kg
Bupivacaine 0.5% (Marcaine[b])	1.3 mg/kg
Articaine 4% (Septocaine[c]) with epinephrine	7 mg/kg
Mepivacaine 3% (Carbocaine[d])	2 mg/kg
Ropivacaine 0.5% (Naropin[e])	2.5 mg/kg or 300 mg
Epinephrine	10 µg/kg or 1 mg

[a]AstraZeneca, LP, Wilmington DE.
[b]Abbott Laboratories, Abbott Park, IL.
[c]Novocol Pharmaceuticals, Cambridge, Ontario, Canada.
[d]Cooke-Waite Dental Anesthetics, Carestream Dental, Rochester, NY.
[e]APP Pharmaceuticals, Schaumberg, IL.

Local anesthetics have the ability to cross the blood–brain barrier, which can result in generalized CNS toxicity. This effect is dose-dependent. Low doses produce CNS depression, whereas high doses provoke CNS excitation and seizures. Compared with CNS toxicity, much larger doses of local anesthetics are needed to produce cardiovascular compromise. Increased cardiotoxicity is seen with more potent and more lipid-soluble agents, such as bupivacaine and ropivacaine. Bupivacaine is 4 times more potent but 16 times more cardiotoxic than lidocaine.[21,22]

Treatment of systemic toxicity is supportive care. Injection of local anesthetics should be terminated without delay. If not already in place, heart rate, blood pressure, and oxygen saturation should be monitored. Standard resuscitation protocols addressing airway, breathing, and circulation should be implemented. Intubation and positive pressure ventilation may be required. Seizure activity may aggravate hypoxemia and hypercarbia. Intravenous thiopental (50 to 100 mg), midazolam (2 to 5 mg), and propofol (1 mg/kg) are treatment options to help terminate seizure activity from local anesthetic toxicity. Succinylcholine (50 mg) can also be used to stop muscular activity from seizures, so that the patient can be more readily ventilated. Cardiovascular depression may proceed to hypotension and bradycardia, treatable with ephedrine (10 to 30 mg) and atropine (0.4 mg), respectively. Malignant dysrhythmias, most often seen with the more potent and lipid-soluble agents, are often difficult to treat and require aggressive resuscitation with epinephrine, vasopressin, amiodarone, and/or electrical cardioversion.

Although extremely rare, local anesthetics do have the ability to cause neural toxicity to peripheral nerves. In clinical applications, this risk is virtually nonexistent. Studies show that the spinal cord and unsheathed nerve roots are most prone to this type of injury.[5] Alternatively, the theoretical risk of permanent neural damage still exists if intraneural injection occurs.

Minor adverse events related to local anesthetics include pain, bleeding at needle-puncture site, and bruising. Hematomas are infrequent but possible. Neurapraxia of surrounding motor nerves is also uncommon but may be unavoidable, depending on the area to be anesthetized. This temporary paralysis resolves when the action of the local anesthetic subsides. Scar formation at needle-entry site is virtually imperceptible if 25- or 27-gauge or smaller needles are used. For cutaneous nerve blocks, broken needles are a trivial event, but they have the potential to be problematic in intraoral blocks, most typically inferior alveolar blocks. The fractured needle fragment often becomes buried, necessitating radiographic guidance for removal under general anesthesia.[23]

Another phenomenon that deserves special mention is tachyphylaxis to local anesthetics. Tachyphylaxis refers to insufficient local anesthetic induction due to drug resistance. In this clinical circumstance, a decline in efficacy of local anesthetic with repeated injections of the same dose is observed. This is widely believed to be related to dosing interval and pain progression.[5] Both pharmacokinetic and dynamic mechanisms responsible for tachyphylaxis are still poorly understood. Currently there are no reliable treatments to prevent its clinical development.

Finally, vasovagal reactions in response to injection of local anesthetics are not uncommon.[24] Subjective feelings of dizziness and light-headedness during or after the procedure are frequent complaints. These adverse events may even be psychosomatic results of needle phobia, reported to affect 10% of the population.[25] Presyncope and true syncopal episodes do occur, and thus physicians must make preparations to ensure a safe environment so that patients do not suffer inadvertent additional injuries. Anecdotally, young patients are more likely to develop presyncope, with young male patients most prone to true syncope.

■ Conclusion

Any physician involved in aesthetic or reconstructive facial procedures needs to be adept in anesthetizing the face to guarantee high patient satisfaction rates. Topical preparations will relieve only superficial discomforts, whereas heavy sedation is often unnecessary and undesirable. Anatomically based local regional blocks can be performed quickly and are highly consistent in providing effective anesthesia for several hours, depending on the specific agent used. Proficiency in the techniques described here will enhance patient comfort and reach the physician's goal to provide painless plastic surgery.

References

1. Altman AJ, Albert DM, Fournier GA. Cocaine's use in ophthalmology: our 100-year heritage. Surv Ophthalmol 1985;29(4):300–306
2. dos Reis A Jr. Sigmund Freud (1856-1939) and Karl Köller (1857-1944) and the discovery of local anesthesia. Rev Bras Anestesiol 2009;59(2):244–257
3. Fink BR. Leaves and needles: the introduction of surgical local anesthesia. Anesthesiology 1985;63(1):77–83
4. Fleming JA, Byck R, Barash PG. Pharmacology and therapeutic applications of cocaine. Anesthesiology 1990;73(3):518–531
5. Ebert TJ, Schmid PG. Local anesthetics. In: Barash PG, Cullen BF, Stoelting RK, et al, eds. Clinical Anesthesia. 6th ed. Philadelphia, PA: Lippincott Williams & Wilkins;2009:413–433
6. Ellis DA, Gage CE. Evaluation of conscious sedation in facial plastic surgery. J Otolaryngol 1991;20(4):267–273
7. Millay DJ, Larrabee WF Jr, Carpenter RL. Vasoconstrictors in facial plastic surgery. Arch Otolaryngol Head Neck Surg 1991;117(2):160–163
8. Young KD. What's new in topical anesthesia. Clin Pediatr Emerg Med 2007;8(4):232–239
9. Beer GM, Putz R, Mager K, Schumacher M, Keil W. Variations of the frontal exit of the supraorbital nerve: an anatomic study. Plast Reconstr Surg 1998;102(2):334–341
10. Ross G, Taams K. Regional anesthesia on the lacrimal nerve. Plast Reconstr Surg 1999;104(3):876–878
11. Zide BM. Nasal anatomy: the muscles and tip sensation. Aesthetic Plast Surg 1985;9(3):193–196
12. Haribhakti VV. The dentate adult human mandible: an anatomic basis for surgical decision making. Plast Reconstr Surg 1996;97(3):536–541, discussion 542–543
13. Stein P, Brueckner J, Milliner M. Sensory innervation of mandibular teeth by the nerve to the mylohyoid: implications in local anesthesia. Clin Anat 2007;20(6):591–595
14. Kaufman E, Weinstein P, Migrom P. Difficulties in achieving local anesthesia. JADA 1984;108(2):20–208
15. Zide BM, Swift R. How to block and tackle the face. Plast Reconstr Surg 1998;101(3):840–851

16. Blake DR. Office-based anesthesia: dispelling common myths. Aesthet Surg J 2008;28(5):564–570, discussion 571–572

17. Shapiro FE. Anesthesia for outpatient cosmetic surgery. Curr Opin Anaesthesiol 2008;21(6):704–710

18. Iverson RE, Pao VS. MOC-PS(SM) CME article: liposuction. Plast Reconstr Surg 2008;121(4, Suppl):1–11

19. Bonanno PC. Safe dosages of lidocaine for facial analgesia. J Craniofac Surg 1994;5(2):124–126

20. Ramon Y, Barak Y, Ullmann Y, Hoffer E, Yarhi D, Bentur Y. Pharmacokinetics of high-dose diluted lidocaine in local anesthesia for facelift procedures. Ther Drug Monit 2007;29(5):644–647

21. Reiz S, Nath S. Cardiotoxicity of local anaesthetic agents. Br J Anaesth 1986;58(7):736–746

22. Nath S, Häggmark S, Johansson G, Reiz S. Differential depressant and electrophysiologic cardiotoxicity of local anesthetics: an experimental study with special reference to lidocaine and bupivacaine. Anesth Analg 1986; 65(12):1263–1270

23. Pogrel MA. Broken local anesthetic needles: a case series of 16 patients, with recommendations. J Am Dent Assoc 2009;140(12):1517–1522

24. Shalom A, Westreich M, Hadad E, Friedman T. Complications of minor skin surgery performed under local anesthesia. Dermatol Surg 2008;34(8):1077–1079

25. Hamilton JG. Needle phobia: a neglected diagnosis. J Fam Pract 1995;41(2):169–175

5 Superficial Chemical Peels

Phillip R. Langsdon, David W. Rodwell III, Parker A. Velargo, Carol H. Langsdon, and Amanda Guydon

Key Concepts

- Enhanced superficial chemical peels are an important minimally invasive cosmetic technique that can benefit a wide range of patients and can be easily incorporated into an aesthetic practice.

- The success of the enhanced superficial chemical peel can be improved with adequate patient preparation.

- Performance of a series of six to eight adequately frosted trichloracetic acid (TCA) peels (15 to 25%) accomplishes a more advanced form of superficial peeling—which may be considered equivalent to medium-depth peels.

- Enhanced superficial chemical peels can, in some patients, approximate the results of fractionated laser treatments.

■ Introduction

For centuries, man has searched for a "miracle potion" that would reverse aging, wrinkled skin. Ancient topical treatments with milk, wine, and various fruits were used in an attempt to improve the skin. By the early 20th century, "lay peelers" began using a variety of techniques and topical agents that afforded deeper skin penetration. These peels, adopted by some members of the medical community, were often a source of controversy; however, eventually they became an accepted practice. Deep chemical peels became a key procedure in the treatment of the aging face and represented an important component of a successful facial aesthetic practice after Baker and Gordon popularized the classic phenol peel in the

1960s. Since then, there has been continuing interest in resurfacing the facial skin and an evolution of peeling agents, including those for superficial peeling.

In the 1990s, lasers became popular tools to resurface the skin. Whereas some lasers treat more superficially, others, such as the carbon dioxide laser, have the potential to treat deeply. The side effects of deep carbon dioxide lasers (e.g., long-term hypopigmentation) fostered the development of fractionated beams designed to lessen tissue damage and reduce side effects. However, the separation of beams to spare segments of untreated tissue and the reduction of intensity of the fractionated light beam reduced aesthetic results.

Properly structured skin care/peeling protocols utilizing the sequential application of a novel superficial chemical peeling technique may approximate many of the fractionated laser treatments. Peels can be offered as an effective alternative to laser treatments because they are inexpensive. This chapter describes a unique technique that can provide greater improvements than those typically obtained by superficial peels. The technique of "enhanced superficial chemical peeling" has been found to produce excellent results with minimal down time and costs.

■ Background: Basic Science of Procedure

Chemical peeling involves the application of a chemical exfoliant that initiates a controlled wound to the epidermis and/or dermis. In general, results are dependent upon the depth of penetration. Penetration can be altered by the type of agent, the concentration of the agent, the time of contact with the skin, the potential reapplication of the agent, and the resistance of the skin. Peeling may be enhanced by pretreating the skin with an effective daily exfoliation program designed to disrupt a damaged keratin surface, allowing improved penetration of the peel. Pretreating may also stimulate regeneration from the basal layer. Effective peeling may improve surface irregularities and stimulate fibroblast activity and collagen production.

Superficial peeling agents include α-hydroxyl acids (glycolic, lactic, and pyruvic acids), salicylic acid, retinoic acid, resorcinol, and TCA (in lower concentrations). Solutions like Jessner's solution (resorcinol, 14 g; salicylic acid, 14 g; lactic acid, 14 mL; ethanol, 100 mL) have also been formulated to peel at a superficial level.

Most superficial peels are used to improve very fine wrinkles and pigmentary changes. However, some peels are used for other indications. The lipophilic nature and anti-inflammatory properties of salicylic acid make it a popular peel for acne-prone patients.

The concentration of the peel determines whether it is considered superficial or medium. For example, TCA used in higher concentrations may be considered a medium-depth peel. The authors consider TCA peeling above 35% to be unpredictable, and it is known to be associated with scarring when used above 45%.[1,2] The length of application time can also determine if a treatment is superficial or medium. Repeated single-treatment placement of high concentrations of pyruvic or glycolic acids, for example, may cause a medium-depth treatment.[3]

Pertinent Anatomy

The epidermis is composed of several layers of cells that are all generated from the innermost stratum basale. The basal cells continually regenerate the layers of skin cells. The cells migrate up from the stratum basale to the stratum spinosum, stratum granulosum, stratum lucidum (usually found only on the friction-prone areas, such as the palms and soles), and to the outermost stratum corneum (**Fig. 5.1**). Melanocytes can be found in the basal layer.

Beneath the dermal-epidermal junction lies the papillary dermis. Deep to this layer is the reticular dermis, which interdigitates with the papillary dermis above. The papillary dermis is thin, with loose collagen bundles and abundant fibrocytes. The reticular dermis, in contrast, is thicker, with dense collagen and fewer fibrocytes.

As we age, the skin regeneration process slows, the epidermis thins, and the outer stratum corneum layer becomes less organized. The rete pegs and dermal papillae become less pronounced, which results in a flattening of the dermal-epidermal junction. The dermis also thins and the collagen and elastin fibers diminish in volume and organization. The additive effects of this aging process and associated solar damage lead to characteristic findings, including irregular, wrinkled skin with keratosis and pigment changes.

Patient Selection

Perhaps the most important aspect of appropriate patient selection is in a realistic understanding of the limitations of various types of chemical peels. Many of the so-called superficial peels may disrupt the stratum corneum but have limited impact on more advanced skin-aging changes. Some of the more aggressive superficial peels (e.g., the higher concentrations of glycolic acid) may be an appropriate option

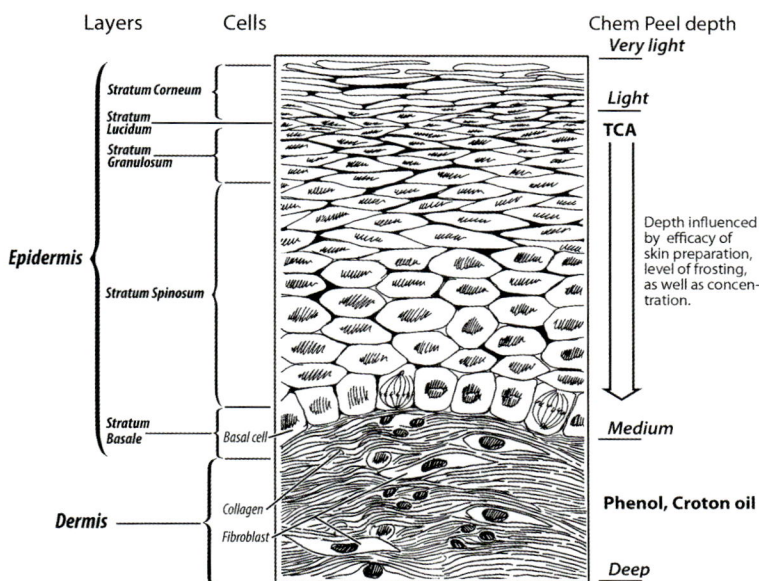

Fig. 5.1 Schematic of skin cross-section showing cellular layers and approximate depth of penetration of commonly used peeling agents.

for improving overall skin quality, such as rough texture and some solar damage. Photoaging to a Glogau I or II level may respond well to some types of superficial chemical peeling.

Acne may sometimes be improved with superficial chemical peels. Superficial pigmentary dyschromias, such as solar lentigines and melasma, can also be treated. However, deeper vascular abnormalities may not be addressed.

Although it has been taught that multiple superficial peels are not equivalent to medium or deep peels, in the experience of the authors a sequential application of enhanced superficial chemical peels can be effective in reducing fine rhytids. Enhanced improvement is attainable using a lower level of TCA, with adequate skin pretreatment and a series of more aggressive peels that are applied to the proper frosting level. The immediate reapplication of the peel, in the opinion of the authors, can increase the depth of treatment and improve a significant portion of superficial rhytids when used with this protocol.

A careful patient history should focus on any skin disorders, such as various forms of dermatitis, rosacea, acne, or herpes simplex virus infection. History of radiation exposure, immunosuppression, autoimmune disease, and collagen vascular disease is also important to elicit. These factors can impact wound healing. Additionally, there is the potential for chemical peeling to exacerbate an underlying skin disorder.

The physician, as with all cosmetic procedures, should understand the patient's desire and communicate realistic expectations of the refined superficial chemical peel. The patient should also understand the importance of the role that he or she will play in the pre- and posttreatment skin-care regimen. Standardized photographic documentation, as always, may help record most conditions. However, some details may not be captured by photography, especially with slight changes due to the limits of lighting, exposure, and camera capabilities.

■ Technical Aspects of Procedure

Pretreatment

The success of the enhanced superficial chemical peel can be improved with adequate patient preparation. Pretreatment preparations may be separated into two categories: antecedent and immediate. Antecedent pretreatment preparations include the use of sunscreen, glycolic acid, tretinoin, and/or hydroquinone prior to the superficial chemical peel.

During the pretreatment and posttreatment periods, patients should comply with limitations to sun exposure and the daily use of sunscreen. Sunscreen with a sun protection factor (SPF) of 30 or greater is preferred and should be used not only prepeel but also for at least the first several months postpeel. The use of sunscreen reduces the incidence of hyperpigmentary changes after chemical peeling.

Antivirals may be recommended as prophylaxis for superficial medium-peel patients with a positive history of herpetic outbreaks. If indicated, antivirals are started 1 day prior to the procedure and are continued for 1 to 2 weeks posttreatment. The authors do not routinely recommend prophylactic antibiotic therapy for these techniques.

The prepeeling skin preparation includes the daily use of a facial exfoliation cream containing an effective concentration of glycolic acid, for 1 to 2 weeks prior to the process. The cream is usually stopped 2 days before the procedure. Glycolic acid is an α-hydroxy acid derived from sugarcane that initiates keratinocyte dyscohesion and increases type I collagen and hyaluronic acid deposition in the skin.[4] The tightening properties of collagen and the hydrophilic characteristics of hyaluronic acid may give the skin a fuller and less-wrinkled appearance.

Tretinoin (e.g., Retin-A) not only thins the stratum corneum in thick-skinned individuals but also helps prepare the skin for chemical peels by activating dermal fibroblasts and stimulating increased collagen deposition. This product is also used for 1 to 2 weeks prior to the improved superficial chemical peel.

Hydroquinone may be used in the pretreatment regimen, especially in patients with significant pigmentation, spotty hyperpigmentation, and melasma. Hydroquinone blocks the production of melanin precursors and subsequent epidermal neopigmentation during the healing phase by inhibiting the enzyme tyrosinase. The authors recommend 4% hydroquinone cream for patients with Fitzpatrick type III skin or greater or for patients with pigmentary dyschromias. If indicated, this product is used for 1 to 2 weeks prior to the enhanced superficial chemical peel and then is resumed for a short period of time after healing.

Immediate pretreatment preparations include facial cleansing with soap and water or an antiseptic solution, followed by the use of acetone to "degrease" the skin.

Peeling

Several catalysts are available for use with superficial chemical peels. The aesthetic services of the authors include glycolic and salicylic acid peels; however, the authors achieve enhanced results with a slightly more detailed program. Their protocol is based upon aggressive skin pretreatment and a series of TCA peels that reach a refined frosting level. Recall that TCA causes keratocoagulation with precipitation of proteins as it penetrates deeper into the skin. The depth of penetration is dependent on skin cleansing and preparation, the concentration used, and the technique of application. The prepeeling skin preparation and modified TCA application used by the authors improve the impact of the weaker TCA concentrations, while avoiding the unpredictability of using higher concentrations as well as the thermal tissue damage associated with laser treatments.

By rigorously pretreating the skin, as outlined above, and following with a series of six to eight adequately frosted TCA peels, a more advanced form of superficial peeling—which may be considered equivalent to medium peels—is accomplished. This technique achieves results commensurate with some fractionated laser treatments in only one or two treatments.

The depth of the peel is dependent on the concentration of the agent, application duration, and number of applications. The authors prefer peels at 15, 20, and 25% TCA. In the experience of the senior author, TCA concentrations greater than 35% are more unpredictable and potentially more prone to postoperative scarring. Although increased concentrations of TCA are often safely used by others, the authors find that lower concentrations can attain equivalent benefits without the increased unpredictability of the higher concentrations. The authors increase the depth of the treatment program by proper pretreatment and cleansing and either increasing TCA contact time or immediately reapplying the peeling catalyst until the proper frosting has occurred. Frosting is carried to at least level II. A series of six to eight peels performed every 6 to 8 weeks can produce excellent results.

Typically, neither local anesthesia nor sedative medications are required for the enhanced superficial chemical peel. The process begins with 15% TCA for patients with superficial defects or sensitive skin ▶ Video 5.1. Treatment may begin with 20% TCA for damaged or more wrinkled skin. After cleansing and "de-greasing," the solution is evenly applied to the forehead, cheeks, nose, and chin using a saturated cotton ball. The eyelids are usually treated using cotton-tipped applicators. The exercise should take no longer than 1 to 2 minutes and the solution is reapplied until frosting has reached the expected level. The procedural end point is at least level II frosting (appearance of erythema and streaky whitening on the surface) and often the treatment is at level III. The timing of this end point varies from patient to patient. It may occur as early as 1 minute after application in thin, dry skin. It may take longer in thicker, severely aged, or weathered skin. Reapplication of the peel may be required in patients with resistant skin. The level of frosting needed is determined by the condition of the skin. Patients with more severe damage may require more advanced frosting. The frosting will be associated with a mild stinging/burning sensation. Once the required level of frosting manifests, the solution is washed off with tap water.

Postoperative Care

The patient can expect to have mild desquamation and erythema that begin to resolve within the first 5 days after a superficial peel. However, with increasing frosting, the initial healing process may last up to 7 days, with resolution of erythema in another week or so. Beginning the day after the peel, the face should be gently washed with a mild soap and water several times a day. The frequent application of fragrance- and color-free moisturizers, such as Aquaphor (Beiersdorf Inc., Hamburg, GE) cream, will aid in the healing process. Once re-epithelialization has occurred, the patient can apply a water-based or mineral makeup. Long-term sunscreen use is of critical importance to protect the newly healed skin.

Expected Results

Enhanced superficial chemical peels can improve overall skin texture and smooth superficial pigmentary abnormalities. Acne control may also be improved for many patients. Fine rhytids may show some improvement in select patients after one treatment. However, continued use of a strong daily skin exfoliation program combined with a series of TCA peels can obtain better long-term results. The concentration of TCA is often increased in the second and subsequent peels, and continued improvements should occur in subtle increments. The maximum benefit is seen after a series of enhanced superficial chemical peels over a period of several months, with an appropriate healing time between each peel session. This treatment program can effectively achieve deeper results and skin regeneration comparable to medium-depth peels. However, the healing time and side effects are usually less than that of deeper treatments. Sequential improvements may be difficult to visually appreciate from peel to peel. Proper photography may help demonstrate the long-term changes (**Figs. 5.2a,b**).

Complications and Their Management

Enhanced superficial chemical peels have relatively few complications in comparison to the deeper peel techniques or deep laser treatments. Pigmentary changes after superficial peels do occur and can be difficult to address. Erythema lasting longer than 3 to 4 weeks after an enhanced superficial chemical peel is unusual. Avoidance of sun exposure in the post-treatment period is helpful in decreasing hyperpig-

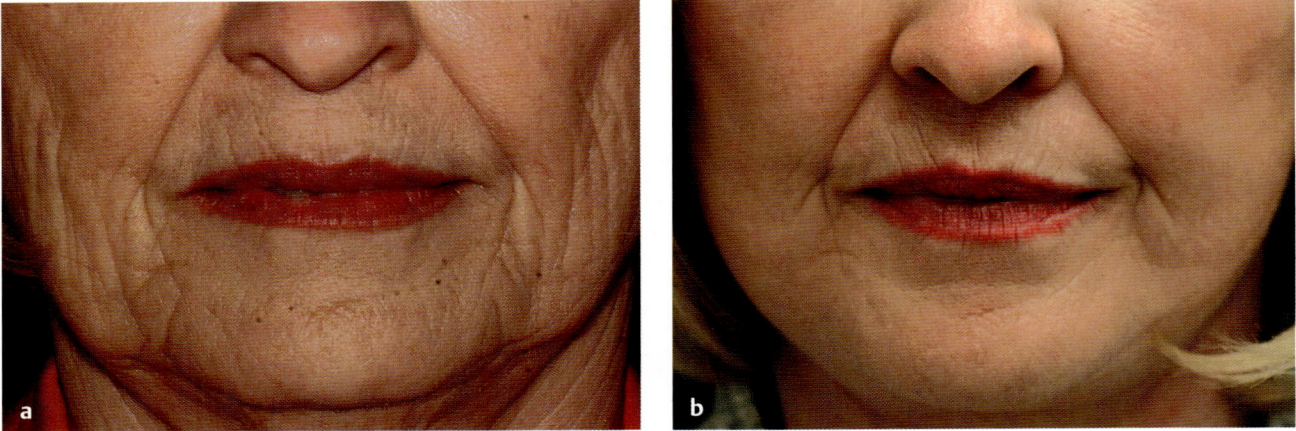

Fig. 5.2 **(a)** Prepeel. Note the fairly deep rhytids. **(b)** Postpeel. Status postenhanced superficial chemical peeling and rhytidectomy. The patient received a total of three peels spaced 6 to 8 weeks apart with increasing TCA concentrations with each peel (15 → 20 → 25%). Note the tremendous improvement in the rhytids.

mentation. Hydroquinone represents an additional option in treating hyperpigmentation. Occasionally, topical steroids may be used for prolonged erythema. Vitamin C serum may also decrease erythema.

Hypopigmentation is rarely seen after enhanced superficial chemical peels. This is typically due to melanocyte destruction and is known to be more problematic with deep peels or carbon dioxide laser treatments. Milia often develop after chemical peels. These areas sometimes resolve spontaneously but when they do not, management consists of mild exfoliation or unroofing of the milia.

The skin creates an important barrier of protection. When there is loss of this natural barrier by the use of a resurfacing agent, the potential for infection is increased. Careful cleansing of the skin and the use of moisturizers to create a moist occlusive dressing should prevent most infections. Bacterial infections are rare with appropriate wound care. As previously discussed, antiviral medications may be recommended in patients with a history of herpes simplex virus outbreaks. For patients with a strong history and recent outbreaks, the medication is started during the prepeel phase and is continued until re-epithelialization occurs.

Scarring and systemic complications are not usually seen with this enhanced superficial chemical peel technique. If these were to occur, treatment would be similar to that of more aggressive peeling programs.

■ Conclusion

Enhanced superficial chemical peeling is well tolerated by patients and offers an exceptional improvement in skin quality with little down time and few associated complications. When combined with an appropriate skin-care regimen, a series of sequential peels of increasing concentrations of TCA has the ability to produce results better than those seen with traditional methods of superficial chemical peeling. Refined superficial chemical peels are an important minimally invasive cosmetic technique that can benefit a wide range of patients, can be easily incorporated into an aesthetic practice, and can, in some patients, approximate the results of fractionated laser treatments.

References

1. Kotler R. Chemical Rejuvenation of the Face. St. Louis, MO: Mosby–Year Book, Inc.; 1992:65
2. Stegman SJ. Medium-depth chemical peeling: digging beneath the surface. J Dermatol Surg Oncol 1986; 12(12):1245–1246
3. Kotler R. Chemical Rejuvenation of the Face. Personal communication with Dr. Griffin. St. Louis, MO: Mosby–Year Book, Inc.; 1992:68–69
4. Bernstein EF, Lee J, Brown DB, Yu R, Van Scott E. Glycolic acid treatment increases type I collagen mRNA and hyaluronic acid content of human skin. Dermatol Surg 2001; 27(5):429–433

6 Medium-Depth Chemical Peels

Fred G. Fedok and Dhave Setabutr

Key Concepts

- Both the potential benefits and the potential deleterious side effects of resurfacing are directly related to the depth of skin injury created by the resurfacing modality.

- It is frequently better to be more conservative rather than more aggressive in the utilization of resurfacing techniques.

- It is usually best to use antiviral prophylaxis in all patients for full-face and perioral resurfacing.

◼ Introduction

Facial enhancement through the use of chemical peels has existed since at least 1550 BC, when Egyptians used caustic preparations for skin-peeling procedures.[1] Originating from these archaic formulations have evolved more modern agents developed to denature the protein framework of the skin and produce controlled wounding of the papillary/upper reticular dermis for cosmetic and noncosmetic indications.[2] In 1882, Paul G. Unna described the actions of salicylic acid, resorcinol, trichloracetic acid (TCA) and phenol on the skin.[1] "Skinning" or peeling of the face continued to be practiced using several agents and, by the 1960s, the modern era of peeling advanced with the development of modified phenol solutions by Baker and Gordon.[3] This integral aspect of cosmetic surgery has subsequently grown to include the use of a number of modified phenol preparations, various TCA concentrations, and α-hydroxy acids.[1]

◼ Background: Basic Science of Procedure

Photoaging principally refers to the effects of long-term ultraviolet (UV) exposure and sun damage superimposed on intrinsically aged skin.[4] The negative effects of sun exposure on the skin can be exhibited by dyspigmentation, laxity, sallow color, wrinkles, telangiectasia, leathery appearance, and cutaneous malignancies.[4,5] Histopathologically, there are abnormalities in collagen and elastin and ground substance breakdown and resynthesis.[5] The cell population increases and becomes disorganized, with an abundance of collapsed and elongated fibroblasts, whereas elastin quantity decreases (**Figs. 6.1a,b**).[6] Chemical peeling addresses this disorganization through limited wounding and subsequent healing, with collagen and elastin synthesis and cellular reorganization that ultimately result in more youthful and appealing skin. If the wounding proceeds to the epidermal basement membrane, where melanocytes lie, the wounded skin heals with a lighter, more even pigment. As wounding continues through the papillary dermis to the upper reticular dermis, deposition of new collagen, elastin, and glycosaminoglycans can result in a reduction of fine rhytids.[7] Results become more pronounced the deeper the peel progresses.

Chemical peels can be used to treat a variety of cosmetic and noncosmetic skin issues. They can alter the effects of skin aging, stimulating neocollagenesis and correcting pigment.[1] The desquamating properties of chemical peels can assist in acne treatment.[8] The removal of melanin is effective in managing melasma and lentigines.[9] Other indications for chemexfoliation include actinic keratoses, rhinophyma, xanthelasma, and syringoma (**Table 6.1**).[10]

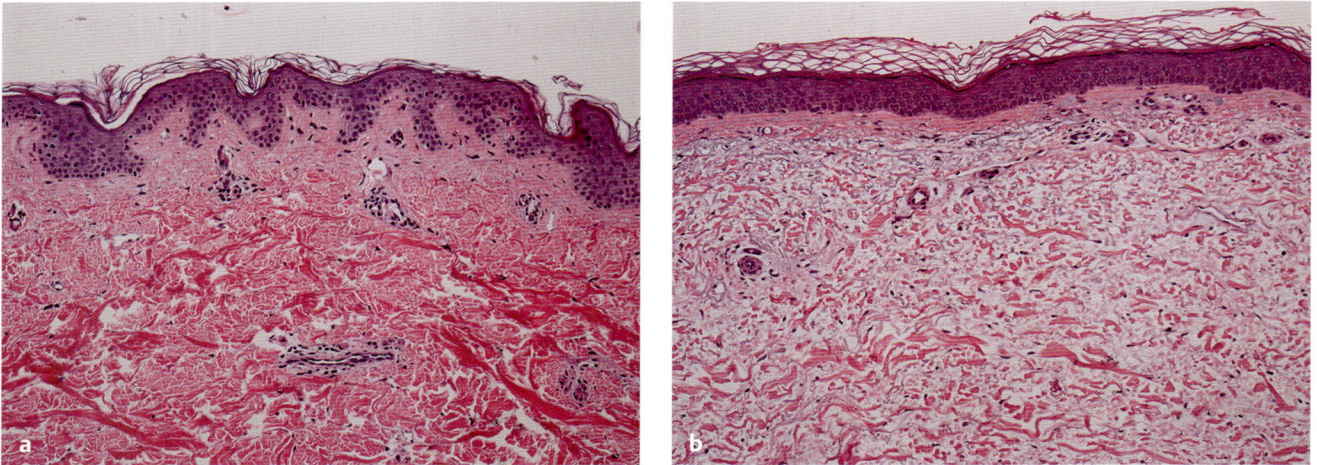

Fig. 6.1   (a) Photomicrograph of normal skin with orderly progression of epidermis, and normal dermal architecture. **(b)** Photomicrograph of sun-damaged skin and subsequent alteration of normal skin architecture with disorganized epidermis and lack of normal dermal architecture.

Table 6.1 Common indications for chemexfoliation

Rhytids (fine, medium, deep)

Scars (traumatic, acne, varicella)

Xanthelasma

Pigmentary irregularities (i.e., melasma)

Actinic keratosis (i.e., rhinophyma)

Syringoma

Classification of Peels

The expected depth of wounding is one way to categorize chemical peels. Superficial peels principally affect the epidermis (**Fig. 6.2**), acting as exfoliants and removing the stratum corneum and superficial aspects of the epidermis. There is little cellular necrosis or stimulation of epidermal growth. Medium-depth peels typically extend to the papillary dermis and the upper part of the reticular dermis (**Fig. 6.3**). Induction of inflammation within the papillary dermis occurs down to a depth of 0.60 mm. Deep peels generally extend down to the midreticular dermis[11,12] and create an inflammatory response that induces production of new collagen and ground substances (**Fig. 6.4**). The increase in ground substance results in an increased dermal volume and younger-looking skin. Reduced melanocyte activity and new col-

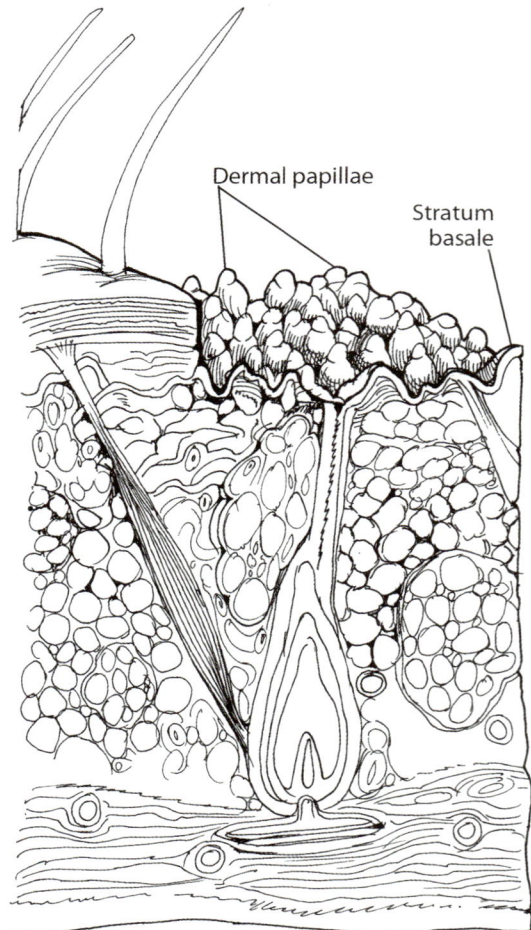

Fig. 6.2   The effect of a superficial chemical peel with penetration to the stratum basale.

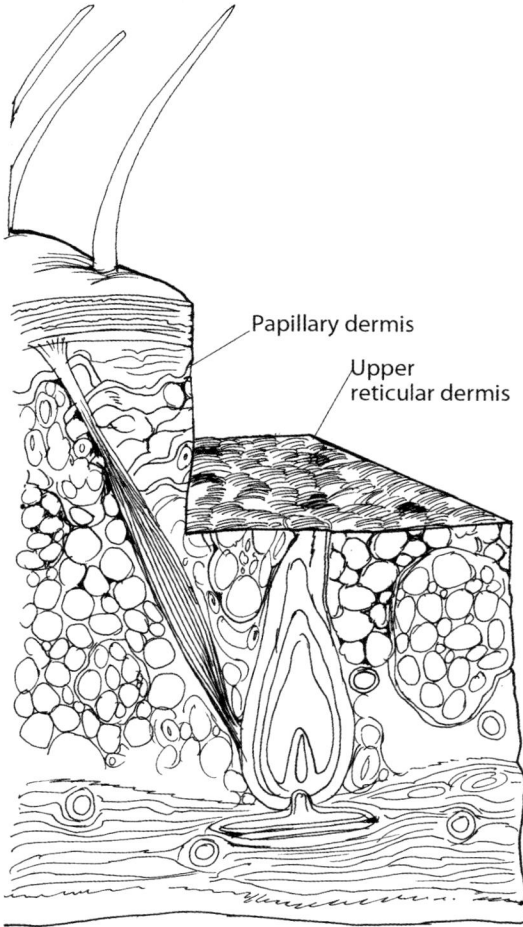

Fig. 6.3   The effect of a medium-depth chemical peel with penetration to the papillary dermis and the upper reticular dermis.

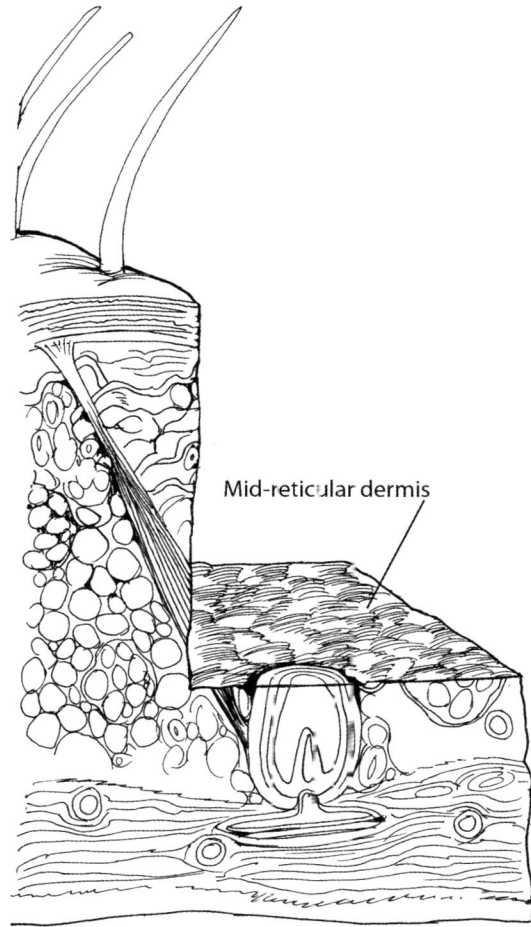

Fig. 6.4   The effect of a deep chemical peel with penetration to the midreticular dermis.

lagen and anchoring fibril deposition result in a reduction in wrinkling and skin roughness.[5] These depths of penetration are approximate and will vary depending on patient factors, the surgeon's application technique, and the pre- and posttreatment of the skin.

The Medium-Depth Peel: 35% Trichloracetic Acid and Jessner's Solution

TCA is a frequently used agent for chemical resurfacing of the face,[10] treating a wide array of facial conditions in varying concentrations. At sufficient concentrations, the application of TCA will result in the disruption of the epidermis and dermis, thus stimulating regeneration of the dermal and epidermal elements.[7] This catalyst is frequently used in combination with other agents that enable a deeper penetration, particularly Jessner's solution. Composed of salicylic acid, ethanol, lactic acid, and

resorcinol, Jessner's solution is a keratolytic that breaks intracellular bridges between keratinocytes (**Table 6.2**).[13,14] TCA can be used as a superficial-, medium-, or deep-peeling instrument depending on the concentration employed.[14,15] This chapter specifically addresses the use of the 35% TCA and Jessner's medium-depth peel.

Table 6.2   Typical components of Jessner's solution to make 100 mL

Salicylic acid 14 g
Resorcinol 14 g
Lactic acid (85%) 14 mL
95% Ethanol (sufficient to make 100 mL)

Source: Data from Alam et al.[14]

■ Pertinent Anatomy

The layers of the facial skin include the epidermis and the dermis. The deepest component of the epidermis is the basal cell layer, or stratum basale, which consists of undifferentiated proliferating cells and melanocytes (**Fig. 6.5a,b**). As cell migration advances upward, the process of cell differentiation is noted. Above the basal layer lies the stratum spinosum, which is composed of keratinocytes. Photoaged skin is characterized by loss of the orderly maturation of these keratinocytes.[4] As cells differentiate further, they form the stratum granulosum, where additional keratin is synthesized. Also known as the granular cell layer, this layer has lamellar granules that contain polysaccharides, glycoproteins, and lipids that hold the stratum corneum cells together. The major physical barrier, or stratum corneum, lies most superficially and consists of devitalized, keratin-filled cells.

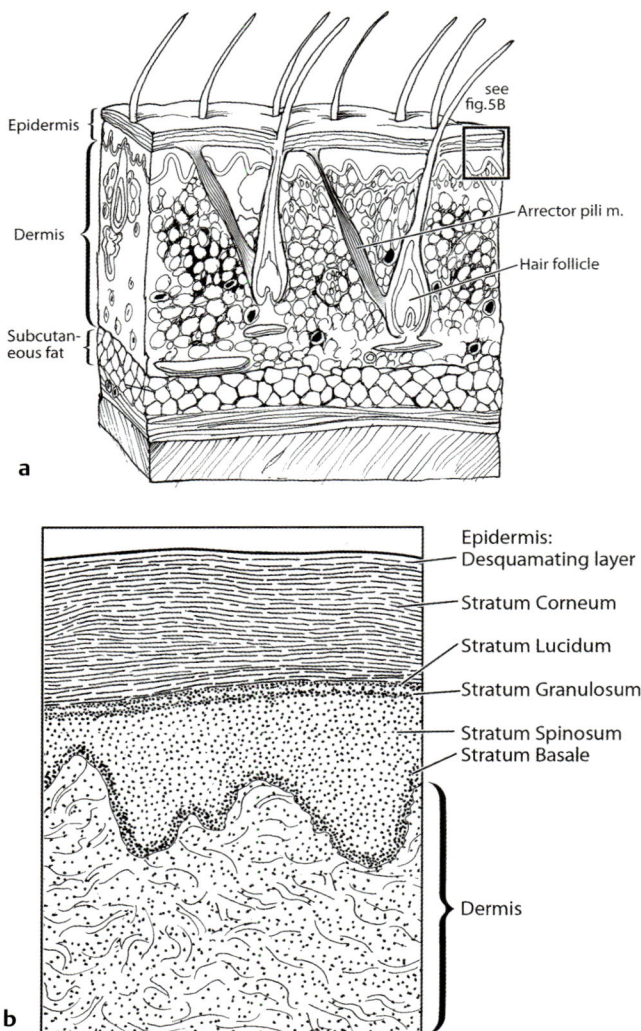

Fig. 6.5 **(a)** Anatomical layers and adnexal structures of skin. **(b)** Drawing depicting closer view of epidermis.

The reticular dermis is the deepest layer of the dermis and has thick and densely packed collagen fibers and the highest content of elastic fibers in the skin.[16] Above the reticular dermis lies the papillary dermis, which consists of fine and loosely arranged collagen fibers. Collagen fibrils in the papillary dermis become disorganized in aging skin. The resultant fine wrinkles are a prominent feature of both aged skin and photoaged skin.[4] Scarring from acne can result in thicker and more abundant collagen that is disorganized and stretched.[17]

■ Patient Selection

Proper patient selection is important to obtain cosmetically superior results and minimize complications. The photoaging classification system developed by Glogau[18] (**Table 6.3**) and the Fitzpatrick skin-type classification[19,20] (**Table 6.4**) are valuable references when assessing patients. These classification systems guide what depth peel is optimal and can predict the risk of postoperative complications. Specific complications are of concern when addressing patients with advanced Fitzpatrick skin types; patients with Fitzpatrick skin types III through VI may become hyperpigmented after peeling with superficial and medium-depth peels, but hypopigmented after undergoing deep peels.

Potential contraindications to chemical peeling of the face include pregnancy, breastfeeding, peeling within 6 months of isotretinoin treatment, skin infection, and active herpetic lesions (**Table 6.5**). The level of peel must also be taken into consideration when judging risks. Relative contraindications to chemexfoliation include patient compliance issues, postoperative and preoperative care, sun exposure, smoking habits, and other compromising comorbidities. The experience of the physician in managing patient characteristics and expectations will aid in achieving optimal results.

Table 6.3 Glogau photoaging classification

I "No wrinkles" (20s–30s)	Mild pigmentary changes, no keratoses, minimal wrinkles; minimal to no makeup
II "Wrinkles in motion" (late 30s or 40s)	Early senile lentigines visible, keratoses palpable, parallel smile lines; some makeup foundation
III "Wrinkles at rest" (50s or older)	Obvious dyschromia, telangiectasia, visible keratosis, wrinkles even without moving; heavy foundation makeup
IV "Only wrinkles" (60s–70s)	Yellow-gray color of skin, prior skin malignancies, wrinkled throughout; can't wear makeup, "cakes and cracks"

Source: Adapted from Glogau.[18]

Table 6.4 Fitzpatrick skin types

Type	Hair Color	Skin Color	Eye Color	Tan?
I	Red	Light	Blue/green	Always burns, never tans
II	Blonde	Light	Blue	Usually burns, tans with difficulty
III	Brown	Medium	Brown	Sometimes mild burn, tan average
IV	Brown/black	Medium/dark brown	Dark brown	Rarely burns, tans with ease
V	Black	Dark brown	Dark brown	Very rarely burns, tans very easily
VI	Black	Black	Dark brown	No burn, tans very easily

Source: Data from Fitzpatrick.[19,20]

Table 6.5 Potential contraindications to chemexfoliation

Darker Fitzpatrick skin types (III–VI)

History of keloid

History of herpes infections

History of diabetes mellitus or prior facial irradiation

Unrealistic patient expectations

Telangiectasias

Anticipation of inadequate photo protection

Significant hepatorenal disease

Human immunodeficiency virus (HIV)

Immunosuppression

Poorly treated emotional instability or mental illness

Ehlers-Danlos syndrome

Scleroderma or collagen vascular disease

Accutane treatment (within 6–12 months prior)

Breastfeeding

■ Technical Aspects of Procedure

Pretreatment

To diminish morbidity and accelerate healing, many preoperative regimens can be implemented. Pretreatment with retinol, hydroquinone, kojic acid, and azelaic acid can benefit patients and is routinely recommended. Optimally, pretreatment skin conditioning is implemented for 6 weeks. The authors recommend a regimen of hydroquinone 4% be applied twice daily to the area to be resurfaced a minimum of 2 weeks prior to the procedure. Retinol is recommended nightly for

at least 2 weeks prior as well. The agents are stopped 2 days before the chemical-peel procedure. This skin conditioning can improve skin tolerance, regulate fibroblast and melanocyte function, and enhance wound healing.[7] Preoperative sun avoidance is also recommended. The pretreatment skin conditioning will vary depending on skin types and can be patient and physician specific.

Two Days before the Procedure

Oral antiherpetics are routinely initiated preoperatively starting 2 days before the procedure. Acyclovir (Zovirax, GlaxoSmithKline, Research Triangle Park, NC) 200 mg 5 times daily or valacyclovir hydrochloride (Valtrex, GlaxoSmithKline) 500 mg twice daily is recommended and is continued for 2 weeks after the process. Other topical skin treatments are stopped.

One Day before the Procedure

Cephalexin (Shionogi, Inc., Atlanta, GA) 500 mg 4 times a day is started the day before the procedure. This is continued for 1 week postoperatively.

The Day of the Procedure

The peel is generally performed in the senior author's clean-office setting using either mild oral sedation or no sedation. There is no intravenous access. If it is judged that the particular patient will benefit from sedation, either oral lorazepam and/or a fast-acting oxycodone preparation is given. To help with pain and swelling, patients can be started on a Medrol dose pack (Pfizer Pharmaceuticals, New York, NY).

Topical or injected anesthesia is patient-dependent and has been rarely used when performing this particular peel. When necessary, local nerve blocks have been executed using 1 to 2% lidocaine with 1:100,000 epinephrine. LMX cream (Ferndale Laboratories, Inc., Ferndale, MI) (4% lidocaine) can be used at the nerve block sites. Most patients, however, require no local anesthesia, and their oral sedative medication suffices.

The equipment necessary for peeling includes: a recommended balanced eye flush readily available for an emergency, sterile saline, gauze sponges, cotton-tipped applicators, 35% TCA solution, Jessner's solution, and acetone. The steps to perform the peel are as follows ▶ **Video 6.1**:

1. The face is cleansed with a bacteriostatic cleanser. Septisol (Steris, Mentor, OH) or other low-residue soap is ideal.
2. The skin is then treated with acetone to "degrease" it. This is done by firmly rubbing the skin with a folded 4 × 4 gauze pad and acetone. This can be done quickly and without necessarily conforming to an aesthetic unit. Note that the thoroughness and pressure applied during this step will actually create a mild abrading effect on the skin and will influence the penetration of the chemical peel solution (**Fig. 6.6**).
3. Jessner's solution is applied next. The entire face can be treated in less than 2 to 3 minutes and the solution will be only mildly irritating for the patient. This process is done with a folded 4 × 4 gauze pad or a sterile cotton-tipped applicator. The goal is to apply the solution evenly and to have total coverage from hairline to hairline and down to the mandibular border. This coverage is described in further detail below. If instead of a gauze pad, a cotton-tipped applicator is used, the operator can get an even coverage by "rolling" the swab, rather than by wiping. The applicator will be particularly helpful in addressing the periorbital and perioral regions. A translucent mild "frost" should be uniformly obtained.
4. The TCA solution can be utilized almost immediately after the Jessner's solution has been applied. Although the 35% TCA solution can be

applied with the use of 2 × 2 or folded 4 × 4 gauze placed between the thumb and middle and index fingers, there may be more control of application of the solution if a cotton-tipped applicator is used with a rolling technique (**Fig. 6.7**). This is most useful for the less-experienced surgeon and in critical areas such as the eyelids. Again, the use of cotton-tipped applicators with the side of the cotton tip rolled over the skin and light pressure are recommended in the perioral area, near the philtral columns, and on the upper and lower eyelids.

Patient discomfort is usually apparent and most report a burning sensation at this stage of the process. A white frost becomes evident and indicates the coagulation of proteins in the skin (**Fig. 6.8**). It is generally recommended that the face be treated one region or subunit at a time, pausing between regions to allow any discomfort to subside. Incomplete or uneven frosting may necessitate touch-ups and reapplication in certain areas. A few minutes should be allowed to ensure an adequate frosting response. The 35% TCA/Jessner's combination should be spread from hairline to hairline and down to the mandibular border. The neck should not be treated with this concentration to avoid scarring. The eyelids should only be treated to within 3 mm of their margins; the TCA solution should be "feathered" at the mandibular border to avoid a sharp demarcation (**Fig. 6.9**).

5. For the less-experienced surgeon, one application with production of an even frost is a reasonable goal. More-experienced users will reapply the solution to achieve the desired depth, guided by both the color and density of the frost. Those beginning their practice in peeling should use a timed format of waiting 2 to 5 minutes after TCA solution placement and then to "neutralize or

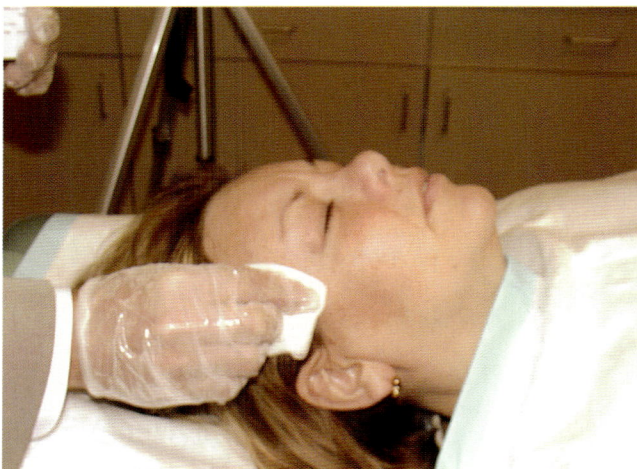
Fig. 6.6 "De-greasing" of the skin using medical-grade acetone.

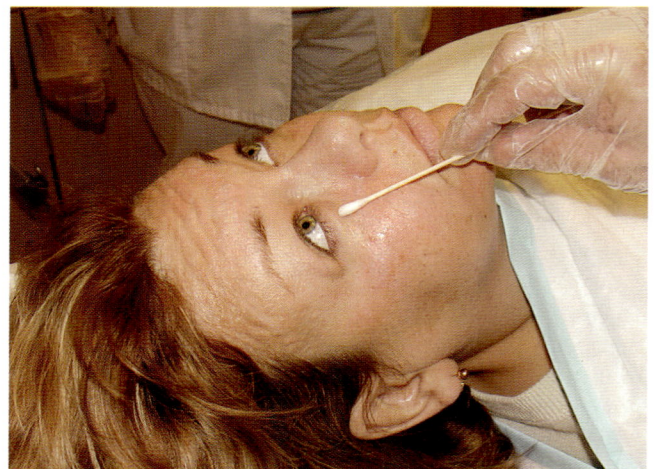
Fig. 6.7 Application of 35% trichloracetic acid solution to the lower eyelids using a cotton-tipped applicator. Jessner's solution has been applied previously.

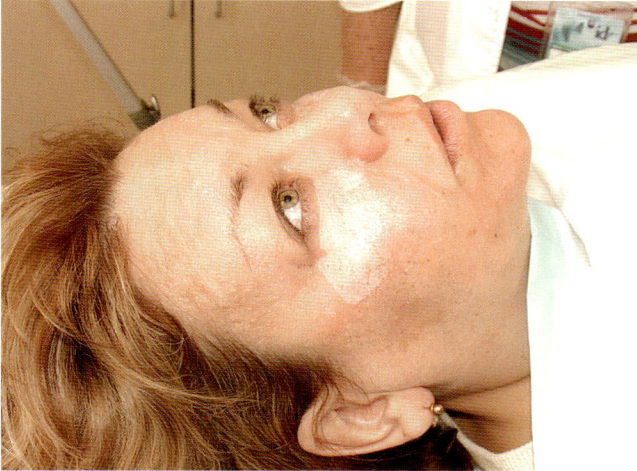

Fig. 6.8 The "frost" that can be obtained using the Jessner's/ 35% TCA chemical peel.

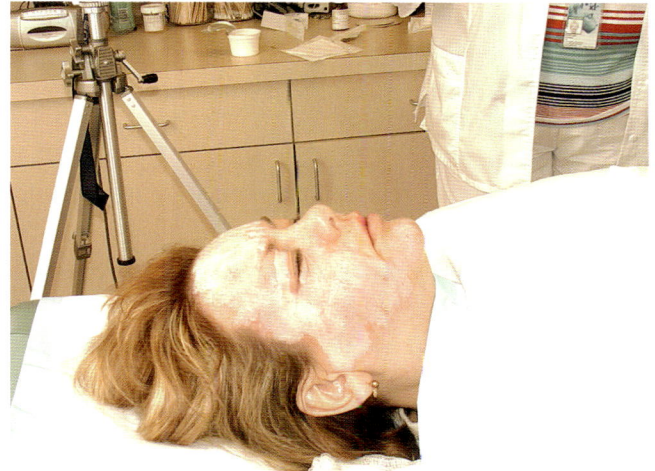

Fig. 6.9 "Feathering" of the chemical peel solution at the mandibular border.

dilute" the peeled area with cool sterile saline. Cool saline compresses, with frequent changes, are applied immediately after wait period for patient comfort (**Fig. 6.10**). Fanning the area with an electric fan is helpful.

6. Patients are discharged without a dressing, although some clinicians use various commercial and over-the-counter ointments before discharge.
7. Patients who are new to peeling are seen the following day.

■ Postoperative Care

An adequate postoperative plan for your patients will help ensure a positive and pleasing outcome (**Table 6.6**). Patients are instructed to continue an-

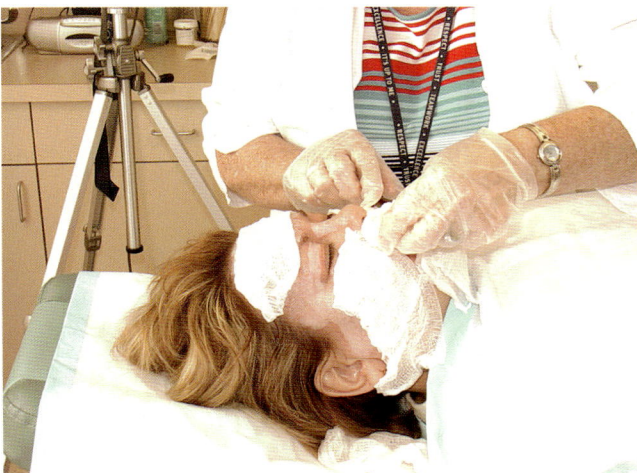

Fig. 6.10 "Dilution" of the chemical peel solutions by using cool saline-soaked gauzes.

tivirals for 2 weeks and an antistaphylococcal antibiotic for 7 days postoperatively (Cephalexin 500 mg 4 times daily unless the patient has an allergy to the medication). Cool compresses and anxiolytics provide initial patient comfort in the office and can be continued at home. Postoperative stinging or burning usually stops within a few hours. Occlusive petroleum-based creams such as Aquaphor or Eucerin (Beiersdorf, Inc., Wilton, CT) may be applied for up to 10 days while the skin sloughs and re-epithelializes.[7] These moist occlusive dressings promote faster re-epithelialization, at the same time reducing pain. The authors have found Preparation H (Pfizer, New York, NY) to be beneficial in reducing discomfort and preventing crusting. The rate of re-epithelialization is faster than with nonocclusive dressings and may increase collagen synthesis. Continued avoidance of sun exposure and adequate sun protection may prevent hyperpigmentation and erythema postoperatively. After re-epithelialization, depending on the clinical course, hydroquinone topical steroids, and retinols may be used.

■ Expected Results

The potential improvements—as well as the potential morbidity and healing time associated with chemical peels—are largely related to the depth of the peel. Within 24 hours, postoperative erythema, pain, and edema typically improve. The authors have observed healing times to be ~ 6 to 9 days for these medium-depth peels. Overall, patient selection, antiviral prophylaxis, and proper postoperative instructions can diminish morbidity associated with the chemical peeling (**Figs. 6.11a,b**; **Figs. 6.12a,b**; **Figs. 6.13a,b**; **Figs. 6.14a,b**; **Figs. 6.15a,b**).

Table 6.6 Fred G. Fedok's postoperative care instructions given to patients after chemical and laser resurfacing procedure*

Week 1	Spray plain lukewarm water six times daily on affected areas while using fingertips to pat skin. Pat skin dry with unscented tissues. Apply occlusive moist dressing.
Week 2	Continued cleansing as described above if crusts are still present. Keep areas "moisturized" with recommended cream. If no crusts are present, use Neutrogena (Johnson & Johnson, Los Angeles, CA) to cleanse skin. Rinse thoroughly to remove soap film.
Week 3	Continue Neutrogena to cleanse skin. Rinse thoroughly to remove soap film. You may initiate water-based hypoallergenic makeup if skin is free of crusts and smooth. Continue recommended cream under base makeup as moisturizer.
Week 5	Oil-based makeup may be initiated. If tolerated, use #30 sunscreen to protect face against sun exposure.

*Note: Patients are advanced in this regimen as allowed by their individual healing and depending on the depth and type of resurfacing procedure. For the Jessner's/35% TCA peel, patients are usually reepithelilized within two weeks.

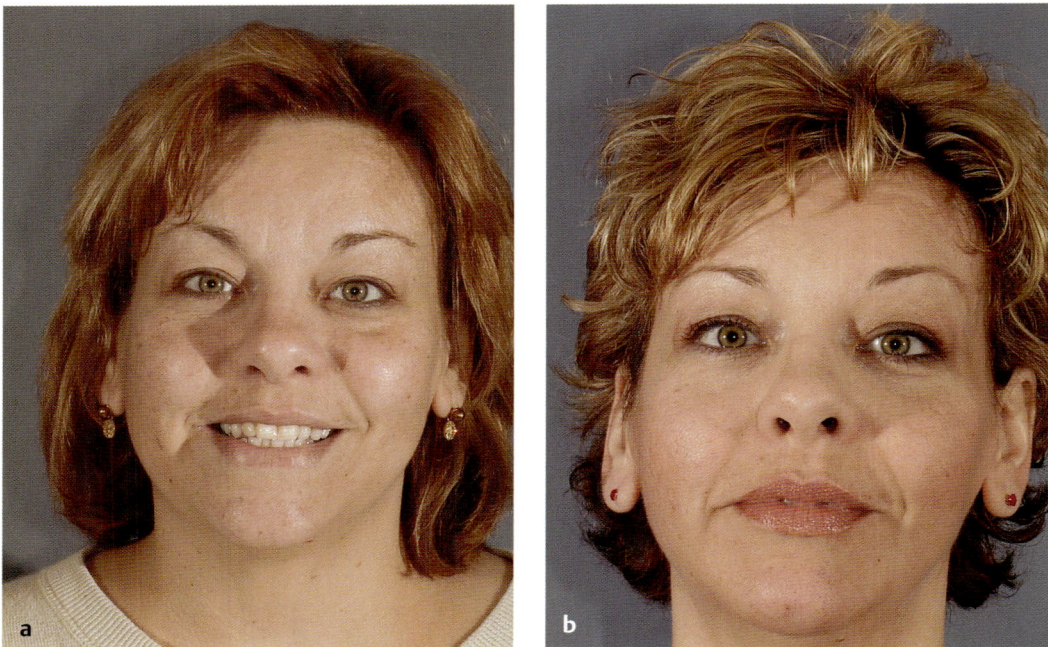

Fig. 6.11 **(a)** Patient preoperatively and **(b)** postoperatively after Jessner's/35% trichloracetic acid peel. Note improvement in skin texture, reduction of rhytids, and reduction of lentigines.

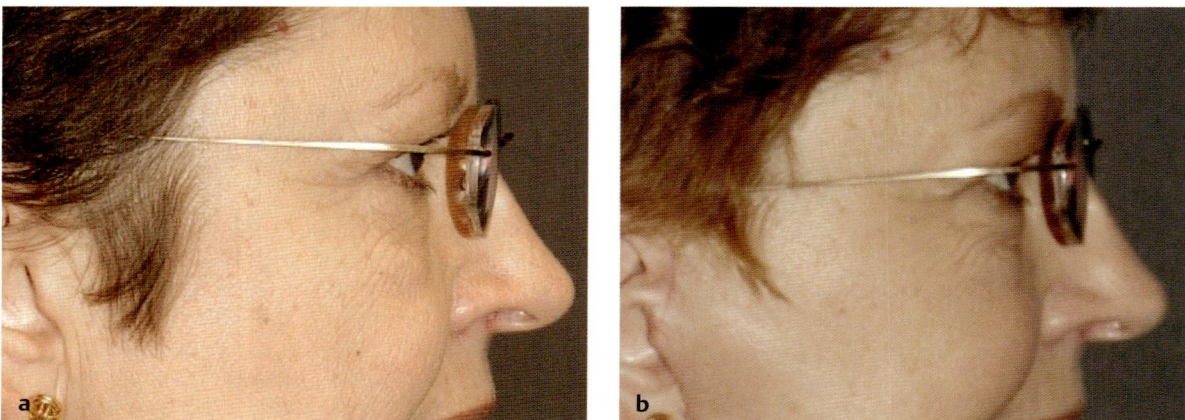

Fig. 6.12 **(a)** Patient preoperatively and **(b)** postoperatively after Jessner's/35% trichloracetic acid peel. Note improvement in skin tone and reduction of rhytids.

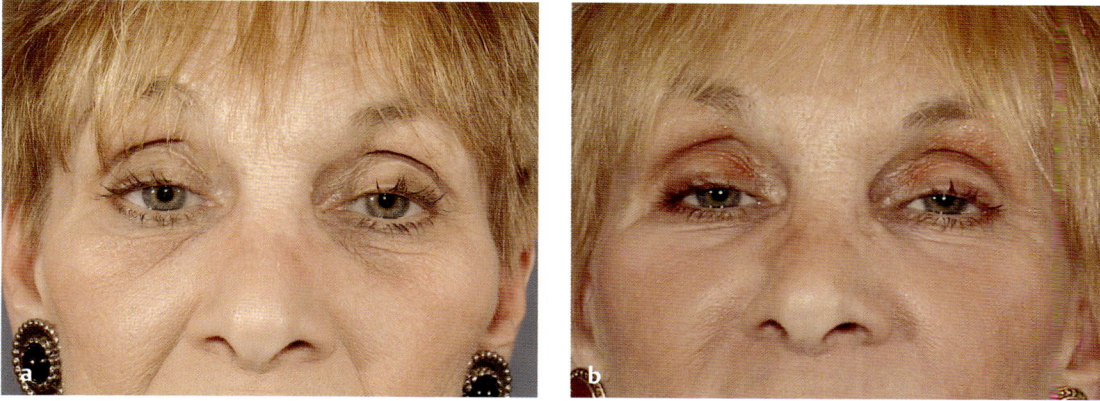

Fig. 6.13 **(a)** Patient preoperatively and **(b)** postoperatively after combination peel procedure. Baker-Gordon formula was used in the periorbital area, and Jessner's/35% trichloracetic acid was used on the cheeks, forehead, and other facial areas outside of the periorbital area. Note improvement in the skin texture and skin tones and reduction of rhytids.

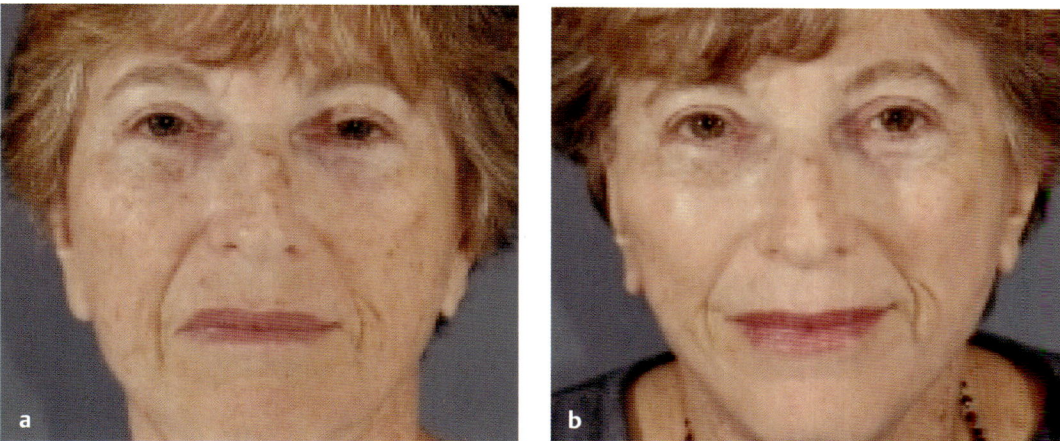

Fig. 6.14 **(a)** Patient preoperatively and **(b)** postoperatively after Jessner's/35% trichloracetic acid peel. Note improvement in skin texture and skin tones and reduction of rhytids and lentigines.

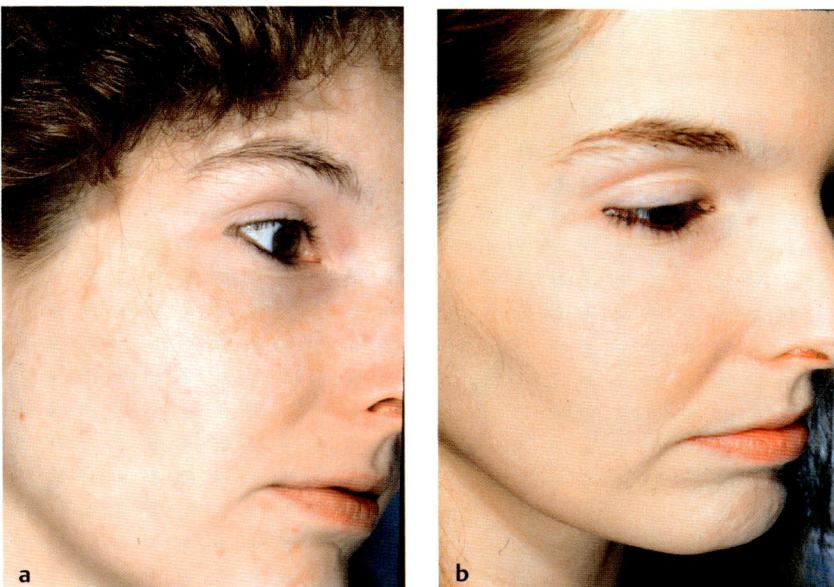

Fig. 6.15 **(a)** Patient preoperatively and **(b)** postoperatively after Jessner's/35% trichloracetic acid peel. Note improvement in melasma and skin pigmentation.

■ Complications and Their Management

Potential complications of chemexfoliation increase as the depth of peel deepens.[1] Fortunately, complications following superficial peels and medium-depth peels are uncommon and primarily include postoperative erythema and hyperpigmentation. The assessment of risk for pigmentation problems through selective screening of skin types is helpful in the initial evaluation. Postoperatively, these problems are usually managed with the use of bleaching preparations and topical steroid creams. Photoprotection, including the use of sunscreens, is imperative for several months postprocedure. Bacterial and fungal infections are uncommon and are managed according to the offending organism. Herpetic flare is among the most generally cited postoperative complication and routine administration of antivirals should be performed for all patients. If there is a postoperative outbreak, the antiviral dosage will have to be increased appropriately.

Although hypertrophic scarring has been a concern when executing TCA peels at higher concentrations and in conjunction with other facial processes,[7] the authors have not found this to be a problem with medium-depth peels. If deeper scarring occurs, intralesional steroid injections, topical Silastic gels, or pulsed dye laser therapy may be necessary.

■ Conclusion

The medium-depth chemical peel provides an effective treatment of facial rhytids, melasma, lentigines, and other signs of photoaging. It is a cost-effective modality that provides a low-risk alternative for the patient seeking facial rejuvenation.

References

1. Fischer TC, Perosino E, Poli F, Viera MS, Dreno B; Cosmetic Dermatology European Expert Group. Chemical peels in aesthetic dermatology: an update 2009. J Eur Acad Dermatol Venereol 2010;24(3):281–292
2. Friedman S, Lippitz J. Chemical peels, dermabrasion, and laser therapy. Dis Mon 2009;55(4):223–235
3. Baker TJ. Chemical face peeling and rhytidectomy. A combined approach for facial rejuvenation. Plast Reconstr Surg Transplant Bull 1962;29:199–207
4. Rabe JH, Mamelak AJ, McElgunn PJ, Morison WL, Sauder DN. Photoaging: mechanisms and repair. J Am Acad Dermatol 2006;55(1):1–19
5. Rachel JD, Jamora JJ. Skin rejuvenation regimens: a profilometry and histopathologic study. Arch Facial Plast Surg 2003;5(2):145–149
6. Kligman LH. Photoaging. Manifestations, prevention, and treatment. Clin Geriatr Med 1989;5(1):235–251
7. Herbig K, Trussler AP, Khosla RK, Rohrich RJ. Combination Jessner's solution and trichloroacetic acid chemical peel: technique and outcomes. Plast Reconstr Surg 2009;124(3):955–964
8. Kessler E, Flanagan K, Chia C, Rogers C, Glaser DA. Comparison of alpha- and beta-hydroxy acid chemical peels in the treatment of mild to moderately severe facial acne vulgaris. Dermatol Surg 2008;34(1):45–50, discussion 51
9. Gupta AK, Gover MD, Nouri K, Taylor S. The treatment of melasma: a review of clinical trials. J Am Acad Dermatol 2006;55(6):1048–1065
10. Monheit GD. The Jessner's + TCA peel: a medium-depth chemical peel. J Dermatol Surg Oncol 1989;15(9):945–950 PubMed
11. Monheit GD. Chemical peels. Skin Therapy Lett 2004;9(2):6–11 PubMed
12. Langsdon PR, Milburn M, Yarber R. Comparison of the laser and phenol chemical peel in facial skin resurfacing. Arch Otolaryngol Head Neck Surg 2000;126(10):1195–1199
13. Fulton JE. Jessner's peel. In: Rubin MG, ed. Chemical Peels. Philadelphia, PA: Elsevier Saunders; 2006:57–71
14. Behl DS, Tung R. Chemical peels. In: Adam M, Gladstone HB, Tung RC, eds. Requisites in Dermatology: Cosmetic Dermatology (Vol. 1). Edinburgh: Elsevier Ltd.; 2009:81–101
15. Park SS, Khalid AN, Graber NJ, Fedok FG. Current trends in facial resurfacing: a survey of American Academy of Facial Plastic and Reconstructive Surgery members. Arch Facial Plast Surg 2010;12(1):65–67
16. Marks JG, Miller JJ. Structure and function of skin. In: Lookingbill DP, Marks JG, eds. Principles of Dermatology. Philadelphia, PA: Saunders; 2000:5–9
17. Rivera AE. Acne scarring: a review and current treatment modalities. J Am Acad Dermatol 2008;59(4):659–676
18. Glogau RG. Chemical peeling and aging skin. JGD 1994; 2:30–35
19. Fitzpatrick TB. Soleil et peau. J Med Esthet 1975;2:33–34
20. Fitzpatrick TB. The validity and practicality of sun-reactive skin types I through VI. Arch Dermatol 1988;124(6): 869–871

7 Hetter Chemical Peels

Devinder S. Mangat

Key Concepts

- Phenol peels the skin more deeply with increased concentrations, and the resultant peel is deeper with elevating mixtures of croton oil.

- The dilution of croton oil, in a constant phenol content, shortens the healing time and incurs a more shallow depth of penetration.

- Hetter peels allow different depths of peeling in individual subunits of the face by varying solutions of croton oil in different facial regions.

- The depth of the peel is dependent upon the amount of solution on the cotton tip and the uniform application of the mixture, as well as the number of applications.

- Experience reveals that 0.8% croton oil Hetter solution works well in areas of deeper rhytids and thicker skin, such as the perioral, glabellar, and lateral periorbital regions.

- Intermediate areas, such as the inferior periorbital zone, should be treated with 0.4% croton oil Hetter concentration.

- A simple 88% USP (United States Pharmacopeia) phenol solution is used for all other facial sections to even out the appearance.

■ Introduction

As medical advancements have increased not only our life span but also our quality of life, it is natural to expect a greater public desire to undo the untoward effects of sunlight, aging, and genetics. This desire has spawned a myriad of unsubstantiated skin-care products and practitioners of "wonder" technologies promising unrealistic end results. Chemical peeling has withstood the harshest critics of both safety and results. Starting with "lay peelers" in the early 20th century, chemexfoliation has provided not only a stalwart treatment for practitioners of skin rejuvenation, but also the standard by which other modalities are judged. The various formulations have provided treatment for rhytids, lentigines, dyschromias, and actinic damage. The goal of this chapter is to address some recent changes in our overall knowledge base regarding chemical peels; to uproot some old, outdated tenets; and to discuss the versatility of Hetter chemical peels.

■ Background: Basic Science of Procedure

The history of chemical peeling did not begin in the hands of physicians, but rather in those of the "lay peelers." Hollywood, California, in the 1920s was fertile ground for these early practitioners because the stars of early motion pictures wished to maintain both a youthful appearance as well as career longevity. In the 1950s and 1960s that physicians began not only to learn these practices but also to "wrestle" them away from prominent "lay peelers" trained by Jean DeDesly and Antoinette LaGasse. Gregory Hetter, in his four-part series in 2000,[1,2,3,5] eloquently laid out a detailed history of the passing of the chemical peeling art from the "lay peelers" to the plastic surgeons of the 1950s and 1960s.

With the entry of chemical peeling into the realm of medical science, many reports appeared in the literature regarding the experiences of plastic surgeons. Not all accounts were matched with scientific scrutiny. Instead, in some cases, dogma was written and adhered to for decades. Much of this dogma came from the use of the Baker-Gordon phenol-croton oil formulation (**Table 7.1**), the earliest formula widely used by physician peelers.

Several insular suppositions were reported repeatedly, for years, in the literature regarding the phenol-croton oil peel. These assumptions date back to the late 1950s and early 1960s, when the phenol-croton oil formulas were introduced to the plastic surgery arena. It was from "lay peelers" in Hollywood in the 1920s and the Miami, Florida, area in the 1950s that plastic surgeons were able to "tease away" secret, long-used phenol-based peeling solutions.[1] Most formulas contained similar concentrations of croton oil. Litton was the first to present one of these formulas to the American Society of Plastic and Reconstructive Surgeons (ASPRS) in the late 1950s. However, it was Baker who was credited for the formula he presented in November 1961 and then modified to his "classic" formula in 1962.[2]

Around the same time that Baker's "classic" formula was described, Adolph Brown presented three doctrines of phenol peeling. First, increased concentrations of phenol (80 to 90%) prevented deeper peels by causing an immediate keratocoagulation that blocked its further penetration. Second, addition of saponin increased the depth of penetration of phenol. Third, croton oil's role was simply to "buffer" the solution.[3,4] The literature regarding chemexfoliation in the 1960s quickly adopted these assertions and created further claims (i.e., phenol was the one and only active ingredient within the Baker formulation; phenol in lower concentrations penetrated more deeply than in higher concentrations). It was believed, as a result of these pronouncements, that lower phenol concentrations were more dangerous due to their deeper penetration. It was supposed, as well, that Septisol (Steris, Mentor, OH) caused a deeper penetration and that croton oil had no physiological role in the peel. Since Brown's assertions in the early 1960s, there had been neither animal nor human scientific studies that supported his postulates. Gregory Hetter questioned these claims in the late 1990s and, more importantly, questioned croton oil's role, or supposed lack there of, in Baker's formula.

Croton oil is pressed from the seeds of *Croton tiglium*, a small shrub found in India and Ceylon. The oil consists mainly of oleic, linoleic, myristic and arachidonic acids.[5] Less than 5% of the oil is made up of a resin that has been known in scientific literature since 1895 to possess irritant and toxic properties. In 1935, Joseph R. Spies isolated this toxic resin and applied it to a volunteer's arm, creating severe vesiculations of the skin and a resultant wound that took almost 3 weeks to heal.[5] Spies also showed that croton oil was soluble in ethanol and benzene, and that it had poor solubility in a 50:50 phenol-to-water solution.[5] Hetter theorized that this might create the need for the surfactant, Septisol, in the Baker formula.

To refute Brown's postulates and to help elucidate the role of croton oil, Hetter found a patient who was willing to undergo multiple chemical peels at different concentrations of phenol and croton oil. His findings contradicted what had been previously assumed. At the lowest concentration of phenol, 18%, there was minimal postpeel effect. Mild keratolysis occurred with 35% phenol but there was no clear dermal effect. Hetter noted some desquamation with mild dermal effect after the 50% phenol peel. It was only with 88% phenol that Hetter saw an obvious upper dermal effect, which took 4 to 5 days to heal. A more profound dermal effect ensued with the addition of croton oil; and with different croton oil concentrations, there were varying healing times. A 0.7% croton oil concentration application required a 7-day healing time, whereas a 2.1% croton oil concentration—equivalent to that of the classic Baker formula—resulted in an 11-day healing period.[5] From his experience with this one patient, Hetter deduced: phenol peels more deeply with increased solutions; higher concentrations of phenol (88%) without Septisol peel more deeply than lower mixtures (35% and 50%); and the resultant peel is deeper with increasing concentrations of croton oil.

Table 7.1 The "classic" Baker or Baker-Gordon formulation

Ingredients	Baker-Gordon Solution	Original Baker Formulation
Phenol USP 88%	3 mL	5 mL
Distilled water	2 mL	4 mL
Croton oil	3 guttae[b]	3 guttae
Septisol[a]	8 guttae	8 guttae

Source: Used with permission from Baker TJ. Chemical face peeling and rhytidectomy. A combined approach for facial rejuvenation. Plast Reconstr Surg Transplant Bull 1962;29:199–207.

Abbreviation: USP, United States Pharmacopeia.

Note: Published in 1962 following the original initial formulation from November 1961.

[a]Steris, Mentor, OH.
[b]27 guttae = 1 mL.

Hetter used this case to guide his treatment of five additional patients with varying croton oil concentrations. The results from these five cases allowed him to arrive at some generalizations about phenol-croton oil peeling. First, the dilution of croton oil in a constant phenol solution shortens the healing time, suggesting a more shallow depth of penetration. Second, phenol concentration has little to do with depth of injury. He confirmed the observation of Stegman in 1980,[6] reiterated by Stone in 2001,[7] that multiple coats will increase the depth of injury. Obagi[8] first described the need for different depths of peeling for individual subunits of the face. Hetter translated this to his use of varying concentrations of croton oil in diverse regions of the face. Although he found that the lower nose could tolerate croton oil concentrations up to 1.2%, the cheeks and forehead tolerated mixtures up to only 0.8%; and the upper nose, temple, and lateral brow could withstand concentrations up to only 0.4%—before the risk of complications rose. Last, Hetter believed 1% croton oil solutions were the upper threshold for safe use to avoid serious risk of hypopigmentation.

Initially, Hetter performed his preliminary work using phenol as a "vehicle" at 33% for the croton oil with 1-drop (0.35%), 2-drop (0.7%), and 3-drop (1.1%) formulations. Later, he believed it would be optimal to have a more standardized means of measuring the croton oil concentrations, rather than relying on inherently inconsistent droppers. He converted drops to cubic centimeters by having 25 drops equal 1 cubic centimeter. Using this conversion, he created a stock solution of 0.04 cc (now mL [milliliter] would be used) of croton oil per 1 cc of phenol. From this—needing only Septisol, phenol, and water—he could make varying croton oil concentrations of 0.4, 0.8, 1.2, and 1.6% in a constant phenol mixture. Using Hetter's formulations, the practitioner can decide between a phenol concentration of 35 or 48.5%. **Table 7.2** shows the formulas for the varying croton oil mixtures of the Hetter peels using a phenol concentration of 35%.

Hetter demonstrated that the depth of penetration is partially dictated not only by the components of the peeling solution, but also by the concentrations of the components. Stone emphasized the importance of how application of these different solutions must be controlled to create desired results. Stone tested Hetter's postulations by performing peels on three sample patients. He used Hetter's varying concentrations; the "classic" Baker formula with and without croton oil; and different phenol concentrations without croton oil.

In the first patient, Stone showed on successive biopsies that the "classic" Baker formula with and without croton oil created the same depth of penetration and injury with repeated rubbings and occlusive taping. In the second case, he peeled the patient with both alternating concentrations of phenol (50 and 88%) and solutions of croton oil (2.2 and 0.4%) on the thick forehead skin and the thinner nasojugal trough skin. Stone varied the number of rubs on the nasojugal trough as well, using wrung-out gauze. He found, on biopsy, that all formulas—when applied with 50 rubs—created equal histological results and similar fibrosis. However, by decreasing the number of rubs, Stone confirmed Hetter's findings that the depth of penetration increases with increasing phenol concentration. These results suggest a threshold of injury that can be achieved with phenol and croton oil in varying concentrations, when enough applications are employed. This was confirmed in the third patient, on whom he used lower phenol concentrations with 2.2, 0.4, and 0% croton oil. He found that the injury threshold can be met with all three solutions, but with different numbers of applications. Stone concluded that croton oil serves to lower the threshold number of applications.[7]

Stone's work emphasizes the important point addressed but not stressed in Hetter's work—*how* the peeling solution is applied to the skin is as crucial as *what* active agents are present within the concentration. In the author's opinion, this is where the experience of the peeler and the "art" of peeling become significant.

Table 7.2 The Hetter peel formula

Croton oil (%)	0.2	0.4	0.8	1.2	1.6
Water	5.5 mL	5.5 mL	5.5 mL	5.5 mL	5.5 mL
Septisol[a]	0.5 mL	0.5 mL	0.5 mL	0.5 mL	0.5 mL
Phenol 88%	3.5 mL	3.0 mL	2.0 mL	1.9 mL	0.0 mL
Stock solution	0.5 mL	1.0 mL	2.0 mL	3.0 mL	4.0 mL

Source: Adapted from Hetter.[5]
[a]Steris, Mentor, OH.

Patient Selection

Defining the patient's suitability for a chemical peel is paramount for the cosmetic surgeon. The individual needs to be physically suitable for the peel and, as well, must have appropriate expectations of what the peel can and will accomplish. Rhytids and photodamage must be distinguished from age-related gravitational changes, jowling, and facial fat volume loss.

The ideal chemical peel patient is one with fair skin, blue eyes, and mild, shallow rhytids. However, these characteristics represent only a minority of the individuals who will present seeking treatment for rhytids and photodamage. To help define a patient's skin type, the Fitzpatrick scale (see **Table 6.4**) is most often employed. Patients can be rated by their skin type, complexion, skin texture, thickness, and photoaging. A useful categorizing scale is the one described by Glogau (**Table 7.3**).

The patient's medical history and lifestyle must be thoroughly discussed prior to the planning stages of the peel. Relative contraindications for any resurfacing procedure include cutaneous radiation history, smoking, active or frequent herpes simplex

Table 7.3 Glogau classification scale

Skin Class	Description
I	"Early wrinkles" * Patient age: 20s–30s * Early photoaging • Mild pigment changes • Minimal wrinkles • No "age spots"
II	"Wrinkles in motion" * Patient age: 30s–40s * Early to moderate photoaging • Appearance of smile lines • Early brown "age spots" • Skin pores more prominent • Early changes in skin texture
III	"Wrinkles at rest" * Patient age: 50s and older * Advanced photoaging • Prominent brown pigmentation • Visible brown "age spots" • Prominent small blood vessels
IV	"Only wrinkles" * Patient age: 60s or 70s * Severe photoaging • Yellow-gray skin color • Prior skin cancers • Precancerous skin changes (actinic keratosis)

virus (HSV) outbreaks, diabetes, and hypertrophic scar or keloid history. Birth control pills, exogenous estrogens (including soaps and cosmetics containing lavender oil), and photosensitizing drugs are to be avoided due to risks of hyperpigmentation. The patient should not have plans to become pregnant within the first 6 months after the chemical peel, due to elevated estrogen levels of pregnancy.[9]

Lifestyle and habitual activities, more specifically sun exposure and smoking, should be addressed. A chemical peel for a chronic smoker can lead to poor tissue healing and cosmetic results, due to the ensuing microvascular damage. Practitioners should be honest and open regarding the risks, and a smoking cessation program should be recommended. Smokers should stop smoking 1 month prior to and at least 6 months after the peel. Ultraviolet (UV) light exposure can be equally problematic in the postoperative period. A patient's habitual sun exposure should be assessed prior to proceeding with the peel, and the individual should be advised that chronic or frequent sun exposure should be avoided after the chemical peel. If this is unacceptable, the practitioner should consider other options and not perform a peel.

Isotretinoin (Accutane, Roche Laboratories, Rotkreuz, Switzerland) use is an absolute contraindication to chemical peeling or any other resurfacing procedure. Postpeel re-epithelialization relies upon the epidermis within hair follicles and sebaceous glands. Isotretinoin prevents re-epithelialization from these locations. Most recommendations include a cessation period of 12 to 24 months prior to the peel.

The patient's expectatations should be clarified and agreed upon with the practitioner. The axillary skin can often well predict the final product of a chemical peel, if that area has not had excessive UV light exposure over a lifetime.[10]

Technical Aspects of Procedure

Prepeel Preparation

Proper skin preparation must be employed, once the patient has been defined as suitable. The skin preparation helps to prevent complications and allows the best healing and results. Sunscreens, including both ultraviolet A (UVA) and ultraviolet B (UVB) block, should be started to prevent prepeel burns or tanning. This helps to decrease melanocyte activity prior to the peel. Sunscreen usage should begin 3 months prior to the peel in combination with minimal sun exposure.

Topical tretinoin (Retin-A) is recommended for 6 to 12 weeks prior to the peel. Animal studies have demonstrated both the clinical and histological healing benefits of pretreatment tretinoin prior to dermabrasion. Synergistic qualities of pretreatment tretinoin and trichloracetic acid (TCA) peels have been shown to sustain the effects of the chemical peel.[11,12] Tretinoin aids in re-epithelialization[13] and leads to increased melanin distribution. After tretinoin treatment, the thickened epidermis displays decreased corneocyte adhesion, decreased stratum corneum thickness, and neocollagen production, all of which are beneficial to the peel and the postoperative result. The thickened and uniform epidermis aids in the uniform application of the peeling agent.[14]

The patient should begin nighttime tretinoin treatments 6 weeks prior to the peel and continue them after the postpeel re-epithelialization is completed. The dose range recommended is from 0.025 to 0.1%. However, there is no literature describing an improved benefit with the higher dosing, indicating that lower concentrations might be just as effective. This becomes important in those patients who may be sensitive to tretinoin use. They should be warned of the potential side effects, including irritation, erythema, and flaking of the skin; the dose should be decreased; or it should be discontinued altogether.

Also beneficial in the pretreatment of all peel patients, hydroquinone is most effective in those patients with lentigines, dyschromias, and Fitzpatrick type III, IV, V, and VI skin types because of the higher risk of postpeel postinflammatory hyperpigmentation (PIH). Hydroquinone blocks the conversion of tyrosine to L-dopa (Ajinomoto, Eddyville, IA) by tyrosinase, thus decreasing melanin production. In a concentration of 4 to 8%, hydroquinone should be started 4 to 6 weeks prior to resurfacing. Like tretinoin, hydroquinone should be re-started after the peel, as soon as the patient's skin can tolerate its application.

Although they may have no recollection of prior herpetic vesicle occurrence, all patients should be warned of the possibility of HSV outbreaks. Patients can have a latent infection even in the setting of a negative history. Common and advisable practice is to start anyone with a negative history on a prophylactic dose of antivirals (Acyclovir, Yanan Changtai Pharmaceuticals, Ltd., Shaanxi, China), 400 mg 3 times a day, 3 days prior to and continued for at least 7 days after the peel. For those patients with a positive history of active HSV infections, a therapeutic dose of antivirals, such as valacyclovir (Valtrex, GlaxoSmithKline, Philadelphia, PA) 1 g, must be employed three times a day for the aforementioned time period. Postpeel herpetic outbreaks can be unnerving for the practitioner but devastating for the patient; therefore, all precautions should be taken to avoid them.

To maintain appropriate and uniform depth of penetration of the peeling agent, avoidance of waxing, dermabrasion, and electrolysis should be strictly maintained for 3 to 4 weeks prior to peeling.

Peeling Technique

Application of the peeling solution should always be done on properly prepared skin. The preparation begins with vigorous cleaning with Septisol or an acne wash the evening before and the morning of the procedure ▶ Video 7.1.

Preoperative oral sedation of 10 to 15 mg of diazepam and 100 mg of Dramamine (McNeil Consumer & Specialty Pharmaceuticals, Fort Washington, PA) helps relieve the patient's anxiety regarding the intravenous (IV) catheter placement and the upcoming process. The antihistamine also reduces oral secretions and aids in airway protection during periods of deeper sedation. IV fluids should be initiated prior to the patient's entering the operating room. At this point, additional IV benzodiazepine can be administered if anxiety continues. The patient should have cardiac monitoring.

With the patient in a seated position, the patient's submandibular shadow is marked. This step is important to avoid obvious postoperative delineation between peeled and nonpeeled areas at the jawline. The patient is then placed in the supine position. After administration of a sedating dose of propofol, the nerve blocks (supraorbital, infraorbital, and mental) and field blocks are performed with an equal mixture of 2% lidocaine and 0.5% bupivacaine. Avoid epinephrine use, even in the nerve blocks, to allow maximal clearance of phenol. While waiting for maximal anesthesia to occur, the face is thoroughly de-greased with an acetone-soaked gauze. Any residual oil on the skin will cause an uneven peel. Repeat the acetone cleaning throughout the procedure if necessary.

Both Obagi and Hetter recommend using wrung-out cotton 2-inch × 2-inch gauze for the application of the peeling agent.[3,5] However, in the author's opinion, wide cotton-tipped applicators are superior for control of application. As previously mentioned, the depth of the peel depends upon the amount of solution on the cotton tip, the uniform application of the mixture, and the number of strokes applied.

One of the benefits of using a phenol-based solution is that the resultant frost is almost immediate, as compared with TCA, where the practitioner must safely wait 3 to 4 minutes before assessing a peeled area for needed repeat applications.[15] The quality of the depth is quickly and readily apparent with the phenol-croton oil peel and areas in need of reapplication can be immediately treated. Medium-depth peels should give a level II to level III frosting (**Table 7.4**).[15]

The subunits of the face should be divided by degree of rhytids, lentigines, and photodamage as well as inherent thickness. The author's experience has been to use 0.8% croton oil Hetter solution in areas of deeper rhytids (Glogau III and IV) and thicker skin, such as the perioral, glabellar, and lateral periorbital areas. The intermediate regions (Glogau II and III),

Table 7.4 Classification of the degree of frosting obtained with chemical peels

Level I: Erythema with stringy or blotchy frosting

Level II: White coat with erythema showing through (should be used for eyelids and areas of bony prominences, i.e., zygomatic arch, malar, chin— higher rate of scarring)

Level III: Solid white frost with little or no background erythema

such as the inferior periorbital area, are treated with 0.4% croton oil Hetter solution. To even the appearance of the face, a simple 88% USP phenol solution is used for all other areas.

A period of 10 to 15 minutes must be allowed between each subunit peeled to allow for proper clearance of the phenol. The entire face should be peeled from 90 to 120 minutes. In the event that a minor supraventricular arrhythmia occurs, the peel should be stopped, and the practitioner should wait for a return to normal sinus rhythm. The peel should be carried into the hairline because phenol and croton oil will not affect pigment of the hair follicles. The edge of each peeled area will have a line of reactive hyperemia. This does not represent peeled skin but rather an unpeeled skin reaction. This line of hyperemia (**Fig. 7.1**) should

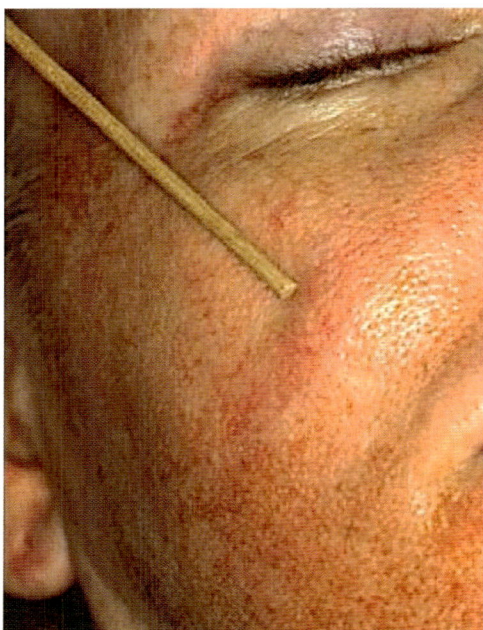

Fig. 7.1 The clear line of hyperemia that occurs at the periphery of a peeled area is shown. This hyperemic skin has not been peeled. Care must be taken to peel the area to avoid a discrete line of unpeeled skin.

be included and adequately peeled, when peeling the adjacent areas, so as not to create obvious lines of demarcation. Similarly, the peel should be carried over the vermilion border. The practitioner can stretch wrinkled skin to allow an even peel over these areas. For deep perioral rhytids, the cotton-tipped applicator can be broken and the wooden edge used to apply the peeling agent in the rhytid.

There is no need for solution neutralization because the frost represents a completed reaction, which is precipitation of the keratin by the phenol. Great care must be taken around the lower eyelid margin. The peel should be performed to within 3 mm of the ciliary line and stopped. There should be no excess solution on the lower lid. The patient may develop tearing during the procedure. Any tearing should be dried to avoid the tears pulling the peeling solution into the eye. If not adequately anesthetized, the patient will experience an immediate burning sensation for 15 to 20 seconds. However, this sensation will return in 20 minutes and can last up to 4 to 8 hours. The longer-lasting effect of the bupivacaine will greatly aid in minimizing this burning sensation in the postoperative period. Therefore, it is essential to perform adequate nerve and field blocks. Even with all precautions in place, accidents may happen. In case of patient or staff excess phenol exposure, propylene glycol, glycerol, olive, castor, or cotton-seed oil should be poured onto the site to solubilize the phenol. If exposure to the eyes occurs, mineral oil should be immediately applied to the eyes using a dropper.

■ Postoperative Care

Postoperative care begins immediately after the last subunit is peeled. The patient should have been preoperatively warned regarding the burning that may last up to 8 hours. Preoperative awareness will aid in analgesia provided by IV and oral narcotics. The patient should be prescribed an oral narcotic for the postoperative period and should also expect considerable edema, erythema, and eventual desquamation.

When the frost subsides and only erythema persists, a thick layer of bland emollient should be applied to all peeled areas, leaving no peeled skin exposed. The author prefers Eucerin (Beirsdorf, Inc., Wilton, CT) cream, but Elta (Steadmed Medicals, Fort Worth, TX) or Bacitracin (Fera Pharmaceuticals, Locust Valley, NY) ointments may be used. None of these acts as an occlusive dressing and they will not increase the depth of penetration. Starting with postoperative day 1, the patient should apply the cream 3 to 4 times a day to those areas that are exposed. The peeled skin can be monitored with greater ease on a day-to-day basis by using the emollient.

The healing process takes place in four stages.[15] First, inflammation occurs and increases during the first 12 hours. Next, the epidermis begins to change in appearance, becoming leathery and separating from the dermis. The underlying dermal injury becomes necrotic and sloughs. The emollient aids in clearing this necrotic tissue from the underlying dermis, which is then recovered with the emollient. Desquamation occurs over 4 to 7 days, exposing the underlying erythematous dermis. The re-epithelialization, which typically begins in 48 to 72 hours, continues through days 7 to 10 (**Fig. 7.2**), depending on the depth of the peel.[15] This re-epithelialization will be represented by a conversion of bright red erythema to a lighter shade of pink. The benefit of the peel comes out of the fourth and final stage. This final stage of fibroplasia begins within the 1st week and continues for 12 to 16 weeks after the peel. This period is marked by neoangiogenesis, new collagen formation, and reorganizing of the collagen.

In the first 12 weeks after the peel, the patient is susceptible to UV light exposure and a resultant hyperpigmentation. Strict avoidance of direct, prolonged, sun exposure should be encouraged for that 12-week period. It has been the author's experience that sunscreens should also be avoided for the first 6 weeks. Para-aminobenzoic acid, found in many sunscreen preparations, can cause an undesirable reaction, including irritation, increased erythema, and induration. **Figs. 7.3, 7.4, 7.5, 7.6,** and **7.7** demonstrate the exceptional results that are obtained from Hetter peels in the treatment of dyschromia and rhytids.

Women of childbearing age should avoid birth control pills or pregnancy. Increased circulating estrogens can result in hyperpigmentation following chemexfoliation.

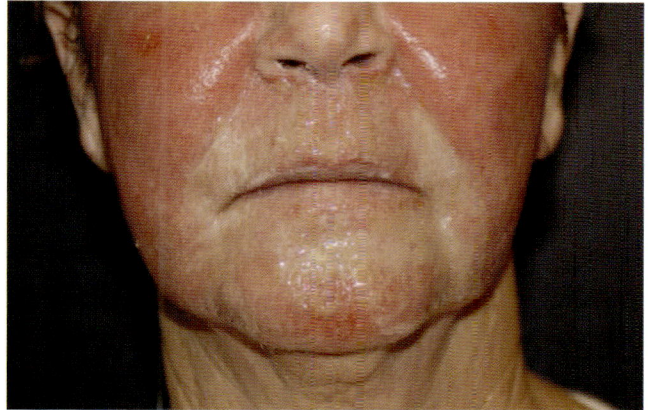

Fig. 7.2 Erythematous neoepithelialization has replaced the sloughed chemexfoliated skin in a patient who underwent a Hetter chemical peel ~ 7 days earlier.

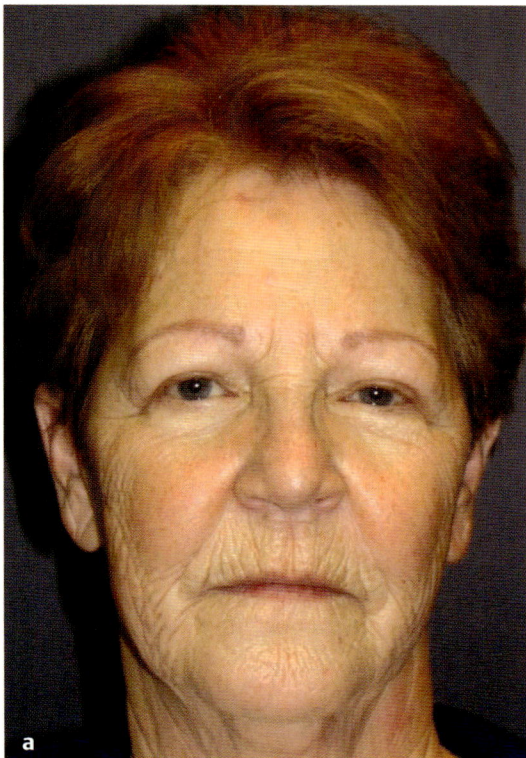

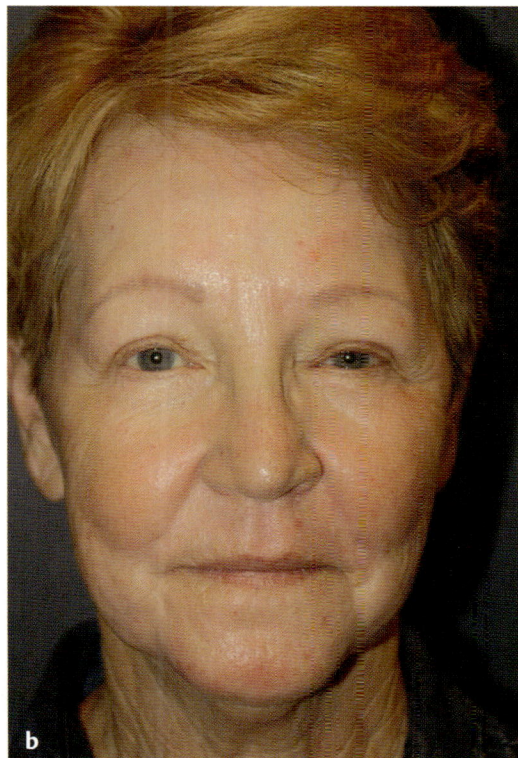

Fig. 7.3 **(a)** Prepeel and **(b)** postpeel. Dramatic improvement in rhytids can be appreciated in a patient who underwent a full-face Hetter chemical peel.

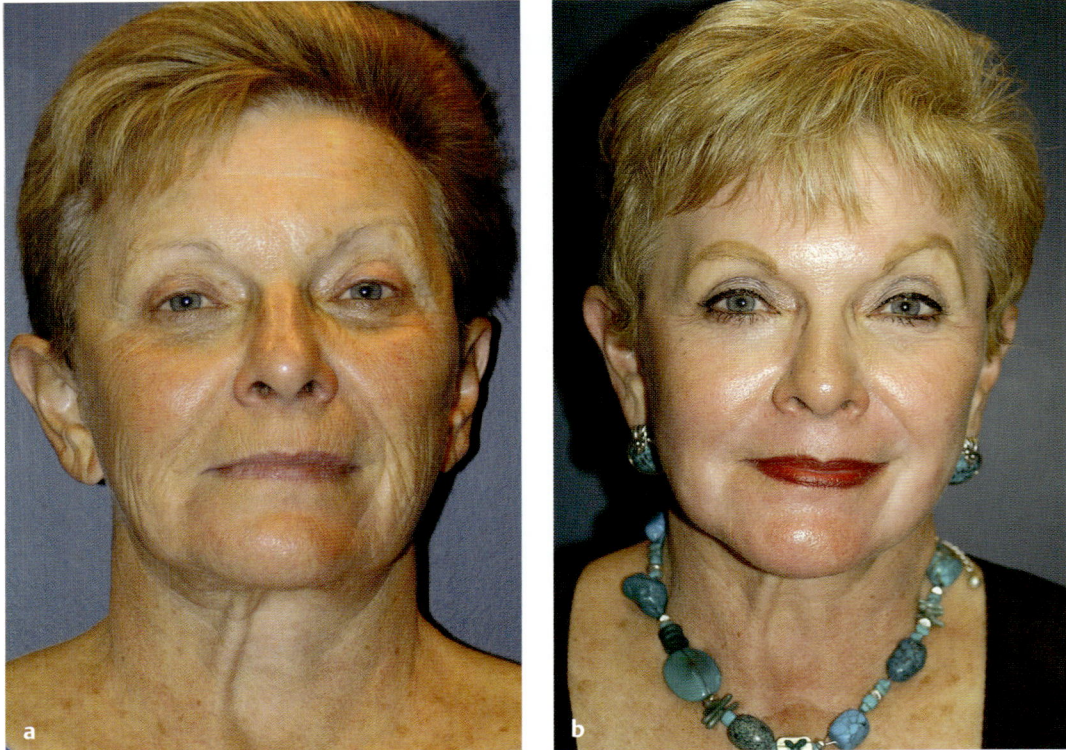

Fig. 7.4 **(a)** Prepeel and **(b)** postpeel. Another example of typical expected results in rhytids and dyschromia after a full-face Hetter chemical peel.

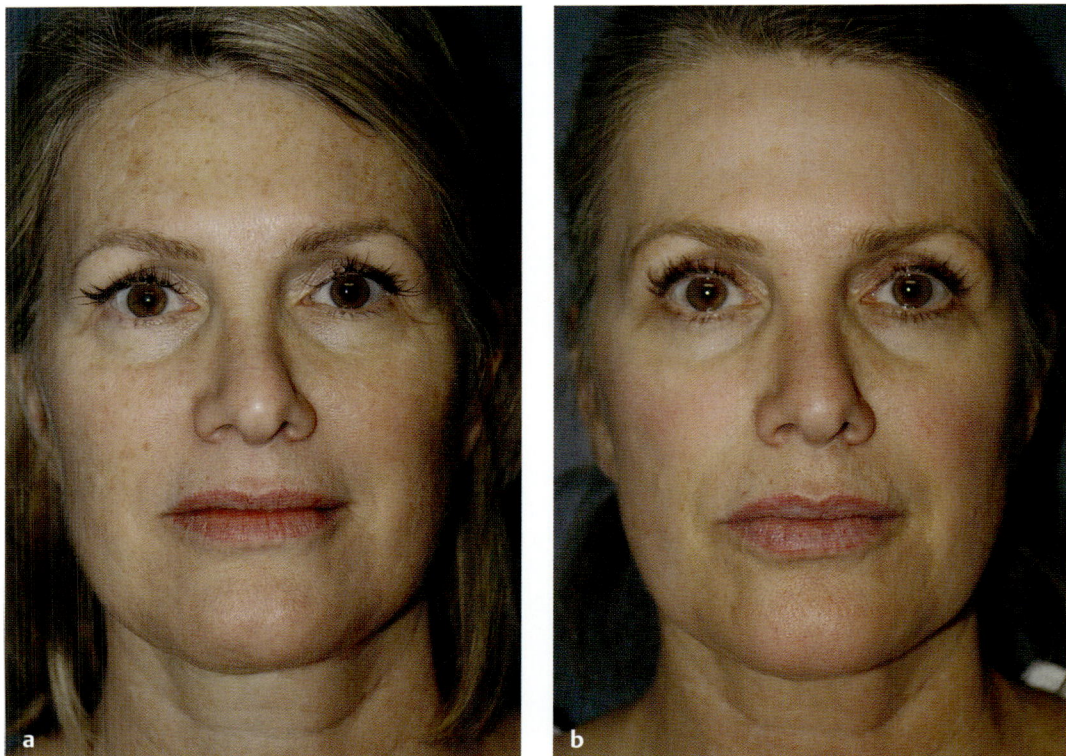

Fig. 7.5 **(a)** Prepeel and **(b)** postpeel. A lower croton oil concentration Hetter peel formulation was used here to improve facial dyschromia.

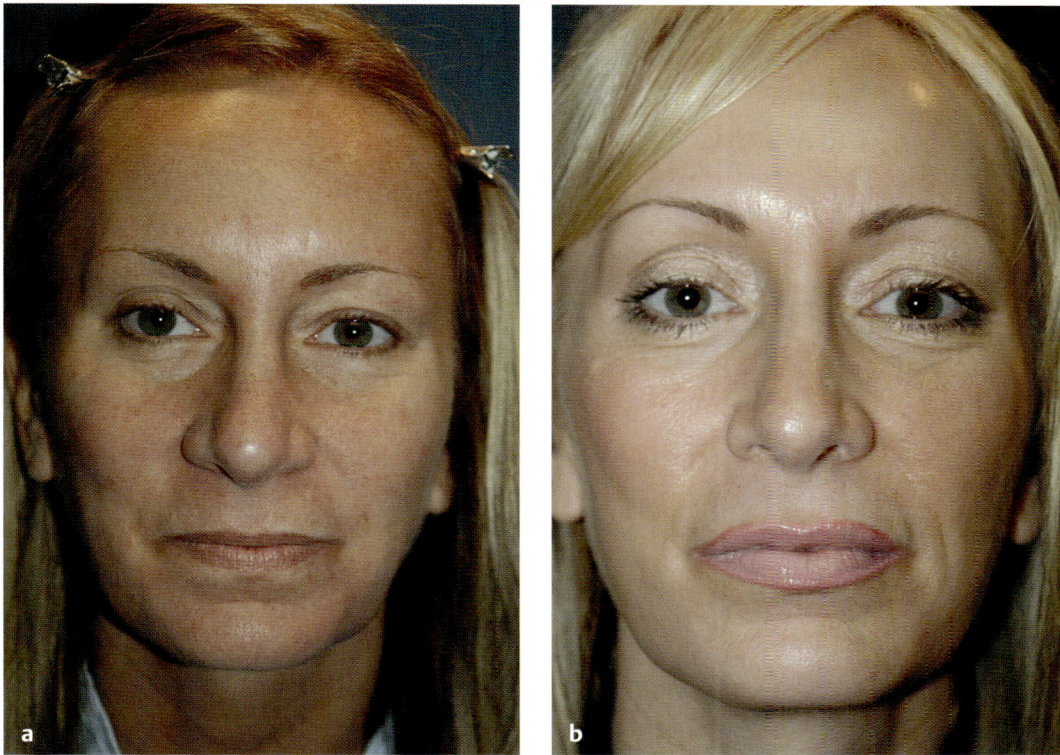

Fig. 7.6 **(a)** Prepeel and **(b)** postpeel. Another example of the use of a lower croton oil concentration Hetter peel formulation to improve facial dyschromia.

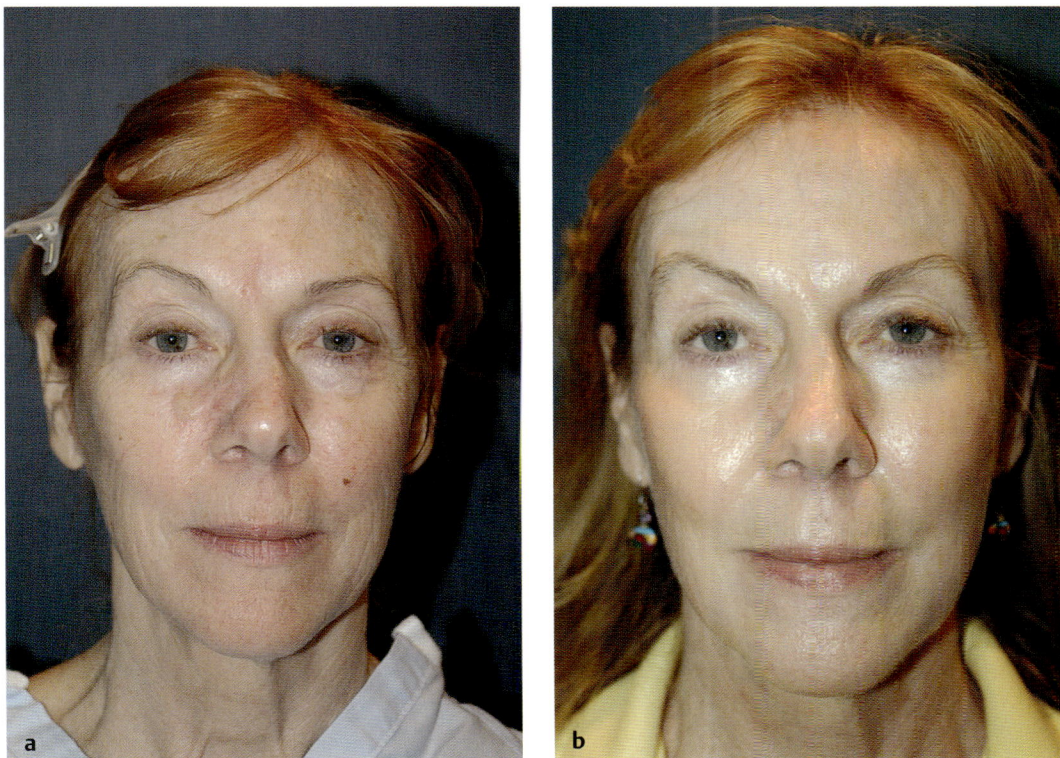

Fig. 7.7 **(a)** Prepeel and **(b)** postpeel. A mid-to-higher croton oil concentration was used here to improve both facial dyschromia and rhytids.

■ Complications and Their Management

Despite taking all necessary preoperative precautions and measures, the practitioner may encounter postoperative complications. A comprehensive understanding of these complications and the means by which to correct them can serve the peeler well. Proper management of these complications, both minor and major, can make the difference between undesirable and optimal results.

Probably the most feared complication of phenol peels is cardiac arrhythmias. Although no death due to phenol peeling has been described in the literature, the specter of a potential cardiovascular crisis has led to great alarm regarding the use of phenol. A reversible arrhythmia can occur, even in patients preoperatively screened and well hydrated, especially in those with undiagnosed myocardial sensitivity. These patients will develop a supraventricular tachycardia within 30 minutes of the onset of the peel, which, if exacerbated, can progress to paroxysmal ventricular contractions, paroxysmal atrial tachycardia, ventricular tachycardia, and possibly atrial fibrillations. The key is not to allow this progression to take place. Once an irregular rhythm is noted, the peeling should be halted and adequate hydration continued; the patient's rhythm will return to baseline as the phenol is cleared. At this point, the chemical peeling can proceed, but with vigilant observation of the cardiac rhythm. In the extremely rare case that the rhythm does not return to normal, proper measures should be employed for the aberrant rhythm.

Although not of as much concern as arrhythmias, prolonged healing times are a nuisance for both the patient and the practitioner. Any area that does not re-epithelialize by day 10 should be considered prolonged. This is more common with medium-depth TCA and deeper phenol peels.[16] The wounds should be checked daily. The practitioner must rule out the presence of infection or contact irritants and treat accordingly. The areas should be treated promptly or they will incur an increased risk of scarring.

In the event that scarring occurs, it will arise most often in the perioral area, specifically the upper lip. Scarring is frequently the result of too deep a peel or poor postoperative care. The risk of scarring is increased in isotretinoin users. Again, after discontinuing isotretinoin, the practitioner should wait until the patient is clearly developing skin oil. These scars can be treated with Silastic (Dow Corning, Midland, MI/Barry, UK) (cross-linked polydimethylsiloxane polymer) sheeting and intralesional steroid injections (Kenalog [E. R. Squibb & Sons, Princeton, NJ] 20 mg per mL) every 2 to 3 weeks. Overuse of steroids can result in dermal atrophy; therefore, judicious use is recommended. If the scars are erythematous, multiple treatments with flash-lamp pumped dye lasers are helpful.[2]

A bacterial pyoderma can aggravate wound healing and lead to scarring. In the rare case of a bacterial or fungal infection, appropriate antimicrobials should be initiated and continued for a 7- to 10-day course. Similarly, a herpetic outbreak can be devastatingly uncomfortable for the patient. If, despite prophylaxis, such an infection occurs, a maximal antiviral course of Valacyclovir 1 g three times a day for 10 days should be used.

The postoperative erythema that is typical in all peeled patients may last longer than expected. This is more prevalent with patients with sensitive skin or in cases of contact dermatitis. Topical hydrocortisone (2.5%) lotions are helpful for accelerating the resolution of the erythema.

As the erythema subsides, some patients, as a result of inadvertent sun exposure or darker skin type, can develop postinflammatory hyperpigmentation. This usually occurs weeks after the peel and is most readily seen in skin overlying bony prominences, such as the lateral malar regions. Postinflammatory hyperpigmentation is more common in Fitzpatrick III to VI skin types. A combination of 0.05% retinoic acid, 8% hydroquinone, and hydrocortisone cream is effective in reducing or eliminating this pigmentation. Glycolic acid lotion has been noted to be effective as well.[2]

More problematic than hyperpigmentation is hypopigmentation. Classically, this is more typical in phenol-based peels. Phenol is thought to eliminate the melanocytes' ability to produce melanin. This can be much more noticeable when single facial subunits are peeled. Hypopigmentation occurred with much greater frequency in the past, with the Baker formulation and postoperative occlusive taping or thymol iodide masks. The concentration of the phenol and croton oil, the skin type, and taping are all factors contributing to the risk of hypopigmentation—a complication that is irreversible. Patients should be counseled regarding the possible need for makeup use.

■ Conclusion

With the advent of CO_2 laser resurfacing followed by erbium:YAG laser resurfacing, chemical peeling was marginalized as an outdated practice supplanted by technological advances. Also, phenol-croton oil peeling became considered a deep, dangerous peel that had an all-or-none effect at best, and was riddled with complications at worst. Much like the outdated assertions of Adolph Brown and his contemporaries, neither of the aforementioned could be further from the truth. Chemical peeling should be considered the "standard" because it is an effective and safe tool for the facial cosmetic surgeon. Furthermore, with our relatively new understanding of the role of croton oil, the modified phenol-croton oil peeling formulations offer a modality that can be tailored for different skin types, thicknesses, and rhytid depth. A thorough understanding of this peel can greatly expand the options a practitioner is able to offer his resurfacing patients.

References

1. Hetter GP. An examination of the phenol-croton oil peel: Part II. The lay peelers and their croton oil formulas. Plast Reconstr Surg 2000;105(1):240–248, discussion 249–251

2. Hetter GP. An examination of the phenol-croton oil peel: Part III. The plastic surgeons' role. Plast Reconstr Surg 2000;105(2):752–763

3. Hetter GP. An examination of the phenol-croton oil peel: Part I. Dissecting the formula. Plast Reconstr Surg 2000;105(1):227–239, discussion 249–251

4. Brown AM, Kaplan LM, Brown ME. Phenol-induced histological skin changes: hazards, technique, and uses. Br J Plast Surg 1960;13:158–169

5. Hetter GP. An examination of the phenol-croton oil peel: Part IV. Face peel results with different concentrations of phenol and croton oil. Plast Reconstr Surg 2000;105(3):1061–1083, discussion 1084–1087

6. Stegman SJ. A comparative histologic study of the effects of three peeling agents and dermabrasion on normal and sun-damaged skin. Aesthetic Plast Surg 1982;6(3):123–135

7. Stone PA, Lefer LG. Modified phenol chemical face peels: recognizing the role of application technique. Facial Plast Surg Clin North Am 2001;9(3):351–376

8. Johnson JB, Ichinose H, Obagi ZE, Laub DR. Obagi's modified trichloroacetic acid (TCA)-controlled variable-depth peel: a study of clinical signs correlating with histological findings. Ann Plast Surg 1996;36(3):225–237

9. Brody HJ. Complications of chemical peeling. J Dermatol Surg Oncol 1989;15(9):1010–1019 PubMed

10. Brody HJ. Complications of chemical resurfacing. Dermatol Clin 2001;19(3):427–438, vii–viii

11. Vagotis FL, Brundage SR. Histologic study of dermabrasion and chemical peel in an animal model after pretreatment with Retin-A. Aesthetic Plast Surg 1995;19(3):243–246

12. Kim IH, Kim HK, Kye YC. Effects of tretinoin pretreatment on TCA chemical peel in guinea pig skin. J Korean Med Sci 1996;11(4):335–341

13. Popp C, Kligman AM, Stoudemayer TJ. Pretreatment of photoaged forearm skin with topical tretinoin accelerates healing of full-thickness wounds. Br J Dermatol 1995;132(1):46–53

14. Hevia O, Nemeth AJ, Taylor JR. Tretinoin accelerates healing after trichloroacetic acid chemical peel. Arch Dermatol 1991;127(5):678–682

15. Monheit GD. Medium-depth chemical peels. Dermatol Clin 2001;19(3):413–425, vii

16. Szachowicz EH, Wright WK. Delayed healing after full-face chemical peels. Facial Plast Surg 1989;6(1):8–13

8 Deep Chemical Peels

E. Gaylon McCollough

Key Concepts

- *New* is not necessarily *better*.

- A tool is just that . . . *a tool.*

- If the only "tool" one knows how to use is a hammer, everything begins to resemble a nail.

- The nature of machines is to malfunction . . . at the worst possible time.

- The more complex the machine, the more apt it is to malfunction.

■ Introduction

Often referred to in nonphysician circles as a "nonsurgical facelift," chemical exfoliation remains the gold standard for treating advanced wrinkling and solar elastosis of the face. Creative ways to apply peeling solutions and modifications in formulations and concentrations do not change the fact that the materials cause a separation of the upper layer of skin, which peels or sheds within a few days. The amount of peeling or shedding is directly related to the depth of injury, a factor that is dependent on the kinds—and caustic nature—of chemicals used.

Although other methods of exfoliation are effective in removing superficial signs of aging and sun-damaged skin, in the author's experience, level II and III peeling with the *original* Baker-Gordon peel formula (**Table 8.1**) has proven to stand the test of time; therefore, the author has seen no reason to modify the formula. It has also been the author's experience that the depth of injury depends upon several factors, only one of which is related to the chemicals chosen and the formulation of such chemicals with other agents. Penetration can also be affected by adjusting the mechanical act of degreasing the skin that is to be peeled, the number *of times* that a peeling solution is applied to the treated area, the amount of solution applied with each application, and how well a patient complies with good wound healing principles and instructions following the procedure. Using the same formulation (Baker-Gordon formula), it is possible to do a level II or level III peel on the same patient; it all depends on the factors mentioned in the preceding sentence.

In short, chemical peeling is both an art and a science. There is no one-size-fits-all formulation or application method for all skin types. The treatment plan for each patient must be individualized. Even on the same face, skin thickness varies, requiring more—or less—aggressive treatment. In this regard, the outcomes of treatment are very much determined by the skills and experience of the surgeon as well as patient compliance.

Table 8.1 Chemical peeling, Baker-Gordon solution

Phenol 88% USP	3 mL
Croton oil	3 guttae[b]
Septisol[a]	8 guttae
Distilled water	2 mL

Source: Baker TJ. Chemical face peeling and rhytidectomy: a combined approach for facial rejuvenation. Plast Reconstr Surg Transplant Bull 1962;29:199–207. Used with permission.
Abbreviation: USP, United States Pharmacopeia.
Note: A proven formula for more than 30 years.
[a]Steris, Mentor, OH.
[b]27 guttae = 1 mL.

■ Background: Basic Science of Procedure

With all peels, dermabrasion, and laser resurfacing techniques, outer layers of the skin are removed. However, only with more penetrating (levels II and III) procedures are new collagen and elastic fibers produced in the deeper layers of the skin. As a result, some tightening of facial tissues occurs (more with level III peels than with level II peels), but, in either case, not to the extent that can be achieved with conventional facelifting and eyelid-lifting techniques.

As a rule, light (level I) peels do not produce long-term improvement in the quality and texture of the skin but may be used as adjuncts to the methods herein described for continued maintenance.

Neither a facelift, eyelid surgery (blepharoplasty), nor a brow lift will remove wrinkles that have been etched into weather-beaten skin, transverse creases of the forehead, "crow's feet" around the eyes, or vertical wrinkles of the upper and lower lips. A good principle to remember is: *surgery improves sags and bulges, whereas resurfacing improves wrinkles*. And, with respect to skin resurfacing techniques, it has been the author's experience that dermabrasion is the treatment of choice for acne scarring or for the second and third stages of surgical scar revisions that required excision and wound resuturing. The author has had extensive experience in laser skin resurfacing and has found it to be helpful but not as effective in treating deeper facial rhytids with chemical peeling, nor in treating acne scarring as with wire brush dermabrasion.

To assist the profession in clearing some of the confusion regarding depth of treatment, the author developed a classification system (based on depth of injury) that applies to peels, dermabrasion, and laser resurfacing:

- **Level I—Superficial** (Spa peels, commercially available topicals such as glycolic and salicylic acid peels, etc.). Level I peels are temporary *skin polishers* and do not effectively rejuvenate wrinkled, scarred, or cancer-prone skin, no matter how often they are repeated.
- **Level II—Medium Depth** (TCA-based or modified phenol-based peels). Level II peels are more effective than level I peels in that more layers of damaged and wrinkled skin are removed. Healing time generally requires about a week. Level II procedures are generally recommended for patients less than 50 years old or those with minimal to moderate sun damage and wrinkling.
- **Level III—Deep** (Wire brush abrasion and Baker-Gordon phenol-based, croton oil peels).

Level III peels are the most effective methods of removing severely sun damaged, blotchy skin and deeper wrinkles. Healing time is longer—generally 2 weeks or more. However, results are long-lasting and often dramatic.

■ Patient Selection

As mentioned in a previous paragraph, different areas of the face require different types of treatment. In full-face resurfacing, the author often combines level II and level III peeling. Level II peeling is effective in treating eyelid rhytids and in blending from treated into nontreated regions (i.e., from the skin overlying the mandible into the shadow line below or into the hairline). And, using the Baker-Gordon formula, it is not necessary to change formulations from one region to the other. Simply modifying the technique of application provides transition from level II to level III. An experienced surgeon will know how to vary the depth of the treatment to meet the patient's specific needs.

The author's Facial Rejuvenation Classification System allows surgeons to quantify the condition of each patient's skin, eyelids, and face (**Tables 8.2; Table 8.3**).[1] Abbreviations have been assigned to each of the regions and structures of the face. A score of 0 through 5 is then assigned to each abbreviation, with 0 being the ideal and 5 being the most advanced signs of aging. Once the condition of each region is determined, it is a matter of choosing the most appropriate technique of either surgery and skin resurfacing or both and performing the procedure(s) in a precise and reliable manner. **Fig. 8.1a–d** demonstrates how the McCollough Facial Rejuvenation Classification was applied in one patient's total facial rejuvenation.

Anyone performing facial exfoliation must understand and remind patients—*in advance of treatment*—of the length of time required for healing, especially for level II and III resurfacing procedures. Regardless of the source of injury (peeling, dermabrasion, laser), unless it takes a minimum of 2 weeks to heal, results will generally fall short of the doctor's and patient's expectations. In that regard, "no downtime equals no long-term improvement."

Relative contraindications for phenol-based chemexfoliation include active herpes infections, unrealistic expectations, unreliable patient, the skin of the neck, and diseased state of any organ system that breaks down—or is sensitive to—phenol (liver, kidney, and heart). In the end, the decision to perform chemical peeling lies with the surgeon, who must weigh the potential risks against the benefits of any procedure.

Table 8.2 The McCollough Facial Rejuvenation Classification System

Stage I: The Less than Thirty Facelift	For the younger individual who has little or no loose skin and may require only liposuction to remove unwanted fat and bulges
Stage II: The Thirty-Something Facelift	For the patient who is beginning to notice sagging of the brows and cheeks, *but not the neck*. Whenever sagging tissues are present, facial muscles and fat must be repositioned into their more youthful relationships. In such cases, a small amount of loose skin is removed.
Stage III: The Forty-Something Facelift	For the patient who exhibits sagging brows, cheeks, and neck. Some of these patients may or may not need liposuction for contouring jowls and fullness under the chin. All, however, require suspension techniques to muscles and fat.
Stage IV: The Fifty-Something Facelift	For the patient with *generalized* facial and neck sagging, with or without jowls and wrinkles around the mouth. With more obvious muscle, fat, and skin laxity, more suspension of these structures is required.
Stage V: The Sixty-Plus Facelift	For the patient with *advanced* aging, coupled with sagging of all facial areas, including the forehead, brows, cheeks, and neck. At this stage in the aging process, deep folds develop in the groove between the nose and face, jowls droop below the jaw line, and the muscles of the neck often produce string-like bands that run vertically from the chin to the upper chest. Many of these patients are also beginning to exhibit wrinkles and blemishes over most of the face.

Source: McCollough EG. The McCollough Facial Rejuvenation System: a condition-specific classification algorithm. Facial Plast Surg 2011;27(1):112–123. Used with permission.

"Facelift" is the term commonly used to describe a surgical procedure better known in medical circles as rhytidectomy (removal of loose, wrinkled skin of the face and neck). The procedure is designed to re-create the firmer, smoother face of youth. However, not all facelifts are the same—nor should they be! *Not all faces are the same.* And at different ages the same face is a different face. Dr. McCollough's system consists of five general treatment plans, or stages.

Table 8.3 The language of surgical rejuvenation

Facelifting

SQ	Skin quality	T	Temple	PL	Platysmal banding
V	Facial volume status	CH	Cheek	ML	Melolabial groove
FH	Forehead	Ne	Neck	MAR	Marionette grooves

Skin resurfacing

WR	Wrinkling/rhytids	PORB	Complete periorbital resurfacing	UPORL	Upper perioral
FH	Forehead	UEL	Upper eyelids	LPORL	Lower perioral
No	Nose	LEL	Lower eyelids	FF	Full-face skin resurfacing
CH	Cheeks	PORL	Complete perioral resurfacing		

Eyelid and periorbital region

R	Right	LEL	Lower eyelids	NFP	Nasal fat pad
L	Left	B	Bilateral	MFP	Middle fat pad
UEL	Upper eyelids	FX	Fat excess	OFP	Orbital fat pad

Source: McCollough EG. The McCollough Facial Rejuvenation System: a condition-specific classification algorithm. Facial Plast Surg 2011;27(1):112–123. Used with permission.

Note: A number from 0 to 5 should be assigned to each of the above criteria with 0 being the ideal and 5 indicating advanced aging.

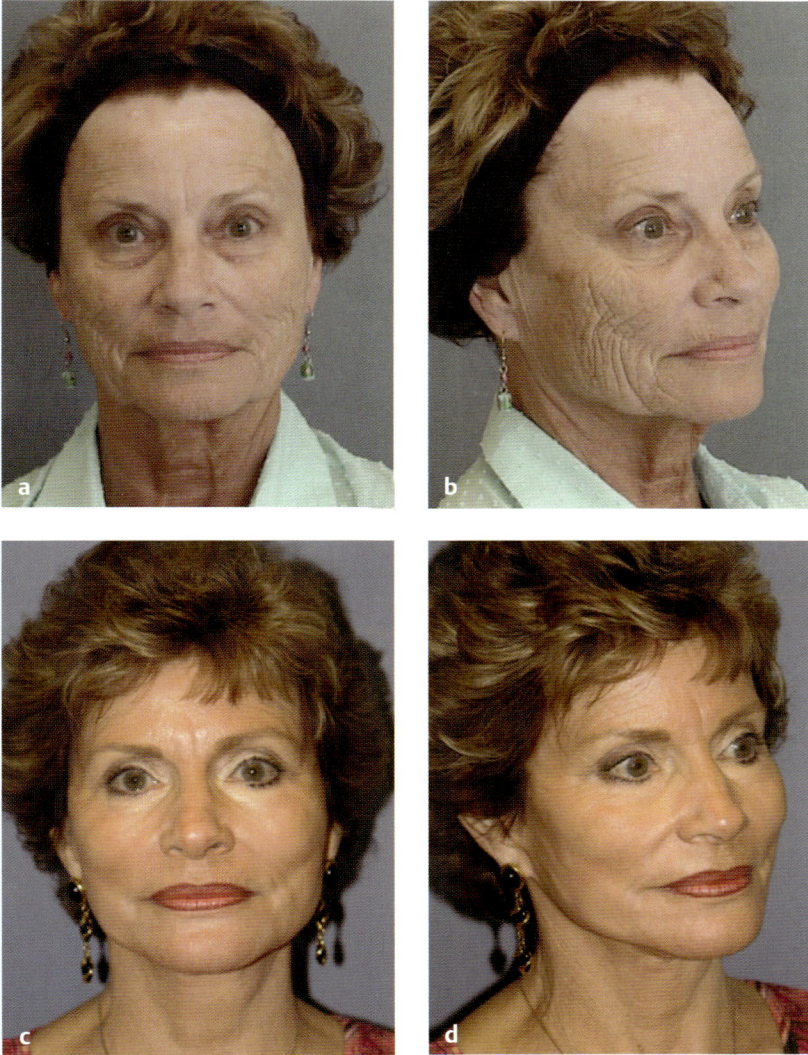

Fig. 8.1 (a–d) This patient exhibits many of the signs of aging that the McCollough Condition-Specific Facial Rejuvenation System is designed to address. Using the previously described criteria, her preoperative code would be: SQ-4 V-2, FH-2,T-2,CH-3,MI-2,MAR-0,Ne-4,PL-4,FX-2, WR-5 (FF),BUEL-2,BLEL-4. (See **Table 8.3**.)

■ Technical Aspects of the Procedure

With all levels of chemical exfoliation, successful outcomes depend on several factors, including patient selection, depth of injury, the skill and experience of the operating surgeon, blending at the perimeters, a thorough understanding of exfoliative healing, knowledge of potential irritants to healing skin, detailed printed instructions, and patient compliance.

A variety of chemicals and formulations have been used for chemical exfoliation of facial skin; however, for almost 40 years, the author has used the same formulation. It is the one developed by Baker and Gordon and published in the *Journal of the Florida Medical Association* in 1961 (**Table 8.1**).

When mixed, the formula becomes an emulsion; if left standing, it will break down into layers of the component parts. Therefore, it is important to agitate and mix the solution before and during the entire peeling procedure.

The solution is applied to the skin, using applicators that have been dipped and swirled into the solution. The solution-soaked tip of the applicator should be swirled against the neck of the amber-colored glass bottle to eliminate dripping ▶ **Video 8.1**.

The process of applying the solution to the skin is an art form and requires rolling the semisaturated applicator over the areas to be treated in a uniform manner (**Fig. 8.2a,b**). Depth of injury can be controlled by modifying the degree of saturation of the applicator used for application. A *more saturated* applicator is used in areas requiring deeper treatments (level III, such as the deep vertical creases of the lips), and a *less saturated* applicator is used in regions that require lesser depths (level II, thinner skin of the eyelids).

The natural oils of facial skin and topically applied oily materials act as a barrier to chemical exfoliates. Removing these oils from the skin allows the solu-

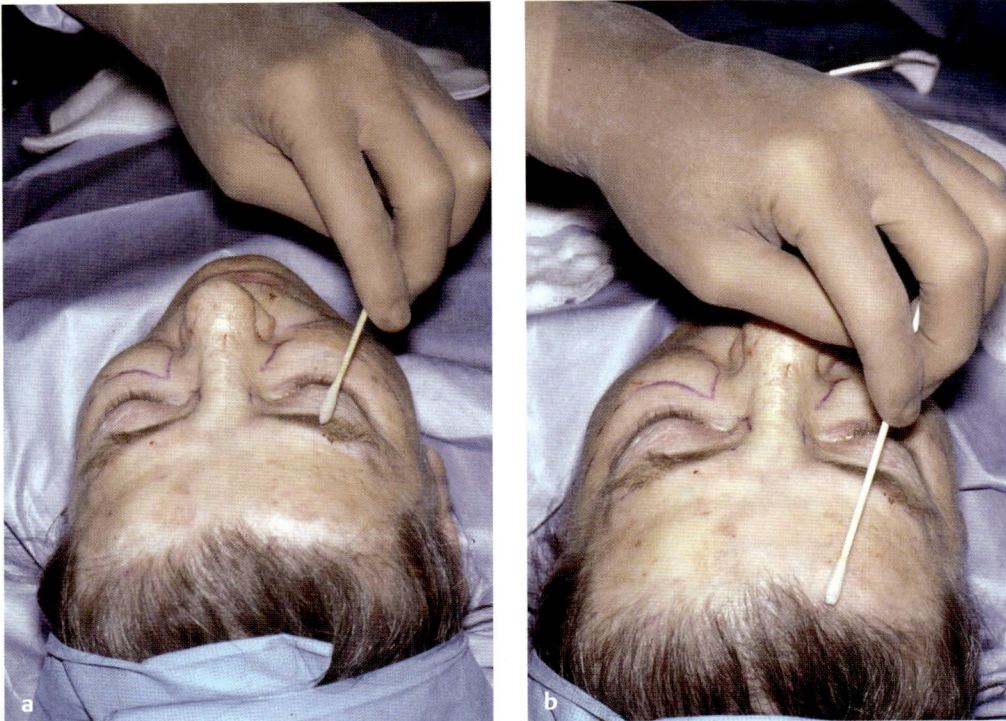

Fig. 8.2 Application of solution into the brow hair using the "rolling" technique **(a)**. Blending into the frontal hairline prevents sharp lines of color demarcation **(b)**.

tion to penetrate more deeply and is another method of varying the depth of treatment to the desired levels. To limit deeper penetration, one would be less aggressive in removing the oily barrier.

The author has seen no reason to modify the formula or to use any solution other than the one already described (the classical Baker-Gordon formula).

Fig. 8.3a–f demonstrates the application of peeling solutions to various regions of the face. Contrary to the method described by Baker and Gordon, the author ceased taping over peeled areas with adhesive tape in the late 1970s and published his work in the *Otolaryngology Clinics of North America* in 1980.[2] Since that time, he has resorted to "wet-dressing" techniques, employing a myriad of topical emollients and sheeting.

Postoperative Care

In 2007, the author developed a topical treatment that he currently favors after chemical peeling. This consists of a dimethicone gel impregnated with lavender oil and plantain oil (DermalAID, MediStat, Foley, AL). The author has noted a 30 to 40% reduction in healing time, shorter periods of postoperative erythema, and a considerable reduction in posttreatment milia formation since the initiation of use of this product,

making it the "dressing" of choice. This has been important because many topicals, especially those that are petrolatum based, can promote milia. The gel should be applied to peeled areas once blisters rupture—usually on postoperative day 2. Detailed instructions should be given to patients following treatment. Environmental conditions and avoidance of irritating products are crucial to healing.[3]

Postoperative management of peeled skin is crucial to optimal wound healing, avoidance of complications, and a speedy recovery. With level II and III peels, erythema slowly subsides over the ensuing weeks (2 to 4 weeks for level II peels, 4 to 6 for level III peels).

Expected Results

Skin resurfacing can often be the "icing on the cake" for comprehensive facial rejuvenation. Patients undergoing blepharoplasty or rhytidectomy should be informed that surgery will not eradicate deeper rhytids and may require level III skin resurfacing. Level II and III peel procedures are much like sunburns or blisters in that the top layer of skin begins to shed over a 4- to 5-day period, revealing the fresh, new, deep pink layer underneath. **Fig. 8.4a–e** demonstrates the appearance of a face following levels II and III chemical peeling. **Fig. 8.4f** demonstrates

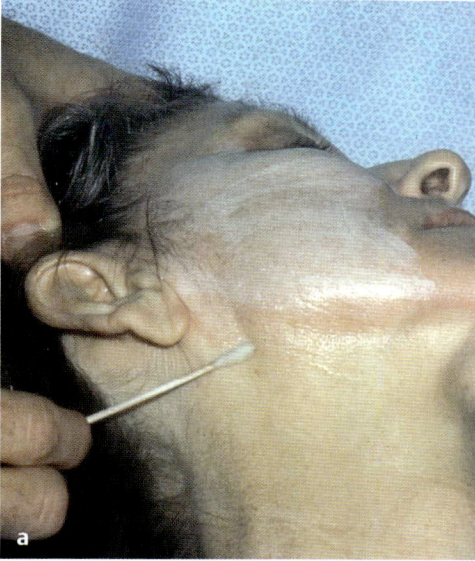

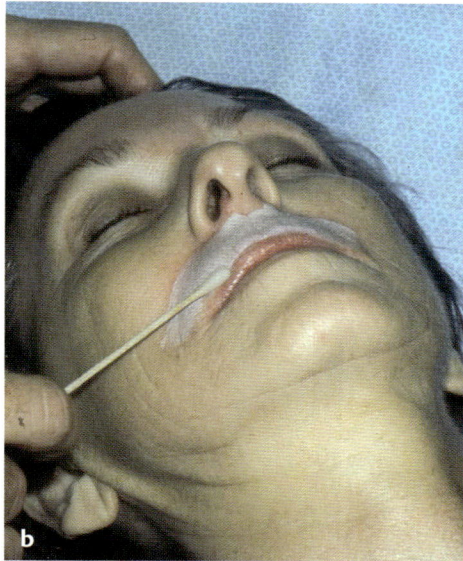

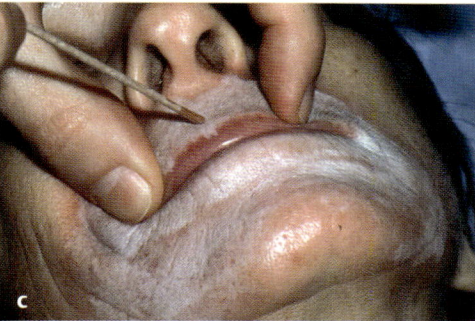

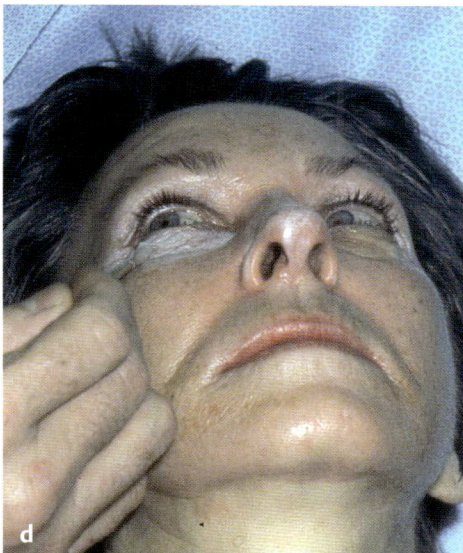

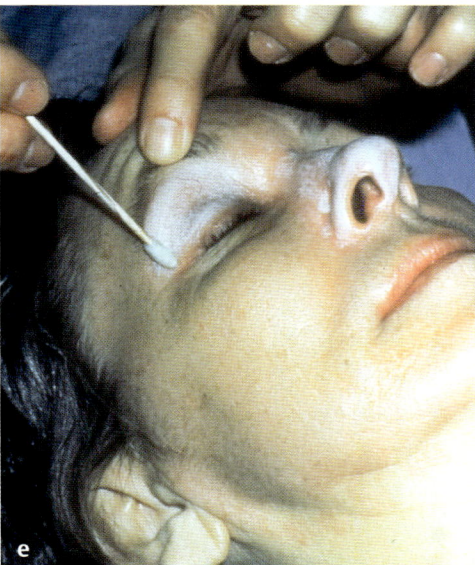

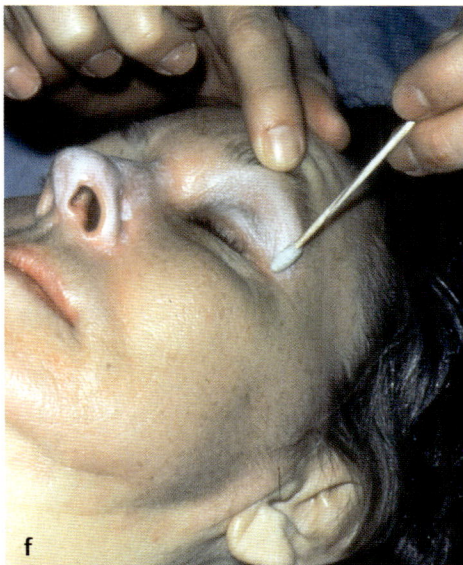

Fig. 3.3 (a) Feathering from the cheeks and across the mandibular margin with a semimoist applicator provides a gradual transition from treated to untreated areas. (b) Crossing the vermilion border of the lips for ~ 2.0 mm is helpful in minimizing wrinkles on membranes. (c) Deeper rhytids can often be improved with pinpoint application of additional solution. Stretching the skin in such cases allows for more accurate application. (d) When peeling the lower lids, it is advisable to have the patient sit in an elevated position. Solution can be brought to within 2.0 mm of the lash line. Lid skin is best peeled with a semimoist applicator tip, thereby creating a level II peel. (e) Upper lids can be peeled to within 2.0 mm of the lash line, which is best performed with the patient in a more level position. (f) Note that the skin on the nose can also be treated with a level II peeling technique.

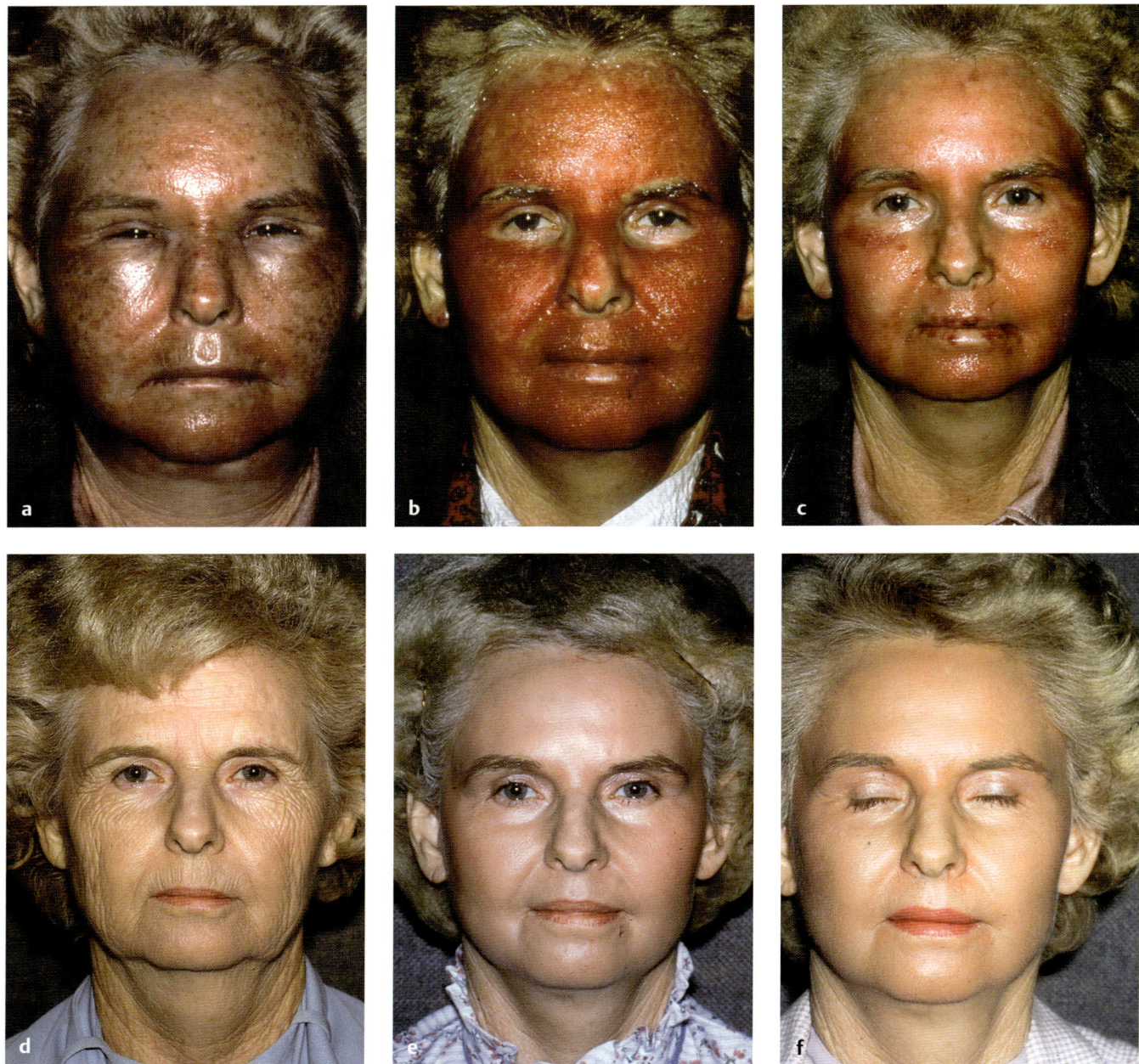

Fig. 8.4 **(a)** Photograph of a patient on the first postpeel day. Note the significant amount of edema and the beginning of blister-like vesicles over the entire face. **(b)** With the use of topical occlusive gels, the top layers of skin peel off within 4 to 5 days leaving a deep red appearance. Once vesicles rupture, swelling begins to subside. **(c)** In approximately 1 week, most crusting has disappeared and newly regenerating skin begins to emerge. Note that the lower lids often take a bit longer to heal. Also note the appearance of a perioral herpetic outbreak in this patient. It can be controlled with oral and topical antiviral medication. **(d)** The same patient shown in the previous photographs before a full-face (level III) peel. **(e)** Approximately 3 full weeks after a full-face (level III) peel. **(f)** When treated areas no longer demonstrate a *deep* pink color, mineral makeup may be applied to camouflage any residual erythema.

longer-term healing and the ability to camouflage erythema with makeup. Even though longer healing times are often looked upon as a negative for level III resurfacing techniques (peels, lasers, and dermabrasion), the end result is well worth the inconvenience. Results are often dramatic (**Fig. 8.5a,b**; **Fig. 8.6a,b**; **Fig. 8.7a,b**; **Fig. 8.8a,b**).

As a rule, peeling over the same skin that has been surgically freed from underlying tissues during facelifting or blepharoplasty puts added strain on the healing process of both procedures and is not generally recommended. However, if a layer of muscle has been left between the skin surface and undermined areas (i.e., subgaleal forehead lifting or a skin muscle lower lid blepharoplasty), a level II peel can often assist with improving some rhytids that surgery alone will not eliminate. Areas far removed from undermined areas (i.e., the perioral region) are safe to peel at the same time of facelifting, even if the plane of dissection in cheek regions is superficial to facial muscles. Full-face resurfacing over superficially undermined areas may be best delayed for 2 to 3 months (**Fig. 8.9a,b**).

■ Complications and Their Management

As is the case with any surgical procedure (including skin resurfacing), complications can occur. Problems can be minimized or prevented by paying close attention to detail and following trusted protocols and formulations. The following are potential problems that need to be considered by surgeons and their patients, particularly with phenol croton oil level II and III peels.

Cardiac Arrhythmias

When large amounts of phenol are absorbed into the bloodstream, premature atrial and ventricular contractions can occur. These arrhythmias may be reduced or eliminated by making sure that patients are well hydrated before peeling begins and by using lidocaine infiltrated into the areas to be peeled. Epinephrine added to lidocaine tends to increase the

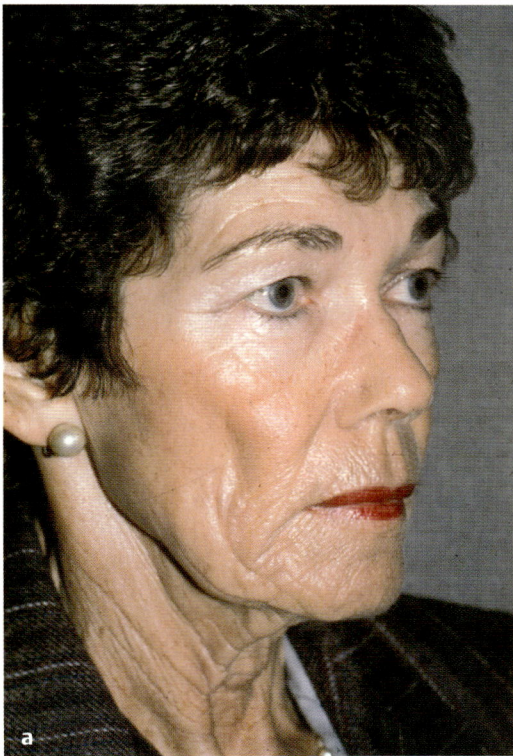

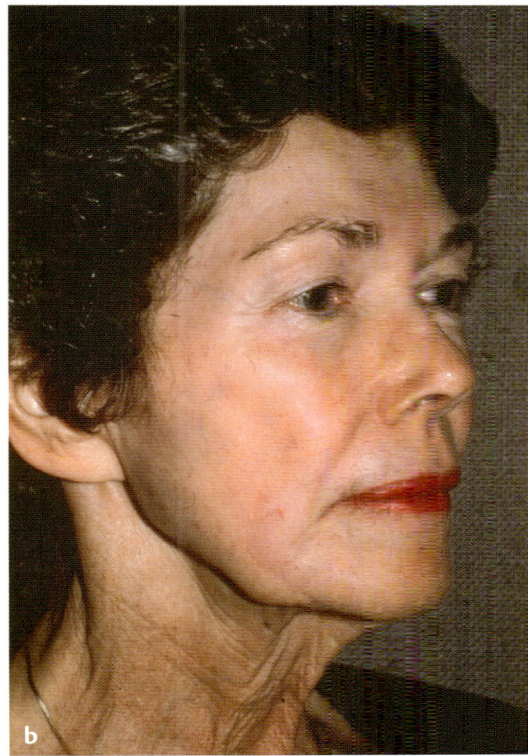

Fig. 8.5 Before (**a**) and after (**b**) level III chemical peel. No other procedures were performed. Note the texture and tightening of the facial and eyelid skin.

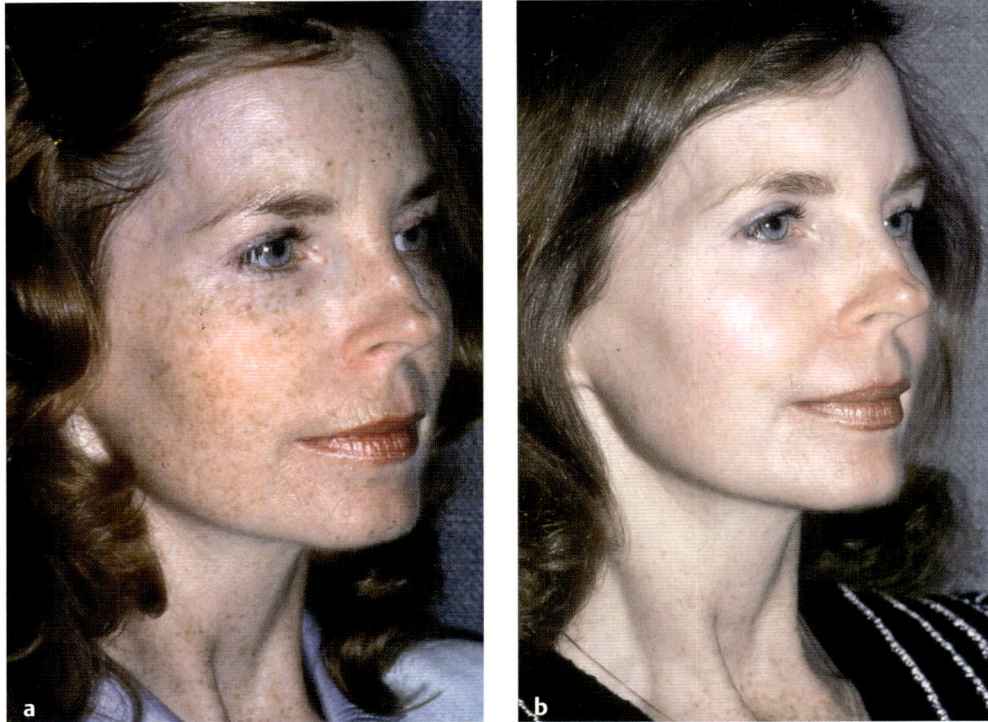

Fig. 8.6   Before **(a)** and after **(b)** of a patient who underwent level II chemical peeling to diminish facial freckles.

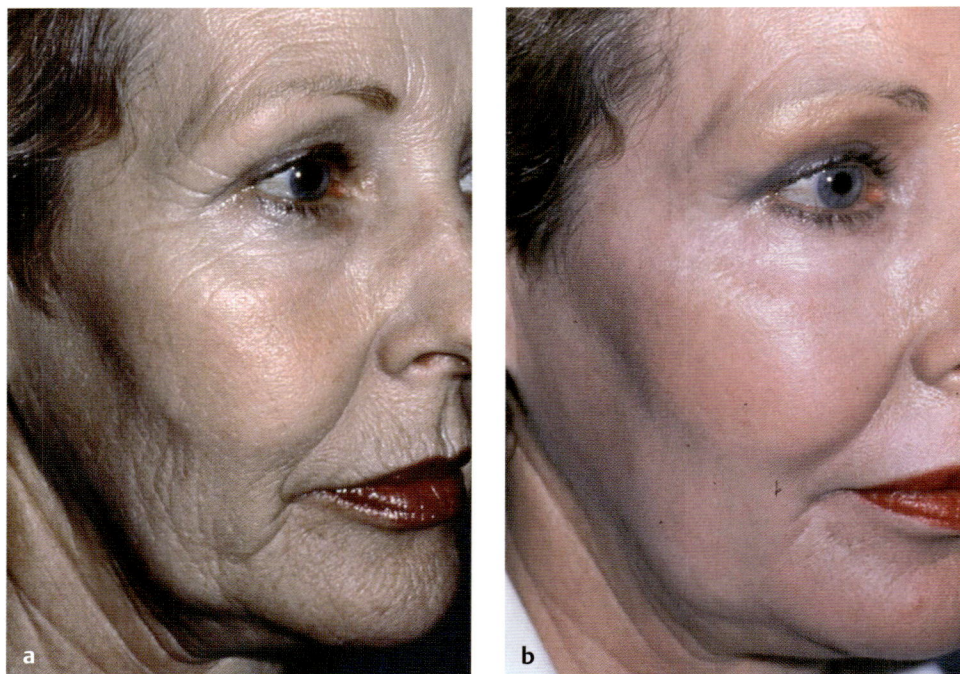

Fig. 8.7   Before **(a)** and after **(b)** level III chemical peeling. Note the improvement in the texture of the skin and reduction in rhytids in all regions.

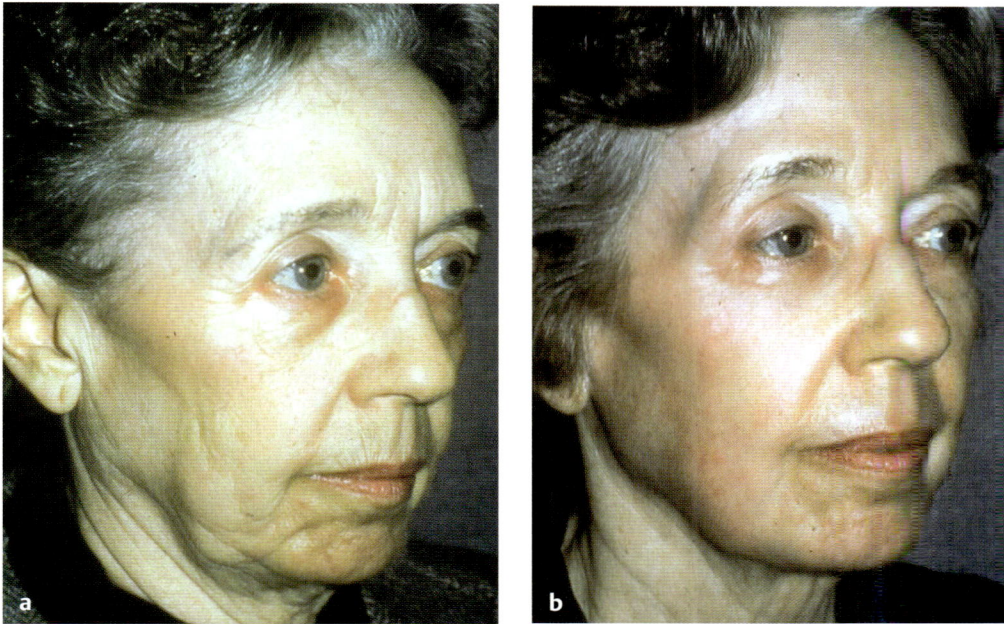

Fig. 8.8 Another patient before **(a)** and after **(b)** *only* a level III chemical peel. No other procedures were performed. Note the amount of skin tightening along the jaw line and in the neck. The peel extended only 2.0 mm below the mandibular margin

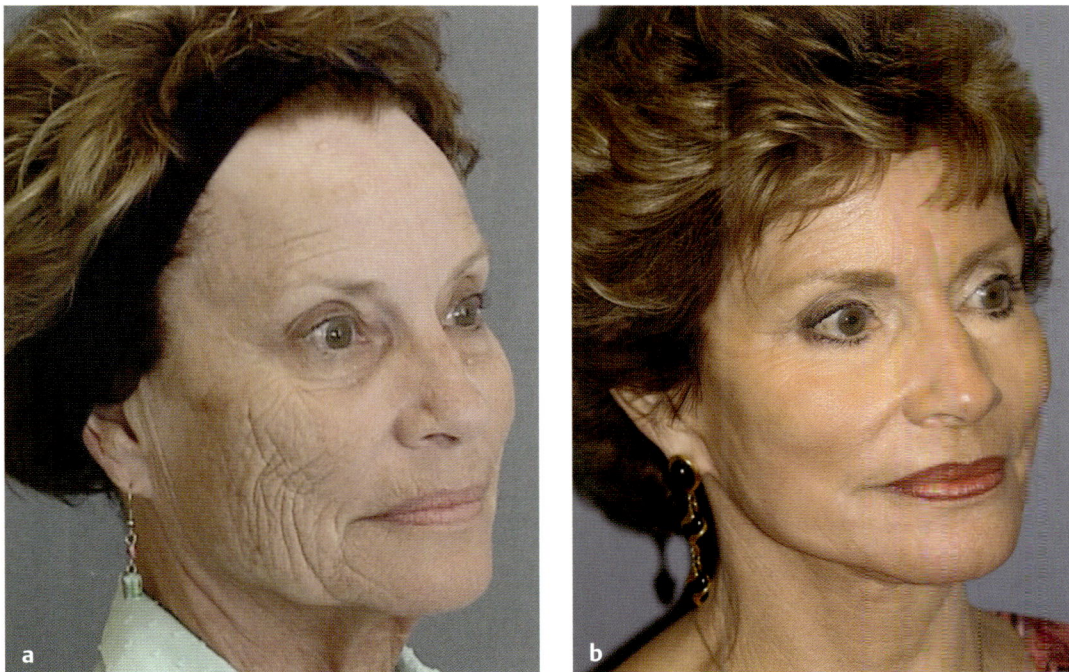

Fig. 8.9 Closer views of the patient shown in **Fig. 8.1**. Full-face resurfacing using level III chemical peeling in the periorbital and perioral regions and level III dermabrasion in the cheeks, nose, and forehead was performed ~ 1 year following stage V face lift and stage IV blepharoplasty. **(a)** Before treatment. **(b)** After treatment.

possibility of arrhythmias. Plain lidocaine not only provides anesthesia during the immediate postoperative period but reduces the heart's sensitivity to absorbed phenol. One should plan on peeling no more than one fourth of the face at a time and waiting 10 to 15 minutes before peeling another fourth.

Exacerbation of Herpes Lesions

In patients with a prior history of herpetic outbreaks, a pre- and posttreatment regimen of antiviral agents is recommended. Should outbreaks occur, topical antiviral agents can also be helpful. If patients have previously experienced herpes conjunctivitis, or lesions occur around the eye, ophthalmic antiviral prophylaxis is recommended. To minimize or avoid scarring, it is important to keep crusty herpetic lesions moist with gels or ointments until healed.

Pigmentary Aberrations

Any level II or III resurfacing procedure affects melanocytes. Level II treatments tend to stimulate melanocytic activity, leading to *hyper*pigmentation, which can be effectively treated with compounded formulations of tretinoin and hydroquinone. Level III treatments tend to destroy a certain number of melanocytes, thereby producing varying amounts of *hypo*pigmentation. Extreme areas of hypopigmentation can be camouflaged with temporary—or permanent—makeup. The experienced resurfacing surgeon will learn how to blend peeling solutions to minimize pigment aberrations and lines of demarcation. Streaking (irregularly pigmented areas) can be avoided with proper application and often can be corrected with additional peeling or dermabrasion techniques over *hyper*pigmented regions.

Posttreatment Erythema

Perhaps one of the most disconcerting sequelae for patients and surgeons alike is persistent redness following level II and III peels. The sensitive "new" skin that replaces sun-damaged, wrinkled skin must go through a maturation process before it can withstand products and environmental conditions that it will ultimately tolerate with ease. Many patients become impatient during the early stages of healing and use lotions, creams, moisturizers, sunscreens/blocks, and makeups that can irritate the delicate new skin before the skin is resilient enough to tolerate these products, resulting in prolonged erythema. In 1998, McCollough and Monheit et al reported that, in 236 consecutive chemical phenol peels, 11% of patients developed prolonged postpeel erythema. Topical irritants were the most common etiology. All patients had complete resolution of skin change with avoidance of irritating products and environmental conditions.[4]

A good rule to remember is this: as long as the skin is pink, all topical products should be avoided. When the newly resurfaced skin no longer exhibits a pink color, it is generally resilient enough to withstand products that were used *prior to treatment*. Skin care programs that include exfoliating agents should be avoided for approximately 3 months following level II and III peels. In virtually every case of prolonged erythema, the author has been able to identify the irritating agent (**Fig. 8.10a,b**). Because of the care that newly resurfaced skin (treated with level II and III peels) requires, it is imperative that the surgeon provides patients *with written instructions and precautions*. On occasion, a course of intense pulsed light (IPL) treatments can "calm down" areas of erythema. Naturally, every patient's skin is different and responds to the same treatments in different ways.

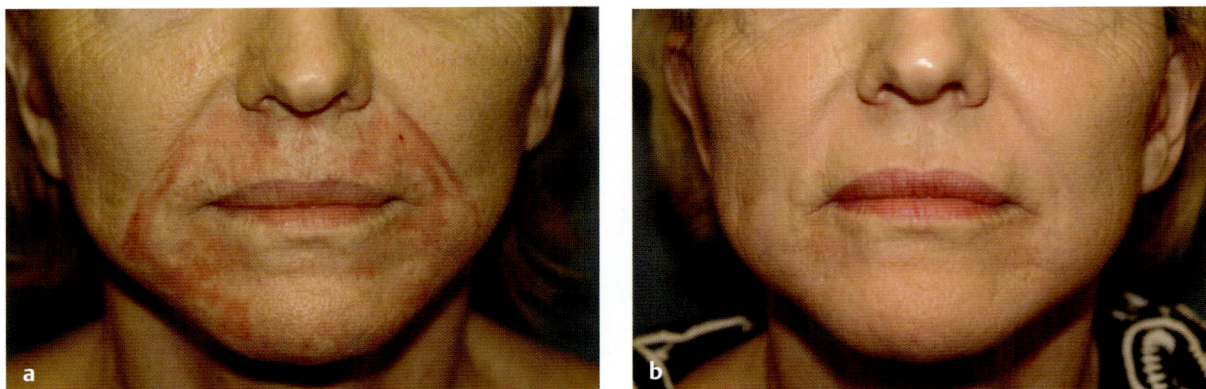

Fig. 8.10 A patient demonstrating the "postpeel erythema syndrome" as a result of allowing irritants to come in contact with peeled areas before the skin was "mature" enough to handle such products **(a)**. With time, the erythema subsided **(b)**.

Hypertrophic Scarring

Scarring following well-performed level II and level III chemical peels is rare. If scarring occurs, it is generally the result of secondary infection or trauma. Patients should be counseled not to pick at loosening skin or crusts. Doing so could convert a second-degree injury to a third-degree injury, ensuring that some scarring could result. If newly healing skin comes in contact with caustic irritants (ammonia, chlorine, alcohols, and fragrant products), additional chemical damage could occur. This is why printed postoperative instructions and compliance counseling are crucial to avoidance of problems.

Milia

Milia are generally the result of occluded oil gland outlets that have been obstructed either by topical treatment products (i.e., petrolatum-based products) or rapid healing when a new layer of skin grows across an oil gland outlet. In most cases, milia subside in time without treatment. If needed, severe milia may be uncapped with the tip of a sharp, sterile needle.

Subtotal Removal of Rhytids

Residual wrinkling or keratoses should not be considered a complication of chemical peeling—or any level III resurfacing procedure. Persistent rhytids may simply need to be touched up with a small amount of peel solution applied directly into the depths of the crease.

■ Conclusion

Chemical and/or abrasive exfoliation of aging, photodamaged, or scarred skin is a proven method of improving quality and texture. Healing time and pigmentary changes for chemical, abrasive/laser exfoliation procedures are the same . . . so long as the depth of injury for each procedure is equal. Varying the depth of injury *in different regions of the face—and blending—*are the best ways to achieve extraordinary results *and* the safest way to avoid postoperative complications, such as residual defects, pigmentary discrepancies, and scarring.

Chemical exfoliation techniques are cost-efficient, care-effective methods of treating aging skin of the face and should be taught *and practiced* by contemporary facial plastic surgeons. Chemexfoliation is compact and does not require storage rooms, maintenance, finance charges, or periodic replacement with more expensive equipment. Chemical exfoliation (individually or in combination with other facial procedures) often provides the "icing on the cake" for facial rejuvenation and should be part of a long-term treatment/maintenance plan.

As new technology comes into practice, facial plastic surgeons must not forget that the skill and judgment with which tools are used are of prime importance. This is what always has, and always will, distinguish the artist from the mere technician.[5]

References

1. McCollough EG. The McCollough Facial Rejuvenation System: a condition-specific classification algorithm. Facial Plast Surg 2011;27(1):112–123

2. McCollough EG, Langsdon PL. Dermabrasion and Chemical Peel. New York, NY: Thieme 1988

3. McCollough EG. The Appearance Factor. Gulf Shores AL: Compass Press; 2009

4. Maloney BP, Millman B, Monheit G, McCollough EG. The etiology of prolonged erythema after chemical peel. Dermatol Surg 1998;24(3):337–34

5. Baker TJ, Gordon HL. The ablation of rhytids by chemical means: A preliminary report. J Fla Med Assoc 1961;47:451

9 Skin Rejuvenation for Patients with Fitzpatrick Skin Types IV, V, and VI

Jennifer Parker Porter

Key Concepts

- Avoid being overly aggressive. Progress in a stepwise fashion to a predetermined goal.

- Improvement in the skin tone is most important for these patient populations.

- Properly prepare the skin for more intensive treatments (e.g., 20% trichloroacetic acid peel or 30% salicylic acid peel).

- Ensure the patient has realistic expectations of the outcome.

- Photodocumentation is paramount; often both the provider and the patient forget where they started. Photos are taken even if the patient is only starting on a new skin care regimen.

■ Introduction

Skin rejuvenation involves improvement of the skin texture and tone that have deteriorated as the skin ages. Skin that has been damaged by sun, environmental exposure, and gravitational forces frequently manifests the following common changes: rhytids, telangiectasias, and dyschromias. The degree to which we see these changes depends on the Fitzpatrick skin type (see **Table 6.4**). For Fitzpatrick skin types I, II, and III, the skin becomes ravaged with rhytids, lentigines, and telangiectasias, the major signs of both photodamage and skin aging. We have an arsenal of techniques to improve these concerns, from aggressive lasers to light chemical peels. Fitzpatrick skin types I, II, and III are fairly resilient to treatments that involve marked edema, erythema,

and prolonged recovery. However, for patients of Fitzpatrick skin types IV, V, and VI, the process of aging is a bit different, with fewer concerns regarding rhytids and telangiectasias and more concerns regarding dyschromias and textural changes.

Although the Fitzpatrick classification is very helpful in stratifying patient populations based on their reaction to sun exposure, placing a patient into a discrete category is not straightforward. Traditionally, olive-tone Caucasians of Mediterranean descent were considered Fitzpatrick skin type IV. At the present, due to mixing of ethnic backgrounds, we see patients of African American, Asian, and Latino descent that one can classify as a Fitzpatrick IV: light skin that rarely burns. The ability to tan or burn cannot be determined solely by asking patients about their ethnic background because there are many patients with lighter skin who are of Latino, Asian, or African descent. Regardless of how light their skin is, do not discount their ethnicity by opting for a more aggressive treatment. Their ability to produce melanin in response to injury is significant.

Patients within the Fitzpatrick IV skin type have some concerns with rhytids; the concern lessens as the skin becomes more deeply pigmented and progresses to Fitzpatrick skin type VI. Patients in the Fitzpatrick IV through VI categories are more concerned with gravitational changes, including prominent furrows and folds. Injectables such as neurotoxins and dermal fillers do a superb job in treating these concerns for these patient populations because they typically do not have the superficial rhytids associated with the folds. Because these changes tend to appear ~ 10 years later than they do in their Fitzpatrick I through III counterparts, they are more accepted as the normal process of aging.

Skin rejuvenation for Fitzpatrick skin types IV through VI typically focuses on treating dyschromias. The goal is to treat the skin and improve these conditions without causing harm to the skin in the process. Through the use of a variety of chemical peels, microdermabrasion, and at-home skin care, improvement can be realized with a methodical, graduated approach that is not overly aggressive. As such, this chapter focuses on these techniques, as well as the skin care regimens that work in concert to achieve the desired results.

■ Background: Basic Science of Procedure

Chemical peels and microdermabrasion are designed to be chemical or mechanical exfoliative treatments that remove skin cells from the surface of the skin. The depth to which the skin cells are removed depends on the type of peel used or the aggressiveness of the microdermabrasion (**Fig. 9.1**). Superficial peels affect the skin through the level of the epidermis; some peels and microdermabrasion are very superficial, affecting only the stratum corneum. Medium-depth chemical peels penetrate, causing injury in the papillary and upper reticular dermis.[1]

In the superficial category are the 20 to 40% glycolic acid peels, Jessner's peels, 10 to 30% trichloroacetic acid peels, salicylic acid peels, and microdermabrasion. The mechanism of action is different for each peel type. The more common α-hydroxy acid peels are glycolic acid and lactic acid peels. These peels produce a keratinocyte dyscohesion that promotes the shedding of the stratum corneum and thickening of the epidermis as a whole.[2] Additionally, α-hydroxy acid can promote collagen synthesis in the dermis, causing a thickening of the dermis as well. Glycolic acid peels vary based on concentration, 20 to 70%, and pH, buffered and unbuffered. The lower the pH the more epidermal and dermal impact.[3]

Salicylic acid peels, also known as β-hydroxy acid peels or β peels, are safely used in two concentrations, 20% and 30%. This peel functions by breaking the intercellular lipid bonds that encompass the stratum corneum.[3] As will be discussed salicylic acid administered in high concentrations is to be avoided because it can result in salicylism. This also applies to Jessner's solution, because one of its key ingredients is salicylic acid.

Jessner's solution has three different components: resorcinol, lactic acid, and salicylic acid (**Table 9.1**). The modified Jessner's solution is our preference for all patients because there are occasional patients with resorcinol sensitivity. Additionally, the resorcinol can cause postinflammatory hyperpigmentation in this patient population.[4] Alpha hydroxy acids and β-hydroxy acids affect corneocyte adhesion.[4] Epidermolysis results when there is a complete detachment of the keratinocytes. From a clinical standpoint, this appears as a graying of the skin that progresses to vesiculation. Several days after the peel, these areas can appear as darkened eschar. Improperly managed, this can result in postinflammatory hyperpigmentation as well.

The mode of action of trichloroacetic acid is precipitation of epidermal proteins and resultant sloughing of the skin.[3] As the concentration of the solution increases, the depth of penetration and potential for complications increase dramatically.

Microdermabrasion is a mechanical exfoliation of the skin that typically affects the stratum corneum. There exists the ability to penetrate to the level of the papillary dermis, which is ill advised in this patient population.

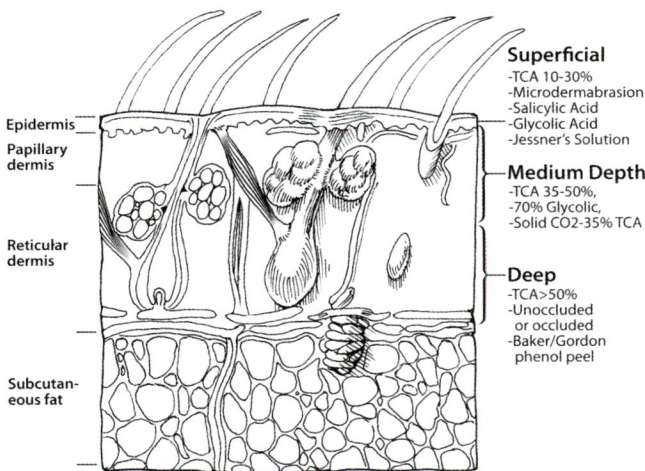

Fig. 9.1 Layers of the skin, with the focus on the epidermis for superficial chemical peels and microdermabrasion.

Table 9.1 Jessner's and Modified Jessner's formulations

Jessner's Solution	Modified Jessner's Solution
Salicylic acid, 14%	Salicylic acid, 14%
Resorcinol, 14%	Citric acid, 8%
Lactic acid	Lactic acid, 17%
Ethanol solution	Ethanol solution

Source: Grimes PE. Aesthetics and cosmetic surgery for darker skin types. Philadelphia: Wolter Kluwer/Lippincott Williams & Wilkins, 2008.

■ Pertinent Anatomy

An understanding of the anatomy of the skin is paramount to using skin treatments in a safe manner. The skin can be thought of as a layered structure. Starting with the outermost layer of the epidermis, the stratum corneum is the horny outside layer. This is the skin that sheds with very superficial skin treatments.

The epidermis is composed of four other layers, with the lowest layer being the basal layer. The melanocytes are present within the basal layer. Keratinocytes found in the basal layer connect the dermis and the epidermis. Within the dermis are blood vessels and collagen. Therefore, when performing microdermabrasion or any other resurfacing procedure, the onset of pinpoint bleeding signifies penetration into the dermal layer of the skin.

The melanocytes produce melanin. Although we all have the same number of melanocytes, the amount of melanin in the skin determines the phenotypic appearance of the skin. Patients with more melanosomes, housed in keratinocytes, produce melanin that appears darker. Furthermore, the melanocytes in those of the higher Fitzpatrick skin types are more labile and produce exaggerated amounts of melanin in response to a stimulus.[3] This accounts for the increased incidence of melasma and postinflammatory hyperpigmentation in these patients.

Encouraging the skin to turn over skin cells will help to reduce the amount of excess melanin in the skin. Mechanical or chemical exfoliation hastens the normal process of cellular turnover, helping patients realize their goals sooner. The addition of a home skin care regimen that targets the reduction of melanin production with the use of products that enhance exfoliation further accelerates the process.

■ Patient Selection

Almost any patient is a candidate for a chemical peel or microdermabrasion. The strength of the peel or aggressiveness of the microdermabrasion treatment is the decision that needs to be made. Additionally, certain categories of peels are more appropriate for particular skin conditions.

Glycolic acid peels are commonly used peels that will enhance exfoliation without significant peeling. This α-hydroxy acid in a strength of 30% is appropriate for almost all skin types but still must be monitored closely for early neutralization in patients who are more sensitive to peels. These peels will also improve hyperpigmentation and fine lines. Buffered glycolic acid peels produce less inflammation, less

tingling, and less peeling. Unbuffered solutions with a low pH tend to produce more exfoliation. Salicylic acid peels are the go-to peel for patients who are bothered by acne vulgaris. They also improve areas of hyperpigmentation, so are ideal for patients of color with postinflammatory hyperpigmentation due to acne. Modified Jessner's peels are preferred over the traditional Jessner's peel due to the replacement of the resorcinol with citric acid or other more universally tolerated compound. The modified Jessner's peel is helpful for patients with acne, dyschromias, enlarged pores, and textural concerns. Microdermabrasion is appropriate for the patient who has acne, textural concerns, and acne scars. Almost any patient can undergo microdermabrasion, though it is not recommended for patients with significant telangiectasias or pustular acne.

Patient selection also involves asking about medical history. Isotretinoin usage in the past year, salicylic acid or aspirin allergy, or known resorcinol sensitivity should be elucidated in addition to the usual questioning to obtain the history. Prior to the first chemical peel or microdermabrasion, patients are given a consent form to read and a printed periprocedural care form to take home and read. The periprocedural form is reviewed with patients before the procedure to ensure that they understand the required postprocedural care. The form also confirms that they have not been on isotretinoin in the past year.

■ Technical Aspects of the Procedures

The technical aspects of glycolic acid peels, Jessner's and modified Jessner's peels, salicylic acid peels, and microdermabrasion are variable based on the treatment. The overarching theme in treating patients of color is conservatism. Avoid being overly aggressive. It is better to do a series of lighter, safer treatments than it is to do one aggressive treatment. A home skin care regimen often enhances the cosmetic result.

Skin preparation is necessary prior to all skin treatments and begins with a thorough cleansing of the skin. In most instances, we use a glycolic acid cleanser with water to cleanse the entire face. In Fitzpatrick IV patients, we use a mechanical cleansing brush to enhance the peel application. In Fitzpatrick V and VI patients, this may deepen the peel to an undesired level. Next, the skin is wiped clean with water-soaked gauze and then patted dry with more gauze. Subsequently, the skin is degreased with alcohol on gauze or a cotton ball and allowed to dry. At this point, the skin is ready to proceed to the chemical peel or microdermabrasion of choice.

Glycolic Acid Peel

Glycolic acid chemical peels are the workhorse peel for many patients. They are in the family of α-hydroxy acid peels, which also include lactic acid. For Fitzpatrick V and VI patients, 30% and 40% glycolic acid peel concentrations are effective without increased risk of complications. For Fitzpatrick IV patients, a 50% glycolic acid peel concentration is the maximum strength; peels are always used in a stepwise manner. However, for some Fitzpatrick IV patients who experience a significant amount of tingling or even a gray patch, epidermolysis, with the administration of the 40% peel, a 50% peel is not recommended.

In preparation for the peel, the neutralizer and timer should be made readily available. The timer should be set for 5 minutes just prior to application of the peel. This is the maximum time that the peel will stay on the skin. Apply the peel solution in a nonoverlapping manner with uniform pressure to the skin. The solution can be obtained from a bottle or premade peel pads. The gauze or pad should not be dripping wet so as to avoid pooling in areas of dependency or running away from the intended area of application. This should be done as efficiently as possible so that the entire face has a relatively similar exposure period. The skin is monitored for markedly increased erythema and gray areas that signify epidermolysis.

Peel neutralization occurs based on symptoms of marked tingling/burning, areas of excessive erythema, or when the timer has reached 5 minutes. The peel is neutralized with a base solution, typically of sodium bicarbonate, prepared in advance so that it is ready and available prior to the application of the peel. The base solution is applied to the area to which the peel was first applied or the area that is burning the most. The solution typically foams when sprayed or applied with solution-soaked gauze to the skin; it will feel slightly warm to the patient due to the exothermic reaction. The foaming and warmth subside when the peel has been neutralized. After complete neutralization, water-moistened gauzes can be placed on the skin for a soothing effect. The skin is observed for any issues or concerns. Antioxidant and sun protection factor creams are applied prior to departure. Questions regarding any of the written post-peel instructions are answered at this point.

Salicylic Acid Peel

Salicylic acid peels are most commonly produced in 20% and 30% concentrations. For the patient who has never experienced a peel, it is best to start with the 20% salicylic acid peel and advance to the 30% peel if the 20% was well tolerated. For darker skin types, Fitzpatrick V and VI, skin preparation with hydroqui-none and an exfoliant, such as tretinoin or glycolic acid, for several weeks prior to the peel helps with the outcome through downregulation of melanin production and prevents postinflammatory hyperpigmentation due to excessive inflammation after the peel. If patients are using these products, they should cease approximately a week prior to the peel. Additionally, patients should be asked about aspirin or salicylate allergy prior to the peel.

After the skin is cleansed and degreased, it is allowed to dry. A petrolatum ointment can be applied to areas where the peel should not be placed: oral commissures, alar groove, and lips. The peel solution should be applied in nonoverlapping strokes on the facial skin with a 2 × 2 gauze or prepackaged peel pads. A white precipitate forms over the skin, during which time moderate stinging and burning of the skin occurs. Fanning the skin during this period improves tolerability of the treatment. The peel is left on the skin for 5 minutes and is self-neutralizing. For tolerant patients, a second coat can be applied in areas of more concern.

At the completion of the peel, water can be applied to the face with moist gauze to soothe the skin and remove the precipitate. At this point, the skin may feel tight, and a light emollient is applied to the skin. The patient is given written instructions on skin care. Of note with salicylic acid peels, the peel solution should be limited to a relatively small surface area of the body, that is, no more than the face and neck in one sitting. This helps avoid such complications as salicylism, discussed later in this chapter.

Jessner's Peel

Jessner's peels are very effective at exfoliation. They are layered on the skin with one to several coats until the desired end point is reached. The modified Jessner's solution is the author's preferred formulation because it does not contain resorcinol. Some patients experience an intense burning sensation when the resorcinol formulation is applied. If one is using the traditional Jessner's peel, a patch test can be done prior to application to the entire face, or the resorcinol-free formulation can be used instead.

After the skin preparation, the skin is allowed to dry, and the peel solution is applied to the face in nonoverlapping strokes using a moist 2 × 2 gauze. Firm pressure is used during the application. After application, a burning or stinging sensation is noticed. During this period of time, the skin is noted to be faintly erythematous, and a white precipitate of the peel solution may form in places. Five to six minutes should pass before considering application of subsequent coats. Areas of the face that have thickened or oily skin are noted to have very little change in the appearance of the skin.

A second coat is appropriate for most patients if the first coat was tolerated. With successive coats, the degree of erythema and the amount of precipitate increases. Typically, no more than two coats are applied to Fitzpatrick skin types V and VI, and three coats to Fitzpatrick IV. Although the patient may appear to tolerate the peel and want to have a higher degree of exfoliation, applying more coats will increase the erythema and edema, thereby potentially increasing the risk of postinflammatory hyperpigmentation.

Trichloroacetic Acid Peel

Trichloroacetic acid peels can be of superficial or medium depth. The superficial peels, ranging from 10 to 30%, produce a superficial wounding of the skin. Medium-depth peels range from 35 to 50% in concentration and can reach the upper reticular dermis. For Fitzpatrick skin types IV, V, and VI, trichloroacetic acid peels should be used with extreme caution due to the increase in complications with increasing concentration. A 20% peel can be used in the compliant patient without complications. The patient must agree to strictly follow the postpeel instructions to achieve the desired outcome. When treating at concentrations of 20% or higher, one must use prophylaxis against viral and bacterial infections due to the deeper penetration of the peel. Additionally, preparation with lightening agents, exfoliants, and sun protection readies the skin for the treatment.

With regard to application of the superficial trichloroacetic acid peels, there is less intensity in the peel itself, and injury can occur down to the level of the basal layer with concentrations up to 30%. In the Fitzpatrick IV patient, a 25 to 30% peel may be appropriate. For the Fitzpatrick V patient, a 20% peel is best. The Fitzpatrick VI patient should stay with the very superficial peels in the 6 to 10% concentrations. Higher concentrations are not recommended for Fitzpatrick VI or noncompliant patients due to the potential for poor recovery.

The peel is applied after cleansing and degreasing the skin. The peel, in concentrations of 15 and 20%, can be administered segmentally in the facial subunits, allowing the intensity of the burning to crescendo and decrescendo prior to application to the next subunit. A light frost, which is precipitated protein from the skin, should be evenly distributed across the skin. The peel application usually takes no more than 20 minutes to perform and depends on patient tolerance. Patients who have undergone a series of superficial peels prior to this peel application yield more even frosting and results.

For the 20% peel, heavy- to medium-weight emollients are applied postpeel for 4 to 5 days to allow for controlled exfoliation of the skin. Patients are instructed to stay away from the sun and to wash their face two to three times per day. During cleansing, the focus is not to remove all of the emollient or scrub off flaking skin. Once the skin has completed the exfoliative process, patients should continue using a bland cleanser and sun protection for several weeks prior to resuming their prepeel skin care regimen.

Microdermabrasion

Microdermabrasion provides a gentle exfoliation of the skin with use of either a wand with a diamond fraise or a machine that uses crystals for abrasion. Both types of machines have the ability to adjust the vacuum pressure with which the treatment is performed. The author, having owned both an aluminum oxide crystal machine and a crystal-free system, prefers the crystal-free system based on the lack of crystal mess and perceived improved results.

With use of a crystal-free machine, the skin is cleansed, and the appropriate wand is chosen based on the skin type. The medium wand is preferred for most patients. The coarse wand is reserved for patients with coarse rhytids, typically not patients in the Fitzpatrick IV through VI categories. The fine wand is recommended for sensitive skin types. The suction on the machine is set to an average setting, approximately –15 mm Hg.

The skin of the cheek is grasped with the thumb and forefinger to spread the skin and keep the skin taut during the treatment. The wand is applied to the skin between the fingers, dragged across the skin, and lifted at the end of the stroke. The patient is questioned regarding comfort level, and necessary adjustments are made before proceeding. Parallel strokes are made across the skin, covering one subunit of the face at a time. The treatment progresses around the face, treating areas that are supported by bone—cheeks, chin, upper lip, and forehead. Perpendicular strokes are then made in all of the previously treated areas, with a third pass made using random circular strokes. When treating the lip area, the lips are brought together in the fashion that a woman uses to blot her lipstick to put tension on the treated skin. Microdermabrasion is not performed on the skin of the eyelids. The entire treatment should take anywhere from 20 to 30 minutes. After the treatment, the skin is cooled with water-moistened gauzes. Antioxidant and sunscreen are applied.

Combination Peels

Several companies have designed effective yet safe peel combination treatments. By combining the aforementioned peeling agents, peels are designed to affect the skin in several different ways in one sitting without causing undue irritation. These peel combinations are used after the patients have undergone a "test" peel with 30% glycolic acid. If the peel was tolerated well during application and there were no untoward sequelae, then more targeted peels are utilized. Subsequent to these combination peels, every patient goes home with written directions and a postpeel kit designed by the company that produces the peels. Within the kit are a bland cleanser, balms, emollients, and hydrocortisone to effect optimal healing.

Three effective formulations are an enhanced Jessner's peel with hydroquinone, a 20% L-lactic acid and 10% trichloroacetic acid combination, and a 20% L-lactic acid and 6% trichloroacetic acid formulation. These formulations are produced by Physician's Choice of Arizona and have been very helpful in improving hyperpigmentation in these patient populations. Many companies that have derived their own formulations that may work just as well. Using the enhanced Jessner's peel followed by the 20% lactic acid/10% trichloroacetic acid has helped the most with lentigines and postinflammatory hyperpigmentation.

Postoperative Care

All patients are given written instructions detailing exactly what they should be doing postprocedure. There are a few rules that all patients must abide by, including avoiding sun exposure for the next week and wearing sunscreen at all times. This prevents the appearance of postinflammatory hyperpigmentation, to which this patient population is highly susceptible. Additionally, for the next 3 to 4 days, patients should avoid exercise, sweating, and shower spray directly on the face. Exercise can cause moderate erythema and inflammation of the skin, which increases the chance of postinflammatory hyperpigmentation. Patients should also avoid picking or rubbing the peeling skin on the face, as well as any unnecessary touching of the face. Patients are also encouraged to sleep on their back for the first several days to avoid accidental irritation to the flaking skin.

For skin care, patients are asked to wash their face with a mild cleanser that contains no active ingredients. After the skin is cleansed with lukewarm water and the desired cleanser, the skin is patted dry without rubbing, and a moisturizer is applied to the skin twice daily. Sunscreen should be applied in the morning after moisturizing. Moisturizer should be applied liberally between washings if the skin is flaky or peeling. As previously stated, some of the chemical peel systems have postpeel kits with several products that can be used in the 3 to 4 days after the peel. This ensures that patients are using products designed to enhance the results. Treatments can be spaced 2 to 4 weeks apart.

Home Skin Care

Determining the proper home skin care regimen depends on the age of the patient, the condition being treated, and the patient's willingness to comply with the regimen. The condition being treated dictates the recommended skin care products, and the products are typically recommended in a sequential approach (**Table 9.2**). The product choices in the table are offered sequentially from left to right. For instance, if the patient is hesitant to use any products, a sunscreen only is recommended, as many patients of color do not feel that they need protection from the sun.[5] If they will tolerate using two products, then an exfoliant is added in the form of an α-hydroxy acid cleanser. This approach is also beneficial in the patient with known sensitive skin. Adding products one at a time, separated by a period of 4 weeks, helps to elucidate what the skin will tolerate.

The table is helpful for most patients concerned with rejuvenation. However, patients with acne vulgaris will often need more intensive treatment with antimicrobials, topically or orally. The use of skin care products in combination with the prescribed skin treatments, chemical peels, or microdermabrasion will facilitate improved results.

Expected Results

Results can be variable in patients of color desiring rejuvenation of the skin. As discussed, rejuvenation generally involves improvement in the texture and tone of the skin. Treatment with dermal fillers and neurotoxins greatly enhances the outcomes. Administering treatments that can enhance the skin reduce the signs of aging.

Table 9.2 Skin care regimen for common skin conditions in Fitzpatrick skin types IV, V, and VI

Condition	Skin Care Options
Dyschromia	Sunscreen + exfoliant + lightening agent + antioxidant
Photodamage	Sunscreen + collagen stimulant + exfoliant + lightering agent + antioxidant
Acne	Tretinoin/Tazorac + α-hydroxy acid cleanser + spot treatment (salicylic acid) ± skin lightening agent + sunscreen

Source: Data from Fitzpatrick TB. The validity and practicality of sun-reactive skin types I through VI. Arch Dermatol 1988;124(6):869–871.
[a]Allergan, Irvine, CA.

Generally, we approach patients in a stepwise fashion. Prior to embarking on a treatment plan with chemical peels and microdermabrasion, the patients are started on a skin care regimen that targets their primary problems. For most, there is some component of dyschromia involved. Typically, the patients are started on a regimen of an exfoliant, a skin lightener, and UVA and UVB sun protection. Although there are many exfoliants available, we have had great success with glycolic acid cleansers, retinols, and tretinoin. The decision as to which product the patient uses is based on patient history of reaction to other products. If the patient is able to tolerate tretinoin, it is generally the first choice. Additionally, there is a wide variety of skin lighteners. Products such as kojic acid, azelaic acid, glycolic acid, and antioxidants are popular choices. Frequently, these are not as powerful as hydroquinone, which is typically used at the 4% level. The sun protection should be used on a daily basis so as to prevent further darkening of the inflamed areas. Furthermore, tretinoin, antioxidants, and glycolic acid are indicated for treatment of the general signs of aging.

The effects of using a skin care regimen alone to improve dyschromia are illustrated in the first patient (**Fig. 9.2a,b**). This patient is of Asian descent and has lentigines and telangiectasias on her cheeks. She is shown after 16 weeks of using an α-hydroxy acid cleanser, 4% hydroquinone, phytic acid cream, and UVA and UVB sun protection (**Fig. 9.2c,d**). Note that, although some dyschromia remains, the darkness of the lentigines is greatly improved. However, there is no improvement in the telangiectasias.

The next patient, an African American woman in her mid-forties, desired improvement in her overall appearance. She wanted to look younger and have a more even skin texture and tone. On examination, she was noted to have diffuse signs of mild photodamage with hyperpigmentation of her facial skin in comparison to her neck (**Fig. 9.3a,b**). She began a skin care regimen that incorporated a glycolic acid cleanser, 4% hydroquinone, and sunscreen with UVA and UVB protection, and she underwent a series of 30 and 40% glycolic acid peels. She is shown after a series of six chemical peels (**Fig. 9.3c,d**) with skin that is improved in texture and tone similar to the skin of her neck. Additionally, she underwent injection with hyaluronic acid filler in the nasolabial folds and marionette folds to soften the look in this area.

This patient is of East Indian descent, with obvious signs of photodamage manifest by diffuse hyperpigmentation of her face (**Fig. 9.4a,b**). In comparison to her neck skin, there was significant darkening of the skin. Additionally, she was plagued by acne and consequential postinflammatory hyperpigmentation. She is shown after treatment with a series of six alternating microdermabrasion and combination chemical peels. The peels consisted of a modified Jessner's peel with hydroquinone followed by a 20% L-lactic acid/10% trichloroacetic acid peel. She had improvement in her overall skin tone but was still bothered by occasional acne and postinflammatory hyperpigmentation (**Fig. 9.4c,d**).

The next patient is of Asian descent and had numerous lentigines of the cheek skin on both sides (**Fig. 9.5a,b**). She was placed on a skin care regi-

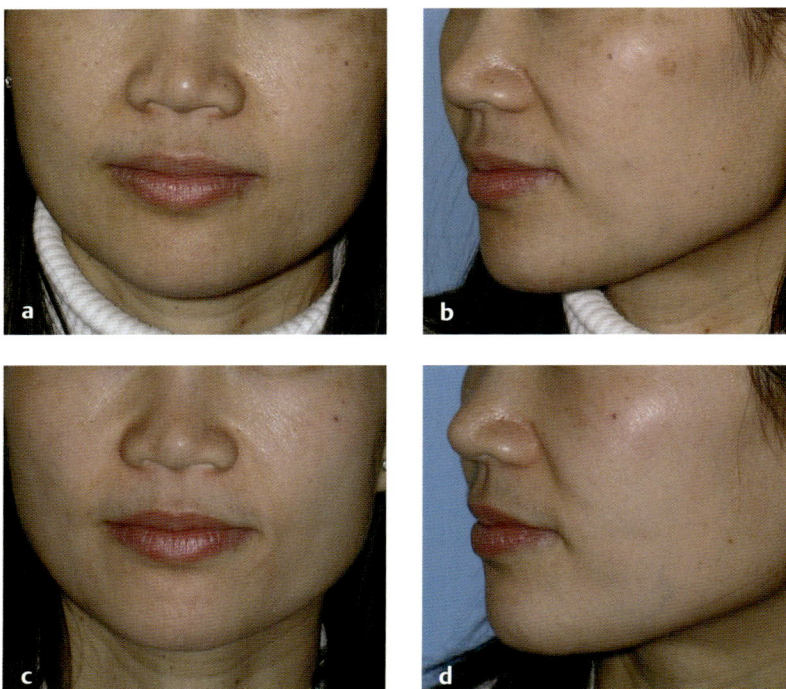

Fig. 9.2 Asian woman with signs of photodamage manifest by lentigines and telangiectasias **(a,b)**. She is shown after using a home skin care regimen alone **(c,d)**. Typical results show improvement without complete eradication of the problem.

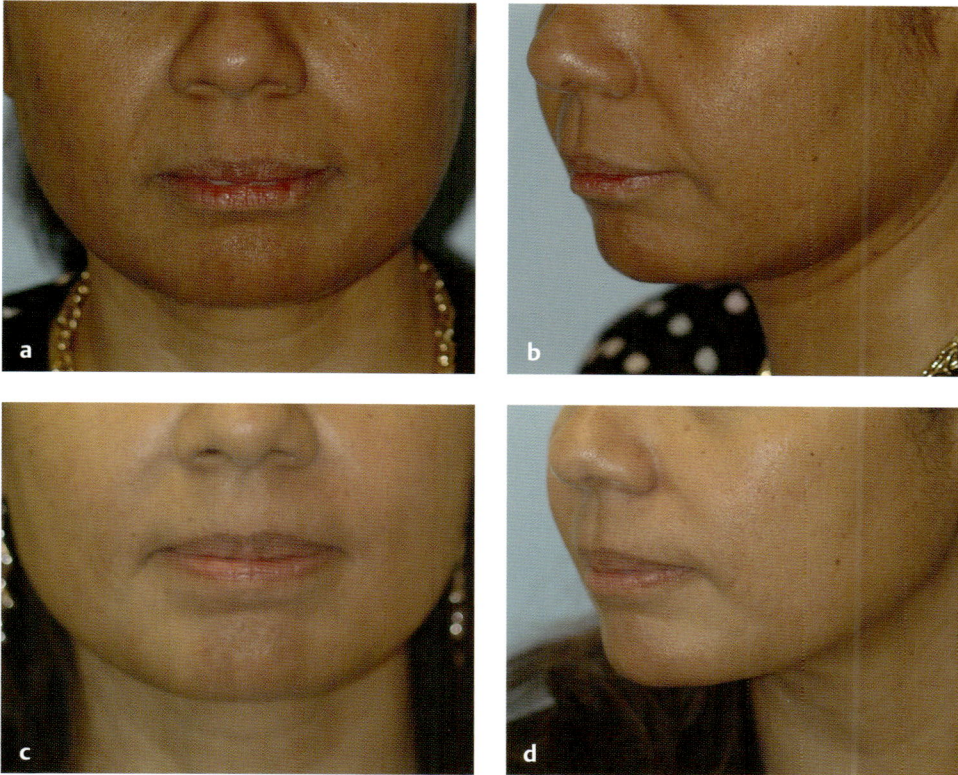

Fig. 9.3 African American woman with mild photodamage manifest by diffuse hyperpigmentation; facial skin is much darker than neck skin (a,b). After using a home skin care regimen and undergoing a series of monthly glycolic acid peels (c,c).

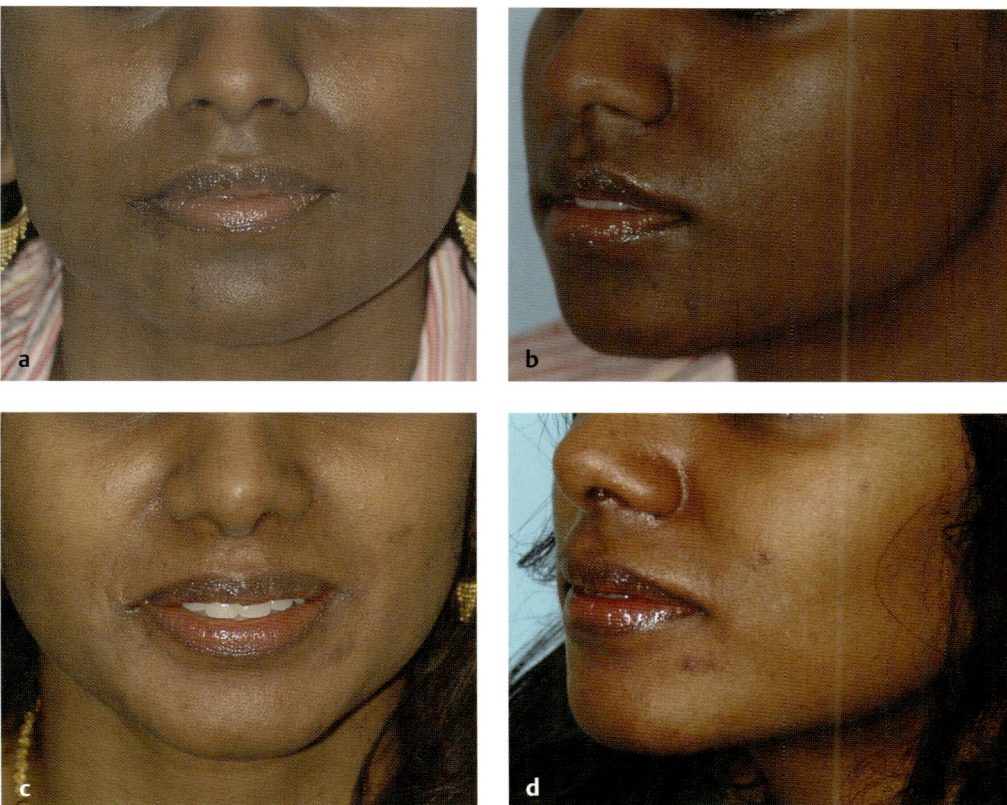

Fig. 9.4 Skin with diffuse hyperpigmentation as well as areas of postinflammatory hyperpigmentation (a,b). After home skin care and a series of modified Jessner's peels with hydroquinone (c,d).

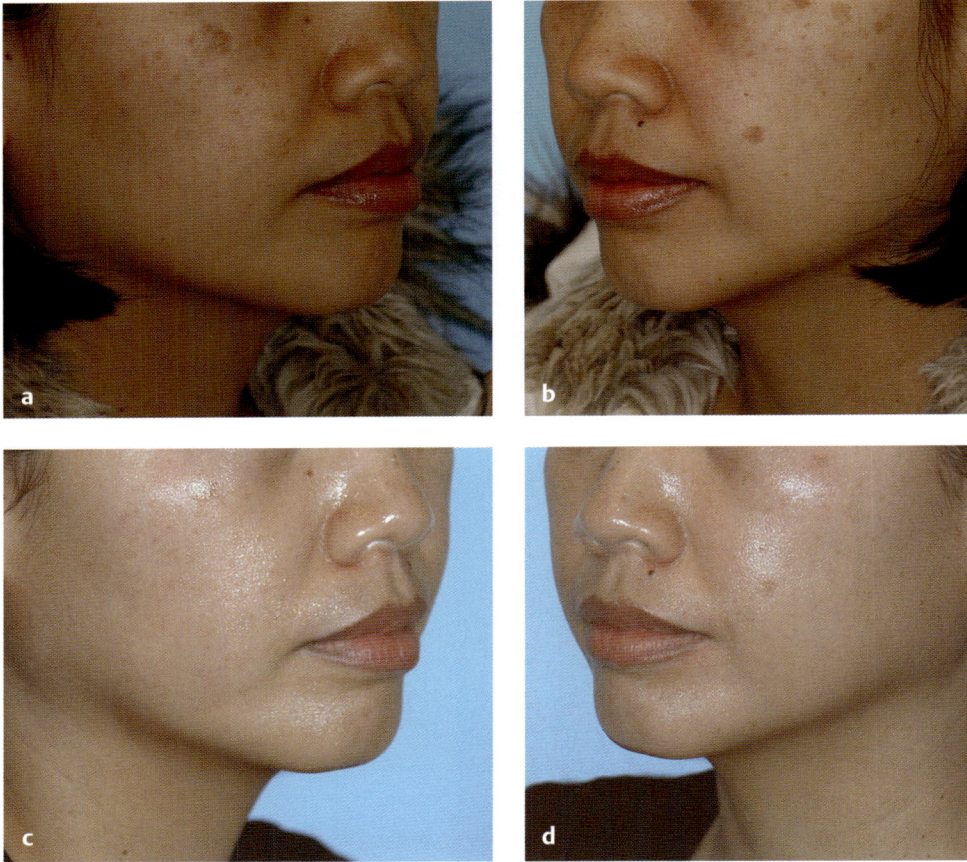

Fig. 9.5 Photodamage manifest by lentigines and telangiectasias (a,b). After home skin care and a series of six monthly modified Jessner's peels with hydroquinone (c,d).

men based on the usage of hydroquinone, tretinoin, α-hydroxy acids, and sunscreen. She is shown 6 months later after a series of six same-combination chemical peels (**Fig. 9.5c,d**). Ironically, the patient perceived no change in her skin until she was shown the before pictures.

The last illustration is of an African American woman who presented with postinflammatory hyperpigmentation that resulted after using a mud mask at home immediately after a microdermabrasion treatment elsewhere (**Fig. 9.6a**). She was placed on a regimen of 4% hydroquinone, glycolic acid cleanser, and sunscreen in addition to undergoing a series of alternating microdermabrasion and chemical peel treatments. At the conclusion of this series, she continued to have prominent hyperpigmentation surrounding her chin region (**Fig. 9.6b**). She subsequently underwent a 20% trichloroacetic acid peel and had tremendous improvement in her skin (**Fig. 9.6c**).

■ Complications and Their Management

Postinflammatory Hyperpigmentation

Postinflammatory hyperpigmentation is one of the more common complications after superficial chemical peels and microdermabrasion. This can be caused by several factors, including pooling of the peel solution, peeling too harshly for the skin type, overlapping the peel, aggressive pre- or postpeel care, and excessive sun exposure in the immediate postpeel period. Pooling of the peel in troughs and overlapping of the peel are easily avoided by paying careful attention to the application of the peel and avoiding overly wet gauze. Patients who have been using tretinoin or started on a more aggressive skin care regimen during the middle of a series of peels

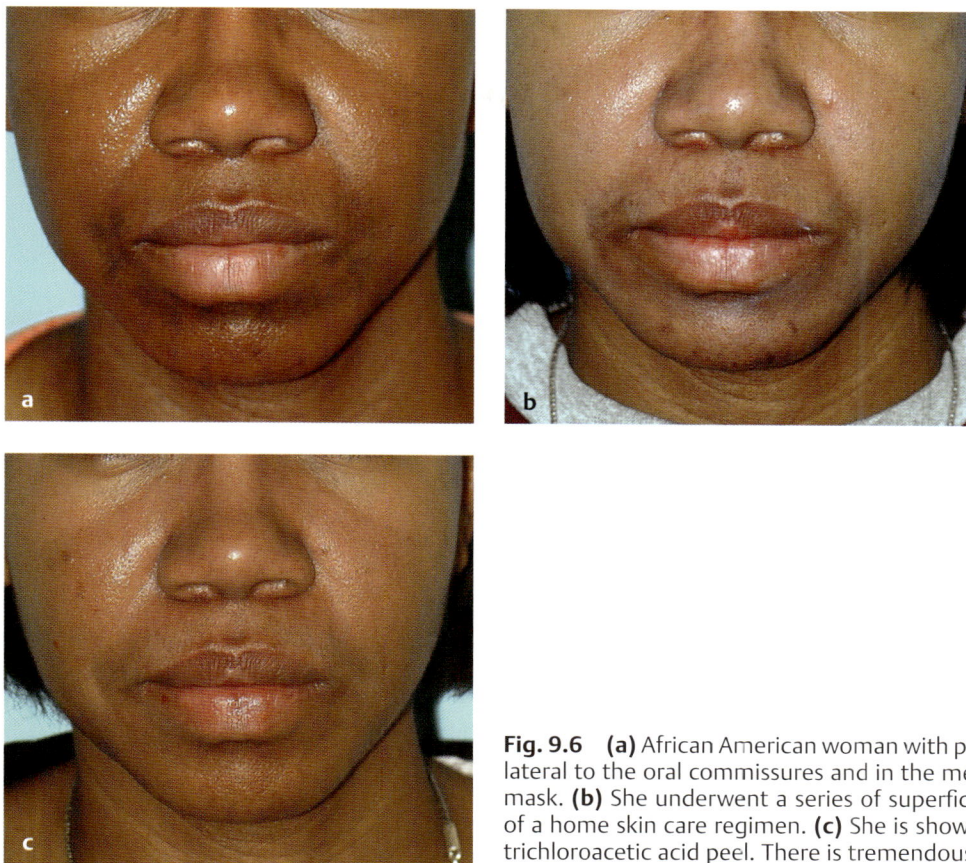

Fig. 9.6 **(a)** African American woman with postinflammatory hyperpigmentation lateral to the oral commissures and in the mental crease after using a home mud mask. **(b)** She underwent a series of superficial chemical peels in addition to use of a home skin care regimen. **(c)** She is shown after ultimately undergoing a 10% trichloroacetic acid peel. There is tremendous improvement in her dyschromia.

or microdermabrasion should probably take a step back in the concentration of the peel because these changes will increase the depth of the peel.

In the instance that the patient experiences an area of increased inflammation or erythema postpeel, the first line of defense consists of a mild steroid cream applied for a few days along with emollients and sunscreen. Should hyperpigmentation appear, the triad of a skin lightener, exfoliant, and sunscreen can usually resolve the hyperpigmentation over time. This trio of products should be instituted once the skin inflammation has subsided.

Hypopigmentation

This is a rare finding after superficial chemical peels because the level of wounding is usually limited to the epidermis. Trichloroacetic acid peels of higher strength can produce areas of hypopigmentation in patients who try to aggressively scrub the dead skin off of the surface of the skin. From a treatment standpoint, it is best to prevent such an occurrence by encouraging strict adherence to the postpeel instructions. Additionally, limiting excessive inflammation in the postpeel period can reduce the chances of such an occurrence.

Salicylism

Salicylism can become a problem when salicylic acid is administered in high doses. Application of either the salicylic acid peel, Jessner's peel, or any peel containing salicylic acid to large surface areas at one time (e.g., face, back, neck, and chest) can result in toxicity. The toxicity is manifest by tachypnea, tinnitus, dizziness, abdominal cramps, hearing loss, and central nervous system disturbances. This should be avoided by limiting the surface area treated in one day to 20% or less. If symptoms occur, the patient should be admitted to the hospital immediately and treated.

Resorcinol

Resorcinol toxicity is a possibility when the medication is used in high concentrations of 40% or more.[2] Allergic reactions can occur, and some patients develop a marked burning sensation and erythema when it is applied. Avoidance of products that use this ingredient alleviates this problem.

■ Conclusion

Skin rejuvenation of the Fitzpatrick IV through VI patient targets improvement of the skin tone and texture. A combination of superficial chemical peels and microdermabrasion is enough to improve hyperpigmentation and fine rhytids. Adjunctive procedures using injectables such as dermal fillers and neurotoxins address the gravitational aspects of the aging process. A conservative stepwise approach will help prevent complications. Avoid succumbing to the desires of patients who insist their skin is tough and can take more than usual. A home skin care regimen that uses an exfoliant, a skin lightener, and UVA and UVB sun protection on a daily basis helps lessen the degree of hyperpigmentation. The skin care procedures exfoliate, increasing the speed at which the skin cells turn over. Because the population of patients in these Fitzpatrick groups is predicted to increase, all physicians will need to become savvy about treating these skin types in a safe manner.

References

1. Mangat DS, Garlich PH. Advances in chemical peels: modified phenol-croton oil medium depth peels. In: Thomas JR, ed. Advanced Therapy in Facial Plastic and Reconstructive Surgery. Shelton, CT: People's Medical Publishing House; 2010:561–572
2. Rubin M. Manual of Chemical Peels: Superficial and Medium Depth. Philadelphia, PA: Lippincott, Williams & Wilkins; 1995
3. Grimes PE. Aesthetics and Cosmetic Surgery for Darker Skin Types. Philadelphia, PA: Wolters Kluwer/Lippincott Williams & Wilkins; 2008
4. Baumann L. Cosmetic Dermatology: Principles and Practice. McGraw-Hill; 2009
5. Leverette K, Moore YL. Skin care for patients of color. In: Matory WE, ed. Ethnic Considerations in Facial Aesthetic Surgery. Philadelphia, PA: Lippincott-Raven; 1998

10 Intense Pulsed Light (with and without Photodynamic Therapy)

J. Randall Jordan

Key Concepts

- Intense pulsed light (IPL) is similar in clinical effect to a variety of medical lasers.

- IPL can be used to treat a wide variety of skin conditions.

- IPL can be used for photodynamic therapy (PDT).

- The combination of IPL and PDT may provide enhanced results for some conditions.

■ Introduction

Goldman and Eckhouse first described intense pulsed light (IPL) for use in medical therapy in 1990.[1] Since that time, IPL has undergone multiple transformations to become the technology used commonly today. IPL devices use a xenon flashlamp to generate an intense polychromatic pulse of light energy in the spectrum of 400 to 1,300 nm. This polychromatic light can then be passed through various cutoff filters to eliminate undesired portions of the spectrum, yielding a band of wavelengths for clinical use. The concept of selective photothermolysis, as proposed by Anderson and Parrish,[2] states that a target tissue has a particular absorption curve, and that this curve can be exploited to cause thermal damage of the target tissue without damaging surrounding tissues. This concept was originally proposed for laser tissue interactions, but it is also applicable to IPL.

The major difference in the two technologies is that laser light energy is monochromatic (1 wavelength, such as 1,064 nm) versus polychromatic (such as 480 to 550 nm) for IPL. Tissue absorption curves are not monochromatic, and nature has no requirement for light to be monochromatic for biological interaction. There are advantages and disadvantages to the use of polychromatic as opposed to monochromatic light. Monochromatic light will more accurately target a limited part of the tissue chromophore's spectrum and may be less likely to cause collateral damage and hence side effects. However, polychromatic light can be used to treat a wider variety of skin conditions with a single device. IPL has been used successfully to treat several different skin conditions and lesions.[3] This chapter focuses on the common applications of this technology in a facial plastic surgery practice.

Photodynamic therapy (PDT) is a group of therapies utilizing certain chemicals that are taken up by living cells and can then undergo molecular alteration when exposed to light energy, typically transforming them into metabolically active molecules. In its most basic form, PDT consists of any treatment that uses light energy to activate a chemical for medical treatment. Early treatments date back thousands of years to treatments for vitiligo used by the Egyptians.[4] The current commonly used PDT chemical, aminolevulinic acid (ALA), was introduced into clinical practice in 1990 by Kennedy et al.[5] Although ALA PDT has been used for a multitude of clinical problems, it is still not commonly employed in everyday practice. The focus here is on the application of PDT in a facial plastic surgery practice.

■ Patient Selection

The approach to the patient is similar when considering any light-based treatment: correct diagnosis of the condition, assessment of the individual's skin type, and evaluation of potential complicating factors, such as medical conditions. Diagnosis of many lesions is possible by examination and history alone, but a biopsy should be considered for any lesion lacking a clear diagnosis. This is particularly true for pigmented lesions. Medical conditions that would preclude the use of IPL include conditions resulting in photosensitivity, pregnancy, breastfeeding, photosensitizing medications, and current oral retinoids. Relative contraindications include diabetes, coagulopathies, previous problems with IPL or light-based therapy such as pigmentary alterations, implants in the treatment area, and presence of a pacemaker. If the patient has a history of herpes simplex in proximity to the treatment area, antiviral prophylaxis should be considered.

IPL can be used to treat individuals with any Fitzpatrick skin type, but the darker skin types are much more difficult to treat and require particular caution. Tanned patients or patients with a history of postinflammatory hyperpigmentation will also require caution. Test spots are recommended for all patients at the initiation of treatment but are clearly advisable for patients with type II or darker skin. Test spots should be placed in a location with skin color and UV exposure similar to those of the area to be treated. Careful recording of the exact location of each test spot and the associated treatment parameters is mandatory. Assessment should be made of the immediate response to the test spot, and treatment parameters adjusted as necessary and repeated. The test spot(s) are evaluated at 4 to 6 weeks for pigment alterations or lack of effect and treatment parameters selected accordingly, or another series of test spots may be performed.

Once treatment parameters are selected, the areas to be treated are assessed for obstacles, such as hair, tattoos, and pigmented nevi. Hair will need to be shaved, and the patient should be informed that hair growth in the treatment area may be affected by the treatment. This may be problematic in the male beard or scalp in either sex. Hair loss may be permanent but is usually temporary. Nevi or tattoos may be covered with a white, damp, similar-sized piece of paper or cloth.

Pain associated with IPL treatments, while universal, is not typically severe, and if the patient complains of significant pain, one should reassess treatment parameters for overfluence. Some patients are less tolerant of treatments, and topical anesthetic creams may be used. Care should be taken in the application of these so as to avoid any potential for overdose with transcutaneous absorption. There have been several reports of lidocaine toxicity associated with the use of these topical agents in this setting. Cooling the skin with ice, chilled contact gel, or refrigerated air delivery devices such as the Zimmer Chiller (Zimmer Medizinsysteme GmbH, Ulm, GE) can also be helpful. Most devices have an integrated cooling tip that can be adjusted to the desired temperature.

After the treatment is complete, patients must avoid UV exposure for 4 weeks. Most patients will require more than one treatment, and this is discussed before treatment is started. For lentigines and photodamage, one or two treatments are typically sufficient, whereas vascular lesions will often require five or more treatment sessions. Hair removal will require more than five in almost all patients and many more in darker-skinned individuals. Typically, a minimum of 4 weeks between treatments is recommended, and in the case of hair removal, after the initial series of three or four monthly treatments, it is recommended to wait 2 to 3 months between treatments.

In selecting patients for PDT, all of the same considerations for IPL also apply to PDT, with a few additional ones. In general, PDT is most effective for photodamage and lentigines in patients with Fitzpatrick type I and II skin. Contraindications to PDT are disorders that cause increased photosensitivity, porphyria, and the patient's current use of photosensitizing medications. PDT is also contraindicated in patients who cannot comply with UV avoidance for 48 hours after therapy. The discomfort associated with PDT is mildly greater than that with IPL alone, and the posttreatment sequelae of erythema, edema, and crusting are more pronounced.

Once the decision has been made to use IPL, a thorough discussion and documentation of the risks and benefits must take place. Specific detailed consent forms listing both common and uncommon posttreatment problems are helpful. The discussion should include both the expected posttreatment course of erythema and mild edema as well as the possibility of blistering, crusting, bruising, pigmentary alterations, burns, scars, and possible lack of effectiveness necessitating alternative therapy.

■ Technical Aspect of Procedure

Intense Pulsed Light

IPL devices can treat multiple types of lesions, which makes IPL an attractive first choice for light-based technology for many practitioners. It is challenging to select an IPL unit because there are multiple models available, most of which are stand-alone, but many are part of a multidevice platform that may contain a wide variety of other lasers or laser-like devices. The marketing for medical lasers is designed to convince potential customers that by purchasing a laser (or other device) they will be able to attract new patients to the practice. Unfortunately, this is often overstated. One must carefully appraise the potential clinical uses in one's practice when considering these devices in general. Comparison of all the units available is not readily possible and is a moving target at best because new devices are introduced every year if not more frequently. In general, it is important that the IPL device have adequate ability to generate a stable square-wave pulse at the desired wavelength and fluence. This is dependent on the xenon light source and the capacitor bank that supplies the current for the flash. In other words, the device must be adequately powered to produce a constant current to the flashlamp so that power is not lost during the generation of the entire pulse. This is particularly important when multiple pulses are used back to back in "stacking." Several device manufacturers also couple the light energy with other forms of energy, such as radiofrequency current. Whether or not this is important clinically is still debated.

The xenon light source of each IPL unit will have a designated lifespan that may range from 200,000 to several million pulses. The handpiece or treatment head contains the flashlamp as well as the light guide and cooling system and is susceptible to more wear and tear than other parts of the device. Almost all IPL devices have a sapphire contact crystal and require coupling to the skin with a gel for adequate function. The crystal may break or otherwise become non-functional, so a warranty or service contract should be considered when purchasing a device. One would want to examine the history and stability of the device maker as well as the reputation of the product. Although it may seem financially attractive to purchase a used device, the buyer should beware of the fact that most manufacturers will require the purchase of a service contract to work on used equipment, and this may offset some of the savings in the used device market. It is strongly recommended that several models be used in the office for a trial period before the decision is made to purchase.

The size of the contact crystal and treatment spot is another consideration because a larger surface area will allow the operator to cover more area with fewer pulses. However, too large a contact head may prove difficult to use in tighter spots, such as the upper lip. Larger spot sizes also require more power to deliver the fluences needed. The ability to adjust both wavelength, fluence and pulse width is critical to obtaining maximum effect from an IPL unit. Many units have preset parameters for treating specific conditions and skin types that are helpful for less experienced users, but the ability to adjust the settings is equally important as one gains experience. Many units now allow for "stacking" of pulses, which is the coupling of pulses back to back. Integral cooling of the tip is a common and important feature of almost all machines. Essentially all IPL units require the use of a gel, such as standard ultrasound gel, for optical coupling to the skin. This gel can be prechilled to add additional cooling if desired.

Routine photodocumentation is advisable before, during, and at the completion of a series of treatments. Documentation of Fitzpatrick skin type in the medical record is also essential. It is also wise to document the lack of tanning in the treatment area, as well as the discussion of the importance of UV protection after treatment.

Safety of both the patient and the treating professional is of paramount importance in all light-based therapy. The most easily injured organ is the eye due to the high pigment content, and opaque protective eye shields are used for the patient. Any treatments close to the eye must be very carefully delivered so as not to move the shields. The author believes the best ones for this application are metal, and they can be obtained from multiple vendors and are easily cleaned and reused. Protection of the treating professional's eyes is more difficult. The broad spectrum of IPL requires very dark green lenses for protection. One should only purchase and use lenses labeled for IPL use. These lenses can pose some difficulty in assessing treatment end points and may have to be removed for adequate visualization of the biological response between treatments. There is no readily available solution to this issue.

Pigmented Lesions

IPL can be an effective treatment for superficial pigmented lesions, particularly solar lentigines (**Fig. 10.1a,b**). As mentioned previously, the correct diagnosis is critical in all uses of IPL but particularly so for pigmented lesions. Biopsy should be considered for any lesion if the diagnosis cannot be made with a high degree of certainty. IPL is not effective for melanocytic nevi or seborrheic keratoses. Although there are several reports of the treatment of melasma with IPL,[6] in general IPL is not very effective for treating melasma.

Lentigines, in general, are often a component of photodamaged skin, and in this situation IPL can be a very effective tool for clearing a larger area. For an isolated lentigo, a white piece of paper or plastic with a fenestration similar to the size of the lentigo can be used to shield the surrounding skin and increase the effectiveness of the treatment. Most lentigines will respond to a single treatment episode, and multiple treatments are not usually required. Darker lentigines respond better than lighter ones,[7] and some authors find a Wood's light useful to identify lesions more likely to respond, but with some practice it is not too difficult to identify lentigines that have a high rate of response. With IPL treatment, the typical immediate response for a lentigo is mild erythema and edema with some darkening of the lesion after treatment, progressing to significant darkening over 24 hours ▶ Video 10.1. Treatment parameters vary somewhat between IPL units, but in general a 560 to 590 nm filter is used with pulse duration of 5 to 10 msec and fluence of 30 to 40 J/cm^2. If pulses are to be stacked, a delay of 25 to 40 msec is used. Again, test spots are recommended at several settings before treatment parameters are chosen.

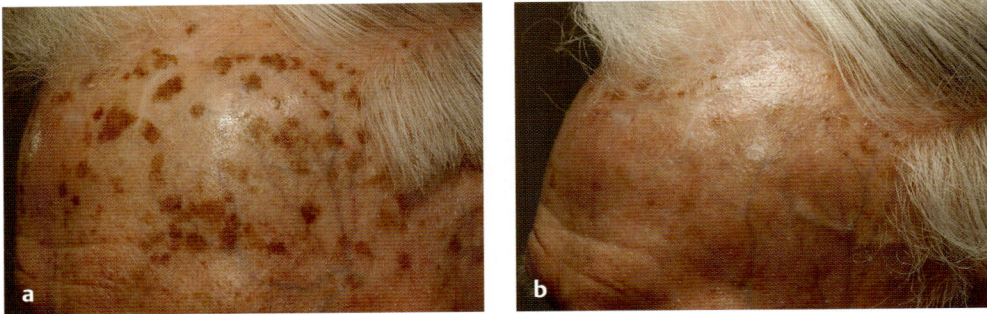

Fig. 10.1 Multiple lentigos of the forehead. **(a)** Before intense pulsed light (IPL) treatment. **(b)** After two IPL treatments.

After delivery of the selected treatment, the coupling gel is removed and the area inspected. A typical response is immediate darkening of the lesion followed by mild erythema and edema at the periphery of the lesion. If this is not noted, the area is re-treated at slightly higher fluence. Once the desired effect is obtained and the treatment is complete, a bland moisturizer with a sunscreen is applied. As mentioned earlier, the treatment is not painless, but it is well tolerated without topical anesthesia by most patients. The use of the cooling tip before delivery of the pulse, and immediately after, can be helpful in increasing comfort levels. If there is significant pain, one should suspect a too-high delivered energy level (overfluence). In this case, if the skin reveals more than mild erythema, immediate cooling should be applied for several minutes. The patient should be instructed to return if there is any evidence of blistering or crusting.

If the lesions revealed the expected response as already described, one can expect the lesion to darken further over 24 hours and begin to flake off at 7 to 10 days, revealing a mild erythema beneath that typically resolves in less than a week. UV precautions are recommended for 30 days after treatment. One can expect recurrence of many of the successfully treated lentigos over time, typically several years. This is somewhat dependent on the individual's skin type and UV exposure, with lighter skin types with more UV exposure faring worse.

Telangiectasia/Vascular Lesions

The treatment of vascular lesions is one of the main indications for IPL. There is very good evidence for the effectiveness of IPL in the treatment of the erythrotelangiectasia of rosacea, port wine stain, essential telangiectasia, angioma, and spider angiomas.[3] Vessel diameters up to 1 mm may be successfully treated with IPL. Larger vessels typically respond better to neodymium:yttrium-aluminum-garnet (Nd:YAG) or PDL devices than to IPL.[8]

The most common vascular lesion treated with IPL in our practice is the erythrotelangiectasia of rosacea. IPL is fairly effective for this, and patients are advised that they can expect a marked decrease in both overall redness as well as flushing (**Fig. 10.2a,b**). Acneiform lesions do not respond as well as erythrotelangiectasia, and these are treated with either topical or oral medications, preferably prior to starting treatment with IPL. Patients are advised that multiple treatments will be required, and the complete clearance of all areas is unlikely. They are also informed that over time there will be some recurrence of the erythrotelangiectasia and that follow-up treatments will likely be necessary. Patients will experience erythema and some transient edema for the first 24 hours after treatments, especially the first several treatments. In general, it is helpful if the patient is somewhat flushed at the time of treatment, and gently rubbing the skin may be useful. Standard photographs are taken before treatment.

Even though almost all patients with rosacea have Fitzpatrick skin types I or II, test spots are still advisable. Typical settings for treatment vary between devices, and one should always consult the manual for the specific device to be used, but in general, a 560 filter with fluences of 18 to 30 J/cm² and a pulse width of 3 to 6 msec are used for this application. Small telangiectasias are treated in a similar fashion to rosacea, but with vessel size > 1 mm or high flow, IPL may not be effective.

Port wine stain has been treated successfully with several different lasers as well as IPL, and some authors have found IPL to be superior.[3] In general, incomplete clearance is expected no matter which device is used. Typically, a 550 filter is used with a fluence of 10 to 20 J/cm² and a pulse width of 8 to 10 msec.

Hair Removal

Hair removal is currently one of the more common uses for IPL technology. Multiple studies have reported the efficacy of IPL as compared with the more

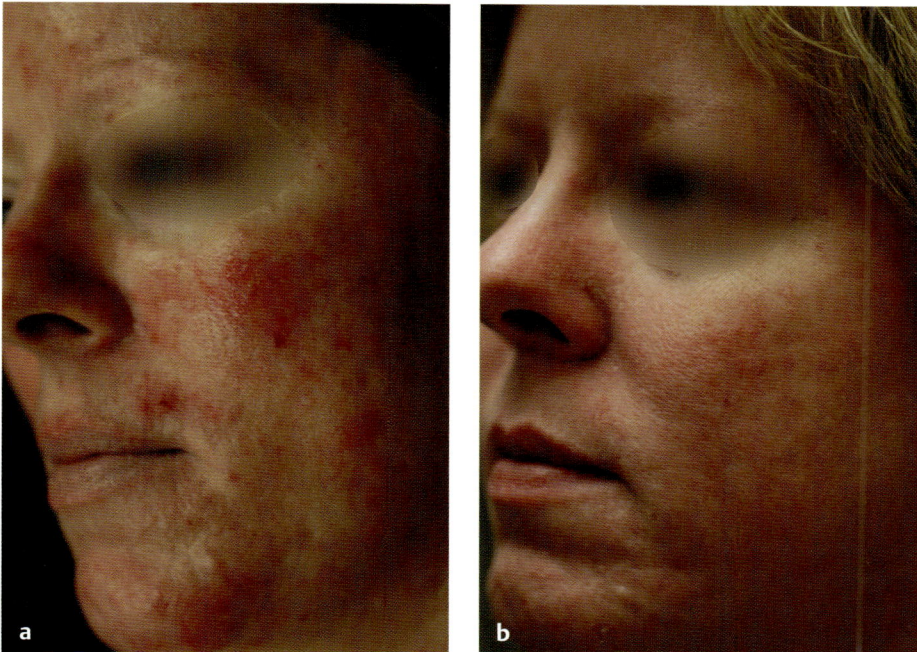

Fig. 10.2 Rosacea of the face. (**a**) Before intense pulsed light (IPL) treatment. (**b**) After five IPL treatments.

specific dedicated hair removal lasers. Many of these studies have found them to be similar in effectiveness, although only a few controlled, randomized trials are available. An evidence-based review from 2006 found no reliable evidence that treatment with IPL results in permanent hair reduction.[9] In the author's experience of using both IPL devices and dedicated hair removal lasers, the major drawback to IPL is that it is slower to use than some of the so-called fast hair removal devices, and it is more painful than the longer-wavelength lasers, such as the 810 nm and 1064 nm devices. Without question, IPL can suppress hair growth, but the permanency appears not to be as good as with the dedicated hair removal lasers. IPL is functional for treatment of facial hair and smaller areas of body hair, but for larger areas, one would want to consider a faster device.

Patient selection for IPL is similar to that for other light-based devices for hair removal, in that skin types I and II with thick black hair are considered the best candidates. Very fine, light red or gray hair does not respond well if at all to IPL. Darker skin types can be treated, but great care must be taken to avoid burns and hyper-/hypopigmentation. Long pulse durations and lower fluences are the mainstays of treating darker skin. Test spots are mandatory. There are multiple lawsuits involving severe burns, scarring, hypo- and hyperpigmentation from hair removal in darker-skinned individuals. Most authors consider tanned skin to be a contraindication for treatment with IPL devices.[3] Patients who are ideal candidates (types I and II skin, coarse black hair) will require a

minimum of five or six treatments, many more for darker-skinned individuals. For type IV through VI patients, one can consider it more of a maintenance treatment than a permanent solution. It is my policy to discuss all alternative treatments for unwanted hair at the initial consultation, and to promote the use of these treatments to those patients I do not consider to be ideal candidates for laser hair removal. A 3-month trial of eflornithine hydrochloride (Vaniqa, SkinMedica, Carlsbad, CA) along with agents for reduction of hyperpigmentation is appropriate in this group.

Discussion of informed consent for this procedure should cover the risk of injury from burns despite adequate test spots, should clarify the expectations with respect to permanent hair removal or lack thereof, and should include the risk of paradoxical hair growth. Paradoxical hair growth is new hair appearing in areas surrounding the treatment area and occurs most commonly on the face in women of skin types III through V, particularly in those of Asian or Indian heritage. This may occur in as many as 10% of patients in this class.

Once the decision is made to treat and informed consent is documented, photographs are taken of the area to be treated. Care should be taken to use reproducible settings, light, focal length, and so forth, as in other medical photography. As already discussed, test spots are utilized for all areas. Treatment then begins according to the test spot parameters. The patient shaves the area for the first few treatments and is then advised not to shave before the next treatment so that the remaining hair can be more easily identified. Treatment parameters vary between devices, and one should always consult the manual for the particular device before use, but in general, use a 600 to 1,200 nm filter, 15 to 30 J/cm² fluences, and pulse durations of 2 to 20 msec. For darker hair, a higher filter, such as 695 nm, and longer pulse width and/or stacking of pulses are used. For lighter hair, a 640 nm cutoff filter is preferred. Fluences are determined by skin type and initial hair density, with lower settings for darker skin and denser hair. The fluence may be increased gradually as hair density decreases. The clinical end point is mild perifollicular edema and erythema. Most patients will experience some degree of folliculitis for 1 to 2 weeks after treatments, especially on nonfacial areas. Skin care aftershave products can reduce the tendency and length of this inflammation. If the reaction is more than mild, a short course of a mild topical steroid cream will also help. All patients are advised that some touch-up treatments will likely be needed in the future.

Photodynamic Therapy

Although PDT in a variety of forms has been used therapeutically for many years, the last decade has seen significant expansion of this therapy in many areas of medicine. With regard to the treatment of skin disorders, the introduction of the topical application of 5-aminolevulinic acid (ALA) has brought a once experimental therapy into the mainstream of everyday clinical medicine. Currently in the United States, the only Food and Drug Administration (FDA)-approved formulation of 5-ALA is the Levulan Kerastick (DUSA Pharmaceuticals, Wilmington, MA). This device is a prepackaged dispenser containing two glass ampoules and an applicator tip. One ampoule contains the 5-ALA powder and the other an alcohol–water solution. Crushing of the two results in a solution of 20% 5-ALA.

PDT involves the absorption of a chemical compound into the cell (in this case 5-ALA), which is converted by normal intracellular metabolism into a photosensitizing compound (protoporphyrin IX in this case). Exposure to light energy then causes the release of cytotoxic intracellular singlet oxygen. Preferential absorption of the compound by highly metabolic cells allows for differential toxicity from normal cells. Topical application has the added benefit of minimal absorption of 5-ALA through normal skin. Activation of 5-ALA can be achieved with a variety of different light sources because it has multiple absorption bands, including 410, 504, 538, 576, and 630 nm. A variety of lasers, IPL, and visible spectrum light sources have been used clinically for activation of 5-ALA.[4] The BLU-U device, which is the recommended light source by the manufacturer of the Kerastick (DUSA Pharmaceuticals), is a fluorescent tube device that emits blue light at a wavelength of 417 ± 5 nm and a fluence of 10 J/cm². The BLU-U is a very potent light source for activation of 5-ALA and probably the most effective device for this. IPL devices emit light in the range of several of the absorption peaks and therefore are also likely candidates for use as a photoactivation source. Multiple studies have confirmed the utility of IPL in this role.[4]

PDT with 5-ALA is FDA approved for the treatment of individual actinic keratosis and is commonly reimbursed by third-party payors for this application. In a facial plastic surgery practice, the application is often mixed ablation of actinic keratosis and rejuvenation of photodamaged skin. There are multiple reports of the use of PDT for a wide variety of cutaneous lesions, including superficial squamous cell carcinoma and basal cell carcinoma. The author has found PDT to be very effective in the treatment of photodamage and lentigines, both of which are considered to be cosmetic applications and not reimbursable by third-party payors. Patients with extensive photodamage and diffuse actinic keratosis are ideal candidates for PDT.

Photodynamic Therapy Technique

Disclaimer: The technique described herein is an off-label use of the Levulan Kerastick (DUSA). The Levulan Kerastick is FDA approved for the treatment of individual actinic keratosis lesions using the BLU-U light source as an activator.

The process for activation of the applicator is fairly specific, and one should either view the demonstration on the DUSA website (http://www.dusapharma .com/levulan-kerastick-preparation.html) or on the DVD that accompanies this text before attempting to use the applicator. The applicator is grasped between the thumb and forefinger and crushed at points A and B as demonstrated. This is then repeated in between the marked letters to be sure all of the ampoules are crushed. Alternatively, one can use a device designed specifically for this, the Kerastick Krusher, which is available from DUSA. Once the ampoules are crushed, the applicator is shaken for a minimum of 30 seconds. This is followed by gentle but continuous pressure of the applicator tip against a gauze or towel. A minute or more is typically required to dispense the liquid preparation. This author finds that a blue or green towel drape helps to visualize the presence of liquid at the tip. Some patience is required here because one will likely think the applicator is not functioning correctly ► **Video 10.1**.

Once the applicator is primed, the Levulan is applied to the treatment area. The skin should be cleansed of any makeup and oil with either soap and water or a mild skin cleanser. The solution is applied liberally over the treatment area by gently rubbing the applicator tip onto the skin surface. It may be necessary to reprime the tip by pressing gently on it with a gloved finger from time to time. One Kerastick will cover ~ 100 cm². After the 5-ALA is applied, a period of time is allowed to elapse before activation by the light source. During this period of time, strict avoidance of sun exposure is essential. For IPL activation, the recommended incubation time is 2 hours. For the BLU-U, it is 14 to 16 hours. Once the patient is ready for activation, if IPL is to be used, the treatment takes place in the standard fashion by the application of the contact gel followed by the IPL head. Pulses are applied over the entire treatment area. The recommended settings are a 560 nm filter, double pulses with a 20 msec delay, and a fluence of 32 to 40 J/cm². Once the treatment is finished, the area is covered with an SPF 60 or better sunscreen, and the patient is advised to avoid direct sun exposure of the treated area for 48 hours.

The typical response to IPL-PDT is nearly immediate onset of mild to moderate erythema followed by mild edema. Any lentigines in the area will darken quickly. Some vesicle formation may be expected in areas with severe photodamage. Mild crusting will follow at 48 to 72 hours, and the application of a moisturizer with sunscreen is advised. At 1 week, erythema and crusting are subsiding. By 2 weeks, the treated area has returned to normal with the exception of some mild erythema.

■ Complications and Their Management

Complications from the use of IPL are fortunately uncommon if the previously stated guidelines are followed concerning skin types and the presence of tanned skin. Use of IPL on patients with Fitzpatrick skin types III through VI or tanned skin may result in burns, crusting, delayed healing, pigment changes, and scarring, even if proper settings and test spots are used. If the patient complains of pain during the treatment, the treatment should be stopped and the area chilled immediately. The treatment tip may become hot as a treatment progresses, and this should be taken into account. If a patient does sustain a burn, treatment with topical antibiotic ointment is advised for the first week. Once epithelial healing has taken place, the patient is observed for signs of hyperpigmentation, which can be treated with a variety of skin lightening agents, such as 4% hydroquinone. As stated previously, adequate eye protection for both the patient and the operator is of paramount importance to avoid eye injury. Patients who are taking photosensitizing medications are not candidates for IPL. Finally, as in many procedures that are performed on the facial skin, patients who have a history of reactivation of herpes simplex are at risk for this when being treated in the perioral area. Prophylactic antiviral treatment is recommended for this group of patients.

Complications specific to PDT are also rare. The most common problem is inadvertent exposure of the treated area to direct sunlight during the 24 hours after the treatment. This may result in an exaggerated skin reaction with blistering and burns. This is best avoided by the immediate application of a potent UV blocking agent (SPF 70 or higher) before the patient leaves the office. Patients should receive both written and verbal instructions for sun avoidance in the immediate posttreatment period. Patients on UV sensitizing medications or those with any of the porphyrias are also at risk for severe reactions and are not candidates for PDT.

■ Conclusion

IPL devices are excellent clinical tools for the effective treatment of a wider spectrum of cutaneous disorders than most other light-based devices. PDT can enhance the effectiveness of IPL in general and is very effective for the treatment of photodamaged skin. Both techniques require experience to obtain optimal results.

References

1. Goldman MP, Eckhouse S. Photothermal sclerosis of leg veins. ESC Medical Systems, LTD Photoderm VL Cooperative Study Group. Dermatol Surg 1996;22(4):323–330
2. Anderson RR, Parrish JA. Selective photothermolysis: precise microsurgery by selective absorption of pulsed radiation. Science 1983;220(4596):524–527
3. Babilas P, Schreml S, Szeimies R-M, Landthaler M. Intense pulsed light (IPL): a review. Lasers Surg Med 2010; 42(2):93–104
4. Choudhary S, Nouri K, Elsaie ML. Photodynamic therapy in dermatology: a review. Lasers Med Sci 2009;24(6): 971–980
5. Kennedy JC, Pottier RH, Pross DC. Photodynamic therapy with endogenous protoporphyrin IX: basic principles and present clinical experience. J Photochem Photobiol B 1990;6(1-2):143–148
6. Li YH, Chen JZ, Wei HC, et al. Efficacy and safety of intense pulsed light in treatment of melasma in Chinese patients. Dermatol Surg 2008;34(5):693–700, discussion 700–701
7. Galeckas KJ, Collins M, Ross EV, Uebelhoer NS. Split-face treatment of facial dyschromia: pulsed dye laser with a compression handpiece versus intense pulsed light. Dermatol Surg 2008;34(5):672–680
8. Fodor L, Ramon Y, Fodor A, Carmi N, Peled IJ, Ullmann Y. A side-by-side prospective study of intense pulsed light and Nd:YAG laser treatment for vascular lesions. Ann Plast Surg 2006;56(2):164–170
9. Haedersdal M, Wulf HC. Evidence-based review of hair removal using lasers and light sources. J Eur Acad Dermatol Venereol 2006;20(1):9–20

11 Laser Resurfacing with an Emphasis on Fractionated Technologies

Louis M. DeJoseph and Paul J. Carniol

Key Concepts

- Fractionated carbon dioxide laser resurfacing has a quicker recovery than carbon dioxide laser resurfacing.

- These technologies can be used for treatment of photodamaged facial skin, rhytids, lentigines, and dermal elastosis.

- Although less frequent than after traditional resurfacing, complications can occur.

- Any surgeon who performs fractional resurfacing should be prepared to diagnose and treat complications.

■ Introduction

Ablative laser skin resurfacing techniques emerged in the mid-1990s amid great fanfare and enthusiasm by the cosmetic practitioning community. The first lasers were high-energy, pulsed carbon dioxide (CO_2) devices. They produced dramatic clinical results in the treatment of photodamaged facial skin, rhytids, lentigines, and dermal elastosis. Their drawbacks came in the form of prolonged recovery and risk of potential complications, which eventually made them less attractive treatment options.[1] This spawned the development of nonablative devices, which solved the issues of prolonged recovery and treatment tolerability, but with less optimal clinical results.

Because of this limited efficacy, a new category of lasers was developed, fractional lasers. The first fractional lasers were nonablative. These were soon followed by ablative fractional lasers. The fractional ablative lasers bridge the gap between full ablative resurfacing and nonablative lasers. They provide clinically significant results with increased tolerability, lower risk of complications than ablative resurfacing, and minimal recovery time.[2]

■ Background: Basic Science of Procedure

Fractional photothermolysis has revolutionized the entire field of laser skin resurfacing by providing significant improvement in clinical results with minimal posttreatment recovery and complications. This concept of fractional photothermolysis was first coined by Manstein and colleagues in 2004.[3] The fractional technique differs from full ablative modalities in that ablative microcolumns are created with intervening skip zones of intact skin. These skip zones allow for adjacent heat dissipation during resurfacing and create the opportunity for horizontal wound healing. These columns are created in the epidermal and dermal layers to a controlled depth, width, and spacing (**Fig. 11.1**). This is in contrast to devices that ablate the contiguous skin surface to a given depth. By ablating only columns of tissue, the healing is more rapid, and the potential for adverse effects, such as new dyschromia, infection, scarring, and prolonged erythema, is diminished. The small surface area of each "micro-wound" also results in rapid healing from the keratinocytes in the surrounding untreated skin.[4]

The fractional laser devices available today can be broken down into two types: ablative and nonablative. The ablative devices include CO_2 (10,600 nm), yttrium-scandium-gallium-garnet (YSGG; 2,790 nm), and erbium-doped yttrium-aluminum-garnet (Er:YAG; 2,940 nm) lasers. The chromophore or target for these lasers is water in the epidermal and dermal skin layers. These high-energy lasers instantly heat the water, causing vaporization of the treated

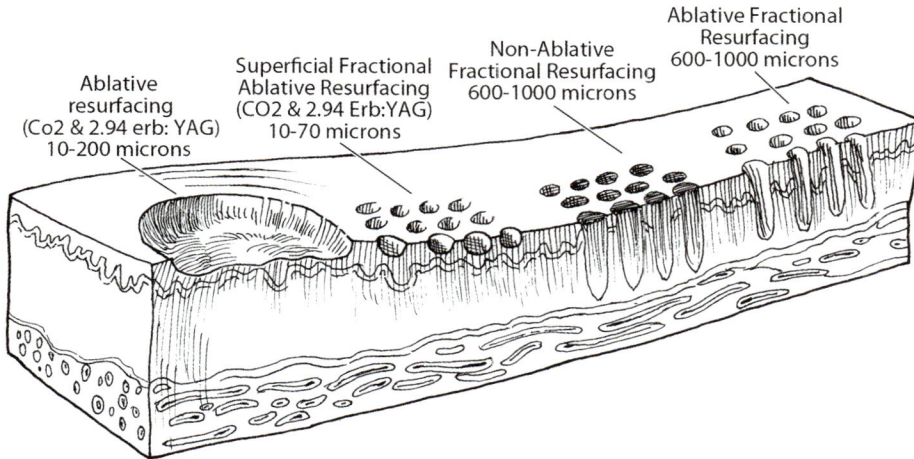

Fig. 11.1 Diagram demonstrating the evolution of resurfacing lasers leading to fractional ablation.

tissue with each pulse. This creates wound columns that can initially have some bleeding, serous drainage, and swelling lasting approximately a week or until reepithelialization is complete. The duration of erythema postfractional ablative resurfacing varies, but it typically lasts from 3 to 7 days.

The nonablative fractional lasers also target tissue water, but without causing an ablative wound. These include 850 to 1,350 nm infrared, 915 nm, 1,440 nm neodymium-doped yttrium-aluminum-garnet, and 1,540 and 1,500 nm erbium lasers. The laser zones created are coagulative in nature, with no epidermal ablation. Recovery is usually more rapid when compared with ablative modalities, and there is a lower risk of adverse events as already mentioned.[5] These advantages are counterbalanced by less significant improvements in clinical outcomes, and multiple treatments may be required to achieve the desired results. Longer-wavelength nonablative fractional lasers can be used to treat some conditions in patients with higher Fitzpatrick skin types, such as melasma and scars. Ablative fractional lasers are usually not used to treat these conditions in patients with higher Fitzpatrick skin types.

■ Pertinent Anatomy

The anatomical subunits of the face are an important concept in all cosmetic procedures of the face (**Fig. 11.2**). Knowledge of these helps guide the physician when deciding on a segmental area of resurfacing versus a full-face procedure. If a segmental resurfacing of the face is planned, such as rhytids in the perioral or periorbital regions, care must be taken to resurface the entire subunit for proper blending. Also, certain areas of the face can be more prone to scarring, such as the malar prominence along the jawline.

Often, the subunits are drawn on the face prior to resurfacing to help guide the practitioner. The authors prefer not to resurface individual facial subunits, but perform a full facial resurfacing encompassing all subunits for balance and blending. The concern, even with fractional ablative resurfacing, is that there may be a noticeable difference if only a subunit is treated. Therefore, if segmental resurfacing is planned, we prefer to resurface at least the entire lower or upper two thirds of the face.

Skin type is also an important variable to consider before a resurfacing procedure. The Fitzpatrick skin typing is based on sun reactivity and tanning response to categorize an individual's skin (see **Table 6.4**). Skin types I through III are usually considered resurfacing candidates because they have less pigmentation, and hence, less chance of dyschromia. However, a Fitzpatrick III skin type with any olive tones to the skin may be at a greater risk for dyschromia. The authors do not routinely perform ablative fractional resurfacing on patients with Fitzpatrick skin types V and VI. Patients with Fitzpatrick skin type IV can have significant variation in skin tone. The authors only perform fractional ablative resurfacing on these patients if they have lighter skin tones.

■ Patient Selection

One of the most important steps in the decision to perform a cosmetic procedure is proper patient selection. Several key points should be addressed in discussions with the patient prior to the procedure: (1) patient's concerns; (2) pertinent medical history; (3) physical examination; (4) treatment options; (5) managing patient expectations; and (6) discussion of the procedure, associated risks and complications. and after care.

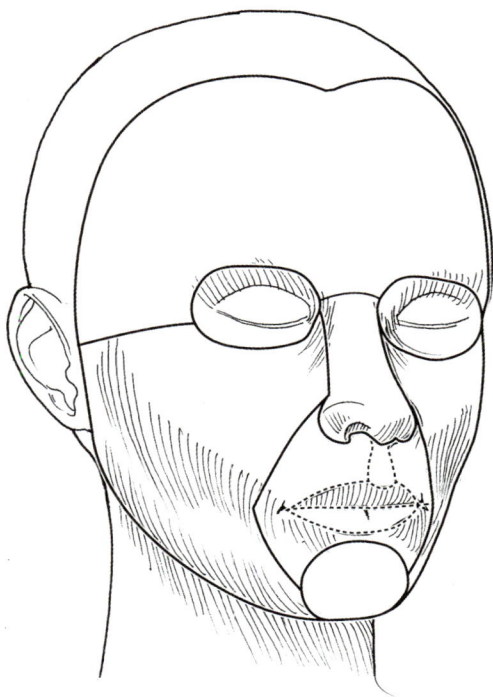

Fig. 11.2 Facial aesthetic units.

These obviously apply to every procedure the authors perform, but some specifics for laser resurfacing need discussion. The first step in the evaluation is the patient's concerns. It is often helpful to have patients stand in front of a mirror with bright lighting and point out the areas on the skin they would like addressed. This creates a general cosmetic skin "wish list" that helps the practitioner understand the patient's desires. This commonly includes rhytids, acne scarring, dyschromia, lentigines, rosacea, and actinic changes.

During this dialogue, a thorough evaluation of the patient's skin should be performed. This includes evaluation of elasticity, pigment, texture, laxity, thickness, scarring, actinic change, and neoplastic processes. All cosmetics should have been removed prior to this portion of the examination. In addition, a full facial examination should be undertaken with focus on areas of concern for laser resurfacing, such as previous surgical and laser procedures, skin cancer resections, radiation therapy, isotretinoin (Accutane, Hoffmann-La Roche, Nutley, NJ) usage in the last year, or history of scar or keloid formation. Patients with a history of radiation therapy, isotretinoin, scleroderma, or burns can have damage to the adnexal structures of the skin, which are vital to skin healing because reepithelialization is initiated from within these structures. The authors recommend a 12-month waiting period after cessation of isotretinoin before resurfacing. Specific attention to the periorbital region and any history of blepharoplasty

is recommended because even a slight lower ectropion or lid contraction can be greatly worsened by resurfacing. This can be evaluated by having the patient look upward while opening the mouth, which will reveal retraction or loss of lid elasticity.

The purpose of the initial patient evaluation is to gain a clear understanding of the patient's expectations so that they can be managed accordingly. It is important to explain the expected result and that results vary from patient to patient. Photos of similar patients before and after the procedure help educate the patients on expected changes. Showing staged photos of patients on immediate postprocedure days to demonstrate the healing and appearance during this period has also proven helpful.

■ Technical Aspects of Procedure

Preoperative Preparation

All patients are instructed to avoid sun exposure for 4 weeks before resurfacing and are taught proper sun protection for the period after the procedure. Some surgeons do not advocate preconditioning for fractional resurfacing. For those who use preconditioning, it can be accomplished with application of retinoic acid 0.025% cream 3 weeks prior to speed reepithelialization.[6] Hydroquinone can also be used 3 weeks prior to decrease the potential for postinflammatory hyperpigmentation, especially in darker skin types. This inhibits tyrosinase, thereby decreasing the formation and increasing the destruction of melanosomes within the melanocytes.[7] If prophylactic antibiotics are used, they are usually started 1 to 2 days before the procedure and continued until most of the reepithelialization has occurred. Antiviral therapy is generally started 2 days prior to the procedure and continued until reepithelialization has occurred. Preoperative photographs are also obtained consisting of a front view and right and left three-quarter lateral views.

Procedure Technique

Patients are asked to cleanse their face before coming in for the procedure and are advised not to apply any makeup, moisturizer, or other topical skin products after cleansing. Further skin cleansing can be performed prior to the procedure with mild soap or glycolic wash.

The type of anesthesia required for ablative fractional resurfacing can vary depending on the specific laser and the surgeon's preference. The authors use a topical anesthesia regimen of 6% lidocaine and 6% tetracaine prior to the procedure. This is applied for 15 to 30 minutes. No occlusion of the topical anesthesia is used. It is then thoroughly removed. Because the laser's chromophore is water, the face should be completely dry prior to starting the procedure. During the procedure, a cool air chiller is used. This regimen provides a good level of anesthesia, and the patients are comfortable. The authors have not found a need for oral sedation for this procedure or injection of any local anesthesia, but there is no contraindication to either if needed for patient comfort. If sedation is utilized, the patient should be carefully monitored.

Immediately prior to commencing the procedure, standard laser safety precautions are undertaken. These include, but are not limited to, blocking of any windows so light cannot go through them and immediate availability of water, a fire extinguisher, and eye protection for the patient and the staff. Staff eye protection should be designed for the type of laser that is being used. The patient's eyes should be covered with metal eye shields, either external or corneal types of shields. Plastic eye shields are not used because there is a risk of melting if struck by the laser.

A multitude of lasers exist for fractional resurfacing. As of this writing, there are no split face studies that clearly demonstrate the superiority of any one fractional resurfacing laser. The first author (LMD) uses a Matrix fractional CO_2 laser (Sandstone Medical Technologies, Homewood, AL). Some patients have extensive superficial actinic changes of their facial skin. These patients may derive greater benefit from combined laser treatment with a fractional CO_2 laser and superficial erbium laser treatment. Two separate laser devices can be used for this or they may be available in the same laser box, such as in the Cortex laser.

The settings used for any given laser vary depending on multiple factors. These include the physician's laser experience and preference, the patient's and physician's goals for the treatment, the recovery time and recovery experience the patient is willing to undergo, potential risk factors for both systemic and local healing problems, and the patient's age and skin thickness. Although the authors rarely do this for fractional resurfacing, if there is any question about the effects of a planned laser treatment, limited test spots can be performed and complete treatment deferred until the results of the test spots are evaluated. Additionally, if during treatment, either the patient's experience or the effects of the laser vary from what was anticipated prior to the procedure, the procedure should be interrupted and an evaluation should be performed as to whether to alter or continue the procedure.

The following settings are those used by the first author (LMD) when treating patients with the Sandstone Matrix laser. With this laser, the surgeon has the ability to control many aspects of the laser process, including density, pulse duration, and fluence. The density of the microspots determines how close the laser ablation columns are on the skin surface. It

can also be viewed as the percentage of the skin surface area that is treated. Pulse duration represents the pulse width or tissue ablation time. Laser power, represented in watts, correlates directly with the laser fluence.

All resurfacing is done in continuous-wave mode for fractional ablation. The pattern is generated in the handpiece and can be used in differing sizes and shapes depending on the surgeon's preference and area being treated. These settings or techniques may not apply to other laser devices. Before using a laser check with the manufacturer for recommended settings and techniques ▶ Video 11.1.

The laser is positioned at the patient's side with the laser arm manipulated by the physician. The first author frequently uses a power of 21 to 23 W, density of 0.8 mm, and duration of up to 3 msec. These settings are not universally used by all treating physicians on all patients. The first author takes care to cover each subunit with a uniformly nonoverlapping square beam pattern beginning at the forehead. Care is taken to feather into the hairline for completeness. The second author (PJC) does not treat by subunits. Rather, he prefers to treat at least the lower two thirds of the face and, depending on the clinical findings, treat or omit treatment to the forehead region. An air chiller is also employed at the time of resurfacing to increase patient comfort. Most physicians use a smoke evacuator to remove the laser plume. Surgical masks with 0.1 µm pore size are also frequently worn by the physician using the laser and any other staff in the procedure room.

If resurfacing is performed in the periorbital area, milder settings should be used. The author does not resurface the skin of the upper eyelid below the upper eyelid fold. This is particularly important because fractional CO_2 laser resurfacing can have a significant penetration depth.

The number of passes that are made and the settings for each pass vary between treating physicians and the patient's particulars. If a second pass is performed, it should be performed starting over at the area that was first treated so that the dermis in this area has had time to cool while subsequent areas were treated. Furthermore, the fractional pattern of the second pass should not overlap the first pass to avoid double pulsing any area.

Resurfacing will, on occasion, extend into the neck and décolleté area. This can be done quite effectively with fractional resurfacing, but the laser settings must be adjusted. Moving to a lower power (16 to 18 W), decreasing density to 1 mm and lowering duration to 1 msec has proven safe and effective in this area for the first author. The neck and décolleté area have a lower sebaceous unit (adnexal structure) count in comparison to the face, a different blood supply, and a greater tendency for scarring. The lower settings are used to allow for these differences.

Only one pass is made in these areas. If treated, these areas should be treated carefully because significant scarring has been reported in the cervical region after fractionated resurfacing.[8]

Two areas that warrant further discussion and caution on the face are the infraorbital and mandibular ridge regions. The skin of the infraorbital region is significantly thinner than the surrounding facial skin. This places it at higher risk for hypertrophic scarring and ectropion formation.[9] Care should be taken in this area with lowered passes or energy settings, especially when laxity or previous surgery is noted. Similarly, the skin of the mandibular ridge is prone to hypertrophic scarring, so fewer passes, lower power, or lower density may be warranted in this area.

The skin will have a patterned appearance after fractional resurfacing with the residual of the vaporized epidermis and dermis at each of the microcolumns. It is not necessary to remove this. Pinpoint bleeding may also be noted in some areas immediately after the procedure or the evening after the procedure. This can occur when the fractional resurfacing extends into the level of the dermal plexus of vessels.

■ Postoperative Care

After the laser procedure is complete, as a comfort measure, the patient can be handed a chiller on a low setting to cool the treated surface. Aquaphor (Beiersdorf, Wilton, CT) or another petroleum-based ointment is then applied with a tongue depressor to all treated areas. There are other topical skin care regimens used by other physicians, including Crisco. The second author has the patients rinse the treated area with a mixture of white vinegar and water (1 teaspoonful of white vinegar to 2 cups of water) at least three times a day and then reapply the Aquaphor. This can be refrigerated and applied to the treated area with moist gauze. In this way, the skin surface is cleaned at least three times a day. Furthermore, the mildly acidic solution can inhibit the possible growth of fungus or some gram-negative bacteria.

The ointment can predispose the patient to milia or acneiform eruptions. Therefore, this is discontinued when possible on the fourth day after the procedure. If a patient still has significant dry crusts after 3 days, it is continued for an additional 1 or 2 days. It is important to emphasize to the patient the importance of avoiding sun exposure. The authors start the patient on daytime use of a micronized zinc oxide sunscreen as soon as the Aquaphor use is diminished. Many patients can start using a mineral-base foundation 5 to 7 days after the procedure.

Patients may experience some pruritus during the first or second week after treatment. It is important to discuss scratching with the patient after the procedure because scratching a resurfaced area, even while sleeping, can lead to hypertrophic scarring. In addition to advising the patient not to scratch, the second author's standard postresurfacing instructions include taking an antihistamine such as diphenhydramine at bedtime, even if there is only minimal pruritus. Wearing white cotton gloves when sleeping is also discussed as an antiscratching measure. The first author also uses a 1% hydrocortisone cream once or twice daily for extreme itching; the second author does not use this routinely.

■ Expected Results

The results obtained from fractional CO_2 laser resurfacing can vary by patient and the condition being treated. Results can be quite dramatic when considering the reduced downtime associated with these lasers. Several treatments spaced 8 to 10 weeks apart may be necessary to achieve the desired results, and this should be discussed with each patient. Acne scarring has always been a difficult issue to treat but can be improved with minimal downtime with fractional resurfacing. Again, several treatments may be necessary.

The molecular biology of full ablative and fractional resurfacing has been shown to be similar in the tissues. Reilly et al[10] demonstrated significant changes in the gene expression of several matrix metalloproteinases similar to full ablative resurfacing. This suggests the same molecular changes are elucidated with fractional ablative techniques to impart beneficial tissue results. These metalloproteinases serve to break down and remove collagen, allowing for replacement with well-organized, new collagen bundles.

Healing after CO_2 laser resurfacing appears to adhere to the well-established phases of wound healing.[11] The literature suggests a combination of collagen denaturation and contraction, physical ablation of photodamaged tissue, and neocollagenesis as the most likely mechanisms of action for skin healing after laser resurfacing.[11-13] The patient in **Fig. 11.3** has photoaging changes of her skin. After fractionated resurfacing, she has visible skin tightening, decreased lentigines, and improvement in her rhytids. Similarly, the patient in **Fig. 11.4** has a noticeable improvement in her eyelids, and the patient in **Fig. 11.5** has a significant improvement in global appearance of her facial skin.

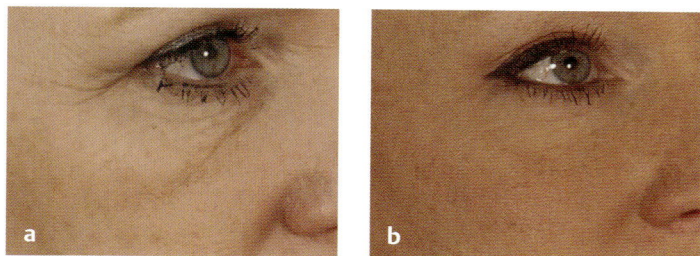

Fig. 11.3 Periorbital segmental fractional CO_2 laser resurfacing. (a) Before. (b) One year after.

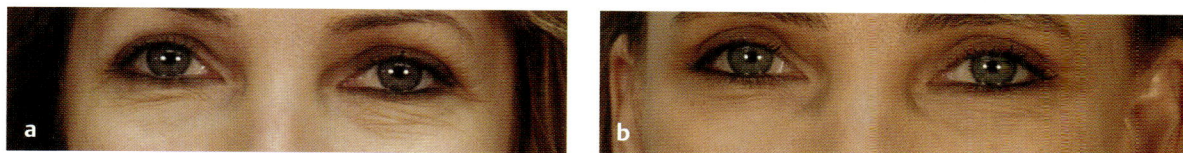

Fig. 11.4 Periorbital segmental fractional CO_2 laser resurfacing. (a) Before. (b) Six months after.

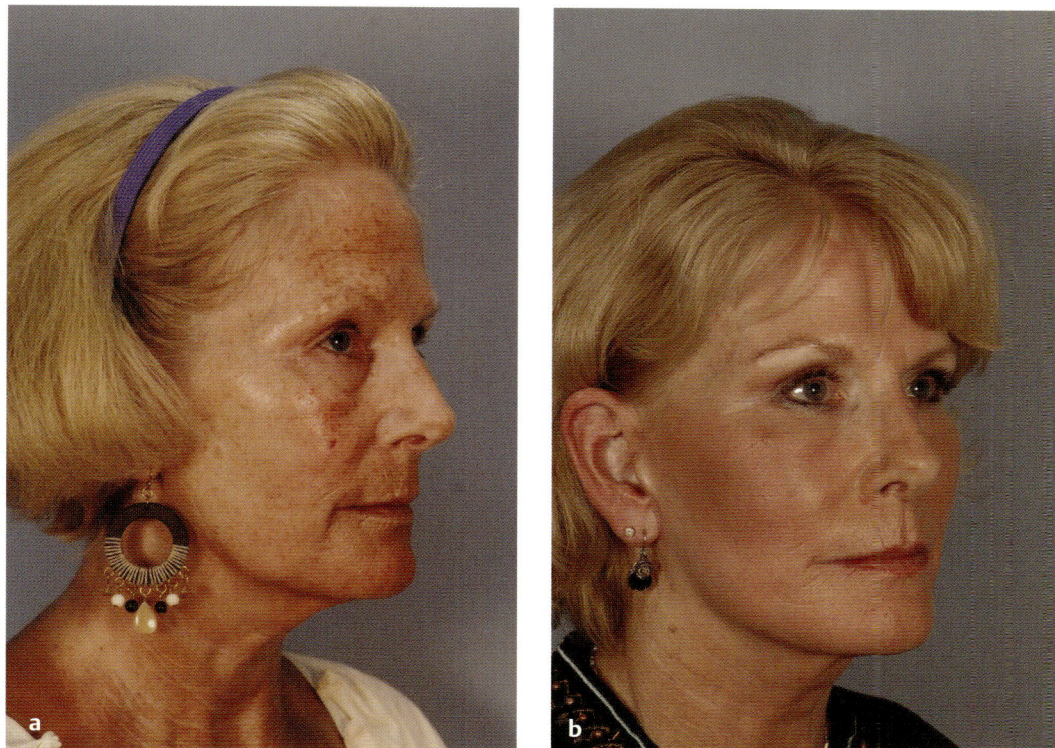

Fig. 11.5 Full-face fractional CO_2 laser resurfacing combined with facelift and upper and lower blepharoplasties. (a) Before. (b) One year after.

■ Complications and Their Management

The risk of complications exists, as with all procedures. Our preoperative planning and preparation lower this risk, but it is not eliminated. Complications do arise, and the surgeon must be knowledgeable, recognize them quickly, and manage them effectively. With laser procedures, there exists a thin line between side effects and complications because some side effects of laser resurfacing are to be expected. These include pruritus, acneiform breakout, immediate posttreatment erythema and bleeding, edema, herpes simplex virus (HSV) outbreak, and transient skin pigment changes. There are also risks of dyschromia and scarring.

Prolonged Erythema

Prolonged erythema after fractional laser resurfacing has been reported in up to 7% of cases of ablative laser resurfacing at 3 months posttreatment.[14,15] Traditional ablative resurfacing tends to carry a higher risk of prolonged erythema, but fractional techniques that employ multiple passes, deep penetration, or pulse stacking also increase the incidence of prolonged erythema.[16] Treatment of this consists of some watchful waiting—most cases resolve within 3 months. Treatment with 590 nm diode laser LED has been reported to reduce the erythema intensity.[17] Ascorbic acid applied topically has also been shown to decrease the duration and intensity of erythema.[18]

Acne and Milia

Acne and milia are relatively common after fractional skin resurfacing, with a reported incidence of 2 to 19%.[19-23] This seems to relate to the use of occlusive moisturizers. In most cases, discontinuing occlusive moisturizers as early as possible postoperatively diminishes the risk of this occurring. Oral antibiotics may also be added.

Pigment Changes

Postinflammatory hyperpigmentation (PIH) is quite uncommon with fractional skin resurfacing in comparison with traditional ablation. It has been reported ranging from 1 to 32%, depending on type of laser, intensity of treatment, and patient skin type.[14,20,24-29] It is more common in patients with higher Fitzpatrick skin types. The authors do not routinely perform fractional ablative CO_2 resurfacing on patients with darker Fitzpatrick IV, V, and VI skin types.

All patients are instructed to avoid sun exposure for 4 weeks before and after the procedure to reduce PIH.[26,30] In general, patients with darker Fitzpatrick skin types (III through VI) carry a higher likelihood of developing PIH. In Asian patients, it is imperative that laser fluencies be reduced, lower density be applied, and longer intervals between treatments be utilized.[26,31] This hyperpigmentation is usually self-limited and resolves with time but can be treated with strict sun precautions, topical lightening agents, and hydroxyl acid skin peels. A UVA and UVB sunscreen is also a mainstay of treatment to reduce pigmentary melanocytic activity. Patients should be reminded to apply this each morning before leaving their house for their regular activities.

At the other end of the spectrum is hypopigmentation, which is rare with fractional skin resurfacing. Hypopigmentation on an area of hypertrophic neck scarring was reported in two patients.[8,9] It persisted for several months and resolved. Care must be taken, especially in the neck region, where scarring can occur.[9] Repigmentation of the area with cosmetic tattooing is a treatment option should this occur permanently.

Infection

Most infections associated with fractional skin resurfacing present within the first week after treatment. This reinforces the need for close follow-up and evaluation so that expedient diagnosis and treatment can be established. HSV is the most common infection with fractional laser resurfacing, with incidence reported from 0.3 to 2%.[20,32] Pretreatment with antiviral prophylaxis is imperative with these procedures. The authors prefer acyclovir for this but have used other antiviral medications. In addition, if the patient has an active herpetic lesion, laser resurfacing needs to be postponed until complete resolution.

Bacterial infection is a rare complication, with 0.1% of cases developing impetigo superficial infection,[20] the common pathogens being *Staphylococcus aureus* and *Pseudomonas*. If these infections develop, scarring may occur, so treatment needs to be prompt. They present with increased pain, erythema, exudates, and erosions with crusts in the 1 to 3 day period posttreatment. Appropriate antibiotic therapy should be started along with wound culture and sensitivity tests. Yeast infection can also present after treatment.[8,9] *Candida albicans* is the most common pathogen and can occur at a later postoperative period (7 to 14 days). Treatment is with appropriate antifungal medications because these infections have been shown to produce scarring.[8,9] The second author believes that rinsing with a dilute acetic acid solution diminishes the risk of *Pseudomonas* and fungal infections postresurfacing.

Scarring

The most feared complication of all resurfacing is scarring. It is relatively uncommon with traditional ablative resurfacing[1,2] and even less common with fractional resurfacing, though it has been reported.[8,9,33] A literature review on the subject demonstrated that 9 of 10 published cases were from treatment on the neck area, resulting in vertical and horizontal hypertrophic scarring.[4]

Patients commonly present with areas of localized erythema and induration at 2 to 4 weeks posttreatment. Prompt diagnosis and treatment are paramount to a successful outcome. It is theorized that the relative paucity of pilosebaceous units, as well as a different blood supply pattern in the neck in comparison to the face, leads to the increased risk of scarring.[34] Also, thin skin architecture adds to the susceptibility to thermal injury in the neck. Therefore, caution must be applied when resurfacing the neck area. The indications for performing fractional resurfacing of this area vary between surgeons. Other areas of known concern are over the mandibular border and the lower eyelids. These areas should also be approached with caution because they are at risk for hypertrophic scar formation.[8]

A history of radiation therapy to an area for which laser treatment is being considered can be an associated risk of a healing problem. Radiation therapy to a different area (such as the breast or prostate) should not affect facial healing. Prior surgery to an area for which laser treatment is being considered may increase the risk of complications but is not a contraindication. With prior lower eyelid surgery there can be a greater risk of an ectropion. Surgery to the face or neck can increase the risk of a healing problem. There are multiple reasons a patient can develop a hypertrophic scar from prior trauma or procedures. If a patient has a history of hypertrophic scarring, the probable cause for this scar should be considered prior to performing an ablative laser procedure. In appropriate circumstances, ablative and nonablative fractional lasers have been used to treat scarring.[35]

If hypertrophic scarring starts to develop, there are several treatment modalities available. These include vascular laser treatments, topical silicone gel products, and topical steroid application. The authors reserve intralesional corticosteroid injection for scars that do not respond to the prior three treatments.

■ Conclusion

Fractional ablative resurfacing has truly changed our way of thinking about skin rejuvenation. It has bridged the gap that has existed between clinical results and postprocedure downtime. These two entities were always at war with each other, in that results always depended on increased recovery times. The first nonablative fractional laser treatment by Manstein in 2004 represented the step leading to a significant improvement in recovery compared with traditional resurfacing.[3]

This first fractional laser awakening utilized nonablative laser technology but demonstrated the concept of focal columns of skin wounding through the epidermis and dermis, surrounded by normal untreated skin. This resulted in quicker skin healing. It also demonstrated a lower incidence of adverse events than traditional CO_2 resurfacing.[5] Although the nonablative fractional modalities showed promise with pigment changes and skin texture,[36] they lagged behind the clinical results of ablative CO_2 and erbium:yttrium-aluminum-garnet (Er:YAG) laser resurfacing. The need for greater clinical results while maintaining the high safety profile spawned the use of ablative lasers utilizing fractional delivery. In 2007, Hantash et al published the first results of ablative fractional laser resurfacing, demonstrating promising results with skin tightening comparable to ablative CO_2 and Er:YAG, but with shorter recovery periods of 7 to 14 days.[37] In general, these ablative fractional lasers were found to give greater results than nonablative fractional lasers for certain conditions, such as acne scarring[38] and facial rhytid reduction.[39]

Although fractional resurfacing is relatively new, it represents one of the most important and exciting discoveries in skin rejuvenation of the prior decade. The technology behind fractional resurfacing should continue to improve as demand for cutting-edge treatments increases. The uses of this technology are already far-reaching and will only expand as research into the technology of fractional resurfacing delves deeper into improving results and defining new uses. It will continue in the coming years to be a powerful tool in the treatment of cutaneous photoaging, facial rhytids, dyschromia, acne scars, and other conditions.

References

1. Alster TS, Tanzi EL. Laser skin resurfacing: ablative and nonablative. In: Robinson JK, Hanke CW, Segelmann FD, et al, eds. Surgery of the Skin. Philadelphia, PA: Elsevier; 2005:611–624

2. Alster TS, Tanzi EL. Complications in laser and light surgery. In: Goldberg DJ, ed. Lasers and Lights. Vol 2. Philadelphia, PA: Saunders Elsevier 2008:99–112

3. Manstein D, Herron GS, Sink RK, Tanner H, Anderson RR. Fractional photothermolysis: a new concept for cutaneous remodeling using microscopic patterns of thermal injury. Lasers Surg Med 2004;34(5):426–438

4. Metelitsa AI, Alster TS. Fractionated laser skin resurfacing treatment complications: a review. Dermatol Surg 2010;36(3):299–306

5. Abbasi NR, Dover JS. Fractional laser resurfacing: why all the fuss? Dermatol Surg 2010;36(3):307–308

6. Mandy SH. Tretinoin in the preoperative and postoperative management of dermabrasion. J Am Acad Dermatol 1986;15(4 Pt 2):878–879, 888–889

7. Ortonne JP, Bose SK. Pigmentation: dyschromia. In: Baran R, Maibach HI, et al, eds. Textbook of Cosmetic Dermatology. Boca Raton, FL: Taylor & Francis; 2005:401–402

8. Avram MM, Tope WD, Yu T, Szachowicz E, Nelson JS. Hypertrophic scarring of the neck following ablative fractional carbon dioxide laser resurfacing. Lasers Surg Med 2009;41(3):185–188

9. Fife DJ, Fitzpatrick RE, Zachary CB. Complications of fractional CO_2 laser resurfacing: four cases. Lasers Surg Med 2009;41(3):179–184

10. Reilly MJ, Cohen M, Hokugo A, Keller GS. Molecular effects of fractional carbon dioxide laser resurfacing on photodamaged human skin. Arch Facial Plast Surg 2010;12(5):321–325

11. Seckel BR, Younai S, Wang KK. Skin tightening effects of the ultrapulse CO_2 laser. Plast Reconstr Surg 1998;102(3):872–877

12. Orringer JS, Kang S, Johnson TM, et al. Connective tissue remodeling induced by carbon dioxide laser resurfacing of photodamaged human skin. Arch Dermatol 2004;140(11):1326–1332

13. Ross EV, McKinlay JR, Anderson RR. Why does carbon dioxide resurfacing work? A review. Arch Dermatol 1999;135(4):444–454

14. Rahman Z, MacFalls H, Jiang K, et al. Fractional deep dermal ablation induces tissue tightening. Lasers Surg Med 2009;41(2):78–86

15. Chapas AM, Brightman L, Sukal S, et al. Successful treatment of acneiform scarring with CO_2 ablative fractional resurfacing. Lasers Surg Med 2008;40(6):381–386

16. Dierickx CC, Khatri KA, Tannous ZS, et al. Micro-fractional ablative skin resurfacing with two novel erbium laser systems. Lasers Surg Med 2008;40(2):113–123

17. Alster TS, Wanitphakdeedecha R. Improvement of postfractional laser erythema with light-emitting diode photomodulation. Dermatol Surg 2009;35(5):813–815

18. Alster TS, West TB. Effect of topical vitamin C on postoperative carbon dioxide laser resurfacing erythema. Dermatol Surg 1998;24(3):331–334

19. Fisher GH, Geronemus RG. Short-term side effects of fractional photothermolysis. Dermatol Surg 2005;31(9 Pt 2):1245–1249, discussion 1249

20. Graber EM, Tanzi EL, Alster TS. Side effects and complications of fractional laser photothermolysis: experience with 961 treatments. Dermatol Surg 2008;34(3):301–305, discussion 305–307

21. Wanner M, Tanzi EL, Alster TS. Fractional photothermolysis: treatment of facial and nonfacial cutaneous photodamage with a 1,550-nm erbium-doped fiber laser. Dermatol Surg 2007;33(1):23–28

22. Alster TS, Tanzi EL, Lazarus M. The use of fractional laser photothermolysis for the treatment of atrophic scars. Dermatol Surg 2007;33(3):295–299

23. Gotkin RH, Sarnoff DS, Cannarozzo G, Sadick NS, Alexiades-Armenakas M. Ablative skin resurfacing with a novel microablative CO_2 laser. J Drugs Dermatol 2009;8(2):138–144

24. Rokhsar CK, Fitzpatrick RE. The treatment of melasma with fractional photothermolysis: a pilot study. Dermatol Surg 2005;31(12):1645–1650

25. Tanzi EL, Wanitphakdeedecha R, Alster TS. Fraxel laser indications and long-term follow-up. Aesthet Surg J 2008;28(6):675–678, discussion 679–680

26. Chan HH, Manstein D, Yu CS, Shek S, Kono T, Wei WI. The prevalence and risk factors of post-inflammatory hyperpigmentation after fractional resurfacing in Asians. Lasers Surg Med 2007;39(5):381–385

27. Hu S, Chen MC, Lee MC, Yang LC, Keoprasom N. Fractional resurfacing for the treatment of atrophic facial acne scars in Asian skin. Dermatol Surg 2009;35(5):826–832

28. Walgrave SE, Ortiz AE, MacFalls HT, et al. Evaluation of a novel fractional resurfacing device for treatment of acne scarring. Lasers Surg Med 2009;41(2):122–127

29. Rahman Z, Alam M, Dover JS. Fractional laser treatment for pigmentation and texture improvement. Skin Therapy Lett 2006;11(9):7–11

30. Izikson L, Anderson RR. Resolution of blue minocycline pigmentation of the face after fractional photothermolysis. Lasers Surg Med 2008;40(6):399–401

31. Kono T, Chan HH, Groff WF, et al. Prospective direct comparison study of fractional resurfacing using different fluences and densities for skin rejuvenation in Asians. Lasers Surg Med 2007;39(4):311–314

32. Setyadi HG, Jacobs AA, Markus RF. Infectious complications after nonablative fractional resurfacing treatment. Dermatol Surg 2008;34(11):1595–1598

33. Ross RB, Spencer J. Scarring and persistent erythema after fractionated ablative CO_2 laser resurfacing. J Drugs Dermatol 2008;7(11):1072–1073

34. Goldman MP, Fitzpatrick RE, Manuskiatti W. Laser resurfacing of the neck with the erbium: YAG laser. Dermatol Surg 1999;25(3):164–167, discussion 167–168

35. Carniol PJ, Meshkov LB, Grunebaum LD. Laser treatment of facial scars. Curr Opin Otolaryngol Head Neck Surg 2011;19(4):283–288

36. Rokhsar CK, Fitzpatrick RE. The treatment of melasma with fractional photothermolysis: a pilot study. Dermatol Surg 2005;31(12):1645–1650

37. Hantash BM, Bedi VP, Kapadia B, et al. In vivo histological evaluation of a novel ablative fractional resurfacing device. Lasers Surg Med 2007;39(2):96–107

38. Chapas AM, Brightman L, Sukal S, et al. Successful treatment of acneiform scarring with CO_2 ablative fractional resurfacing. Lasers Surg Med 2008;40(6):381–386

39. Munavalli G. Single pass fractionated CO_2 laser resurfacing for improvement of lower eyelid rhytids. Abstract presented at American Society for Laser Medicine and Surgery Conference, April 2008, Kissimmee, FL

12 Treatment of Vascular Lesions

William Russell Ries and Joseph E. Hall

Key Concepts

- Appropriate treatment of vascular lesions requires an understanding of the pathophysiology of the lesion and knowledge of the indications for nonsurgical and surgical options.

- Lasers are important tools in the armamentarium of facial plastic and reconstructive surgeons for the treatment of vascular lesions.

- Lasers can allow for targeted treatment of vascular facial lesions.

- Lasers are selected based on the type of lesion, chromophore content of the tissue, desired effect, and characteristics of the laser, including wavelength and energy density.

- Continued advancements in laser technology have improved results of laser treatment of vascular lesions of the head and neck.

■ Introduction

Historical accounts of vascular lesions stem from ancient Greece, Rome, and Europe. The history of vascular lesions is steeped in negative perceptions. For example, the connotation of the term *birthmark*, which is often associated with vascular lesions, has historically implied a direct causal relationship between the emotions, thoughts, or behaviors of the mother and the anomaly of the offspring.[1] The theory that the mother was in some way responsible for vascular lesions was prevalent until the 18th century and was termed maternal impression.[1,2] William Hunter is largely credited with dispelling the unfounded belief in maternal impression.

Advances in medicine have provided understanding of the biological basis for many vascular anomalies. Treatment of vascular lesions has evolved at a rapid pace with increasing knowledge of pathophysiology and technical advancements. One of the greatest strides in the treatment of vascular lesions came with the development of the laser.

Einstein published his paper "On The Quantum Mechanics of Radiation" in 1917, which established the basis for laser theory.[3] Subsequently, the first laser was built by Maiman in 1960 and patient treatment began shortly thereafter.[4] Goldman performed the first cutaneous laser treatment with ruby and neodymium pulsed laser systems,[5] and Patel developed the first CO_2 laser in 1964.[6] The argon laser became popularized in the 1970s for treatment of cutaneous vascular lesions, and by the early 1980s, the argon laser was the treatment of choice for port wine stains. Following these advancements, the flashlamp pumped pulsed dye laser was introduced in the mid-1980s, and the intense pulsed light laser was developed in 1993. Lasers have flourished since the advent of this technology with the development of new lasers with unique characteristics and expanding clinical applications.[7]

This chapter discusses vascular lesion classification, treatment options, laser biophysics, laser-tissue interaction, technical aspects of laser treatment, and complications associated with treatment of vascular lesions in facial plastic and reconstructive surgery. This chapter also provides a detailed understanding of common vascular lesions, laser technology, indications and reasons for employment of specific lasers, and practical knowledge related to the technical aspects of vascular lesion treatment.

■ Background: Basic Science of Procedure

Vascular Lesions

Mulliken and Glowacki are credited with developing the modern classification system for vascular lesions.[8–10] Although the original classification schema has undergone necessary changes with advancements in the understanding of underlying pathophysiology, vascular lesions continue to be categorized based on structural components and biological behavior. The general term *vascular lesion* comprises vascular malformations and hemangiomas.[1]

Vascular malformations are differentiated from hemangiomas based upon their presence at birth, increasing size with patient growth, and normal rate of endothelial cell growth. Additionally, vascular malformations have a propensity to become darker in color and develop surface thickening with time. Vascular malformations are often subclassified based on their vessel components: capillary vascular malformations (port wine stains) and venous, arterial, lymphatic, and combination lesions.[1] Vascular malformations characteristically have large ectatic vessels and lack endothelial hyperplasia.

In contrast, hemangiomas behave like true neoplasms. Hemangiomas have a proliferative phase with rapid growth and endothelial proliferation, followed by an involution phase. Involution of these lesions is a slow process. Hemangiomas are characteristically absent at birth and demonstrate endothelial hyperplasia in ectatic vessels.[1]

Treatment Options

Treatment of vascular lesions has been revolutionized with the development and advancements in laser technology. When considering appropriate management for each patient and individual lesions, one must consider all available options. Common nonlaser treatment options consist of observation, ligation, excision, cautery, sclerosant therapy, chemotherapy, radiation, steroid therapy, embolization, systemic medications, or a combination of treatments. However, laser technology remains a mainstay in the treatment of vascular lesions because laser selection often allows for targeted and selective photothermolysis. Throughout the following discussion regarding laser characteristics and technical aspects of laser treatment, treatment options will be further delineated in relation to specific lesions.

Laser Biophysics

The word *laser* was originally an acronym for *l*ight *a*mplification by the *s*timulated *e*mission of *r*adiation. Lasers produce light that is monochromatic (one wavelength), collimated (little divergence), and coherent (identical temporal and spatial phases). Lasers utilize photon energy to achieve these characteristics.

Lasers start with a source of light energy. The photons present in the light strike atoms in the laser medium, which raises electrons to higher energy states. When an atom in the higher energy state is then struck by an additional photon, two photons are emitted. This process is termed stimulated emission. The photons produced will continue to propagate the energy transfer via mirrors within the system (**Fig. 12.1**). The photons emitted characteristically have the same wavelength, progress in the same direction, and travel in phase.[7]

Laser–Tissue Interaction

Laser energy can have a variety of effects on tissue, ranging from activation of biochemical substances or stimulation of biological tissues at low energy to coagulation or vaporization of biological tissues at

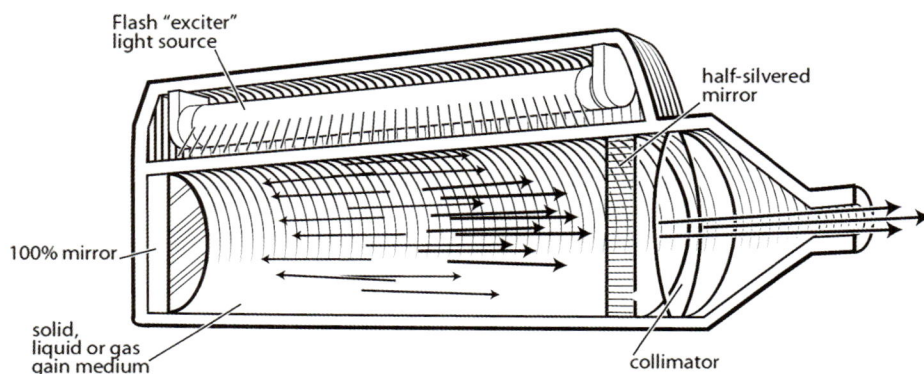

Flash "exciter" light source

half-silvered mirror

100% mirror

solid, liquid or gas gain medium

collimator

Fig. 12.1 Typical laser apparatus. Lasers use a power source to provide light energy to the system while photon energy produces stimulated emission.

high energy.[7] The effect of a laser on a given tissue is a function of the laser wavelength, energy density, and the amount of reflection, scatter, absorption, or transmission of energy that occurs (**Fig. 12.2**).[7]

Chromophores are substances that absorb energy at specific wavelengths. The specific absorption patterns of tissues partly determine the most efficacious laser for a given lesion. The chromophore absorbs light energy, which is then converted to heat. Coagulation of tissues occurs at 60 to 70°C and tissue vaporization occurs at 100°C.[11] Appropriate laser selection allows for targeted thermal damage in tissue components that absorb a specific wavelength of light. This process is termed selective photothermolysis.[11] Another important laser property is wavelength, with deeper tissue penetration occurring with longer wavelengths of light.[11] The peak absorption wavelength for oxyhemoglobin, which is found in high concentrations in vascular malformations and hemangiomas, is 577 to 585 nm. Some lasers are used at the wavelength that corresponds to a chromophore absorption peak, whereas others are designed for use at a wavelength that does not correspond to a chromophore absorption peak.

Two important laser parameters are energy density and power density. Energy density (fluence) is a function of the power (intensity) of the laser and the time of exposure. Power density is a function of the power divided by the cross-sectional area of the laser beam (spot size). Thus, by altering power density or time of exposure, the amount of energy delivered by a particular laser can be altered. Additionally, by decreasing the laser spot size, power density is increased.

Energy density (fluence) = Power density × Time

Power density = Power (watts)/Cross-sectional area of laser beam (spot size)

Pulsed energy can also be utilized. This mechanism incorporates regular periods of irradiation (on period) that are alternated with periods of no irradiation (off period). This alternating delivery of laser energy permits heat dissipation during the off period. Thus thermal heat damage to surrounding tissue is minimized. Duty cycle is defined as the ratio of the on interval to the on plus off intervals. Q-switched lasers release high-energy bursts of light for short time intervals using an electro-optical shutter.[7] Ultimately, one must match the laser wavelength, spot size, energy density, power, and pulse duration to the tissue of interest and desired outcome.[11]

■ Technical Aspects of Procedure

The ideal laser for vascular lesions should have a wavelength that is selectively absorbed by a chromophore in the vascular tissue. The laser should have minimal epidermal absorption to reduce the incidence of scarring and the ability to vary the pulsed laser energy based on the tissue thermal relaxation time. Currently, there are several lasers available for the treatment of vascular lesions based on the key laser characteristics already discussed.

Laser Characteristics

Pulsed Dye Laser

The flashlamp-pumped pulsed dye laser (PDL) was developed in 1989 utilizing the principle of selective photothermolysis. The laser medium is a rhodamine dye, which is excited optically by a flashlamp. Ultimately, this laser produces visible, yellow light.[12] PDLs are currently used to treat hemangiomas, port-wine stains, rosacea, and telangiectasias. These lasers have wavelengths of 585 to 600 nm.[12,13] The more recent versions of the PDL also utilize a dynamic cooling device that reduces the risk of epidermal injury.[14,15]

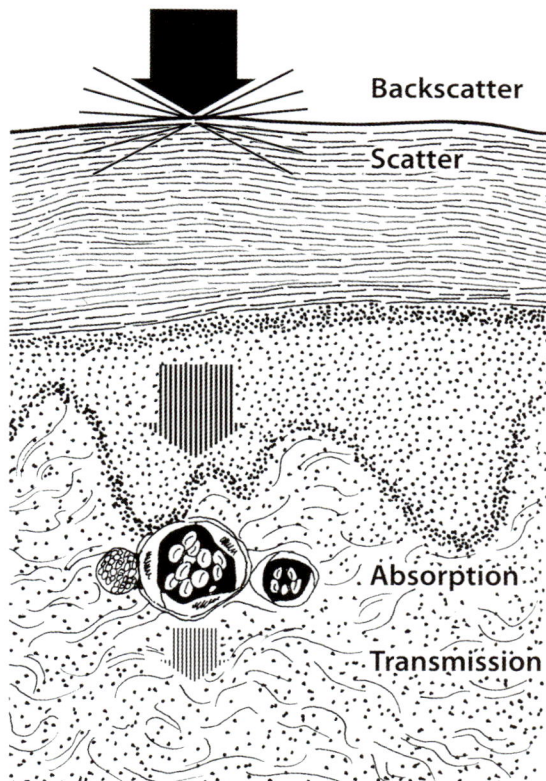

Fig. 12.2 The effect of a laser on a given tissue is partially dependent on the amount of reflection, scatter, absorption, or transmission of energy.

The spot sizes of these lasers vary from 7 to 12 mm and have higher peak fluence potentials. These alterations have been developed for more effective treatment of the deeper vessels found in hemangiomas and port-wine stains.[12,16] Additionally, longer pulse durations of 1.5 to 40 msec have allowed for telangiectasia treatment without the development of significant purpura.[12,16] A new PDL (Perfecta, Candela, Wayland, MA) has incorporated a pulse structure where each macropulse is subdivided into eight micropulses. This technology allows for single-pass treatment with delivery of higher total fluencies with less risk of purpura (**Fig. 12.3a,b**).[17,18]

Most patients develop variable erythema and/or purpura following PDL treatments. This may last for 7 to 10 days. Furthermore, patients may develop hyperpigmentation, hypopigmentation, or scarring.[12]

Intense Pulsed Light Laser

Intense pulsed light (IPL) devices produce 500 to 1,200 nm noncoherent light. Cutoff filters are used to produce wavelengths that target vascular lesions. Likewise, IPL system filters can eliminate shorter wavelengths to allow for greater dermal penetration with light of longer wavelengths.[12] IPL systems have been used to treat port-wine stains, hemangiomas, and telangiectasias.[12,19,20] In comparison with the PDL, IPL treatments require more time and have greater associated risks because additive heating is incurred with successive passes and longer pulse durations.[12]

The primary usage for IPL systems is treatment of telangiectasias. Selected wavelengths between 470 and 1,400 nm corresponding to absorption peaks of oxyhemoglobin are used to specifically target vessels. The range of wavelengths allows for treatment of vessels at various depths and greater energy penetration into the tissue.[12] Newer systems incorporate cooling with chilled sapphire windows.

Potassium Titanyl Phosphate Laser

The potassium titanyl phosphate (KTP) laser is a frequency-doubled (wavelength halved) neodymium: yttrium-aluminum-garnet (Nd:YAG) laser. This is accomplished by passing the laser energy though a KTP crystal. The resultant light is green with a wavelength of 532 nm, corresponding to a hemoglobin absorption peak. The laser energy is delivered to tissue via a fiber. If the fiber is not in contact with the tissue, vaporization and coagulation occur. Lower settings are typically used for coagulation. If the fiber is in semicontact with the tissue, cutting occurs. The KTP laser has a wide range of pulse durations, from 1 to 100 msec. The KTP laser has a shallow penetration depth. Accordingly, this laser is often utilized for vascular lesions given its absorption patterns (e.g., telangiectasias). Additionally, there is low risk of purpura, edema, or crusting.[12,21] Atrophic scarring is a concern with the KTP laser. One of the common KTP lasers in use is the Varilite, a 532 nm KTP and 940 nm diode pumped laser (Iridex, Mountain View, CA).

Red and Infrared Lasers

The alexandrite (755 nm), diode (532 nm, 800 to 940 nm), and Nd:YAG (1,064 nm) lasers are in the red and near-infrared (IR) range. These lasers have been used to treat reticular veins, port-wine stains, and deep vessels in vascular malformations. Red and IR lasers are effective for these lesions because they have wavelengths that target peaks of deoxyhemoglobin in the near-IR range (700 to 1,200 nm), achieve deeper penetration, and allow for higher fluence.[12]

The alexandrite laser is a flashlamp-pumped solid-state laser in the red spectrum of light (755 nm). This laser is absorbed by melanin and achieves deep penetration. The alexandrite laser has been used with

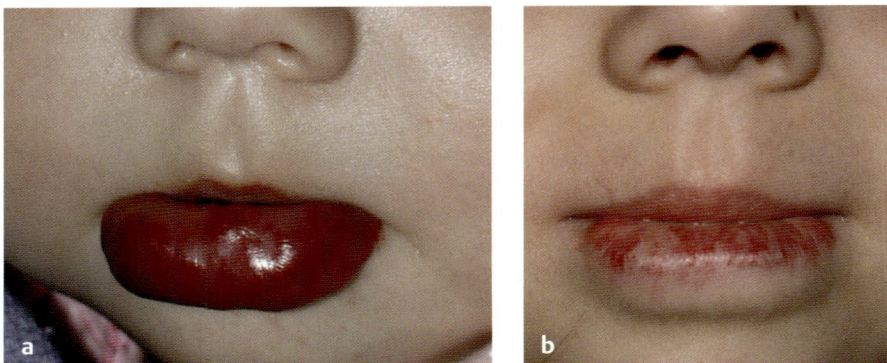

Fig. 12.3 **(a)** Pretreatment appearance of a lower lip hemangioma with extension into the vestibule of the lower lip. **(b)** Appearance following serial excisions for bulk reduction and six pulsed dye laser treatments for surface discoloration over a 2-year period.

significant improvement for hypertrophic port-wine stains. Some authors have reported using settings of 3 mm spot size, fluence range from 30 to 85 J/cm², and dynamic cooling[22]; others have used settings of 8 mm spot size for the initial treatment of deep malformations.[12] Li et al also demonstrated the effectiveness of the long-pulse pulsed alexandrite laser for hypertrophic, purple port-wine stains.[23] The authors did note that this laser can cause dyspigmentation, but no scarring was noted.[23]

The diode laser uses superconducting materials that are directly coupled to fiberoptic delivery devices. These lasers result in varying wavelengths depending on the material used. Diode lasers are efficient, converting electrical power to light at efficiencies of 50%, which allows for less heat production and power input.[21]

The Nd:YAG emits a wavelength of 1,064 nm, in the near-IR spectrum. The laser medium is neodymium:yttrium-aluminum-garnet. Pigmented tissue is selectively targeted with this laser because it penetrates up to 4 to 6 mm for treatment of deeper vessels (**Fig. 12.4a,b**).[24] The depth of penetration of the Nd:YAG is related to its scatter, which is much greater than that with the CO_2 laser. Yang et al found the long-pulsed Nd:YAG laser to be equally effective as PDL for the treatment of port-wine stains in a series of 17 patients.[25] The authors found that purpura lasted longer following PDL treatments, but the Nd:YAG caused greater perivascular and epidermal injury with scarring noted in one patient.[25]

Depressed scarring and hyperpigmentation are potential complications associated with the Nd:YAG laser.[12] Cooling devices assist in minimizing these risks. In comparison with the near-IR diode laser, the Nd:YAG laser has deeper penetration, incurs less surrounding epidermal injury, and may be used more safely in darker pigmented individuals.[12]

CO_2 Laser

The CO_2 laser uses CO_2 gas as a medium and a 10,600 nm wavelength. This wavelength is found in the mid-infrared range and is absorbed by water. This laser has been utilized in the past for tissue with high water content. Effects are typically superficial due to minimal scatter and high absorption rates. This laser seals vessels up to 0.5 mm in diameter and nerve fibers.

A helium-neon aiming beam is utilized with this laser system because the laser beam is invisible. Typically, the beam is delivered to tissue either by a handpiece or by an operating microscope.

Argon Laser

The argon laser has a range of wavelengths from 488 to 514 nm in the visible spectrum. The resonating chamber and laser medium create a band of wavelengths emitted from this laser. Hemoglobin absorbs argon laser energy well, thus allowing for use in vascular lesions. A fiberoptic carrier represents the delivery system. As mentioned previously, the argon laser was initially used in the treatment of vascular lesions and was the treatment of choice for port-wine stains in the early 1980s. Risks associated with the use of this laser include scarring and hypopigmentation.

Laser Applications

Lesion Subtypes

Hemangiomas

Hemangiomas behave like true neoplasms. These lesions typically appear in the few weeks after birth and grow disproportionately with the infant.[26] Hem-

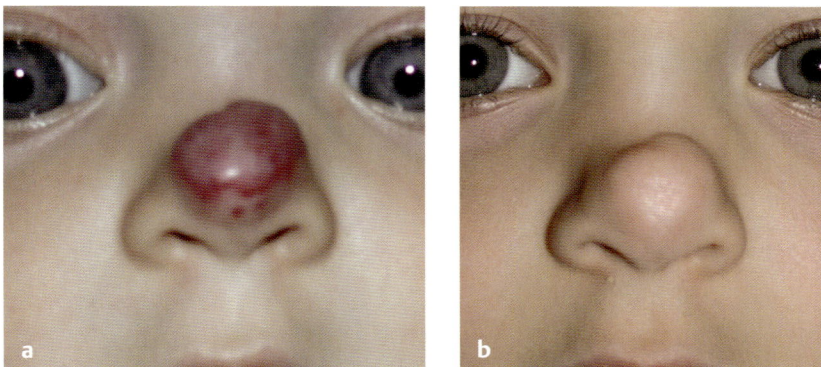

Fig. 12.4 **(a)** Pretreatment appearance of a nasal tip hemangioma. **(b)** Posttreatment appearance following five neodymium:yttrium-aluminum-garnet laser treatments over 1.5 years. Note the decreased lesion thickness and discoloration.

angiomas are more common in Caucasians, with a female to male ratio of 3:1.[27] The proportion of all hemangiomas occurring in the head and neck region is 60%.[28] It has been proposed that these lesions result from growth of placental cells transferred to the fetus in utero.[29] Hemangiomas have a proliferative phase that demonstrates frequent mitoses and plump endothelial cells on histological examination.[30] Involution of these lesions is a slow process with evidence of inactive, normal-appearing endothelial cells in fibrous-fatty tissue.[30] Resolution of these lesions is ~ 50% by age 5 years, 70% by age 7 years, and 90% by age 9 years.[30] Following involution of hemangiomas, 40 to 50% of children will have residual telangiectatic cutaneous vessels, fibrous-fatty tissue, or scarring.[31] Hemangiomas are classified as superficial (capillary), deep (cavernous), or combined (capillary-cavernous).[32]

Treatment of hemangiomas has recently been modified following numerous reports regarding the success of β-blocker therapy for these lesions.[33-35] Recent studies have demonstrated rapid and consistent therapeutic effects of β-blockers on infantile hemangiomas.[35] Buckmiller et al treated over 30 patients with propranolol (2 mg/kg/d, three times a day dosing), and 97% of lesions displayed improvement in the quality of the hemangioma. Side effects noted included somnolence (27%) and reflux (10%).[36] The senior author (WRR) currently offers β-blocker therapy to almost all patients with proliferating hemangiomas. When β-blocker therapy is elected, cardiology is always consulted to administer and monitor the use of this medication.

Although hemangiomas typically undergo spontaneous resolution and have recently been treated with β-blocker therapy, laser therapy continues to be utilized for hemangiomas that alter vital functions, demonstrate ulceration, or cause significant cosmetic disfigurement.[37,38] Pulsed dye lasers have been utilized for superficial lesions to lighten the lesion, induce regression, and possibly halt growth.[11] Early studies found that PDL treatment possibly prevented enlargement and promoted involution.[38] However, recent studies have called into question the ability of PDL to alter the natural course of hemangiomas. For example, a randomized, controlled study by Batta et al found that PDL treatment versus observation in early hemangiomas resulted in similar clearance or residual signs of hemangioma at 1 year.[39] This study also found that PDL treatment increased the likelihood of skin atrophy ($p = 0.008$) and hypopigmentation ($p = 0.001$) compared with observation.[39] Additionally, other studies have noted that early PDL treatment may not decrease deeper hemangioma growth.[40]

The 1,064 nm Nd:YAG laser has been used effectively for deeper hemangiomas that failed to respond to other methods of treatment (**Fig. 12.5a,b**). Clymer et al treated children with hemangiomas with the 1,064 nm Nd:YAG laser using an interstitial technique and found a reduction in size of lesions and achieved good results without lesion reexpansion.[41]

Combined treatment using both the PDL and the Nd:YAG laser can be utilized for hemangiomas with both superficial and deep components. The Nd:YAG laser is often initially used to treat the deep component percutaneously. Settings typically include a 600 µm bare fiber, 10 to 20 J, and 0.5 to 1.0 pulse width. Ultimately, the settings of each laser type depend on the manufacturer and the specific laser utilized. Lesions are treated in a radial fashion to spare the overlying skin and deeper structures. These treatments may be repeated every 6 to 8 weeks. Once the bulk of the lesion is satisfactorily decreased, the superficial component may be treated with a PDL. Postoperative swelling should be expected.

Capillary Malformations (Port-Wine Stains)

Port-wine stains (congenital capillary vascular malformations) are benign lesions within the dermis that are usually present at birth. Port-wine

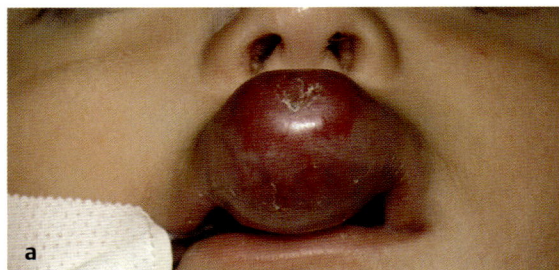

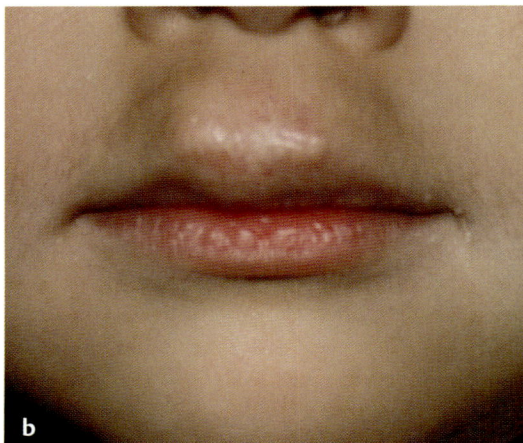

Fig. 12.5 Pretreatment appearance of an upper lip hemangioma **(a)**. Clinical response of this lesion following two neodymium:yttrium-aluminum-garnet laser treatments and serial excisions with adjacent tissue transfer **(b)**.

stains are present in ~ 0.3 to 0.5% of the population, with 5% of the lesions associated with Sturge-Weber syndrome or Klippel-Trenaunay syndrome.[7] The lesions are flat and pink to red in color. With age, the lesions can become darker and thicker, with increased nodularity. The most common location for port-wine stains is within the V2 nerve distribution of the face. Although the lesions are typically not life threatening, capillary malformations have been found to have significant psychological consequences. Troilius et al found that port-wine stains negatively affected the lives of 75% of 259 children with these lesions.[42] Additionally, earlier age at treatment has been associated with improved response rates.[43]

The first treatment popularized for port-wine stains was the argon laser (488 to 514 nm). With limited penetration (0.1 mm), significant melanin absorption, and development of blistering and scarring, this treatment has largely been abandoned. Currently, PDLs with wavelengths between 585 and 595 nm are utilized (**Fig. 12.6a,b**). Treatment response is dependent on location, color, skin type, and age of patient.[11] Two types of lesions have been described: type 1 have ectasias of the capillary loops and have a better response to PDL, whereas type 2 have dilated ectatic vessels in a ring pattern in the superficial horizontal plexus and demonstrate a poor response to PDL treatment.[44]

Treatment of port-wine stains with the PDL is effective with two passes per treatment, with first-pass settings of 5 to 6 J/cm², pulse width of 0.5 msec, and a spot size of 10 mm, and second-pass settings of 0.5 to 1.0 J/cm², pulse width of 2.0 msec, and a spot size of 10 mm ▶ **Video 12.1**. Cooling devices should be used with all treatments.[11] PDL with epidermal cooling has also been used with pulse durations from 0.45 to 3 msec.[11,12] Port-wine stains usually require multiple treatments repeated approximately every 2 to 3 months. IPL treatment has been used with success in port-wine stains, although most believe that patients with port-wine stains respond better to PDL treatment.[19]

Venous Malformations

Venous malformations are treated when they are causing pain or functional problems.[11] Treatment of these lesions typically consists of Nd:YAG laser (1,064 nm) therapy (**Fig. 12.7a,b**). Previous treatment options consisted of sclerotherapy, compression, or surgical resection. Treatment of these lesions can occur intralesionally or superficially.[11,45] The Nd:YAG laser allows for deep vessel coagulation with penetration up to 4 mm. Superficial cooling is used to limit epidermal damage.

The main goal of treatment is to reduce bulk and improve contour. Settings that have been found to be effective for lesions with traceable vessels from 1 to 3 mm in diameter include a 6 mm spot handpiece, 80 J/cm², 50 msec pulse width, and frequency of 1 Hz.[11] For vessels < 1 mm, settings that have been utilized include a 3 mm spot handpiece, 150 J/cm² and 30 msec pulse width.[11] Treatment of these lesions can occur at the earliest 8 weeks following previous treatment. Good results have been noted with Nd:YAG treatment of venous malformations.[11,46,47] Care must be taken with Nd:YAG laser treatment of venous malformations because hypopigmentation, scarring, blistering, or burns can occur. Although sclerotherapy has been used for deep vessels in combination with laser treatments for the superficial vessels, the senior author does not use sclerotherapy for facial lesions.[11]

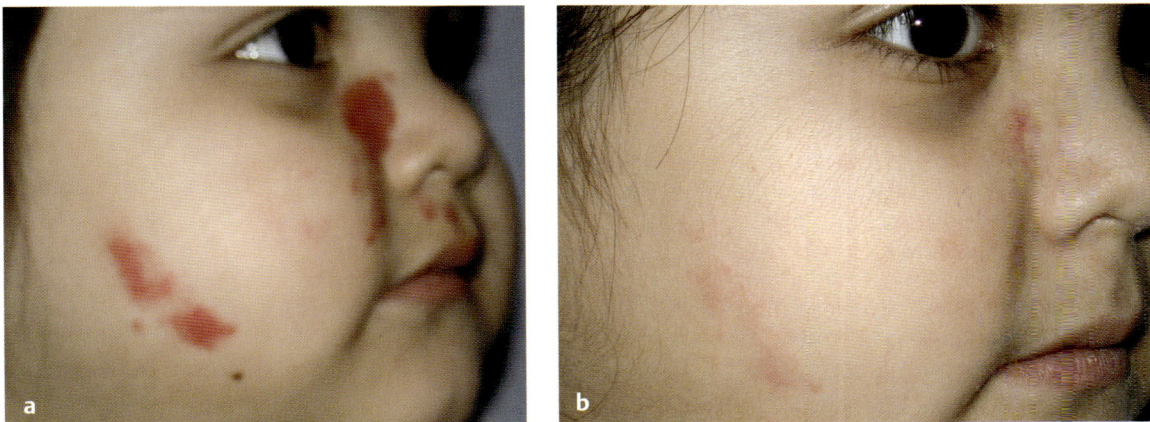

Fig. 12.6 Pretreatment appearance of a port-wine stain of the cheek **(a)**. Appearance of the lesion following multiple pulsed dye laser treatments over 2.5 years. Note the decreased size and discoloration **(b)**.

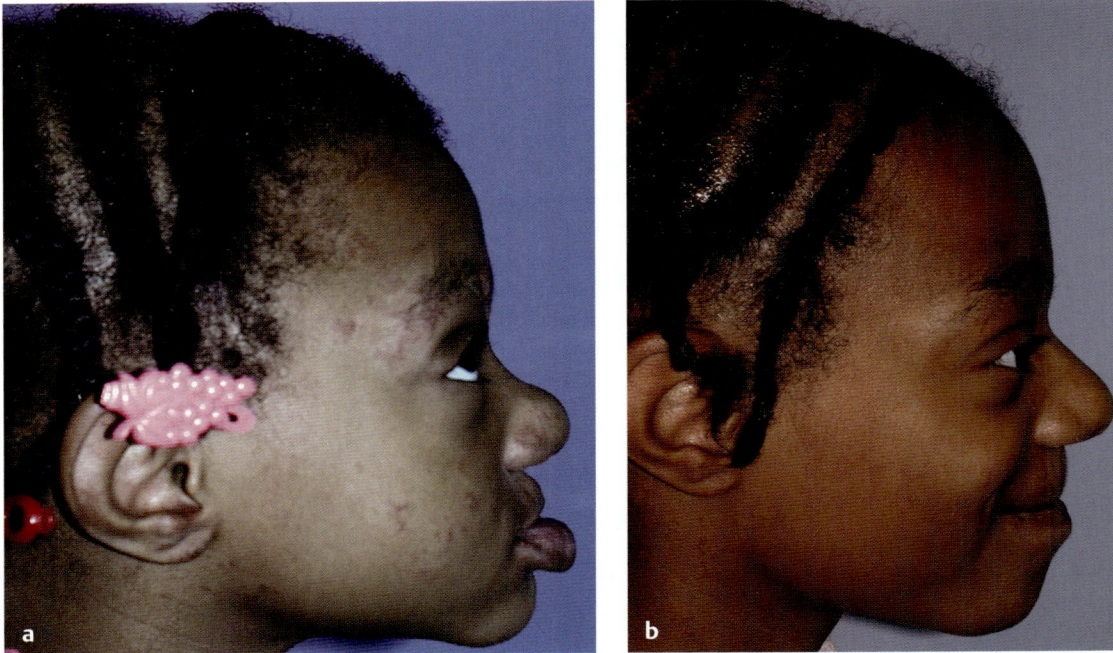

Fig. 12.7 Pretreatment appearance of congenital venous malformations of the nose and lower lip **(a)**. Posttreatment appearance of lesions following application of intralesional Nd:YAG laser treatments combined with serial excisions **(b)**.

Telangiectasias

Telangiectasias are dermal lesions characterized by small ectatic vessels. A variety of subtypes have been described, including linear, arborizing, punctate, and spider (nevi or angiomas). The development of telangiectasias is thought to be related to estrogen, nasal trauma, surgery, and genetic susceptibility.

Facial telangiectasia treatment is based on selective thermolysis of oxyhemoglobin. Common lasers used for these lesions include the 595 nm PDL, 532 nm laser, 940 nm laser, and 520 nm and 1,200 nm IPL.[12] Many surgeons use the PDL with pulse stacking and multiple pass technique with good results.[48] Common settings for the PDL for telangiectasias include 10 mm spot size, fluences of 6.5 to 7.5 J/cm², and pulse duration of 6 to 10 msec.[12] For telangiectasias with surrounding erythema, 532 nm laser treatment has been utilized with single-pass treatments with a 10 mm spot size, 20 to 30 msec, and fluences of 7 to 10 J/cm².[12] Smaller spot sizes are used for smaller lesions. IPL devices with wavelengths of 520 to 1,200 nm have also been used for telangiectasias, especially when significant erythema is present. Epidermal cooling and evaluation of skin pigmentation are important for the successful application of this laser. Given the melanin absorption, hypopigmented patches and blistering can be side effects of using this laser on tanned or highly pigmented skin without selective filter utilization.[12,49]

Generally, when treating telangiectasias, most physicians prefer to use the smallest spot size and lowest power that will obliterate the dilated vessel. This will avoid nonselective, surrounding tissue damage, thereby diminishing the risks of scarring or dyschromia. Treatment ensues by tracing vessels until the dilated vessel disappears. This should be performed using magnification because once a portion of a blood vessel has been injured, it is not necessary to re-treat that area while moving down the vessel. When utilizing magnification, it is possible to observe thermal injury along the vessel, and the next laser pulse can be given where the thermal injury stops.

Spider telangiectasias are treated by obliterating the periphery of the radial vessels and moving toward the center, with treatment of the central vessels last.[7] Treatment of telangiectasias usually occurs at a lower energy density than that needed for treatment of port-wine stains, and re-treatment may be necessary 6 to 8 weeks following previous treatment.

■ Expected Results

As with any procedure, realistic goals should be outlined with the patient or guardian preoperatively. Often, treatment of vascular lesions is not designed for, or even capable of, achieving complete resolution of lesions, and this should be discussed prior to initiation of any therapy. Risks, benefits, and alternatives should also be discussed in a forthright manner. Outlining the expected goals and demonstrating previous, realistic outcomes with patient photographs can be helpful.

Complications and Their Management

Complications in laser surgery are primarily avoided by understanding laser physics and laser–tissue interactions and by selecting appropriate lasers for particular indications. Approved training and safety courses should be attended by all surgeons desiring to perform laser surgery. Additionally, common side effects, including hyperpigmentation, hypopigmentation, blistering, crusting, milia, purpura, scarring, infection, and erythema that can result from laser treatments should be fully discussed with the patient and, as appropriate, the family, preoperatively.

Lasers can cause injury to the eyes or skin. Eye injury may occur via direct intrabeam viewing or reflected laser light.[7,21] Lasers with wavelengths in the 400 to 1,400 nm range can cause retinal damage as a result of the laser beam striking the retina.[21] Wavelengths < 400 nm or > 1,400 nm can produce corneal injury.[21] Goggles protecting against laser-specific wavelengths should be worn at all times by all individuals in the operating room. Eye protection for the patient is also necessary and varies from protective external shields to corneal shields. The eyes of the patient are often protected by taping the eyelids in the closed position with nonflammable, nonmelting tape and covering the eyelids with saline-moistened gauze.[7] Most physicians now use only approved eye shields or devices, as well as additional protective measures. Aluminum foil is then used to cover the periorbital region.[7] Additionally, metallic corneal protectors (instead of plastic) should be used when using lasers in the periorbital region.[50] Furthermore, the patient should have saline-moistened towels draped over all exposed, uninvolved facial skin when the CO_2 laser is in use because misdirected or reflected laser energy can result in burns.[7] These inadvertent burns can also be avoided by placing the laser in standby mode or turning the machine off when it is not being utilized.

Chemical hazards associated with pulsed dye lasers are often related to the dyes used for the laser medium. These dyes should only be changed by properly trained service technicians. Secondary hazards associated with laser usage include fire and noise. The risk of fire is reduced by using moistened towels in the operative field (for CO_2 lasers) and minimizing misdirected laser energy.[7] Management of the side effects and complications associated with laser treatment should address the underlying etiology and typically includes symptomatic treatment.

Conclusion

Treatment of vascular lesions must be individualized for each patient. Nonlaser treatment options consist of observation, ligation, excision, cautery, sclerosant therapy, chemotherapy, radiation, steroid therapy, embolization, systemic medications (β-blockers), or a combination of treatments. Lasers are often important for the targeted treatment of vascular facial lesions. Lasers are selected based on the type of lesion, chromophore content of the tissue, desired biological effect, and characteristics of the laser, including wavelength and energy density. When a surgeon comfortably understands the interplay between vascular lesion pathophysiology and laser characteristics, appropriate treatment and improved patient outcomes will be achieved.

References

1. Ries R, Clymer M, Charous S. Laser treatment of cutaneous vascular lesions. Facial Plast Surg 1995;3(3):307–318
2. Mulliken J, Young A. In: Vascular birthmarks in folklore, history, art, and literature: Hemangiomas and Malformations. Philadelphia, PA: WB Saunders; 1988
3. Einstein A. Zur Quantentheorie der Strahlung. Phys ZS 1917;18:121
4. Zweng HC, Flocks M, Kapany NS, Silbertrust N, Peppers NA. Experimental laser photocoagulation. Am J Ophthalmol 1964;58:353–362
5. Goldman M, Fitzpatrick R. CO_2 laser surgery. In: Goldman M, Fitzpatrick R, eds. Cutaneous Laser Surgery: The Art and Science of Selective Photothermolysis. St. Louis, MO: Mosby-Year Book; 1994:244
6. Stellar S, Polanyi TG. Lasers in neurosurgery: a historical overview. J Clin Laser Med Surg 1992;10(6):399–411
7. Ries W, Clymer M. The appropriate use of lasers in facial plastic surgery. In: Willett J, ed. Facial Plastic Surgery. Stamford, CT: Appleton & Lange 1997:223–241
8. Mulliken JB, Glowacki J. Hemangiomas and vascular malformations in infants and children: a classification based on endothelial characteristics. Plast Reconstr Surg 1982;69(3):412–422
9. Mulliken JB, Zetter BR, Folkman J. In vitro characteristics of endothelium from hemangiomas and vascular malformations. Surgery 1982;92(2):348–353
10. Mulliken JB, Glowacki J. Classification of pediatric vascular lesions [letter]. Plast Reconstr Surg 1982;70(1): 120–121
11. Burns AJ, Navarro JA. Role of laser therapy in pediatric patients. Plast Reconstr Surg 2009;124(1, Suppl):82e–92e
12. Railan D, Parlette EC, Uebelhoer NS, Rohrer TE. Laser treatment of vascular lesions. Clin Dermatol 2006;24(1): 8–15
13. Sommer S, Sheehan-Dare RA. Pulsed dye laser treatment of port-wine stains in pigmented skin. J Am Acad Dermatol 2000;42(4):667–671
14. Chang CJ, Nelson JS. Cryogen spray cooling and higher fluence pulsed dye laser treatment improve port-wine stain

clearance while minimizing epidermal damage. Dermatol Surg 1999;25(10):767–772

15. Waldorf HA, Alster TS, McMillan K, Kauvar AN, Geronemus RG, Nelson JS. Effect of dynamic cooling on 585-nm pulsed dye laser treatment of port-wine stain birthmarks. Dermatol Surg 1997;23(8):657–662

16. Lou WW, Geronemus RG. Treatment of port-wine stains by variable pulse width pulsed dye laser with cryogen spray: a preliminary study. Dermatol Surg 2001;27(11): 963–965

17. Ross EV, Uebelhoer NS, Domankevitz Y. Use of a novel pulse dye laser for rapid single-pass purpura-free treatment of telangiectases. Dermatol Surg 2007;33(12):1466–1469

18. Galeckas KJ. Update on lasers and light devices for the treatment of vascular lesions. Semin Cutan Med Surg 2008;27(4):276–284

19. Raulin C, Schroeter CA, Weiss RA, Keiner M, Werner S. Treatment of port-wine stains with a noncoherent pulsed light source: a retrospective study. Arch Dermatol 1999;135(6):679–683

20. Raulin C, Hellwig S, Schönermark MP. Treatment of a non-responding port-wine stain with a new pulsed light source (PhotoDerm VL). Lasers Surg Med 1997;21(2):203–208

21. Ries W, Powitzky E. Lasers in facial plastic surgery. In: Papel I, Frodel J, Holt G, et al, eds. Facial Plastic and Reconstructive Surgery. 2nd ed. New York, NY: Thieme; 2002: 79–95

22. No D, Dierick C, McClaren M, et al. Pulsed alexandrite treatment of bulky vascular malformations. In: Dermatology/plastic surgery supplement. Lasers Surg Med 2003; 32(Suppl 15):26

23. Li L, Kono T, Groff WF, Chan HH, Kitazawa Y, Nozaki M. Comparison study of a long-pulse pulsed dye laser and a long-pulse pulsed alexandrite laser in the treatment of port wine stains. J Cosmet Laser Ther 2008;10(1):12–15

24. Rogachefsky AS, Silapunt S, Goldberg DJ. Nd:YAG laser (1064 nm) irradiation for lower extremity telangiectases and small reticular veins: efficacy as measured by vessel color and size. Dermatol Surg 2002;28(3):220–223

25. Yang MU, Yaroslavsky AN, Farinelli WA, et al. Long-pulsed neodymium:yttrium-aluminum-garnet laser treatment for port-wine stains. J Am Acad Dermatol 2005;52(3 Pt 1): 480–490

26. Mallucci P. Vascular anomalies must be properly classified. BMJ 1999;319(7214):919

27. Bowers RE, Graham EA, Tomlinson KM. The natural history of strawberry nevus. Arch Dermatol 1960;82:667–679

28. Finn MC, Glowacki J, Mulliken JB. Congenital vascular lesions: clinical application of a new classification. J Pediatr Surg 1983;18(6):894–900

29. North PE, Waner M, Mizeracki A, et al. A unique microvascular phenotype shared by juvenile hemangiomas and human placenta. Arch Dermatol 2001;137(5):559–570

30. Werner JA, Dünne AA, Folz BJ, et al. Current concepts in the classification, diagnosis and treatment of hemangiomas and vascular malformations of the head and neck. Eur Arch Otorhinolaryngol 2001;258(3):141–149

31. Chang CJ, Nelson JS. Cryogen spray cooling and higher fluence pulsed dye laser treatment improve port-wine stain clearance while minimizing epidermal damage. Dermatol Surg 1999;25(10):767–772

32. Waner M, Suen J. A classification of congenital vascular lesions. In: Waner M, Suen J, eds. Hemangiomas and Vascu-

lar Malformations of the Head and Neck. New York, NY: Wiley-Liss; 1999:1–12

33. Léauté-Labrèze C, Dumas de la Roque E, Hubiche T, Boralevi F, Thambo JB, Taïeb A. Propranolol for severe hemangiomas of infancy. N Engl J Med 2008;358(24):2649–2651

34. Siegfried EC, Keenan WJ, Al-Jureidini S. More on propranolol for hemangiomas of infancy. N Engl J Med 2008;359(26):2846, author reply 2846–2847

35. Sans V, de la Roque ED, Berge J, et al. Propranolol for severe infantile hemangiomas: follow-up report. Pediatrics 2009;124(3):e423–e431

36. Buckmiller LM, Richter GT, Suen JY. Diagnosis and management of hemangiomas and vascular malformations of the head and neck. Oral Dis 2010;16(5):405–418

37. Vlachakis I, Gardikis S, Michailoudi E, Charissis G. Treatment of hemangiomas in children using a Nd:YAG laser in conjunction with ice cooling of the epidermis: techniques and results. BMC Pediatr 2003;3:2

38. Garden JM, Bakus AD, Paller AS. Treatment of cutaneous hemangiomas by the flashlamp-pumped pulsed dye laser: prospective analysis. J Pediatr 1992;120(4 Pt 1):555–560

39. Batta K, Goodyear HM, Moss C, Williams HC, Hiller L, Waters R. Randomised controlled study of early pulsed dye laser treatment of uncomplicated childhood haemangiomas: results of a 1-year analysis. Lancet 2002;360(9332): 521–527

40. Ashinoff R, Geronemus RG. Failure of the flashlamp-pumped pulsed dye laser to prevent progression to deep hemangioma. Pediatr Dermatol 1993;10(1):77–80

41. Clymer MA, Fortune DS, Reinisch L, Toriumi DM, Werkhaven JA, Ries WR. Interstitial Nd:YAG photocoagulation for vascular malformations and hemangiomas in childhood. Arch Otolaryngol Head Neck Surg 1998;124(4):431–436

42. Troilius A, Wrangsjö B, Ljunggren B. Potential psychological benefits from early treatment of port-wine stains in children. Br J Dermatol 1998;139(1):59–65

43. Tan OT, Sherwood K, Gilchrest BA. Treatment of children with port-wine stains using the flashlamp-pulsed tunable dye laser. N Engl J Med 1989;320(7):416–421

44. Motley RJ, Lanigan SW, Katugampola GA. Videomicroscopy predicts outcome in treatment of port-wine stains. Arch Dermatol 1997;133(7):921–922

45. Rebeiz E, April MM, Bohigian RK, Shapshay SM. Nd-YAG laser treatment of venous malformations of the head and neck: an update. Otolaryngol Head Neck Surg 1991; 105(5):655–661

46. Ulrich H, Bäumler W, Hohenleutner U, Landthaler M. Neodymium-YAG Laser for hemangiomas and vascular malformations—long term results. J Dtsch Dermatol Ges 2005; 3(6):436–440

47. Chang CJ, Fisher DM, Chen YR. Intralesional photocoagulation of vascular anomalies of the tongue. Br J Plast Surg 1999;52(3):178–181

48. Iyer S, Fitzpatrick RE. Long-pulsed dye laser treatment for facial telangiectasias and erythema: evaluation of a single purpuric pass versus multiple subpurpuric passes. Dermatol Surg 2005;31(8 Pt 1):898–903

49. Butler EG II, McClellan SD, Ross EV. Split treatment of photodamaged skin with KTP 532 nm laser with 10 mm handpiece versus IPL: a cheek-to-cheek comparison. Lasers Surg Med 2006;38(2):124–128

50. Ries WR, Clymer MA, Reinisch L. Laser safety features of eye shields. Lasers Surg Med 1996;18(3):309–315

13 Hair Removal

Mark Hamilton and Jaimie DeRosa

Key Concepts

- Laser hair removal is based on the concept of selective photothermolysis.

- Melanin is the hair follicle's only endogenous chromophore and is the target for laser hair removal.

- The use of lasers with longer wavelengths, such as the Nd:YAG, has allowed patients with darker skin to undergo treatment for unwanted hair.

- Adjustment of other laser parameters, such as pulse width, also aids in the reduction of complications and optimizes results.

- Future advancements are needed in the treatment of hair lacking melanin, such as blond or gray hair.

Introduction

The desire to remove unwanted hair is common in both women and men. Temporary methods such as waxing, shaving, and bleaching continue to be used for this purpose, but patients and practitioners have for years sought a more permanent solution. Until the mid-1990s, the only reliable, long-lasting method to remove hair was electrolysis, which, unfortunately, is poorly tolerated by patients and can be expected to achieve only a 15 to 50% permanent reduction in hair.[1,2] Since then, lasers (light amplification by stimulated emission of radiation) have been used for hair reduction, and laser hair removal has taken over as a popular, effective way to achieve a permanent reduction in hair.

Background: Basic Science of Procedure

A reduction in hair was noted with the first lasers and was achieved by epidermal injury.[1] In 1996, Grossman first reported the removal of hair using the ruby laser.[3] There were no significant advances in hair reduction until the method in which lasers worked (selective thermolysis) was understood.

Selective photothermolysis is the selective destruction (or absorption) of a target chromophore using a brief pulse of radiation with preservation of surrounding structures using the appropriate wavelength, fluence, pulse duration, and energy.[4] The chromophore targeted in laser hair reduction is melanin, and the laser parameters used vary according to the specific laser and patient characteristics, including hair color and patient skin type. Various studies over the years have shown that selective removal of hair is possible using a variety of laser systems and intense pulsed light (IPL).

Today, the primary wavelengths used for hair removal range from 755 to 1,100 nm, which absorb melanin well.[5] These correspond to the alexandrite, diode, and neodymium: yttrium-aluminum-garnet (Nd:YAG) lasers. The IPL system can also be used for hair removal but is not a laser. Instead, IPL systems emit a spectrum of light that can be used to direct energy to specific targets such as melanin, by adding filters.[2]

Pertinent Anatomy

As noted previously, laser hair removal is based on the concept of selective photothermolysis. Melanin is the hair follicle's only endogenous chromophore and is found in the bulb and bulge of the hair follicle.[1,6] Absorption of the heat from the laser by the melanocyte damages, and, ideally, destroys, the follicle.[7] The main competing chromophores are melanin within the superficial epidermis and hemoglobin found within superficial capillaries.[1] Being able to target primarily the melanin within the hair follicle without affecting competing chromophores is one of the main struggles as well as the focus for research in this field.

To fully understand the concept of laser hair removal, a review of the normal hair cycle and hair biology is warranted. Hair follicles have a cyclical growth pattern, and the duration of each cycle varies with anatomical subsite.[2] The first cycle is the anagen, or growth, phase; the second stage is called the catagen phase and is the time in which apoptosis occurs; this is followed by the final, quiescent, telogen phase, during which the hair falls out.

It is the anagen phase of the hair cycle during which laser treatments are believed to be the most effective. The anagen phase of hair follicle growth typically lasts for 2 months to 1 year for hair follicles in the face but varies due to factors such as body site, age, sex, hormonal influences, and genetics.[2] In spite of this variation, between 80 and 85% of hair follicles are in the anagen phase of the hair cycle at any given time.[2] Repeated laser treatments are performed every 4 to 12 weeks, with the thought that it is during this time period that there is a burst of rapid hair regrowth.[2]

The depth of each hair follicle varies between 2 and 7 mm from the skin surface, depending on the specific anatomical subunit within the body.[2] Although it is not entirely understood which portion of the hair follicle is responsible for hair growth, it is thought that the major growth center is the matrix. The follicle has an exceptional ability to regenerate and self-repair, which impedes the effectiveness of laser hair removal therapy.[8] Current laser hair removal techniques attempt to permanently damage the entire follicle at an estimated depth; the specific depth chosen is based on the targeted anatomical subunit.[8]

Patient Selection

During the initial consultation with any patient interested in laser hair reduction, it is important to obtain a thorough history and physical examination, as well as have an open discussion regarding the patient's expectations as compared with the potential results. The history should include information such as whether the patient has undergone previous hair reduction treatments because it is prudent to wait 6 weeks prior to performing any additional treatment.

During the examination, the physician should note the patient's Fitzpatrick skin type, hair color/thickness, the presence of tattoos or suspicious moles, and the possible presence of a systemic disorder, such as

hirsutism (the presence of terminal, coarse hairs in females in a male-like pattern).[4] If one suspects hirsutism, a referral to a specialist may be indicated prior to laser hair treatment because it is typically a sign of an underlying endocrine abnormality.[4] Pretreatment photographs of the areas to be treated are taken and can be useful tools for posttreatment comparison and evaluation of whether the treatment was successful.

Patient education is performed prior to the first treatment. It is important that patients understand that they should anticipate needing three to seven treatments to achieve the desired results. We also counsel our patients to avoid tanning or burning prior to the treatment because darker skin will decrease the effectiveness of the treatment and may increase the risk of complications, such as blistering, scarring, and hyperpigmentation.[1] Finally, we also ask our patients to avoid tweezing or waxing on the day of the procedure because these processes can remove the target chromophore (melanin) at the base of the hair follicle.

Technical Aspects of Procedure

Lasers are composed of an energy source, a focusing (or gating) system, and a radiating medium. The medium determines the wavelength emitted, such as 755 nm for an alexandrite laser ▶ **Video 13.1**. The characteristics of the laser itself can be adjusted by changing one or more of the following parameters: fluence (amount of laser energy per unit area [joules per square centimeter]), pulse width (length of time of exposure to the skin), and spot size (surface area of skin exposed to the laser beam).[9]

Laser parameters can be adjusted to more selectively injure the hair follicle.[1] One method is to lengthen the pulse width. When the pulse width is longer than the thermal relaxation time of the superficial melanin but shorter than that of the hair follicle, the hair follicle can be injured without damage to the skin.[1]

Cooling of the skin can also help to protect the skin surface during laser hair removal. In addition, skin cooling may have an added benefit of increased patient tolerance to the treatment because it has been found to help reduce pain.[9] Skin cooling in combination with longer pulse widths has also allowed patients with darker skin to benefit from laser hair removal.[9] Compression of the skin during treatment can also help to push blood out of the capillaries in the area to reduce the absorption by the competing chromophore, hemoglobin.

There are several lasers used for hair removal treatments. The following section reviews the specific technical aspects for the Nd:YAG laser. A brief summary of the other laser systems used to remove hair follows.

Nd:YAG Laser

There are three main parameters that need to be set when using the Nd:YAG laser for hair reduction treatment: cooling temperature, fluence, and pulse width. Each can be adjusted to a specific patient's needs. The common starting settings are discussed here, although there is not a fixed setting appropriate for all patients.

Performing a test spot prior to each treatment can also help to reduce the risk of complications. If any blistering, excessive swelling, or redness is noted, then another test spot should be performed with different laser parameters. Treatment should not be performed until a satisfactory test spot result is seen.[1]

As noted previously, pretreatment discussion with the patient about expectations, possible complications, and pretreatment care is necessary. All patients should have pretreatment photos taken for documentation, and all should give informed consent. A topical anesthetic may be applied to the treatment area 30 minutes before the procedure to decrease patient discomfort. The skin should also be washed with a gentle cleanser and thoroughly dried prior to treatment.

The cooling temperature is typically set on a separate chilling device. Zero to 15°C will usually provide for maximal patient comfort, and most treatments can be done with a cooling temperature of 15°C. A coating of colorless gel is also placed on intended treatment areas to permit better heat removal. Of note, if the fluence is increased, the cooling temperature should be decreased and vice versa.[10]

The fluence used is dependent on the starting surface area temperature of the skin, as well as such factors as whether or not the patient has been treated before and his or her response to treatment. In general, one may start at 65 J/cm^2 and increase fluence by 10% at each subsequent treatment.

The pulse width is set from 15 to 40 msec. Keeping the pulse width shorter or equal to the thermal relaxation time of the hair follicle (~ 10 to 50 msec) helps to limit or prevent collateral thermal damage.[11] The specific setting used is partially determined by the size of the hair shaft and follicle. Coarse hair typically requires a pulse width of 20 msec, whereas in those with darker skin tones, a longer pulse width is used (**Fig. 13.1a–d**). As the hair reduces in size over the course of treatments, the pulse width may also need to be reduced. We typically decrease pulse width by 5 msec at each treatment session. The Nd:YAG laser has been successfully used to remove hair in patients with darker skin types (**Fig. 13.1**).

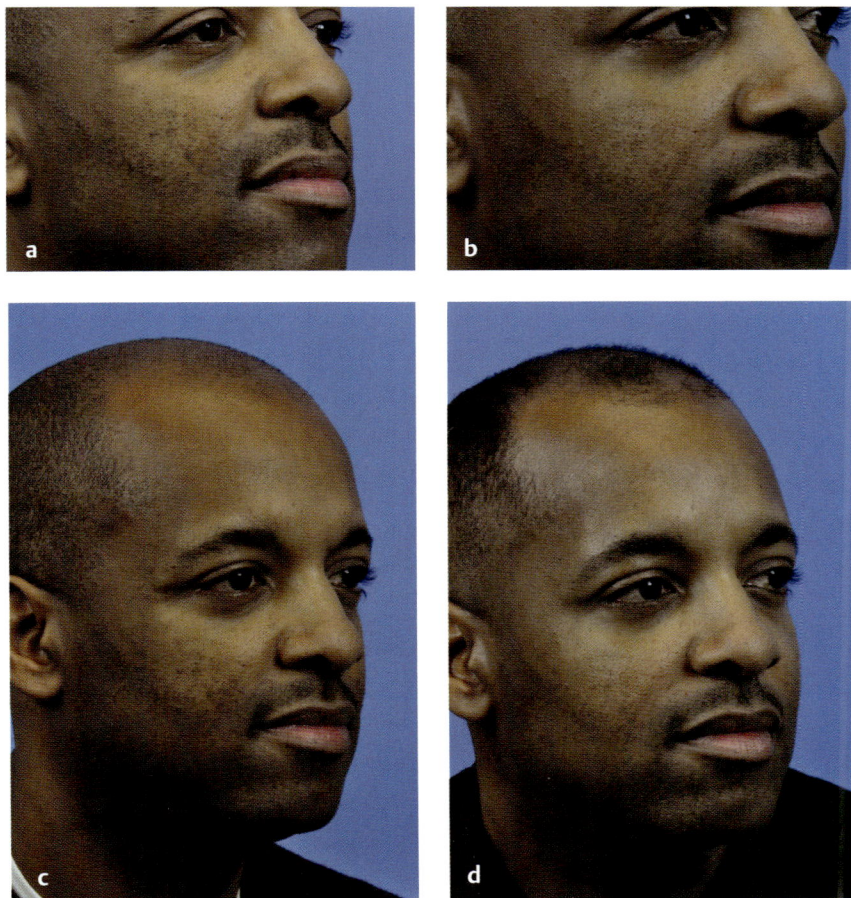

Fig. 13.1 Pre- **(a,c)** and postlaser **(b,d)** hair removal on Fitzpatrick type VI skin with an Nd:YAG laser.

Ruby Laser

The 694 nm wavelength was the first laser that showed permanent reduction in hair growth following treatment.[1] With the addition of a skin cooling device, the ruby laser continues to be a safe and effective laser for the reduction of hair in those with lighter skin types. Unfortunately, in those with darker skin, this laser is less than ideal because there is a high incidence of hypo- or hyperpigmentation.[1,11] In general, darker skin types are more safely treated with longer wavelength systems.[1] In recent years, the ruby laser has become less popular and has been replaced by the alexandrite and diode lasers.

Alexandrite Laser

There are a variety of laser systems that use the 755 nm alexandrite laser for hair removal.[1] It has been shown to be an effective way to remove hair in a safe manner (**Fig. 13.2a–d**). It is safer than the ruby laser for darker skin types.

Diode Laser

The diode laser uses an 800 to 810 nm wavelength and has a treatment profile similar to that of the alexandrite laser. Due to the slightly longer wavelength and lower melanin absorption, this laser is usually safer for patients with higher Fitzpatrick skin types.[1] The current systems have a chill tip in the hand piece to protect the skin surface. With the LightSheer version of this laser (Lumenis, Santa Clara, CA), one can also compress the skin during treatment.[1]

Intense Pulsed Light

Although intense pulsed light (IPL) is not a laser, it has been used for light-based hair removal. IPL systems have a broad wavelength spectrum (515 to 1,200 nm). With filtering of wavelengths so that only those that target melanin reach the skin, it has been able to achieve effective temporary hair removal.[1] The success of IPL for persistent hair removal varies but has been reported to be as high as 90%.[12]

■ Postoperative Care

Prior to treatment, the initial recovery period is discussed with patients. This includes some redness in the areas treated for up to 24 hours (**Table 13.1**). Erythema beyond 24 hours may be treated with a topical steroid. The hair may appear to grow for several days after treatment as the hair is extruding, and then hair should fall out by day 10 to 14. Approximately 6 to 8 weeks later, new hair may appear. At this time, another treatment is performed.

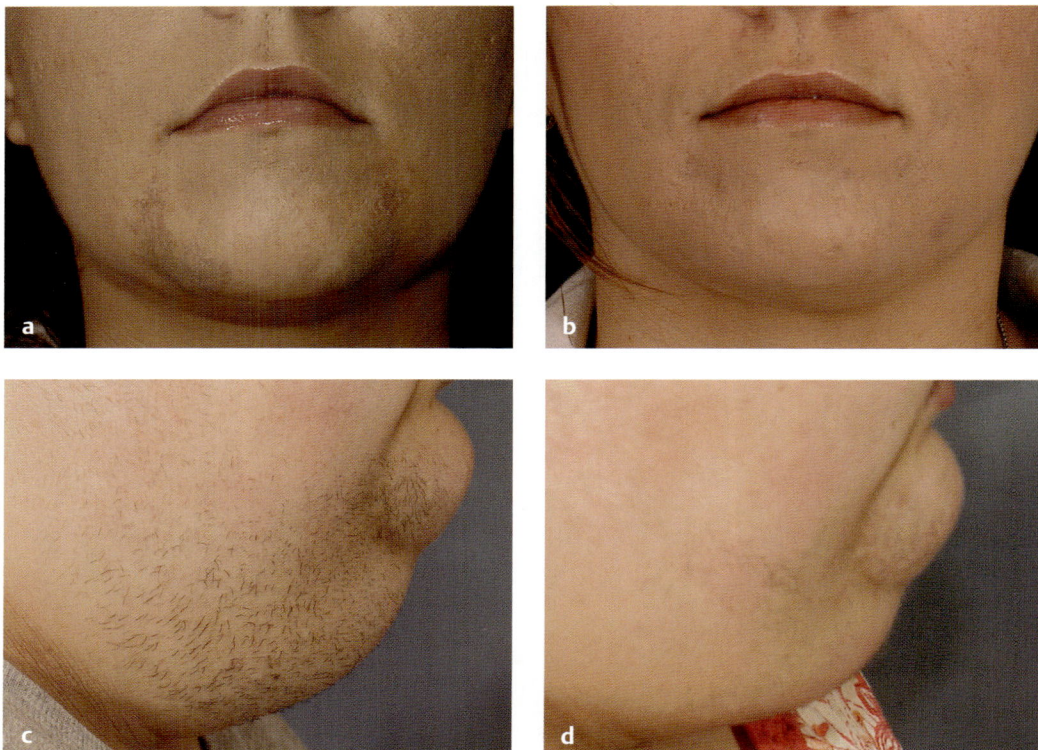

Fig. 13.2 Two different patients treated with a diode laser. Patient number one with polycystic ovary disease: **(a)** pre- and **(b)** postlaser. The second patient with hirsutism of lower central face: **(c)** pre- and **(d)** postlaser.

Table 13.1 Patient instructions

Pretreatment instructions

1. Avoid the sun 4–6 weeks before and after treatment until your healthcare provider allows it. Epidermal melanocytes compete with melanin in the hair.

2. Your provider may ask you to stop any topical medications or skin care products 3–5 days prior to treatment.

3. You *must* avoid bleaching, plucking, or waxing hair for 4–6 weeks prior to treatment. The melanin-containing hair must be present in the follicle because it is the "target" for the laser light.

4. If you have had a history of perioral or genital herpes simplex virus, your provider may recommend prophylactic antiviral therapy. Follow the directions for your particular antiviral medication.

5. If you have a tan or have a darker skin type, a bleaching regimen may be started 4–6 weeks before treatment.

6. *Recently tanned skin cannot be treated!* If treated within 2 weeks of active (natural sunlight or tanning booth) tanning, you may develop hypopigmentation (white spots) after treatment and this may not clear for 2–3 months or longer.

7. The use of self-tanning skin products must be discontinued 1 week before treatment. Any residual self-tanner should be removed prior to treatment.

Intratreatment care

1. The skin is cleaned and shaved prior to treatment. The use of a topical anesthetic is optional.

2. When treating the upper lip, the teeth may be protected with moist white gauze. The gauze also serves to support the lip during treatment, allowing a surface to push against.

3. The CCD (cryogen cooling device), will be used with the laser to cool the skin during treatment.

4. Safety considerations are important during the laser procedure. Protective eye wear will be worn by the patient and all personnel in the treatment room during the procedure to reduce the chance of damage to the eye. In addition, your provider will take all necessary precautions to ensure your safety.

Posttreatment care

1. Immediately after treatment, there should be erythema (redness) and edema (swelling) of each hair follicle in the treatment site, which may last up to 2 hours or longer. The erythema may last up to 2–3 days. The treated area will feel like a sunburn for a few hours after treatment.

2. Your provider may use an optional cooling method after treatment to ensure your comfort.

3. A topical soothing skin care product such as aloe vera gel may be applied following treatment if desired.

4. Makeup may be used immediately after the treatment as long as the skin is not irritated,

5. Avoid sun exposure to reduce the chance of hyperpigmentation (darker pigmentation).

6. Use sunblock (SPF 30+) at all times throughout the course of treatment.

7. Avoid picking or scratching the treated skin. Do not use any other hair removal treatment products or similar treatments (waxing, electrolysis, or tweezing) that will disturb the hair follicle in the treatment area for 4–6 weeks after the laser treatment is performed. Shaving is the preferred method.

8. Anywhere from 10–21 days after the treatment, shedding of the treated hair may occur and this appears as new hair growth. This is *not* new hair growth. You can clean and remove the hair by washing or wiping the area with a wet cloth or Loofa sponge.

9. After the axillae (underarms) are treated, you may wish to use a powder instead of a deodorant for 24 hours after the treatment to reduce skin irritation.

10. There are no restrictions on bathing except to treat the skin gently, as if you had a sunburn, for the first 24 hours.

11. Return to the office or call for an appointment at the first sign of the return of hair growth. This may be within 4–6 weeks for the upper body and possibly as long as 2–3 months for the lower body. Hair regrowth occurs at different rates on different areas of the body. New hair growth will not occur for *at least* 3 weeks after treatment.

12. Call your healthcare provider at _____ with any questions or concerns you may have.

Blistering is uncommon with laser hair removal, but test spots can be performed prior to definitive treatment if there is any question about the optimal treatment settings. If blistering occurs, the patient is instructed to apply ointment to the affected area to prevent drying and crusting. Patients should be followed carefully until they have completely recovered from the treatment. We recommend against shaving the treated area for ~ 1 to 3 days after treatment.

■ Expected Results

Most patients can expect at least a 50% reduction in hair after four to six treatments, with a success rate ranging from 50 to 90%.[1,11,13] There is a small subset of patients who achieve up to 95% reduction in hair, and another 5% of the population will note no change in hair growth. Unfortunately, it is not entirely clear what response a given individual will have prior to treatment. This is another benefit of first performing test spots. If there is inadequate hair reduction in the test spot area, the laser parameters can be adjusted and new test spots performed.

In an evidence-based review of 28 controlled trials of laser hair removal, Haedersdal and Wulf found good evidence for partial short-term hair removal at 6 months using the ruby, alexandrite, diode, and Nd:YAG lasers, as well as the IPL system.[11] Improved outcomes were seen when patients underwent a series of treatments instead of just one. Moreover, long-term (> 6 months) hair removal was found with the use of the lasers described earlier. In this meta-analysis, however, there was not good evidence for long-term hair removal using the IPL.[11]

Interestingly, patient satisfaction may not necessarily be purely tied to the amount of hair that remains at the treatment site. Instead, patients may also be happy with the length of the "hair-free" interval or the time it takes for the hair to regrow. If this is the case, then it would also be ideal to prolong the telogen phase of hair growth for those hairs that remain in the treatment area.[14] A reduction in coarseness in the remaining hairs could also be considered a successful treatment.[14]

Unfortunately, laser hair reduction does not work for all hair types. Since this technology depends on melanin as the target chromophore, any hair that is lacking or deficient in melanin, such as white or blond hair, does not respond well to treatment. Various treatments to address this problem have been investigated, none of which has had great success.

The addition of a liposomal melanin spray to light hairs has been tried.[14] In spite of a clinically significant improvement in the hair reduction with the liposomal melanin spray, the study concluded that this difference was not sufficient to offset the signifi-

cant cost and patient effort required.[15] Others have tried using topically applied carbon particles suspended in mineral oil, which is supposed to add pigment to the hair follicle.[15] Much of future research and advancements in this field may focus on this idea of adding an exogenous chromophore.

Adjunctive treatments to laser hair removal may also improve outcomes and patient satisfaction. Eflornithine hydrochloride cream 13.9% (Vaniqa, SkinMedica, Carlsbad, CA) is U.S. Food and Drug Administration (FDA) approved for the reduction of facial hair in women. It works by reducing the follicular cell growth rate, and hair will regrow after discontinuation of its use. However, concomitant use of eflornithine cream and laser hair reduction treatments demonstrated a statistically significant difference in the onset and degree of reduction of unwanted hair as compared with laser alone.[13]

■ Complications and Their Management

Complications associated with laser hair reduction treatment include erythema, hypo- or hyperpigmentation, blistering, and scarring. As discussed previously, performing a test spot prior to treatment may help to reduce the risk of complications. Temporary erythema is an expected result after laser hair treatment and should be expected to be seen for approximately 4 to 6 hours after treatment. If the patient is counseled appropriately prior to treatment, this redness should not be a significant issue.

The risk of other complications (blistering, pigment changes, and scarring) can be reduced by using the proper parameters during the laser treatment and adding a cooling system during treatment. Some physicians pretreat with 4% hydroquinone to try to reduce the risk of hyperpigmentation. Pigment issues are more likely to be seen in patients with higher Fitzpatrick skin types, so these patients should be made aware of the risks prior to treatment and advised about the importance of sun avoidance.

■ Conclusion

Over the past decade, we have been able to achieve safe reductions in hair growth in all skin types using laser hair removal. The use of lasers with longer wavelengths, such as the Nd:YAG, and using longer pulse widths have permitted the inclusion of patients with darker skin types to also pursue laser hair reduction. Cooling of the skin during treatment helps to reduce the risks of complications, such as blistering. In spite of these advancements, research still needs to be done to understand how to better remove hair with little to no melanin. When understood and used in a safe manner, laser hair removal is a useful addition to any aesthetic medical practice.

References

1. Hamilton MM, Dayan SH, Carniol PJ. Laser hair removal update. Facial Plast Surg 2001;17(3):219–222

2. Warner J, Weiner M, Gutowski KA. Laser hair removal. Clin Obstet Gynecol 2006;49(2):389–400

3. Wu EC, Wong BJF. Lasers and optical technologies in facial plastic surgery. Arch Facial Plast Surg 2008;10(6):381–390

4. Azziz R. The evaluation and management of hirsutism. Obstet Gynecol 2003;101(5 Pt 1):995–1007

5. Davoudi SM, Behnia F, Gorouhi F, et al. Comparison of long-pulsed alexandrite and Nd:YAG lasers, individually and in combination, for leg hair reduction: an assessor-blinded, randomized trial with 18 months of follow-up. Arch Dermatol 2008;144(10):1323–1327

6. Goldberg DJ. Laser hair removal. Dermatol Clin 2002;20(3):561–567

7. Zins JE, Alghoul M, Gonzalez AM, Strumble P. Self-reported outcome after diode laser hair removal. Ann Plast Surg 2008;60(3):233–238

8. Alster TS, Bryan H, Williams CM. Long-pulsed Nd:YAG laser-assisted hair removal in pigmented skin: a clinical and histological evaluation. Arch Dermatol 2001;137(7):885–889

9. Nottingham LK, Ries WR. Update on lasers in facial plastic surgery. Curr Opin Otolaryngol Head Neck Surg 2004;12(4):323–326

10. Medika Farma Ltd. Hair Reduction Protocol. Sciton Profile Laser Configuration Technical Manual. V4 7b

11. Haedersdal M, Wulf HC. Evidence-based review of hair removal using lasers and light sources. J Eur Acad Dermatol Venereol 2006;20(1):9–20

12. Fodor L, Carmi N, Fodor A, Ramon Y, Ullmann Y. Intense pulsed light for skin rejuvenation, hair removal, and vascular lesions: a patient satisfaction study and review of the literature. Ann Plast Surg 2009;62(4):345–349

13. Smith SR, Piacquadio DJ, Beger B, Littler C. Eflornithine cream combined with laser therapy in the management of unwanted facial hair growth in women: a randomized trial. Dermatol Surg 2006;32(10):1237–1243

14. Chana JS, Grobbelaar AO. The long-term results of ruby laser depilation in a consecutive series of 346 patients. Plast Reconstr Surg 2002;110(1):254–260

15. Sand M, Bechara FG, Sand D, Altmeyer P, Hoffmann KA. A randomized, controlled, double-blind study evaluating melanin-encapsulated liposomes as a chromophore for laser hair removal of blond, white, and gray hair. Ann Plast Surg 2007;58(5):551–554

14 Laser Treatment of Facial Scars

Arden Edwards, Jennifer L. MacGregor, and Tina S. Alster

Key Concepts

- Lasers interact with tissue chromophores (hemoglobin, water, and melanin) to selectively target cutaneous structures.

- Lasers induce tissue remodeling to smooth the contour of both hypertrophic (thickened) and atrophic (depressed) scars.

- The vascular-specific pulsed dye laser (PDL) is useful for hypertrophic scars, keloids, and erythematous traumatic and acne scars. The PDL can be combined with fractional laser resurfacing to maximize improvement in skin texture.

- Atrophic scars are best treated by resurfacing with nonablative or ablative lasers. Fractional resurfacing modalities are associated with shorter recovery times and lower risk of complications than nonfractional laser techniques. Clinical efficacy increases as repeat treatments are applied.

- Patients should be carefully selected and treated at appropriate intervals to ensure gradual improvement in their scars with low risk of complications. Meticulous attention to pre- and postoperative care is essential.

■ Introduction

Cutaneous injury from acne, surgery, trauma, or any inflammatory process may result in scarring and disfigurement. Most importantly, scars lower self-esteem and limit a patient's social interaction. Effective treatment for scars is essential because it can greatly improve a patient's quality of life. Treatments for scars have included various physical, chemical, and surgical options and, in the past few decades, laser technology has dramatically improved treatment outcomes for all types of cutaneous scars.

The first lasers used to resurface scars were continuous-wave argon, neodymium:yttrium-aluminum-garnet (Nd:YAG), and carbon dioxide (CO_2) systems. These devices resulted in an unacceptably high risk of tissue necrosis and scar recurrence. In the 1980s, pulsed lasers were developed that allowed for selective absorption of laser light by target chromophores (e.g., hemoglobin, melanin) in the skin to induce temperature-controlled, target-specific injury without damage to surrounding healthy tissue.[1] The first series of clinical studies published in the early 1990s showed sustained improvements in erythematous, hypertrophic scars and keloids using the pulsed dye laser (PDL).[2-6] Additionally, laser skin resurfacing with CO_2 and erbium systems has been used successfully over the past 15 years to improve atrophic scars and other textural abnormalities. Recent improvements in technology have introduced fractionated laser systems that deliver energy in microscopic columns within islands of nontreated skin, thereby maximizing clinical efficacy and improving the recovery time and side-effect profile of earlier pulsed laser skin resurfacing techniques.[7]

Several factors determine the outcome of scar treatment with lasers, notably the type, color, and anatomical location of the scar. Scars are broadly classified as atrophic, flat, hypertrophic, or keloidal. The degree of induration and underlying fibrosis varies, and colors can range from red, purple, and pink to white and brown hues. The scar type and color dictate the appropriate treatment modality, with resurfacing lasers targeting textural abnormalities and PDL systems addressing keloidal, hypertrophic, and erythematous scars. Scars located on the anterior chest, scapula, and mandible are notoriously difficult to treat due to their propensity for further fibrosis, as are patients with Fitzpatrick skin phototypes (SPT) IV through VI because of their susceptibility to dyspigmentation after laser treatment. Other important variables in laser scar revision include operator experience, realistic patient expectations, and compliance with pre- and postoperative care.

Background: Basic Science of Procedure

Cutaneous injury causing interruption of the epidermis, dermis, and/or subcutaneous tissue initiates a cascade of events to repair the wound. The three stages of wound repair are inflammation, proliferation (neoangiogenesis, granulation, reepithelialization), and remodeling or maturation.[8,9] The remodeling phase can last up to a year after initial injury and includes continuous synthesis, degradation, and reorientation of collagen fibers to develop the mature scar. Early wounds are composed of ~ 80% type III collagen and 20% type I collagen, whereas mature scars transition to ~ 80% type I collagen and only 20% type III collagen (similar to unwounded skin).[8,9] Both hypertrophic scars and keloids are results of abnormal fibroproliferative wound repair during the remodeling phase.[10] One important time-dependent cytokine that stimulates fibroblast proliferation and differentiation is fibroblast growth factor (FGF). FGF is upregulated early in the initial injury and quickly decreases to baseline. If it does not decrease, excessive proliferation and collagen production rates may lead to hypertrophic scarring or keloid formation.

There are several mechanisms by which the PDL treats hypertrophic scars and keloids. Kuo et al provide evidence that the 585 nm PDL alters signaling pathways involved with keloid formation by suppressing AP-1 transcription and transforming growth factor (TGF)-β_1 expression via the mitogen-activated protein kinase (MAPK) pathway, thus reducing the proliferation of fibroblasts and type III collagen deposition.[11-13] This induces keloid regression via fibroblast apoptosis during the remodeling phase of wound healing. The heat produced by the PDL may also result in collagenase release and the breakage of disulfide bonds, which initiates remodeling of collagen fibers.[6] By targeting hemoglobin, the PDL causes photothermolysis of the vasculature, leading to local hypoxia and decreased cell function. It has also been shown that mast cells are increased in scar tissue after PDL irradiation, which may account for significant scar remodeling attributed to the effect of histamine and interleukins on fibroblasts that could affect collagen metabolism.[5]

Early pulsed ablative CO_2 erbium lasers yielded impressive improvements in scars not only because of controlled tissue vaporization but because of the presence of residual thermal damage (RTD) that resulted from light penetration of 20 to 30 μm to ~ 100 to 150 μm into the dermis and by stimulation of collagen contracture, remodeling, and skin tightening.[14-17] Newer fractional laser technology delivers laser energy to regularly spaced microthermal zones (MTZs), or columns of skin, with intervening areas of nontreated skin, which initiates the cascade of collagen remodeling while leaving an adequate reservoir of healthy keratinocytes for rapid wound healing.[7] This technology allows delivery of ablative or nonablative wavelengths deep into the dermis (up to 1.5 mm) but maintains a more desirable safety profile by reducing the overall density (or percentage of tissue) treated.

Pertinent Anatomy

The skin is composed of the superficial epidermis; the dermal–epidermal junction, which anchors the epidermis to the deeper dermis; and the underlying subcutaneous (subdermal) fat. The epidermis consists of keratinocytes, melanocytes, and Langerhans cells, whereas the thicker dermis (~ 1 to 2 mm) is composed of mucopolysaccharides, collagen, elastin, and vasculature within a fibrous matrix. The other main components of the dermis are macrophages, fibroblasts, and dermal dendritic cells, which are responsible for inflammation and healing after disruption of the dermis or subcutaneous fat.

The interaction of lasers with tissue is explained by the theory of selective photothermolysis.[1] At a given wavelength, the energy is absorbed by a specific target, or chromophore, in the skin. The pulse duration (time over which the energy is delivered) must be long enough to adequately heat the target but short enough to prevent nonselective heating of surrounding structures. Three cutaneous chromophores govern these interactions—hemoglobin, water, and melanin.

Hemoglobin in the dermal blood vessels strongly absorbs 585, 595, and 1,064 nm wavelengths. The PDL reaches these dermal blood vessels adequately, and the longer-wavelength 1,064 nm Nd:YAG penetrates more deeply to reach larger vessels. Reduction in scar vasculature may reduce erythema, but PDL effects on dermal fibroblasts are likely more important for the treatment of scars than chromophore-specific vascular effects.[11-13] Laser resurfacing of textural abnormalities relies on absorption of laser energy by the chromophore water.[14-20] At laser wavelengths longer than 1,300 nm, there is strong absorption by water-containing tissue. Ablative wavelengths, such as the 2,940 nm erbium or the 10,600 nm CO_2 laser, vaporize skin, whereas nonablative wavelengths, such as the 1,550 nm erbium-doped laser fiber, heat the skin without vaporizing the epidermis.[7,21-23] Both ablative and nonablative lasers induce collagen remodeling to smooth the skin texture. Melanin is located in the basal layer of the epidermis and also in dermal melanophages or traumatic foreign bodies (e.g., gravel, gunpowder) that can be introduced into a scar during trauma. Quality-switched (Q-switched or QS) lasers that deliver short pulses of energy in the nanosecond range are most effective for the destruction of pigment at 694, 755, and 1,064 nm wavelengths.[24]

■ Patient Selection

Before laser treatment of scars, patients must have a complete skin examination as well as a full discussion of the range of laser techniques available. The ultimate treatment recommendation should be based on achieving the best clinical outcome with the lowest possible risk. It is also important to uncover personality traits and lifestyle characteristics that would influence the patient's candidacy for more aggressive procedures. Patients should be questioned about their activities of daily living, including work, childcare, and home responsibilities that could impact or interfere with the healing process. Those who cannot tolerate or schedule for a significant recovery period are better suited for nonablative laser treatments, even if clinical efficacy is somewhat compromised.

Careful assessment of Fitzpatrick SPT, anatomical location, and scar type is essential. Those with SPT IV through VI and scars on more sensitive locations (e.g., chest, scapula, mandible) are at higher risk of complication due to slower wound healing in these areas.[24,25] Finally, classification of scar type will ultimately dictate choice of laser modality. Patients with hypertrophic scars or keloids have scars that are red, thick, and firm. Hypertrophic scars remain confined to the area of original injury and may slowly improve over time, whereas keloids extend beyond the border of the lesion, causing distortion of the original wound. Histologically, keloids are characterized by a unique pattern of haphazard, thickened, hyalinized collagen bundles arranged in whorls. This pattern is attributed to an inherited alteration in fibroblast re-

sponse to stimuli and continued production of excessive collagen. Collagen fibers in hypertrophic scars are arranged parallel to the long axis of the inciting wounds.[10] The vascular-specific PDL remains the first-line laser for treatment of hypertrophic scars and keloids.[26–28] Several studies have shown remarkable improvements in scar color, height, pliability, texture, and symptomatology after one to several treatments using low energy densities and short pulse durations (**Fig. 14.1**).[2–6,29,30]

Atrophic scars appear as indentations in the skin, wrinkled depressions resembling "cigarette paper," or bulges where the subcutaneous fat herniates through the thinned dermis. These scars are the result of inadequate collagen replacement during the remodeling phase of wound healing. The goal of treatment for atrophic surgical and acne scars is to soften the scar borders and blend the texture with the surrounding skin. Acne scars are commonly atrophic and are best classified, according to the system described by Jacob et al,[31] into three types: rolling, boxcar, and icepick. Rolling scars are wide undulating depressions with sloping borders where the depression is often associated with deep fibrous tethering. Boxcar scars have sharply marginated borders with marked "step-offs," and icepick scars are narrow, tapered pits 1 to 2 mm in diameter. Deep boxcar and icepick scars are likely to require surgical revision in addition to laser resurfacing. The 10,600 nm CO_2 and 2,940 nm erbium:yttrium-aluminum-garnet (Er:YAG) lasers allow precise, controlled vaporization of superficial tissue and a deeper zone of RTD to stimulate neocollagenesis, thereby filling depressions and softening irregular scar borders.[14–20] Fractional devices, with their improved safety profile over pulsed ablative lasers, are currently the most popular systems used for resurfacing atrophic traumatic, surgical, or acne scars ▶ **Video 14.1**.[21–23,32–40] An overview of laser resurfacing and fractional devices is presented in **Tables 14.1** and **14.2**.

Prescar is a term used to describe early erythematous wounds in scar-prone skin. During the active healing phase, mild textural change is often present.

Table 14.1 The spectrum of nonfractional cutaneous laser resurfacing

	Ablative		Nonablative	
Laser	Wavelength (nm)	Laser	Wavelength(s) (nm)
CO_2	10,600	PDL	585–595
Erbium:YAG	2,940	KTP	532
Erbium:YSGG	2,790	Nd:YAG (Q-switched, long-pulsed)	1,064
		Nd:YAG (long-pulsed)	1,320
		Diode (long-pulsed)	1,450
		Erbium:glass	1,540

Abbreviations: CO_2, carbon dioxide; KTP, potassium-titanyl-phosphate; Nd, neodymium; PDL, pulsed dye laser; Q-switched, quality-switched; YAG, yttrium-aluminum-garnet; YSGG, yttrium-scandium-gallium-garnet.

Table 14.2 An overview of fractional laser devices

Manufacturer system (trade name)	Laser type	Wavelength (nm)
Ablative		
Alma Harmony High Power Pixel	Er:YAG	2,940
Pixel	CO_2	10,600
Pixel CO_2 Omnifit	CO_2	10,600
Candela QuadraLASE	CO_2	10,600
Cutera Pearl Fractional	YSGG	2,790
Cynosure SmartSkin	CO_2	10,600
Deka SmartXide DOT	CO_2	10,600
Eclipsemed Equinox CO_2 Fractional	CO_2	10,600
Ellipse Inc. Juvia	CO_2	10,600
Focus Medical NaturaLase Er Fractional	Er:YAG	2,940
Fotona SP Plus	Nd:YAG/Er:YAG	1,064/2,940
SP Dualis	Nd:YAG/Er:YAG	1,064/2,940
XS Dualis	Er:YAG	2,940
XS Fidelis	Er:YAG	2,940
Lasering Mixto SX	CO_2	10,600
Lumenis UltraPulse Active FX	CO_2	10,600
UltraPulse Deep FX	CO_2	10,600
Lutronic Mosaic	CO_2	10,600
	eCO_2	10,600
Palomar Lux 2,940	Er:YAG	2,940
Quantel EXEL O_2	CO_2	10,600
FX4 and FX12	Er:YAG	2,940
Sandstone Medical Matrix LS-25$_2$	CO	10,600
Sciton Profractional	Er:YAG	2,940
Sellas Cis F1	CO_2	10,600
Solta Medical Fraxel re:pair	CO_2	10,600
Nonablative		
Cynosure Affirm	Nd:YAG	1,440+/-1,320
Palomar Lux 1,540	Er:glass	1,540
Lux 1,440	Nd:YAG	1,440
Lux DeepIR	Infrared	850–1,350
Sellas True Fractional	Erbium fiber	1,550
Solta Medical Fraxel re:store	Erbium fiber	1,550
Fraxel re:store Dual	Erbium/Thulium	1,550/1,927

Abbreviations: CO_2, carbon dioxide; Er:YAG, erbium-doped yttrium-aluminum-garnet; Nd:YAG, neodymium-doped yttrium-aluminum-garnet; YSGG, yttrium-scandium-gallium-garnet.

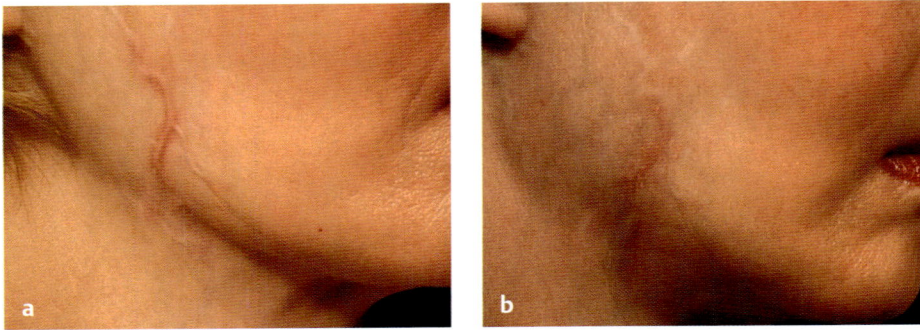

Fig. 14.1 Hypertrophic scar before **(a)** and after **(b)** 585 nm pulsed dye laser therapy.

These prescars have the potential to heal poorly and should be considered for intervention with early laser therapy.[28,29] The 585 nm PDL can be used to treat early scars (prescars) within the first few weeks after wounding. This system is also the treatment of choice for surgical sites, traumatic wounds, or ulcerations to improve the quality of scarring and to prevent excessive scar formation.[41–46] Studies confirm that scars treated early will ultimately heal more favorably than if left untreated.[29,41–43,45,47] New fractional laser systems may also be successful at preventing unfavorable scar formation in surgical patients starting on the day of suture removal.[48] Intraoperative vaporization of wound edges with either a CO_2 or an Er:YAG laser, before primary surgical closure, has also been reported to enhance cosmesis.[49]

■ Technical Aspects of Procedure

Pulsed Dye Laser

PDL is the treatment of choice for hypertrophic scars and keloids, as well as prescars and erythematous shallow boxcar-type acne scars. The 585 nm PDL is slightly superior to the 595 nm PDL for this purpose.[42] Although there appears to be no difference between the 0.45 and 1.5 millisecond pulse durations,[43] it is essential to use short pulse durations, low fluences, and longer treatment intervals (every 6 to 8 weeks) to avoid scar worsening or aggravation of the scar.[26]

Scar revision with the PDL is typically performed in an outpatient setting without anesthesia. If topical anesthesia is desired, a lidocaine-containing cream or gel can be applied to the areas to be treated 15 to 30 minutes before laser irradiation. The skin should be cleansed with soap and water to remove makeup, powder, or creams that could potentially interfere with laser penetration. Flammable solutions, such as alcohol, should be avoided, and skin must dry thoroughly before the procedure is initiated. Wet gauze may be used to protect hair-bearing areas during treatment and to protect nontargeted skin. All in-

dividuals present in the treatment room must wear protective eyewear capable of filtering the appropriate wavelength to avoid retinal damage.

The entire surface of the scar should be treated with adjacent, nonoverlapping laser pulses. The fluences chosen are determined by the skin phototype of the patient, the type of scar, and previous treatments applied to the area. In general, hypertrophic scars and keloids are treated with low-energy densities ranging from 6.0 to 7.5 J/cm^2 with a spot size of 5 or 7 mm and 4.0 to 5.5 J/cm^2 with a spot size of 10 mm.[26] Pulse durations ranging from 0.45 to 1.5 milliseconds are most effective.[43] Energy densities should be lowered by at least 0.5 J/cm^2 or more in patients with darker skin and for scars in more delicate or thin body locations (such as the chest or neck).[24,26] It is important to start treatments at the lowest effective energy and only increase when it appears that the outcome of previous treatments is suboptimal. Any concern regarding patient response to treatment should prompt a test spot or patch in a small area before irradiation of the entire lesion. If postoperative oozing, crusting, or vesiculation is observed, the fluence used on subsequent visits must be decreased and retreatment postponed until the skin has completely healed.

Adjunctive use of intralesional corticosteroids, 5-fluorouracil (5-FU) or surgical debulking should be considered for extremely thick (> 5 mm), nodular or rapidly proliferative scars. Use of adjunctive therapy should be considered early for large/aggressive scars because laser energy will not penetrate the lesion. Otherwise, PDL treatment alone has been shown to be sufficient.[30] Intralesional injections of corticosteroids (20 to 40 mg/mL triamcinolone) are more easily delivered immediately after (rather than before) laser irradiation because the treated scar becomes edematous (making infiltration easier). An additional consideration is that when steroid injection is performed before laser irradiation, the skin blanches, rendering the skin a potentially less amenable target for vascular-specific irradiation.

Keloids often require more treatment sessions to achieve significant improvement, but some may prove unresponsive altogether. The CO_2 laser has also been used to vaporize keloids, particularly on the earlobes and posterior neck, but scar recurrences are common.[50]

Laser Resurfacing

Successful recontouring of atrophic scars has been achieved with pulsed CO_2 or Er:YAG or erbium lasers,[14–20,25] and these have long been considered the gold standard for ablative laser skin resurfacing. The photothermal tissue effect of ablative lasers accounts for collagen shrinkage and stimulation of neocollagenesis, which leads to collagen remodeling, noticeable clinical skin tightening, and marked reduction of skin textural irregularities. Despite their well-proven clinical efficacy, they have been associated with prolonged recovery and risk of complications during healing.[51] Safer nonablative infrared devices were subsequently developed to thermally alter dermal collagen and induce its remodeling while preserving epidermal integrity. After a series of treatments, the nonablative 1,064 and 1,320 nm Nd:YAG and 1,450 nm diode laser systems have been shown to produce mild improvement in scars with virtually no postoperative recovery time.[52–59] Although the improved safety profile of nonablative resurfacing is a distinct advantage, the clinical improvement obtained is typically much less significant (**Fig. 14.2**).[60]

Both ablative and nonablative devices have been further improved in recent years by fractionated technology.[7] Ablative fractionated lasers can deliver excellent clinical results with decreased recovery rates (compared with pulsed lasers), whereas nonablative fractionated devices provide better clinical results than do their nonfractionated precursors and, once again, with minimal recovery time.[61] Fractionated nonablative wavelengths of 1,440, 1,540, and 1,550 nm are associated with mild to moderate discomfort that can generally be controlled with pretreatment application of topical anesthetic and intraoperative use of forced air cooling. Few patients require oral anxiolytics or analgesics for treatment. Prior to laser irradiation, all topical anesthetic cream should be removed and the skin thoroughly dried. Techniques

vary but generally involve a series of multiple-pass, full-facial treatments delivered at 4 to 6 week intervals. To penetrate to the deep sections of atrophic scars, energies should be increased to achieve maximum dermal depth (up to 1.5 mm),[61] and density should be increased gradually as tolerated. Increasing energy and density levels is recommended over the series of treatments if patients recover as expected (1 to 3 day recovery after facial treatment, up to 7 to 10 days after body treatment). Despite the relatively short recovery times, collagen remodeling and scar improvement continue for 6 to 12 months following a series of three or more monthly treatments (**Fig. 14.3**).[21,32]

For more fibrotic moderate-to-deep boxcar, atrophic, and icepick scars, or when more significant skin tightening is the goal, fractional ablative resurfacing is generally recommended (**Fig. 14.4**).[33–40] Systemic anxiolytics, analgesics, or twilight sedation is typically used for these more aggressive (and thus more painful) fractional ablative resurfacing procedures. Age-appropriate preoperative medical evaluation is required, and reliable transportation home after treatment must be arranged. Small, localized areas or single cosmetic units can be sufficiently infiltrated with local anesthetic infiltration prior to fractional ablative resurfacing, although caution is necessary when treating traumatic or burn scars on the extremities due to the risk of compartment syndrome. A smoke evacuator should be used to remove aerosolized debris, and surgical masks are also essential for operating personnel. External eye shields are sufficient for patient protection (with skin retraction and treatment over the bony orbital rim); however, if treatment is to be delivered within the orbital rim, placement of ocular metal shields is required. No flammable solutions or materials should be present in the laser field.

Prior to laser irradiation, the skin is prepped and dried, hair is secured, and Surgilube (Fougera, Melville, NY) is applied to protect the eyebrows and hairline. Test laser pulses should initially be fired on a dampened tongue depressor to ensure proper equipment functioning. The entire cutaneous surface is then treated using either a rolling or stamping handpiece. Multiple, nonoverlapping passes

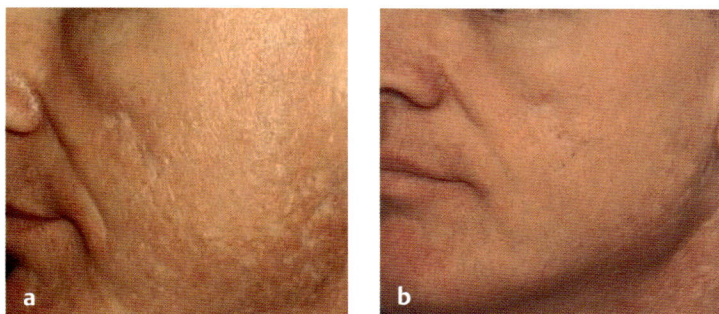

Fig. 14.2 Atrophic acne scarring before **(a)** and after **(b)** nonablative long-pulsed infrared (1,450 nm diode) laser resurfacing.

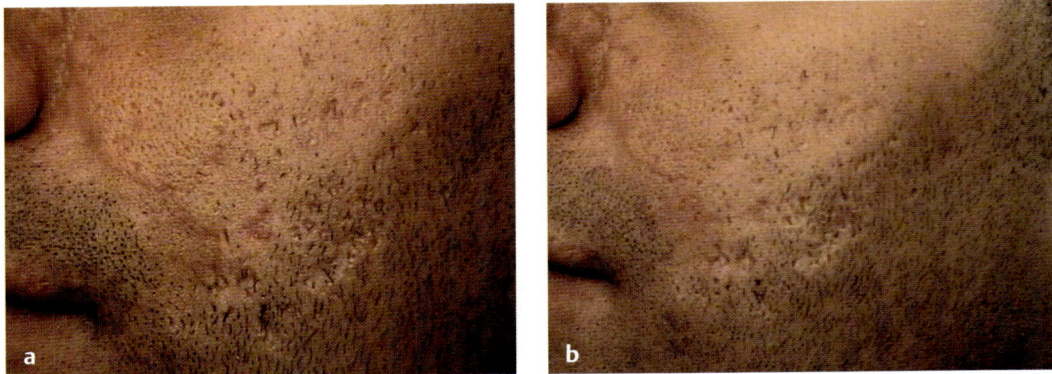

Fig. 14.3 Atrophic acne scarring before **(a)** and after **(b)** fractional nonablative (1,550 nm erbium-doped fiber) laser resurfacing.

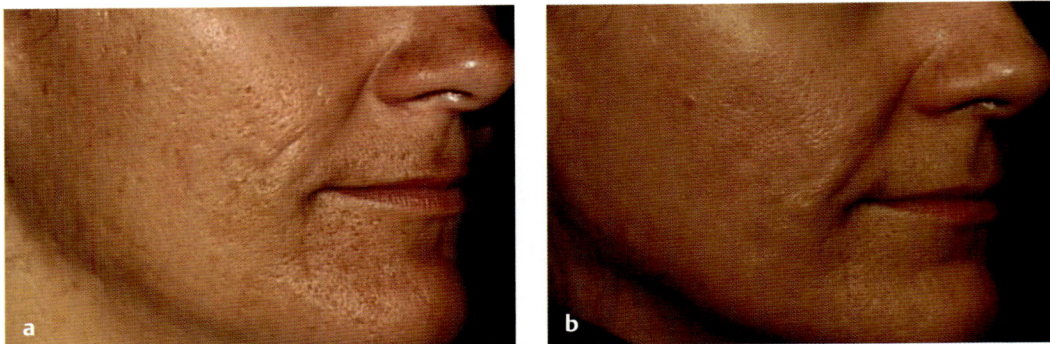

Fig. 14.4 Atrophic acne scarring before **(a)** and after **(b)** fractional ablative carbon dioxide laser resurfacing.

should be used to achieve the target treatment density. For example, 30% density might be achieved with three passes at 10% density to minimize areas of high-density overlap. Periorbital skin is treated with decreased fluences along with a Jaeger bone plate to protect the lashes and brows. The perioral area should be treated with the teeth covered with moist gauze to protect from laser-induced etching of dental enamel. The transition of the mandible to the neck should be feathered with a lower fluence and/or fewer passes to prevent a sharp demarcation line between treated and untreated skin. When treatment is complete, the patient is comforted with cool, moist gauze and forced air cooling or ice packs followed by the application of a petrolatum-based ointment.

Papular scars and those with sharply marginated borders can be sculpted using a pulsed (nonfractional) CO_2 laser with a small spot size. Many fractional devices have a handpiece for this purpose. Prior to treatment of the entire area, the focal sites are marked and sculpted with three to five passes until the scar surface is even with the surrounding skin. It is important for partially desiccated tissue

to be removed with saline- or water-soaked gauze between laser passes to avoid char formation. The development of char indicates excessive thermal damage, which can lead to unwanted tissue fibrosis or scarring; however, after the final laser pass, partially desiccated tissue can be left intact to serve as a biological wound dressing.[62]

■ Postoperative Care

After treatment with the PDL at settings effective for scars, there is often immediate mild to moderate purpura that resolves over the first week and transient erythema and edema that dissipate over 48 hours. After treatment, the skin is cooled and protected from the sun. The patient should be able to return to normal activities immediately and be reevaluated/retreated at 6 to 8 week intervals depending upon response.

Fractional nonablative resurfacing methods require minimal postoperative care.[63] Patients can expect variable amounts of erythema and edema lasting 1 to 3 days after the treatment. If patients have a history of recurrent herpes simplex virus outbreaks, empirical prophylaxis is prescribed for 3 to 7 days. Ice pack application every hour reduces posttreatment edema and aggressive sun protection of the treated area is necessary. Light-emitting diode irradiation has been shown to reduce postoperative erythema following nonablative procedures and can be a useful treatment adjunct.[64]

Recovery following fractional ablative resurfacing requires a clear understanding of postoperative care. Pain diminishes rapidly within the first postoperative hours, and only minimal discomfort is experienced thereafter. Water, saline, or dilute (0.25%) acetic acid–soaked compresses to the treated skin for 15 to 20 minutes assist in the removal of serous discharge and reduce crusting. Compress application should be repeated several times daily followed by a generous application of petrolatum-based ointment.[65,66] Icing regularly and maintaining head elevation helps to minimize edema, but in the case of severe edema, particularly when periorbital swelling is significant enough to impair vision, a 3 to 5 day course of systemic corticosteroids should be prescribed.[65,66] All patients are prescribed prophylactic antiviral medication.[65–68] The postoperative use of prophylactic antibiotics is controversial,[69] but most laser surgeons use intranasal mupirocin ointment and empirical systemic antibiotics for the first postoperative week.[65,66] After a few days, when reepithelialization is nearly complete, the transition from ointment to a cream-based moisturizer is possible. Depending on laser treatment parameters used, one or more follow-up visits are required during the first postoperative week, with regular (e.g., monthly) visits recommended until erythema resolves. Avid sun protection and good nutrition/sleep habits are essential during recovery.

■ Expected Results

Scars vary dramatically based on baseline thickness, pliability, color, growth rate, and individual patient characteristics. Well-designed randomized, controlled trials looking at scar improvement with laser therapy are scarce, and several different methods for evaluating and grading such improvement have been applied. Two scales commonly used to compare scars and quantify improvement include the quartile clinical grading scale and the Vancouver scar scale (**Tables 14.3** and **14.4**). Comparison of methods and predicting clinical improvement for a given patient are nearly impossible, but certain modalities produce clearly positive clinical effects. Patients must be aware that scar improvement is gradual, that multiple treatments applied over time produce the best

Table 14.3 Quartile grading system used for acne scarring

1	< 25% improvement
2	26–50% improvement
3	51–75% improvement
4	> 76% improvement

Table 14.4 Vancouver scar scale

Pigmentation

0	Normal color (resembles nearby skin)
1	Hypopigmentation
2	Hyperpigmentation

Vascularity

0	Normal
1	Pink (slight increase in blood supply)
2	Red (significant increase in local blood supply)
3	Purple (excessive local blood supply)

Pliability

0	Normal
1	Supple (flexible with minimal resistance)
2	Yielding (giving way to pressure)
3	Firm (solid/inflexible, not easily moved, resistant to manual pressure)
4	Banding (ropelike, blanches with extension of scar, does not limit range of motion)
5	Contracture (permanent shortening of scar producing deformity or distortion; limits range of motion)

Height

0	Normal (flat)
1	< 2 mm
2	> 2 mm and < 5 mm
3	> 5 mm

results, and that it is not possible to achieve complete scar eradication. Those with unrealistic expectations or a history of noncompliance should be regarded as poor treatment candidates. Finally, sequential high-quality clinical photographs are necessary to monitor progress and determine scar response.

Hypertrophic scars and keloids from a variety of causes typically respond well to treatment with the PDL.[2-6] A single treatment with the 585 nm PDL has been reported to confer more than 50% improvement, with additional improvement noted on subsequent treatments.[3] Several studies have demonstrated improvement in scars that are treated with the PDL starting on the day of suture removal.[29,41-43] Reported efficacy is based on overall improved cosmetic benefit as well as improvement in the parameters included in the Vancouver scar scale.[43,47] However, multiple treatments are typically needed for fresh surgical scars before an improvement over untreated scars can be appreciated.[45]

Pulsed ablative resurfacing using CO_2 or erbium wavelengths can produce dramatic improvements in facial scars,[16,18,19,70] but newer fractional devices have become even more popular due to their high clinical efficacy and enhanced safety profile.[33-40] Fractional resurfacing is most useful for the treatment of atrophic traumatic, surgical, and acne scars, as well as improving overall texture and color for all scar types.

Nonablative fractional photothermolysis is ideal for the treatment of shallow to moderately deep acne scars, as well as surgical and traumatic scars. In a study using a 1,550 nm erbium-doped fiber laser, 91% of patients with facial acne scarring were reported to have a 25 to 50% improvement after a single treatment, and 87% of patients who underwent a series of three monthly treatments had 51 to 75% improvement.[21] Results were maintained at 6 month follow-up. Another published study using similar laser parameters reported an average level of improvement of 41% after five treatments.[22] A post-treatment questionnaire revealed 100% of patients were satisfied with the treatment, and the perceived improvement was 48%. Following these initial studies, the technology was modified to deliver higher fluences and treatment densities, resulting in deeper dermal penetration. With the use of higher fluences, the majority of patients can achieve a 50 to 75% improvement in facial and back acne scarring.[32]

Nonablative fractional photothermolysis has also been reported to improve hypopigmented surgical scars and fresh surgical thyroidectomy scars.[71,72] The authors currently use nonablative fractional resurfacing alone or in combination with the 585 nm pulsed dye laser for all types of traumatic, burn, surgical, and acne scars (**Figs. 14.5** and **14.6**).

Fractional ablative skin resurfacing is also useful for treating acne scars, burn scars, traumatic and surgical scars. However, postoperative recovery is longer than that for nonablative treatment, though not as prolonged as after pulsed ablative treatment. Although no studies have directly compared the efficacy of nonablative and ablative skin resurfacing, several studies have reported significant textural improvement of moderate to severe acne scars in patients with various skin phototypes.[33-40]

For patients who are not appropriate candidates or are unable to undergo fractional skin resurfacing, nonablative resurfacing may be a suitable option. Mild improvements in acne scarring have been reported in several studies using various long-pulsed infrared (1,064 nm Nd:YAG, 1,320 nm Nd:YAG, 1,450 nm diode) lasers.[52-60] Of course, patients must be made aware that their clinical improvements will be modest compared with the aforementioned modalities.

■ Complications and Their Management

With careful planning and attention to detail, most complications can be prevented. **Table 14.5** summarizes potential complications and the strategies for prevention. Complications following nonablative laser surgery are typically transient and resolve without serious sequelae.[15,63] Fractional ablative resurfacing carries a lower risk of complications than pulsed ablative resurfacing, but complications still occur (**Table 14.6**).[61]

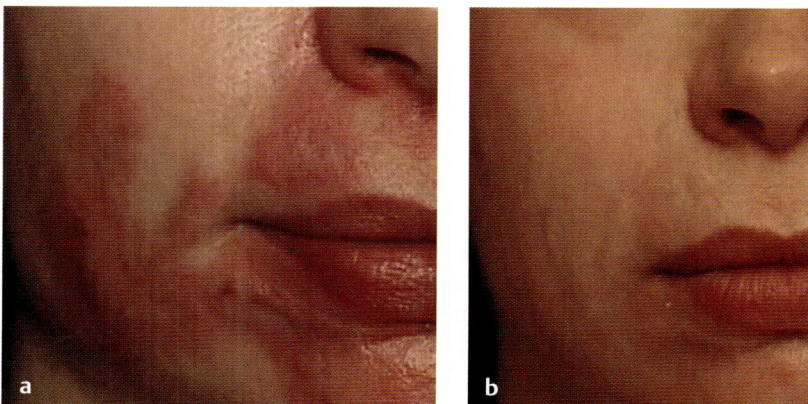

Fig. 14.5 Traumatic burn scars before **(a)** and after **(b)** combination treatment with 585 nm pulsed dye laser and fractional nonablative (1,550 nm erbium-doped fiber) laser resurfacing.

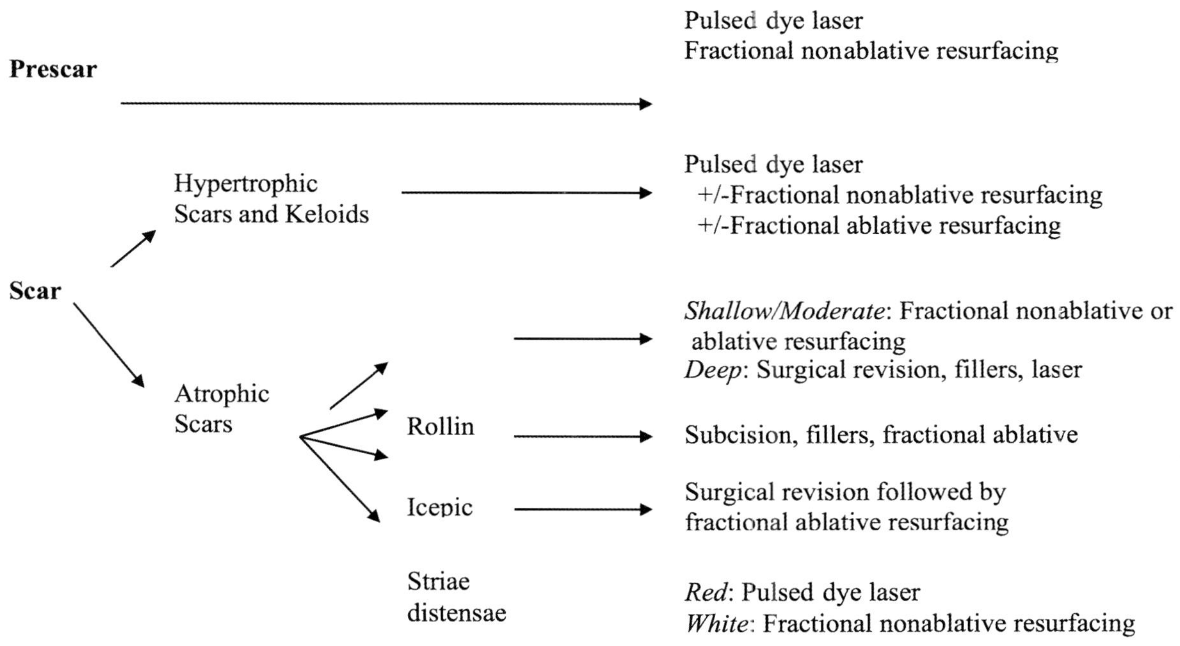

Fig. 14.6 Relating scar type to preferred laser treatments modality.

Postoperative erythema lasts ~ 2 to 3 days following fractional nonablative resurfacing and 3 to 4 weeks following fractional ablative resurfacing. Erythema lasting more than 4 days after fractional nonablative resurfacing is considered prolonged erythema and occurs in less than 1% of treatments.[63] Following fractional ablative resurfacing, prolonged erythema (lasting longer than 1 month) is more common but resolves within a few months. Treatment with a 590 nm wavelength light-emitting diode (LED) has been shown to reduce the intensity and duration of post-fractional laser erythema,[64] and the authors routinely administer this following facial treatment.

Postinflammatory hyperpigmentation occurs in 1 to 32% of patients following fractional laser resurfacing and is highly dependent on the wavelength, device, settings, and skin phototype of the patient.[61,63] The transient dyschromia is less common, less intense, and of shorter duration than that seen with pulsed (nonfractionated) ablative lasers.[51,61,63,65,66] In patients with darker skin phototypes at higher risk for developing this complication, lower treatment densities should be utilized and aggressive posttreatment sun protection should be advocated. Topical hydroquinone, retinoic, azaleic, ascorbic, and glycolic acid, as well as biweekly mild chemical peels can be used to hasten its resolution.

Hypopigmentation most commonly represents the relative color difference between lighter, treated skin and the adjacent photodamaged skin with actinic bronzing. The delayed hypopigmentation that was associated with pulsed (nonfractionated) CO_2 lasers has not been reported following fractional therapy, though it remains a potential risk with application of higher energies and more aggressive laser techniques.[51,61]

Acne and milia are common during the healing phase following laser resurfacing. Patients should have their acne well controlled prior to treatment, and those that are acne prone should be aware that a flare can occur during recovery. The incidence rate of acneiform eruptions (~ 2 to 10%) with fractional resurfacing is much lower than with older resurfacing lasers[61,63] and is likely related to the use of occlusive moisturizers in the postoperative period or to aberrant follicular epithelialization during the recovery process. Outbreaks should be treated with systemic antibiotics to prevent further scarring.

Dermatitis can occur after laser resurfacing of any type because of impaired epidermal barrier function. Most episodes of dermatitis resolve with discontinuance of the offending agents, but topical corticosteroids may be used to speed resolution in more severe cases.[61,63,73]

The incidence of viral, bacterial, and fungal infections is much lower following fractional resurfacing compared with pulsed and scanned ablative lasers.[51,61,63,67–69] Herpes simplex outbreak occurs in

Table 14.5 Preoperative considerations and prevention of complications

Darker skin phototype	Proper wavelength selection, caution regarding postinflammatory pigmentation risk, consider test area
History of herpes simplex virus	Antiviral prophylaxis[a]
Anticoagulant use	Discontinue 2 weeks prior to treatment for pulsed dye and ablative resurfacing
Acne prone	Empirical systemic therapy if recent history of inflammatory lesions, control acne before resurfacing
Smoking	Avoid or reduce smoking following ablative resurfacing
Dermatographism	Consider pretreatment with antihistamines
Rosacea	Consider vascular laser in combination, anticipate flare following resurfacing
Atopic history	Anticipate and control dermatitis
Psoriasis or vitiligo	Consider potential for Koebner phenomenon
Pregnancy/nursing	Delay procedure
Isotretinoin use	Delay treatment 6 months
Concurrent infection	Avoid laser treatment to affected area
Ectropion	Avoid ablative infraorbital treatment, caution in patients with lower blepharoplasty
Previous dermabrasion or phenol peel	Greater risk for poor healing and postoperative hypopigmentation, consider nonablative therapies
Seizures or migraine headache	Possible laser-induced trigger, avoid treatment with visible light wavelengths
Keloids or abnormal scarring	Greater scar risk, avoid ablative resurfacing (exceptions possible)
History of radiation or scleroderma	Greater risk for poor healing, avoid ablative resurfacing (exceptions possible)

[a] All patients (regardless of herpes simplex virus history) receive oral antiviral prophylaxis with perioral or full-face ablative laser resurfacing.

Table 14.6 Complications of ablative and fractional ablative laser resurfacing

Mild/transient	Moderate	Severe/prolonged
Prolonged erythema	Localized infection	True hypopigmentation
Postinflammatory hyperpigmentation	Topical anesthesia toxicity	Disseminated infection
Relative hypopigmentation	Eruptive keratoacanthomas	Scarring
Milia and acne exacerbation		Ectropion formation
Dermatitis		

0.3 to 2% of patients after fractional resurfacing.[61] Despite its low incidence, all patients should be prescribed an oral antiherpetic prior to fractional ablative laser resurfacing regardless of history. Bacterial infection is even more rare (0.1% infection rate); thus empirical antibiotic prophylaxis remains controversial.[69] Close and frequent postoperative follow-up is the best way to ensure early recognition and aggressive treatment of suspected infections and prevent unwanted scarring.

Scarring related to the resurfacing procedure is a potentially devastating complication. This can occur as a result of acne or infections in the postoperative period, but it can also be related to poor intraoperative technique involving excessively high energies, densities, overlapping passes, or a combination of these. Scattered reports of hypertrophic scars on the neck and chest have emerged following treatment with fractional ablative CO_2 laser resurfacing.[74-76] Regardless of the fractional device used, proper technique involves multiple nonoverlapping passes at very low density (5 to 10%). For higher-density treatments, multiple passes are applied in an attempt to reduce the density in small areas of overlap that can occur. This technique minimizes the risk of developing areas of high-density deep ablation that would ultimately induce a scar. Subtle raised areas, papules, or tender areas should raise suspicion of impending scar formation and treatment involves early initiation of corticosteroids and PDL irradiation.

Conclusion

The prognosis for all types of facial scars has improved dramatically with the development of new fractional laser technology. Pulsed dye 585 nm laser remains the preferred laser treatment for hypertrophic scars, keloids, and new surgical scars. Repeat treatments in series at 6 to 8 week intervals and combination therapy with fractional resurfacing enhance efficacy. Textural irregularities and atrophic scars are best treated with nonablative or ablative fractional resurfacing. Operator experience, appropriate patient selection, and meticulous pre- and postoperative care are crucial variables that ultimately determine treatment efficacy, patient satisfaction, and clinical outcome.

References

1. Anderson RR, Parrish JA. Selective photothermolysis: precise microsurgery by selective absorption of pulsed radiation. Science 1983;220(4596):524–527
2. Alster TS, Kurban AK, Grove GL, Grove MJ, Tan OT. Alteration of argon laser-induced scars by the pulsed dye laser. Lasers Surg Med 1993;13(3):368–373
3. Alster TS. Improvement of erythematous and hypertrophic scars by the 585-nm flashlamp-pumped pulsed dye laser. Ann Plast Surg 1994;32(2):186–190
4. Dierickx C, Goldman MP, Fitzpatrick RE. Laser treatment of erythematous/hypertrophic and pigmented scars in 26 patients. Plast Reconstr Surg 1995;95(1):84–90, discussion 91–92
5. Alster TS, Williams CM. Treatment of keloid sternotomy scars with 585 nm flashlamp-pumped pulsed-dye laser. Lancet 1995;345(8959):1198–1200
6. Alster TS, Nanni CA. Pulsed dye laser treatment of hypertrophic burn scars. Plast Reconstr Surg 1998;102(6):2190–2195
7. Manstein D, Herron GS, Sink RK, Tanner H, Anderson RR. Fractional photothermolysis: a new concept for cutaneous remodeling using microscopic patterns of thermal injury. Lasers Surg Med 2004;34(5):426–438
8. Schreml S, Szeimies R-M, Prantl L, Landthaler M, Babilas P. Wound healing in the 21st century. J Am Acad Dermatol 2010;63(5):866–881
9. Monaco JL, Lawrence WT. Acute wound healing an overview. Clin Plast Surg 2003;30(1):1–12
10. Wolfram D, Tzankov A, Pülzl P, Piza-Katzer H. Hypertrophic scars and keloids—a review of their pathophysiology, risk factors, and therapeutic management. Dermatol Surg 2009;35(2):171–181
11. Kuo YR, Wu WS, Wang FS. Flashlamp pulsed-dye laser suppressed TGF-beta1 expression and proliferation in cultured keloid fibroblasts is mediated by MAPK pathway. Lasers Surg Med 2007;39(4):358–364
12. Kuo YR, Wu WS, Jeng SF, et al. Activation of ERK and p38 kinase mediated keloid fibroblast apoptosis after flashlamp pulsed-dye laser treatment. Lasers Surg Med 2005;36(1):31–37
13. Kuo YR, Wu WS, Jeng SF, et al. Suppressed TGF-beta$_1$ expression is correlated with up-regulation of matrix metalloproteinase-13 in keloid regression after flashlamp pulsed-dye laser treatment. Lasers Surg Med 2005;36(1):38–42
14. Alster TS. Cutaneous resurfacing with CO_2 and erbium: YAG lasers: preoperative, intraoperative, and postoperative considerations. Plast Reconstr Surg 1999;103(2):619–632, discussion 633–634
15. Alster TS, Tanzi EL. Laser skin resurfacing: ablative and nonablative. In: Robinson J, Sengelman R, Siegel DM, Hanke CM, eds. Surgery of the Skin. Philadelphia, PA: Elsevier; 2005:611–624
16. Alster TS, West TB. Resurfacing of atrophic facial acne scars with a high-energy, pulsed carbon dioxide laser. Dermatol Surg 1996;22(2):151–154, discussion 154–155
17. Alexiades-Armenakas MR, Dover JS, Arndt KA. The spectrum of laser skin resurfacing: nonablative, fractional, and ablative laser resurfacing. J Am Acad Dermatol 2008;58(5):719–737, quiz 738–740
18. Walia S, Alster TS. Prolonged clinical and histologic effects from CO_2 laser resurfacing of atrophic acne scars. Dermatol Surg 1999;25(12):926–930
19. Tanzi EL, Alster TS. Treatment of atrophic facial acne scars with a dual-mode Er:YAG laser. Dermatol Surg 2002;28(7):551–555
20. Fitzpatrick RE, Rostan EF, Marchell N. Collagen tightening induced by carbon dioxide laser versus erbium: YAG laser. Lasers Surg Med 2000;27(5):395–403

21. Alster TS, Tanzi EL, Lazarus M. The use of fractional laser photothermolysis for the treatment of atrophic scars. Dermatol Surg 2007;33(3):295–299

22. Geronemus RG. Fractional photothermolysis: current and future applications. Lasers Surg Med 2006;38(3):169–176

23. Tanzi EL, Wanitphakdeedecha R, Alster TS. Fraxel laser indications and long-term follow-up. Aesthet Surg J 2008;28(6):675–678, discussion 679–680

24. Shah S, Alster TS. Laser treatment of dark skin: an updated review. Am J Clin Dermatol 2010;11(6):389–397

25. Alster TS, Tanzi EL. Hypertrophic scars and keloids: etiology and management. Am J Clin Dermatol 2003;4(4):235–243

26. Alster TS, Zaulyanov L. Laser scar revision: a review. Dermatol Surg 2007;33(2):131–140

27. Elsaie ML, Choudhary S. Lasers for scars: a review and evidence-based appraisal. J Drugs Dermatol 2010;9(11):1355–1362

28. Sobanko JF, Alster TS. Laser treatment for improvement and minimization of facial scars. Facial Plast Surg Clin North Am 2011;19(3):527–542

29. McCraw JB, McCraw JA, McMellin A, Bettencourt N. Prevention of unfavorable scars using early pulse dye laser treatments: a preliminary report. Ann Plast Surg 1999;42(1):7–14

30. Alster TS. Laser scar revision: comparison study of 585-nm pulsed dye laser with and without intralesional corticosteroids. Dermatol Surg 2003;29(1):25–29

31. Jacob CI, Dover JS, Kaminer MS. Acne scarring: a classification system and review of treatment options. J Am Acad Dermatol 2001;45(1):109–117

32. Chrastil B, Glaich AS, Goldberg LH, Friedman PM. Second-generation 1,550-nm fractional photothermolysis for the treatment of acne scars. Dermatol Surg 2008;34(10):1327–1332

33. Chapas AM, Brightman L, Sukal S, et al. Successful treatment of acneiform scarring with CO_2 ablative fractional resurfacing. Lasers Surg Med 2008;40(6):381–386

34. Tierney EP, Kouba DJ, Hanke CW. Review of fractional photothermolysis: treatment indications and efficacy. Dermatol Surg 2009;35(10):1445–1461

35. Hu S, Chen MC, Lee MC, Yang LC, Keoprasom N. Fractional resurfacing for the treatment of atrophic facial acne scars in Asian skin. Dermatol Surg 2009;35(5):826–832

36. Walgrave SE, Ortiz AE, MacFalls HT, et al. Evaluation of a novel fractional resurfacing device for treatment of acne scarring. Lasers Surg Med 2009;41(2):122–127

37. Cho SB, Lee SJ, Kang JM, Kim YK, Chung WS, Oh SH. The efficacy and safety of 10,600-nm carbon dioxide fractional laser for acne scars in Asian patients. Dermatol Surg 2009;35(12):1955–1961

38. Mahmoud BH, Srivastava D, Janiga JJ, Yang JJ, Lim HW, Ozog DM. Safety and efficacy of erbium-doped yttrium aluminum garnet fractionated laser for treatment of acne scars in type IV to VI skin. Dermatol Surg 2010;36(5):602–609

39. Weiss ET, Chapas A, Brightman L, et al. Successful treatment of atrophic postoperative and traumatic scarring with carbon dioxide ablative fractional resurfacing: quantitative volumetric scar improvement. Arch Dermatol 2010;146(2):133–140

40. Manuskiatti W, Triwongwaranat D, Varothai S, Eimpunth S, Wanitphakdeedecha R. Efficacy and safety of a carbon-dioxide ablative fractional resurfacing device for treatment of atrophic acne scars in Asians. J Am Acad Dermatol 2010;63(2):274–283

41. Nouri K, Jimenez GP, Harrison-Balestra C, Elgart GW. 585-nm pulsed dye laser in the treatment of surgical scars starting on the suture removal day. Dermatol Surg 2003;29(1):65–73, discussion 73

42. Nouri K, Rivas MP, Stevens M, et al. Comparison of the effectiveness of the pulsed dye laser 585 nm versus 595 nm in the treatment of new surgical scars. Lasers Med Sci 2009;24(5):801–810

43. Nouri K, Elsaie ML, Vejjabhinanta V, et al. Comparison of the effects of short- and long-pulse durations when using a 585-nm pulsed dye laser in the treatment of new surgical scars. Lasers Med Sci 2010;25(1):121–126

44. Bowes LE, Alster TS. Treatment of facial scarring and ulceration resulting from acne excoriée with 585-nm pulsed dye laser irradiation and cognitive psychotherapy. Dermatol Surg 2004;30(6):934–938

45. Alam M, Pon K, Van Laborde S, Kaminer MS, Arndt KA, Dover JS. Clinical effect of a single pulsed dye laser treatment of fresh surgical scars: randomized controlled trial. Dermatol Surg 2006;32(1):21–25

46. Chan HH, Wong DS, Ho WS, Lam LK, Wei W. The use of pulsed dye laser for the prevention and treatment of hypertrophic scars in Chinese persons. Dermatol Surg 2004;30(7):987–994, discussion 994

47. Conologue TD, Norwood C. Treatment of surgical scars with the cryogen-cooled 595 nm pulsed dye laser starting on the day of suture removal. Dermatol Surg 2006;32(1):13–20

48. Jung JY, Jeong JJ, Roh HJ, et al. Early postoperative treatment of thyroidectomy scars using a fractional carbon dioxide laser. Dermatol Surg 2011;37(2):217–223

49. Stefani WA. Minimizing scars with excision and immediate laser resurfacing. Aesthet Surg J 1998;18(5):342–345

50. Apfelberg DB, Maser MR, White DN, Lash H. Failure of carbon dioxide laser excision of keloids. Lasers Surg Med 1989;9(4):382–388

51. Nanni CA, Alster TS. Complications of carbon dioxide laser resurfacing: an evaluation of 500 patients. Dermatol Surg 1998;24(3):315–320

52. Rogachefsky AS, Hussain M, Goldberg DJ. Atrophic and a mixed pattern of acne scars improved with a 1320-nm Nd:YAG laser. Dermatol Surg 2003;29(9):904–908

53. Tanzi EL, Alster TS. Comparison of a 1450-nm diode laser and a 1320-nm Nd:YAG laser in the treatment of atrophic facial scars: a prospective clinical and histologic study. Dermatol Surg 2004;30(2 Pt 1):152–157

54. Sadick NS, Schecter AK. A preliminary study of utilization of the 1320-nm Nd:YAG laser for the treatment of acne scarring. Dermatol Surg 2004;30(7):995–1000

55. Fournier N, Mordon S. Nonablative remodeling with a 1,540 nm erbium:glass laser. Dermatol Surg 2005;31(9 Pt 2):1227–1235, discussion 1236

56. Lipper GM, Perez M. Nonablative acne scar reduction after a series of treatments with a short-pulsed 1,064-nm neodymium:YAG laser. Dermatol Surg 2006;32(8):998–1006

57. Keller R, Belda Júnior W, Valente NYS, Rodrigues CJ. Nonablative 1,064-nm Nd:YAG laser for treating atrophic facial

acne scars: histologic and clinical analysis. Dermatol Surg 2007;33(12):1470–1476

58. Chua SH, Ang P, Khoo LS, Goh CL. Nonablative 1450-nm diode laser in the treatment of facial atrophic acne scars in type IV to V Asian skin: a prospective clinical study. Dermatol Surg 2004;30(10):1287–1291

59. Friedman PM, Jih MH, Skover GR, Payonk GS, Kimyai-Asadi A, Geronemus RG. Treatment of atrophic facial acne scars with the 1064-nm Q-switched Nd:YAG laser: six-month follow-up study. Arch Dermatol 2004;140(11):1337–1341

60. Bhatia AC, Dover JS, Arndt KA, Stewart B, Alam M. Patient satisfaction and reported long-term therapeutic efficacy associated with 1,320 nm Nd:YAG laser treatment of acne scarring and photoaging. Dermatol Surg 2006;32(3):346–352

61. Metelitsa AI, Alster TS. Fractionated laser skin resurfacing treatment complications: a review. Dermatol Surg 2010;36(3):299–306

62. Bedi VP, Chan KF, Sink RK, et al. The effects of pulse energy variations on the dimensions of microscopic thermal treatment zones in nonablative fractional resurfacing. Lasers Surg Med 2007;39(2):145–155

63. Graber EM, Tanzi EL, Alster TS. Side effects and complications of fractional laser photothermolysis: experience with 961 treatments. Dermatol Surg 2008;34(3):301–305, discussion 305–307

64. Alster TS, Wanitphakdeedecha R. Improvement of post-fractional laser erythema with light-emitting diode photomodulation. Dermatol Surg 2009;35(5):813–815

65. Horton S, Alster TS. Preoperative and postoperative considerations for carbon dioxide laser resurfacing. Cutis 1999;64(6):399–406

66. Alster TS, Lupton JR. Prevention and treatment of side effects and complications of cutaneous laser resurfacing. Plast Reconstr Surg 2002;109(1):308–316, discussion 317–318

67. Alster TS, Nanni CA. Famciclovir prophylaxis of herpes simplex virus reactivation after laser skin resurfacing. Dermatol Surg 1999;25(3):242–246

68. Beeson WH, Rachel JD. Valacyclovir prophylaxis for herpes simplex virus infection or infection recurrence following laser skin resurfacing. Dermatol Surg 2002;28(4):331–336

69. Walia S, Alster TS. Cutaneous CO$_2$ laser resurfacing infection rate with and without prophylactic antibiotics. Dermatol Surg 1999;25(1):857–861

70. Woo SH, Park JH, Kye YC. Resurfacing of different types of facial acne scar with short-pulsed, variable-pulsed, and dual-mode Er:YAG laser. Dermatol Surg 2004;30(4 Pt 1):488–493

71. Glaich AS, Rahman Z, Goldberg LH, Friedman PM. Fractional resurfacing for the treatment of hypopigmented scars: a pilot study. Dermatol Surg 2007;33(3):289–294, discussion 293–294

72. Choe JH, Park YL, Kim BJ, et al. Prevention of thyroidectomy scar using a new 1,550-nm fractional erbium-glass laser. Dermatol Surg 2009;35(8):1199–1205

73. Fisher AA. Lasers and allergic contact dermatitis to topical antibiotics, with particular reference to Bacitracin. Cutis 1996;58(4):252–254

74. Ross RB, Spencer J. Scarring and persistent erythema after fractionated ablative CO$_2$ laser resurfacing. J Drugs Dermatol 2008;7(11):1072–1073

75. Fife DJ, Fitzpatrick RE, Zachary CB. Complications of fractional CO$_2$ laser resurfacing: four cases. Lasers Surg Med 2009;41(3):179–184

76. Avram MM, Tope WD, Yu T, Szachowicz E, Nelson JS. Hypertrophic scarring of the neck following ablative fractional carbon dioxide laser resurfacing. Lasers Surg Med 2009;41(3):185–188

15 Surgical Treatment of Facial Scars

Maurice Khosh

Key Concepts

- Scarring occurs when injury extends to the deep dermis.

- Unfavorable scar characteristics include excessive width, unfavorable depth, excessive length, and orientation inconsistent with underlying relaxed skin tension lines (RSTLs).

- There are several surgical techniques and technologies that can be used to improve an unfavorable scar.

■ Introduction

Injury to, or disruption of, the deep dermis will result in the formation of scar as the skin heals. The scar appearance following wound healing depends on multiple factors, including genetic predisposition, age of the patient, direction of the scar, depth of the scar and associated tissue loss, technique of wound closure, and wound healing complications, such as infection. The goal in primary wound closure or secondary scar revision is minimizing and camouflaging the scar. The patient should be made aware that plastic surgery will not eliminate scars entirely, but it will help to make them less perceptible.

■ Background: Basic Science of Procedure

Scar formation is the process by which skin heals after injury in the deep layer of the dermis. Epidermal and papillary dermal injuries typically heal without scar formation. When skin injury extends to the deep papillary and reticular dermis, fibroblastic activity and collagen formation result in a scar. Normal wound healing can be categorized into three phases: inflammatory, transitional repair, and maturation. During the inflammatory phase of wound healing, an initial vasoconstriction is followed by vasodilatation secondary to histamine release. White blood cell migration into the site of injury will lead to phagocytosis of necrotic tissue, neoangiogenesis, and fibroblast stimulation.

The transitional repair phase or the fibroblastic phase usually begins a few days after the injury and lasts 4 weeks. Fibroblasts migrate to the site of injury and begin to produce collagen. Inflammation, continued collagen production, and cross-linkage of collagen fibers result in formation of thick, inelastic scar tissue. Some fibroblasts evolve into myofibroblasts, which express smooth muscle actin (s-SMA), causing tissue contraction. Myofibroblasts generally disappear from wounds within 1 month; their persistence has been noted in abnormal wound healing, such as keloids and hypertrophic scars. The final phase, maturation, begins 6 to 12 weeks after injury. During this period, the healing process is a mixture of new collagen formation and breakdown of old collagen.[1]

Nearly all scars improve as they mature over a period of 1 year. During the first 6 months, the most significant improvements occur, and the initial scar erythema tends to subside within this period. The scar itself becomes less indurated and softer, allowing better mobilization of the tissues in its vicinity. Scar hypertrophy often improves within a year. The timing of scar revision should take these factors into consideration. Unfavorable scar characteristics that can be improved by scar revision include the direction of the scar, the width of the scar, and the length of the scar, as well as other negative attributes, such as webbing and bowstringing. In general, scars that are greater than 2 cm in length and 2 mm in width may be improved by scar revision.

■ Pertinent Anatomy

The camouflage of facial scars is most effective when scars can be aligned with the relaxed skin tension lines (RSTLs) or at the junction of the aesthetic subunits of the face. The RSTLs are generally perpendicular to the direction of the facial mimetic muscles. In older patients, the RSTLs are easily visible at rest; younger individuals need to be asked to make facial expressions to demonstrate the direction of the RSTLs. In the forehead and lower neck, the RSTLs are horizontal. In the crow's feet and around the mouth, the lines are radial in direction. The lines are tangential in the cheeks and the lower eyelid region (**Fig. 15.1**).[2]

Aesthetic facial units comprise the different features of the face with unique color, texture, and topography. Certain facial units can then be divided into subunits based on skin thickness and anatomical topography. Scars that are located along anatomical facial subunits are less noticeable (**Fig. 15.2**).

■ Patient Selection

Facial scars are especially distressing to patients because they cannot be covered with clothing. Women who wear makeup can camouflage scars to a certain degree. Facial scars may be noticeable due to their width, orientation, and distortion of facial features. The ideal facial scar is narrow, flat, and a good color match to surrounding tissues, and it does not distort adjacent anatomy. The scar is preferably aligned with the RSTLs or located at the junction of facial subunits. Prior to the start of treatment, the treating physician should present the options and outline the possible need for multiple procedures. The limitations of scar revision need to be discussed so that the patient can have realistic expectations of treatment.

Additionally, patients who seek scar revision may have suffered psychological trauma from the accident or the assault that caused the injury. In most instances, passage of time will allow the patient to adjust psychologically to the presence of a scar. However, when there are signs of a posttraumatic disorder, the patient should be evaluated and treated by a qualified mental health professional, because healthy psychological adjustment will allow the patient to better cope with recovery from scar revision.

■ Technical Aspects of Procedure

The scar revision options to be presented can be used serially or concurrently. Generally, surgical scar revision is followed by nonsurgical scar revision maneuvers. Scar revision should result in minimal tension at the wound edges because wound tension increases the risk of scar hypertrophy or keloid formation.

Surgical Scar Revision

During surgical scar revision, anesthesia choice is dependent on the extent of the procedure, the age of the patient, and the level of anxiety. Most scar revisions

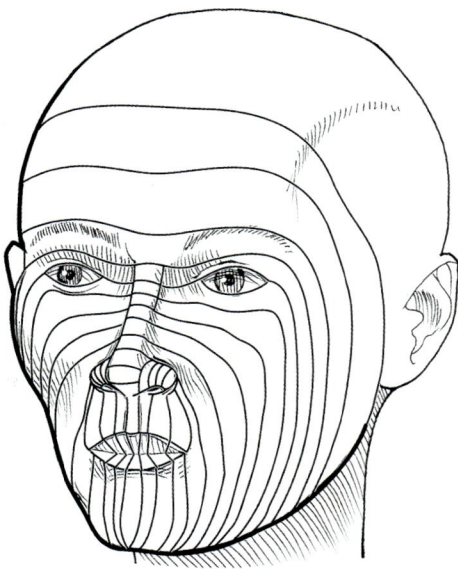

Fig. 15.1 Relaxed skin tension lines (RSTLs) in the face.

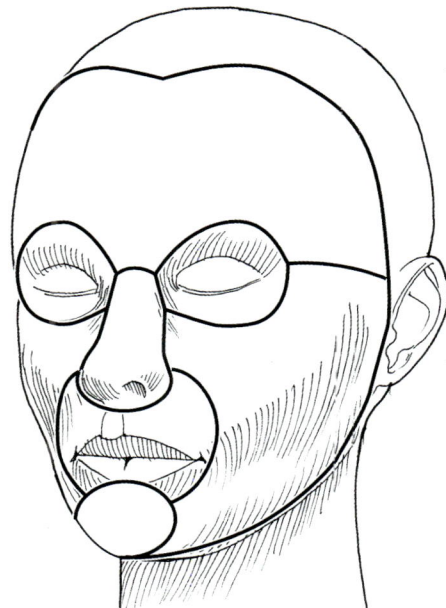

Fig. 15.2 Aesthetic facial subunits.

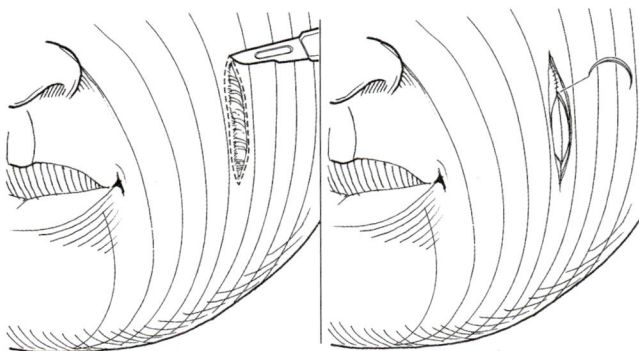

Fig. 15.3 Scar revision by incision parallel to the relaxed skin tension line.

can be safely and comfortably performed under local anesthesia utilizing 1% lidocaine with 1:100,000 epinephrine. In children or anxious patients, general anesthesia or monitored sedation is more appropriate. Prior to infiltration of local anesthesia, the surgical incisions, the RSTLs, and the borders of the facial subunits should be marked with a surgical marker because infiltration of local anesthesia can distort normal anatomy.

Proper instrumentation, including fine tissue forceps, single and double hooks, and delicate scissors and needle drivers, facilitate nontraumatic tissue handling during facial scar revision. Minimal use of cautery is also advised in an attempt to preserve maximal blood supply to the wound edges. Plastic surgical techniques of minimal tissue injury, appropriate wound undermining, layered skin closure, and effective wound dressing should always be used in facial scar revisions.[3]

Direct Excision

Wide scars can be appreciably improved by simple scar excision and skin repair. The scar is removed in fusiform fashion and wound edges are undermined in a subdermal plane. The incision is then repaired in a layered fashion, resulting in a more refined scar. This simple technique is especially useful in treating traumatic scars that are parallel to the RSTLs (**Fig. 15.3**).

In wider scars where fusiform excision would create a wide defect that would be difficult to close directly, serial excision may be used. Serial excision is often used in removal of large, nonmalignant skin lesions. In this technique, a smaller central portion of the scar is removed, and the narrower scar is allowed to heal. Secondary or tertiary excisions will then be performed to remove the entire scar and allow closure under minimal tension. In **Fig. 15.4**, the patient had a tracheotomy scar healed with an excellent result by following the relaxed tension lines of the inferior cervical regions.

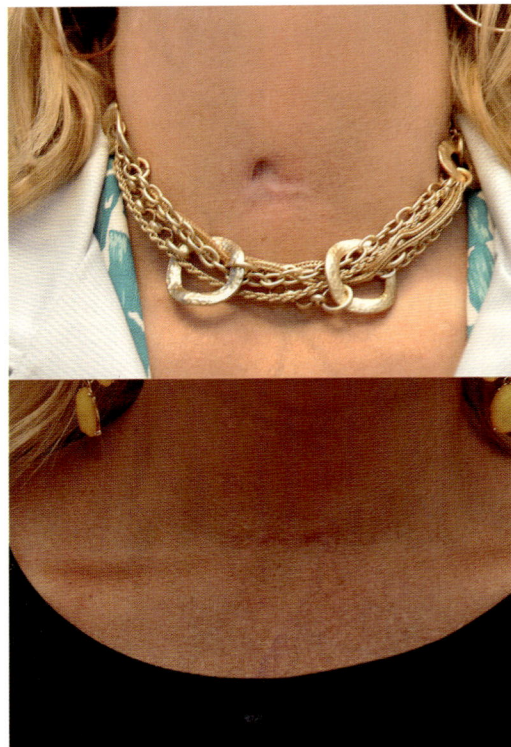

Fig. 15.4 Revision of a tracheotomy scar treated by direct excision.

Z-plasty

Z-plasty is a double transposition flap designed to reorient the direction, increase the length, and disrupt the linear appearance of a scar. Z-plasty is used to treat scars that cross the RSTLs by redirecting the central limb of the scar along the RSTL. This scar revision technique is especially effective in treating contracted scars that cross anatomical subunits, such as the eyelid, medial canthus, vermilion of the lip, or oral commissure.

Z-plasty is accomplished by designing two triangular transposition flaps with a common central limb along the scar. The angle between the central limb and the lateral limb of the triangular flaps is associated to the increase in the length of the scar. Classic z-plasty with a 60-degree angle will increase the length of the scar by 75%. Z-plasties with 45- and 30-degree angles produce 50% or 25% increases in scar lengths, respectively (**Fig. 15.5**).

The design of a z-plasty requires careful analysis and planning. The triangular flaps can be designed in two ways based on the direction of the lateral limbs. The two flap designs are mirror images of one another. The RSTLs have to be studied to decide which design will result in the most aesthetic result once the flaps have been transposed. The flap design should

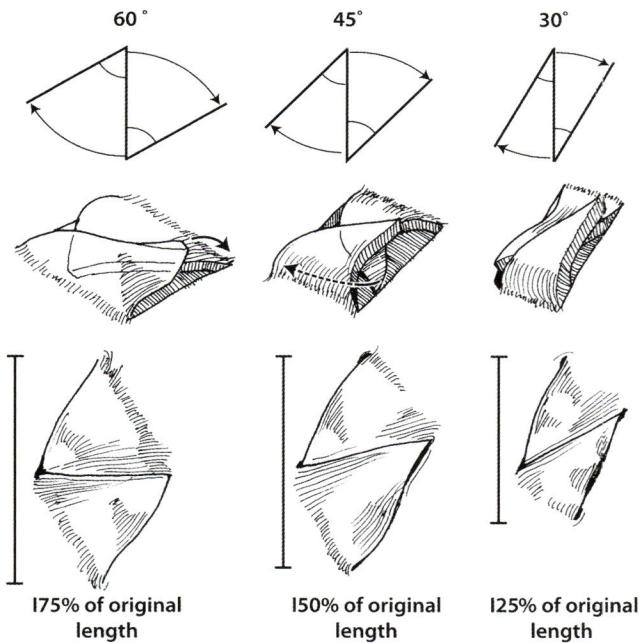

Fig. 15.5 Schematic representation of a z-plasty. Note that the angle of the flap design will impact the gain in length.

then be marked on the skin before infiltration of local anesthetic (**Fig. 15.6a,b**). Once the incisions are made, skin should be undermined widely to allow for transposition of the flaps with minimal tension. Temporary anchoring sutures at the tips of flaps should then be replaced with final sutures. Layered closure of the flaps can be performed when appropriate.

Multiple Z-plasties

The lateral limbs of a z-plasty are typically designed to equal the length of the central limb. The lateral z-plasty limbs can be designed to be shorter if the scar is divided into two or more segments. Multiple z-plasties are useful when long lateral limbs of a standard z-plasty would be too obvious or would violate borders of anatomical subunits. Multiple z-plasties are also used at the perimeter of trapdoor deformities to equalize the height of tissues and redistribute tension. The principles of design and execution for multiple z-plasties are similar to the standard z-plasty technique (**Figs. 15.7** and **15.8a–c**).

W-plasty

Long linear scars that are not parallel to RSTLs are more conspicuous. To make the scar less visible, the straight line can be broken into smaller slanted incisions with techniques known as w-plasty and geometric broken line closure. In w-plasty, small triangular flaps are designed on opposite aspects of the scar. The tissue between the triangles is removed, and the apex of each triangle is placed at the base of the triangle on the opposing side of the scar (**Fig. 15.9**). Unlike z-plasty, w-plasty does not increase the length of a scar. Because w-plasty removes some normal skin, the technique may not be appropriate when there is a dearth of normal skin in the area of the scar.

Geometric Broken Line Closure

Geometric broken line closure is another technique for breaking up a linear scar. Theoretically, geometric broken line closure has an advantage over w-plasty in that the resultant scar is more irregular in its pattern and therefore, less noticeable to the eye. In practice however, the two techniques result in similar outcomes and can be used interchangeably. Geometric broken line closure is more difficult to execute because the various geometric shapes must be matched exactly on the two sides of the scar (**Fig. 15.10**).

Skin Grafts and Flaps

In larger scars that result in more significant facial deformities, other surgical techniques may be necessary. Scar removal and skin grafting may be appro-

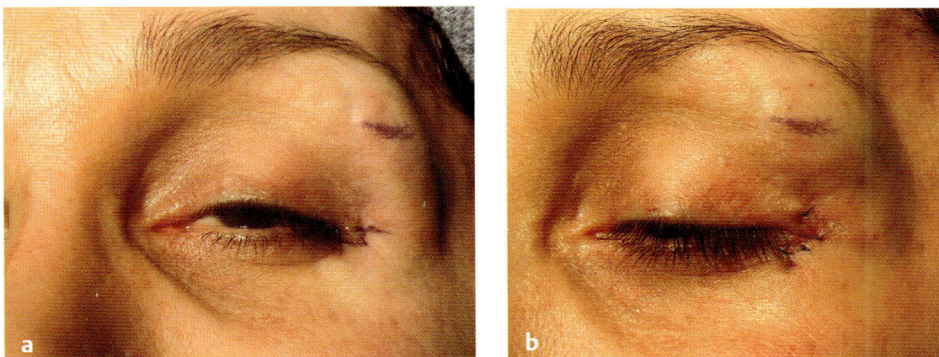

Fig. 15.6 Z-plasty used to treat a webbed canthal lateral scar in the lateral canthus of the left eye. **(a)** Z-plasty planning. **(b)** Final result after rearrangement of the z-plasty triangular flaps.

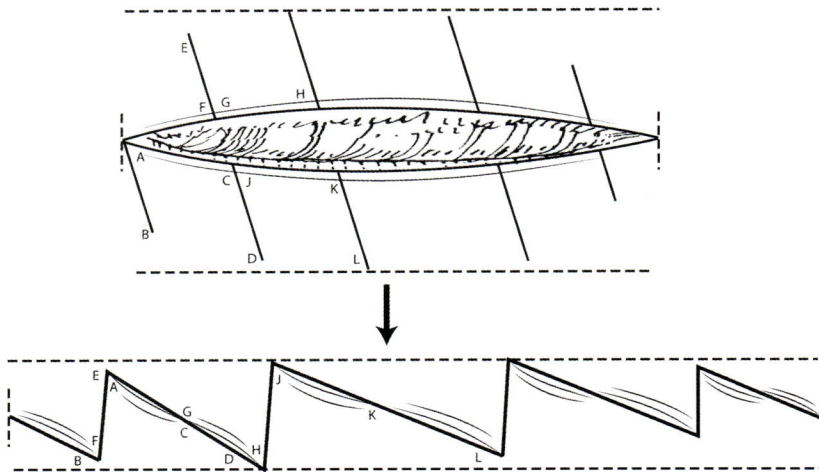

Fig. 15.7 Schematic representation of multiple z-plasties.

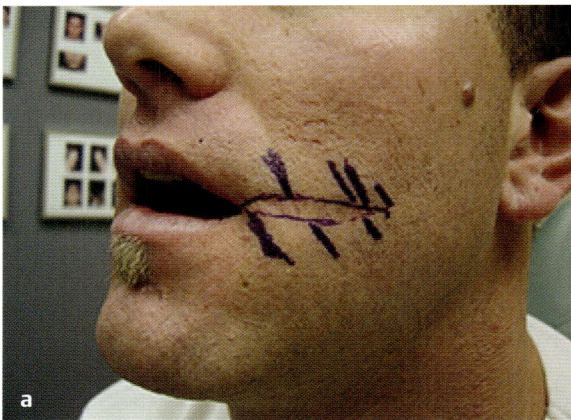

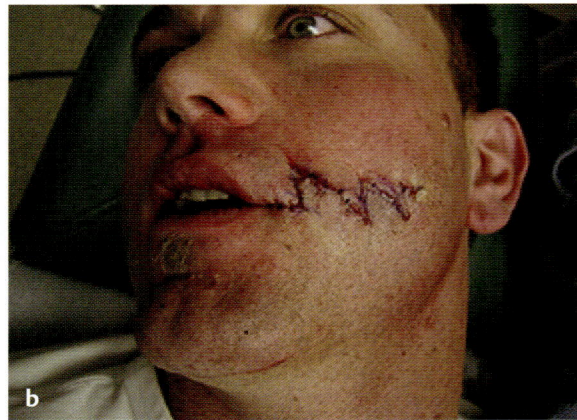

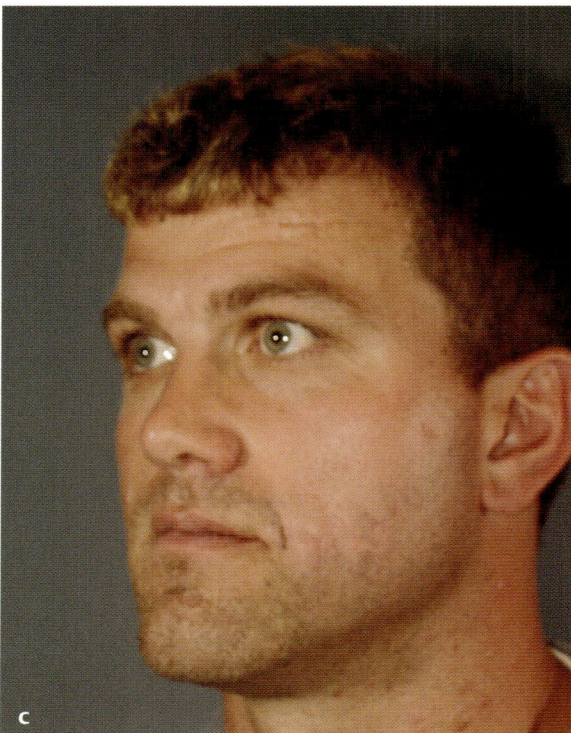

Fig. 15.8 Multiple z-plasties used to treat a traumatic scar extending from the oral commissure. **(a)** Horizontal scar violating the relaxed skin tension lines. **(b)** Multiple z-plasties completed. **(c)** Long-term result.

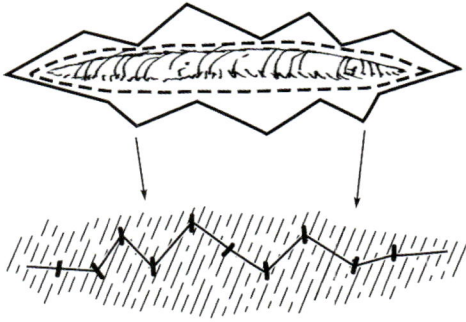

Fig. 15.9 Schematic representation of a w-plasty.

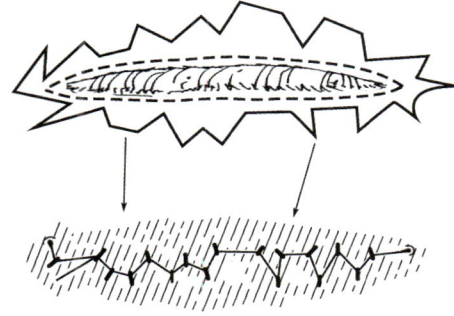

Fig. 15.10 Schematic representation of a geometric broken-line closure.

priate for burn victims or older patients who cannot tolerate longer procedure times or the need for general anesthesia. Skin grafts may be disadvantageous due to their poor skin color or thickness match. Full-thickness grafts exhibit less contracture and appear more natural on the face; split-thickness skin grafts should only be used when an adequate donor site for a full-thickness graft is not available. Full-thickness skin graft donor sites should be chosen as close to the face as possible for best color and texture match. The postauricular and supraclavicular regions represent good donor sites for skin graft harvest.

Tissue transfer techniques may be suitable for wide or distorting scars that are not candidates for the more minor treatment options yet to be presented. Local rotation-advancement flaps or transposition flaps provide additional skin where soft tissue loss and increased wound tension have contributed to undesirable scar formation. Because local flaps necessitate additional incisions, the flap borders must be carefully designed to minimize their visibility.

Flap design should incorporate the incisions into RSTLs or the borders of the facial subunits. During the preoperative consultation, the location and extent of the flap incisions should be clearly discussed with the patient, and the treatment rationale explained (**Fig. 15.11a,b**).

In rare circumstances, scars are unsightly due to extensive tissue loss, and local skin flaps do not provide adequate soft tissue supply. Tissue expansion is an excellent technique in these scenarios. After selection of an appropriately sized and configured expander, the expander is placed through an incision that can be utilized during the secondary reconstruction. The expander is then serially injected during repeated office visits until the desired expansion is achieved. During a second surgical procedure, the expander is removed and the stretched tissue is used as a skin flap to replace missing or scarred tissue (**Fig. 15.12a–c**). Regional flaps or microvascular free tissue transfers may be used as alternatives to tissue expansion.

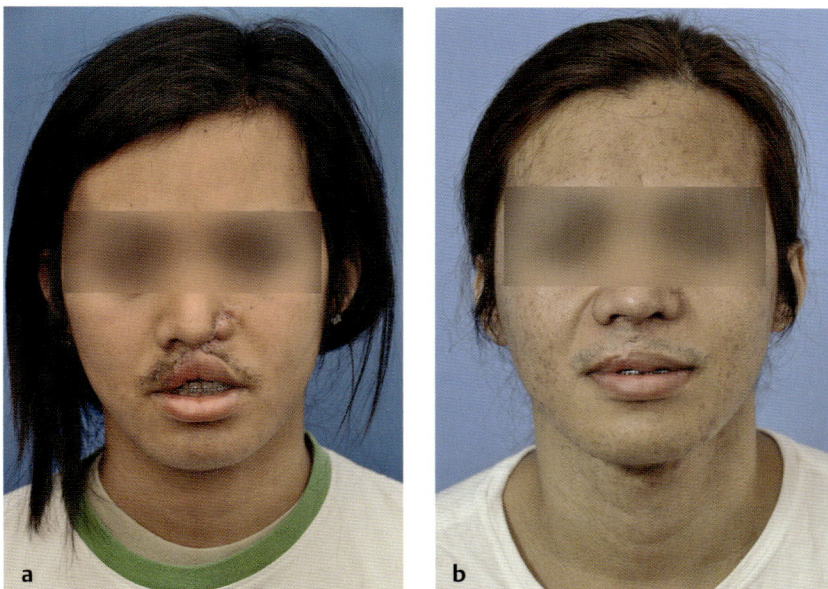

Fig. 15.11 This patient had lost skin from the upper lip with a resultant scar from the lip to the nose. (**a**) The patient before scar revision. (**b**) Adjacent tissue transfer from the upper lip allowed lengthening of the scar and restoration of the upper lip contour.

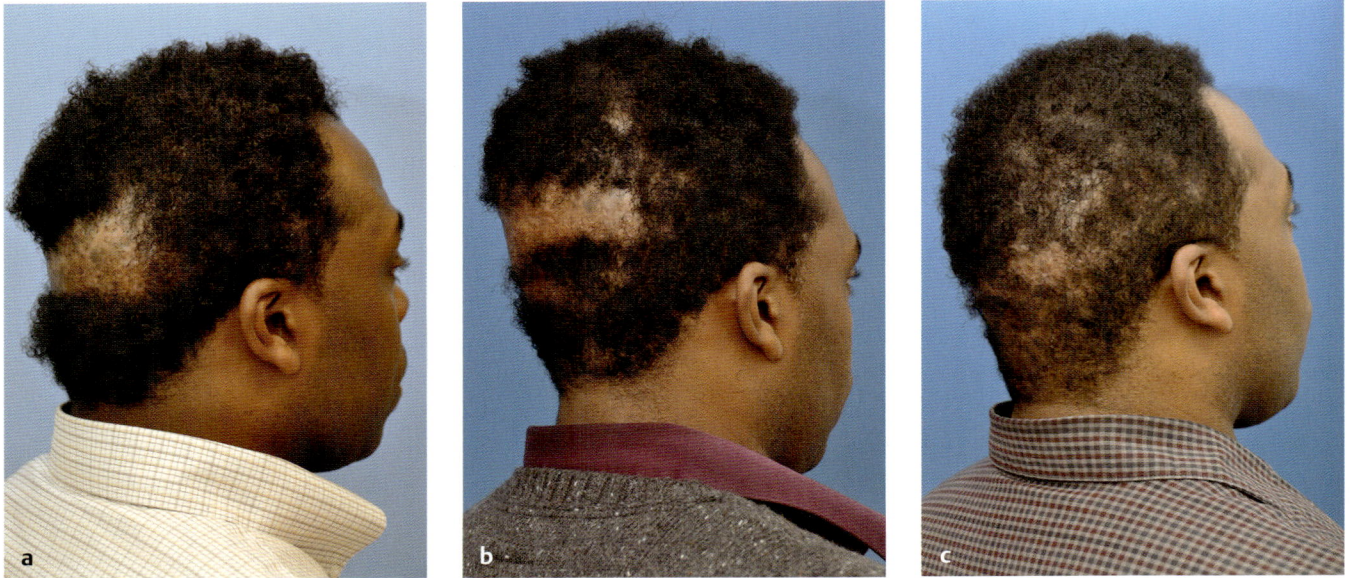

Fig. 15.12 Tissue expansion and subsequent tissue transfer for repair of a wide posterior alopecic scalp scar. **(a)** Wide alopecic scalp scar. **(b)** Expanded scalp with tissue expander in place. **(c)** Final result after removal of tissue expander and excision of alopecic scar.

Nonsurgical Scar Revision

Nonsurgical treatment of scars is an important part of the physician's armamentarium in camouflaging facial scars. The nonsurgical techniques can help to minimize skin erythema, improve contour or texture abnormality of the scar, and diminish fibroblastic activity.

Laser Treatments

Two broad categories of lasers may be used in scar revision. The pulsed dye laser (PDL) with a wavelength of 585 nm is used for treatment of hypertrophic and keloid scars and to address scar erythema. Skin resurfacing lasers such as ablative and fractional CO_2 or erbium:yttrium-aluminum-garnet (Er:YAG) lasers can be used to address atrophic scars by stimulating collagen formation. PDL treatments may be repeated in 6 to 8 weeks. Skin resurfacing may be repeated in 4 to 6 months. Patients with Fitzpatrick skin types I and II represent the ideal candidates for laser treatments. PDL and fractional ablative lasers may also be safely performed in patients with skin type III. Patients with higher degrees of skin pigmentation would be at risk of hypopigmentation following laser therapy (**Fig. 15.13a,b**). A thorough discussion of laser therapy and resurfacing is beyond the scope of this chapter, and the reader is referred to other chapters in this book.

In general, however, laser settings for ablative and nonablative skin resurfacing, as well as PDL treat-ments, are device-specific and vary according to the degree of skin pigmentation. In the postoperative phase, ablative and fractional laser skin resurfacing requires attentive care. The ablated skin remains raw and tends to ooze serous exudate. Keeping the area moist by applying petrolatum ointment or other nonirritating moisturizers helps the skin heal more efficiently. Posttreatment antibacterial and antiviral medications are indicated in some patients who undergo ablative skin resurfacing.[4]

Dermabrasion

Dermabrasion is effective in the treatment of atrophic scars by stimulating collagen formation, similar to the effect of skin resurfacing lasers. The results of dermabrasion depend on the coarseness of the abrading tip, the length of time the tip is applied to the skin, and the pressure used to apply the tip. In general, the abrading tip is applied in smooth strokes to gradually remove the damaged outer layers of the skin until a smooth uniform surface of bleeding tissue remains. The skin is held taut and maintained in a stationary position by the nonoperating hand. An alternate technique employs a freezing spray to create a hard skin surface to facilitate the abrasion. This technique must be employed carefully on the face to avoid eye injury. When reaching the periphery of the area to be treated, feathering is appropriate to avoid a clear demarcation between treated and untreated

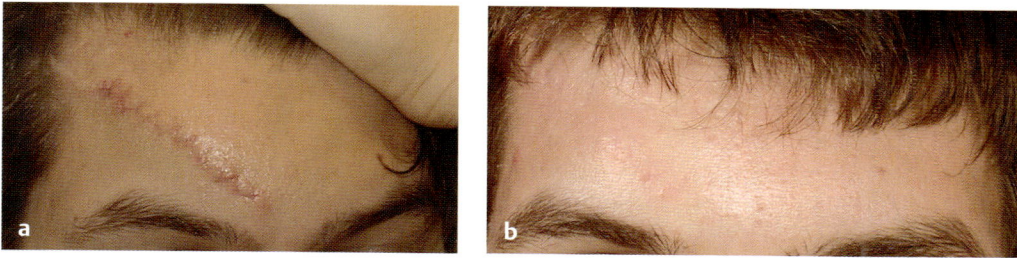

Fig. 15.13 Laser treatment to improve scar appearance after w-plasty **(a,b)**.

regions. Dermabrasion is typically carried to the level of deep papillary dermis or the superficial reticular dermis where collagen fibers appear rougher and there is increased bleeding. Dermabrasion beyond this depth increases the risk of scarring.

Following dermabrasion, the skin is raw and can bleed or ooze serous exudate. Similar to ablative skin resurfacing, maintaining the wound moisture by applying petrolatum ointment or other nonirritating moisturizers helps the skin heal more efficiently.

Injections and Topical Applications

Triamcinolone injections can be quite effective in reducing the thickness of hypertrophic scars and improving small keloid scars. Steroid injections are effective due to their action in diminishing collagen synthesis, decreasing mucinous ground substance, and inhibiting collagenase inhibitors that prevent the degradation of collagen. Triamcinolone 10 mg/mL is injected in small amounts of 0.1 to 0.2 mL into the hypertrophic or keloid scar on a monthly basis. Typically, three to six injections are required. Steroid injections can have secondary adverse effects, including skin atrophy, hypopigmentation, and telangiectasia formation. Adverse effects can be minimized by using small injection volumes and the lower concentration of triamcinolone, as well as by confining the injections to the deeper dermal layer of skin.[5]

Topical application of silicone/Silastic sheeting has shown some beneficial impact on the appearance of scars and has been clinically useful in treatment of hypertrophic scars and keloids. In vitro studies of burn scar fibroblasts have demonstrated decreased contraction of the scars exposed to silicone sheeting. This benefit is postulated to be secondary to downregulation of transforming growth factor (TGF)-β_2 production. The clinical benefit of silicone sheet application is dependent on the duration of use. Silicone sheet use on the face may be challenging depending on the site. The nose, the ears, and the lips do not offer a wide or stable enough platform for application of the sheets. Silicone sheets are more easily used on the forehead and the neck. Silicone creams may offer beneficial effects similar to silicone sheeting while providing ease of use and increased patient compliance.[6]

■ Postoperative Care

In patients who undergo surgical scar revision, suture removal is performed 5 to 7 days after surgery. Swelling begins in the immediate postoperative period and becomes most pronounced at 2 to 3 days after surgery. Ecchymosis is common in surgical patients and tends to last from 7 to 14 days. Once the incisions have healed, postoperative scar erythema typically lasts 4 months.

Postoperative care for ablative laser therapy is similar to skin dermabrasion. Maintenance of a moist wound environment by applying nonirritating moisturizer helps promote reepithelialization of the treated area. Skin healing can take 3 to 10 days to complete depending on the depth of treatment. The resurfaced skin can appear erythematous for 4 months. Sun avoidance will reduce the risk of hyperpigmentation in the treatment area.

During the evaluation of patients with facial scars, the importance of cosmetics in scar camouflage should not be forgotten. Professional cosmetologists can help patients minimize the appearance of their scars before scar revision is accomplished. Cosmetologists can help patients conceal the ecchymosis or the erythema that follows laser treatment or surgical scar revision.

■ Expected Results

Typically, patients appreciate an improvement in the appearance of the scar during the first postoperative visit. Occasionally, the extent of surgical incisions or laser therapy causes patients anxiety during the early postoperative period. In such circumstances, patients should be reminded that wound healing is a dynamic process, and continued improvement can be expected for the first 6 months. The clinician should reassure the patient and see the patient on a frequent basis. It can be very helpful to have anxious patients talk to past patients who have undergone scar revision. Late postoperative results are highly satisfactory to patients because the induration and edema have subsided and wound erythema has resolved.

◼ Conclusion

Scar revision can be highly satisfying to patients and treating physicians. To be successful in revising scars, the physician must be well versed in various techniques of scar revision and their effect on the facial subunits and RSTLs. It is not uncommon that the best results require two or more treatments in tandem. Management of patient expectations should not be underestimated as a major factor in achieving patient satisfaction.

References

1. Goslen JB. Physiology of wound healing and scar formation. In: Thomas JR, Holt GR, eds. Facial Scars: Incision, Revision and Camouflage. St. Louis, MO: Mosby-Year Book; 1989
2. Borges AF. Principles of scar camouflage. Facial Plast Surg 1984;1(3):181–190
3. Thomas JR, Holt GR. Facial scars. In: Facial Scars: Incision, Revision and Camouflage. St. Louis, MO: CV Mosby;1989
4. Martins A, Trindade F, Leite L. Facial scars after a road accident—combined treatment with pulsed dye laser and Q-switched Nd:YAG laser. J Cosmet Dermatol 2008;7(3): 227–229
5. Maguire HC Jr. Treatment of keloids with triamcinolone acetonide injected intralesionally. JAMA 1965;192: 325–326
6. de Oliveira GV, Nunes TA, Magna LA, et al. Silicone versus nonsilicone gel dressings: a controlled trial. Dermatol Surg 2001;27(8):721–726

16 Treatment of Facial Imperfections with Dermal Fillers

Georgann A. Poulos and Suzan Obagi

Key Concepts

- Numerous soft tissue filling agents are available for facial rejuvenation and scar revision.

- Knowledge of the properties of individual soft tissue fillers will guide the aesthetic physician in selecting the appropriate agent for a particular patient and anatomical location.

- It is critical that the aesthetic practitioner recognize an adverse event and initiate appropriate action at the first sign of a complication from a soft tissue filler.

■ Introduction

As the demand for facial rejuvenation continues to rise, the goal for physicians performing aesthetic procedures is to optimize outcomes while minimizing downtime. It has become recognized that successful rejuvenation of most cosmetic patients requires addressing facial volume deficiencies. Therefore, the armamentarium of soft tissue fillers continues to grow, making it more important than ever that the aesthetic practitioner choose the best soft tissue filler for each patient and anatomical location.

This chapter serves as a practical guide for injecting dermal fillers for all practitioners regardless of experience. Agents discussed include the hyaluronic acids: Restylane/Perlane (Medicis Pharmaceutical, Scottsdale, AZ), Juvederm Ultra/Juvederm Ultra Plus (Allergan, Irvine, CA), Prevelle Silk (Mentor, Santa Barbara, CA), and Belotero (Merz Aesthetics, San Mateo, CA); calcium hydroxylapatite (Radiesse, Merz Aesthetics, San Mateo, CA); poly-L-lactic acid (PLLA, Sculptra Aesthetic, Sanofi-Aventis U.S., Bridgewater, NJ); polymethyl methacrylate (PMMA, Artefill, Su-

neva Medical, San Diego, CA); and the technique of autologous fat transfer. Silicone injections are not addressed in this chapter.

■ Background: Basic Science of Procedure

Special factors to take into consideration when selecting the appropriate agent for a patient include longevity of the filler, the anatomical area to be treated, the depth of the defect, the risk of allergic reaction, the risk of delayed (granulomatous) reactions, and the risk of infection.

Hyaluronic Acid Fillers

Hyaluronic acid (HA) is a ubiquitous component of connective and synovial tissues. It is a glycosaminoglycan biopolymer composed of alternating residues of D-glucuronic acid and N-acetyl-D-glycosamine that can bind up to 10,000 times its weight in water. Its affinity for water molecules gives it a unique ability to add to skin turgor and volume. However, injection of unmodified HA results in almost immediate degradation. Therefore, for HA to be a clinically useful injectable filler, it must undergo cross-linking to confer longevity. Currently available HA fillers will vary with regard to particle size and the type of cross-linking used. For example, Restylane has 100,000 particles/mL, and Perlane has 10,000 particles/mL. Although Perlane has fewer particles per milliliter, the particles are much larger than those of Restylane.

HA fillers continue to gain popularity among both practitioners and patients due to ease of use, lower rates of hypersensitivity reactions, longer-lasting effects than traditional human and bovine collagen fillers, and reversibility upon injection with hyaluronidase.[1] Several agents are available, including Restylane and Perlane, Juvederm Ultra/Juvederm Ultra Plus, Prevelle Silk, and Belotero. Although Hylaform (no longer available) is avian derived, the others are derived from *Streptococcus* fermentation.[2,3]

Restylane, Juvederm Ultra, and Prevelle Silk are injected into the mid-dermis. Perlane, Belotero, Juvederm Ultra Plus, and Juvederm Ultra Plus XC are injected into the deep dermis/subcutaneous junction. Mid-dermal injections can be accomplished with the use of a 30-gauge half-inch needle, which allows for easy flow of the filler and minimizes bruising.

Deeper filler placement into the dermal/subcutaneous junction can be accomplished with a 29-gauge, thin-walled needle (Terumo Medical, Somerset, NJ) or a 27-gauge needle. The 29- gauge thin-walled needles have replaced the need for 27-gauge needles in the authors' practice. These needles have a 29-gauge outside diameter and an inside diameter equivalent to a regular 27-gauge needle, thereby allowing the treatment to proceed with less bruising.

Studies indicate that the effects of products such as Restylane last approximately 6 months.[4] Juvederm has been reported in the literature to last for 12 to 15 months in the deeper folds such as the melolabial region.[5] In the authors' experience, Juvederm has proven to last for a shorter duration of approximately 6 months in most patients and up to 18 months in a small subset of patients.

Calcium Hydroxylapatite

Calcium hydroxylapatite (CaHA), which is naturally found in bone, had been used in orthopedics, dentistry, and urology prior to its use as a semipermanent soft tissue filler.[6,7] The CaHA microspheres measure 25 to 45 μm, are suspended in a carboxymethylcellulose gel base, and are capable of augmenting bone structure.

CaHA is a volumizing filler, making it not ideal for finer lines but useful for elevating soft tissue, such as in the malar, buccal, and mandibular regions. The risk of visible nodules makes it unsuitable for augmentation of the periorbital region (unless cautiously placed deep along the periosteum) and the lips.

Prior to injecting, the addition of 0.2 mL sodium bicarbonate and 0.3 mL lidocaine with epinephrine has shown to improve patient comfort. The vasoconstrictive effects of lidocaine with epinephrine help to reduce bruising. The dilution is best achieved with a female-to-female Luer Lock-to-Luer Lock adapter (Sterile Rapid-Fill Connector, Baxter, Englewood, CO) (**Fig. 16.1**).[8] The use of a 28-gauge three-quarter-inch needle and a retrograde injection is the preferred technique. The product is placed into the deep subcutaneous plane or at the level of the periosteum. The material is then massaged immediately after injection to avoid palpable nodule formation. Typi-

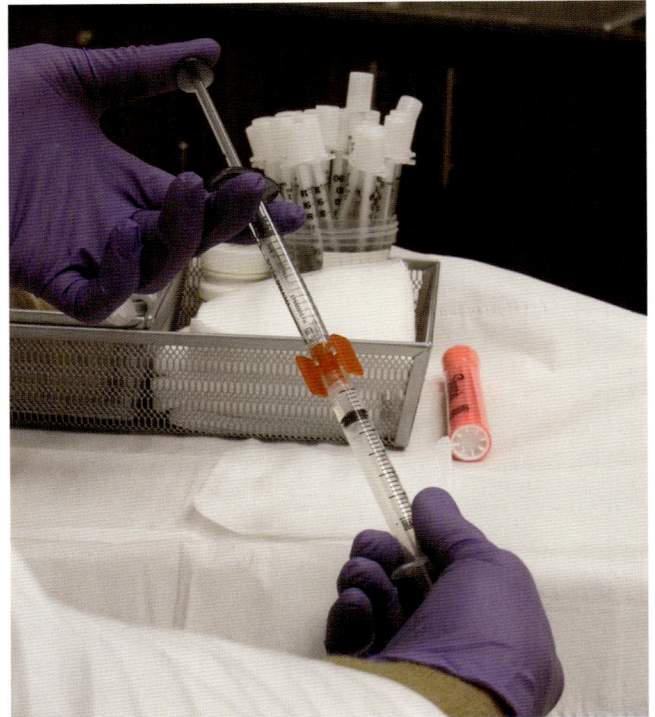

Fig. 16.1 A female-to-female Luer Lock adapter can be used to mix lidocaine with epinephrine and sodium bicarbonate to various fillers.

cally, the effects of CaHA last for at least 1 year and possibly longer.[4]

Poly-L-Lactic Acid

PLLA was originally used for manufacturing absorbable suture material (Vicryl, Dexon) prior to its use as a soft tissue filling agent. Sculptra (Sanofi-Aventis), the powdered form, consists of 40 to 63 μm microspheres[2] suspended in a nonpyrogenic mannitol and sodium cellulose preparation.[9] Placement of PLLA into the deep dermal–subcutaneous plane yields dermal fibroplasia and cutaneous thickening over the subsequent months.[9] Previously published reports indicate that higher dilutions may result in a more uniform mixture with decreased incidence of nodule formation.[9,10,11] The manufacturer suggests diluting PLLA with 5 mL sterile water for injection at least 2 hours prior to planned injection and keeping the reconstituted product for no more than 72 hours.[12] More recently, the authors favor reconstitution with 6 mL bacteriostatic water 7 days prior to the planned injection. On the day of the procedure, 3 mL lidocaine with epinephrine is added to aid in the reduction of bruising. A gentle rolling motion of the vial prior to injection will ensure an even suspension. The PLLA is transferred into 1 mL syringes via a 21-gauge needle immediately prior to injection. The areas to be treated are outlined with a marking pen prior to the injection of PLLA. The authors use a depot (0.1 to 0.2 mL aliquots) and fanning technique with a 25-gauge 1-inch needle for soft tissue augmentation at the level of the upper subcutaneous fat and along the periosteum in certain areas. PLLA has been reported to have its greatest effect at approximately 28 months posttreatment.[4] Bauer has reported the effects of PLLA lasting up to 40 months in some individuals.[13]

Polymethyl Methacrylate

PMMA consists of microspheres suspended in a collagen matrix with 0.3% lidocaine.[14] The 30 to 40 μm microspheres are suspended in bovine collagen derived from a closed herd in the United States.[14] The bovine collagen serves to deliver the microspheres to the soft tissue. The microspheres are left behind to stimulate the deposition of the patient's own collagen in place of the bovine collagen.[14] It is recommended that this product be injected into the deep dermis/subcutaneous junction to prevent surface irregularities. It is important to perform skin testing prior to its injection given the bovine collagen contents. This agent has been shown to provide correction in the highly mobile region of the nasolabial folds for as long as 5 years postinjection.[14] Due to the need for skin testing, patients may find the product less convenient.

Autologous Fat Augmentation

Any discussion of soft tissue filling agents would not be complete without the mention of autologous fat transfer. In most patients of normal to increased body mass index, the donor site is plentiful and holds virtually no risk of immunogenicity.[15] The authors favor a modification of a technique developed by Dr. Sidney Coleman, in which adipocytes are harvested in manual suction via 10 mL syringes.[16] Minute fat parcels (0.05 to 0.1 mL) are placed along multiple facial places using blunt-tip cannulas for a long-lasting restoration of facial volume. The small depot technique is designed to maximize surface area exposure of individual adipocytes and may improve the vascular supply to the newly grafted tissue.[15] Care must be taken to ensure that the fat is harvested, prepared, and infiltrated in a sterile fashion to minimize complications, including infection.[15] The patient is advised that the excess harvested fat will be frozen for 1 year and can be used for touch-ups within that time period.[15]

■ Technical Aspects of Procedure

Autologous fat transfer is the authors' preferred method for full-face soft tissue augmentation. However, not all patients have adequate fat donor sites or are willing to tolerate the 7-day recovery period associated with the procedure. The authors consider the following synthetic filling agents to be the products of choice when autologous fat cannot be utilized. The approach to the patient is broken down by anatomical region, with certain fillers having better filling properties than others for a given area ▶ Video 16.1.

Periorbital Region

The orbital region tends to naturally decrease in volume with age.[17] In addition, some patients have undergone aggressive blepharoplasty procedures that have further exacerbated the orbital hollowing. More attention is being placed on volume restoration of the periorbital region as part of full facial rejuvenation.[18] Patients may find the concept of adding volume to the brow in an effort to augment their appearance difficult to visualize; Lambros proposed injecting a dilute local anesthetic into the brow region to offer the patient a preview of the outcome.[19]

The periorbital region consists of the thinnest skin on the face. Thus care should be taken to use a filler that will result in smooth contour enhancement. Certain large-particle fillers can result in visible nodules in this area and are best avoided.

The authors favor the use of a small-particle HA, such as Restylane, in the periorbital region for brow and tear-trough augmentation. This filler has a very smooth consistency upon injection, can be easily massaged into place, and has the least likelihood of edema. Additionally, the use of an HA filler in the periorbital region has the added advantage of being reversible with hyaluronidase should the patient not like the final outcome.

Although fillers can be purchased with lidocaine premixed in them, the authors prefer to mix the filler with 0.3 mL of 1% lidocaine plus epinephrine and 0.2 mL of sodium bicarbonate. A female-to-female Luer Lock adapter allows for the addition of lidocaine with epinephrine (**Fig. 16.1**).[8] The epinephrine induces vasoconstriction and decreased bruising. The mixing technique also allows for ease of injection and improves malleability of the product.

Brow augmentation is used for patients who have lost volume in the brow fat pad. The deflation of the brow appears as dermatochalasis of the upper eyelid and a bony appearance of the brow. A 30-gauge half-inch needle is used to inject this area in a linear, retrograde fashion along the contour of the upper orbital rim (**Fig. 16.2**). The area is then massaged in a

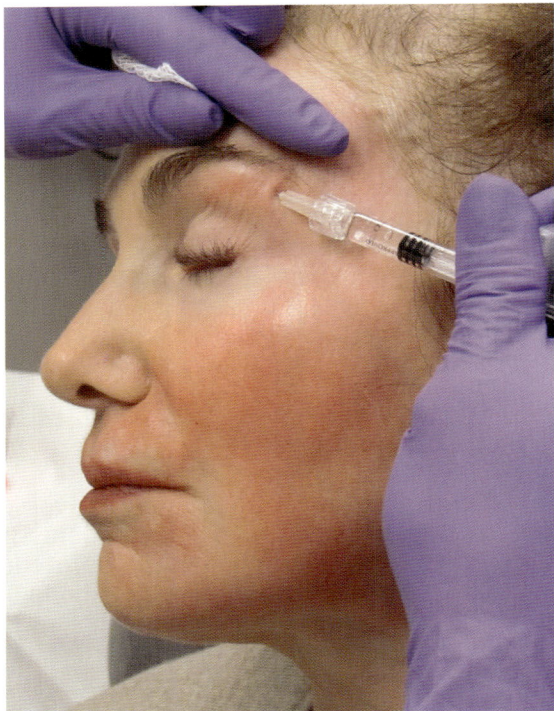

Fig. 16.2 Brow augmentation is accomplished using a linear, retrograde injection along the contour of the upper orbital rim.

in the lower lids and brows can exceed the 2 year mark.[19] The use of a larger particle size of HA, such as Juvederm Ultra Plus, in the lower eyelid can result in prolonged posttreatment edema in some patients and should thus be undertaken cautiously.

Temple Region

Volume loss of the temporal fat pads causes the face to appear skeletonized. This area is relatively easy to correct using either autologous fat augmentation or a larger particle filler that has long-lasting results. The preferred method for addressing temporal hollowing using a synthetic filler involves depot injections of PLLA. A significant improvement can be achieved by using a series of one to three PLLA injections at 6-week intervals. The temple is injected with 0.5 mL to 1 mL of PLLA using a 1 mL syringe with a 25-gauge needle. The injection should be performed perpendicular to the skin, and the needle advanced to the level of the periosteum (**Fig. 16.3**). One or two depots can be placed ~ 1 cm apart if needed. In this plane, there is less risk of intravascular injection, deep enough placement of the filler to allow for a smooth contour, and the least chance of bruising. Placement of PLLA in the dermis or subcutaneous level in the temporal region can result in very long-lasting visible nodules.

linear fashion to smooth out the contour and to identify "skip" areas.

The tear-trough deformity poses a challenge because it may be due to (1) loss of volume along the lid–cheek junction, (2) loss of volume and increased lower eyelid edema in patients with a history of seasonal allergies, or (3) iatrogenic hollowing following lower lid fat resection. The goal of treatment is to blend the lid–cheek junction for a smoother appearance to the area. However, patients with thinner skin should be counseled that it is best to perform this treatment conservatively over a couple of treatment sessions so that one does not create visible nodules.

For tear-trough augmentation, use a 30-gauge half-inch needle to inject small (0.1 mL), submuscular depots of HAs (mixed with lidocaine plus epinephrine) over the bony orbit, followed by massage in the direction of the deformity (i.e., massage toward the nose if trying to fill the medial aspect of the tear-trough deformity). Injection in the submuscular plane will help to avoid the Tyndall effect (or visible blue hue). In thicker-skinned patients, it is adequate to inject submuscularly. However, in thinner-skinned individuals, one may have to inject at the level of the periosteum to avoid visible filler or nodule formation. The area is then massaged along the entire lower orbital rim to ensure a smooth contour and to avoid skip areas. Lambros has reported that the effects of HAs

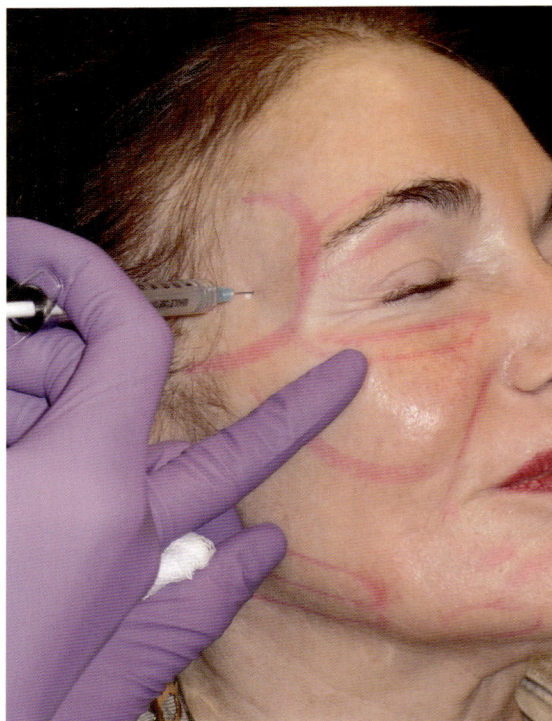

Fig. 16.3 Volume loss of the temporal fat pads can be corrected with poly-ʟ-lactic acid injected perpendicular to the skin and advanced to the level of the periosteum.

Mid and Lower Face Regions

CaHA and PLLA are the preferred soft tissue fillers for buccal cheek atrophy and zygoma augmentation. The mid- and lower face requires lifting or volumizing types of fillers to re-suspend the overlying soft tissue. PLLA is diluted, as described previously, and injected with a 25-gauge needle with both a depot and a fanning technique. The CaHA injections are made in a retrograde fashion with a 28-gauge needle. Injecting the material with small, linear depots combined with a fanning technique yields excellent results with decreased bruising. Both fillers are premixed with lidocaine with epinephrine, as previously described.

The aging mandible displays a wavy or "broken" mandibular arc, as described by Donofrio,[20] and has been shown to undergo significant volume reduction[21] as part of the overall panfacial volume loss that occurs. In many patients, a small dip or depression can be seen and felt with one's fingers along the border of the mandible (**Fig. 16.4a**). This bony recession contributes to the prominence of the jowls, the appearance of the prejowl sulcus, and an overall weak cheek/neck definition. The authors' preferred method of restoration of the youthful primary arc is via autologous fat transfer (**Fig. 16.4b**). However, the preferred synthetic filler for this area is either PLLA or CaHA. The filler is placed in a depot technique at the level of the periosteum and then in the dermal/subcutaneous junction using a fanning technique to restore the youthful mandibular arc.

Perioral Region

When addressing strictly the perioral region, an HA such as Juvederm Ultra Plus is the filler of choice for correction of the melolabial and melomental folds and the perioral region. One needs a filler that can give some degree of "lift" to the deeper folds while being "thin" enough to allow use in the finer perioral lines.

The melolabial and melomental folds are addressed at the level of the dermal–subcutaneous junction using a fanning and cross-hatching technique that is parallel to the fold as well as crossing the fold perpendicularly. Depot placement at the prejowl sulcus at the level of the periosteum can improve the jawline definition.

A retrograde, fanning and cross-hatching technique can result in significant improvement of the perioral rhytids and enhancement of the oral commissures. In fact, perioral lines can be treated with HA fillers placed first very superficially in the upper dermis (**Fig. 16.5**). The needle should then be redirected with filling of the rhytid at a slightly deeper dermal level. Additional filler should be fanned out a little beyond the line to allow for a "smoothing out" of the cutaneous lip. Results with this technique can be quite dramatic (**Fig. 16.6a,b**). Adding volume in a fanning technique to a commonly overlooked site, the lateral cutaneous upper lip, can significantly improve cosmesis (**Fig. 16.7a,b**). The adjunctive use of botulinum toxin in the area is often necessary to maximize perioral rejuvenation by either targeting

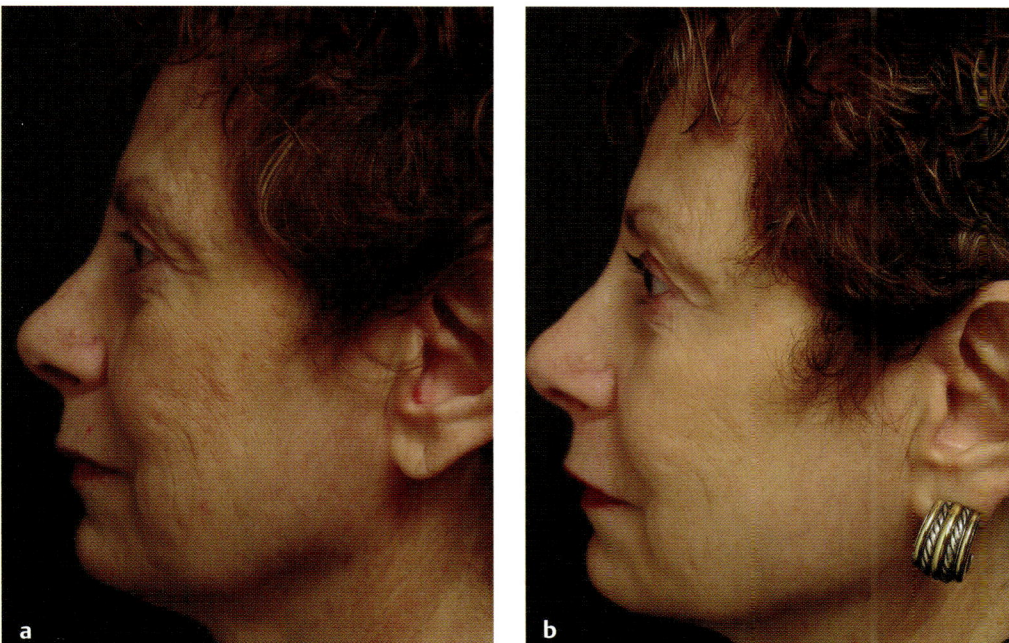

Fig. 16.4 Autologous fat transfer. **(a)** Patient prior to autologous fat transfer to the jawline. Note the wavy mandibular arc. **(b)** Patient post–autologous fat transfer to the mandible displaying improved jawline.

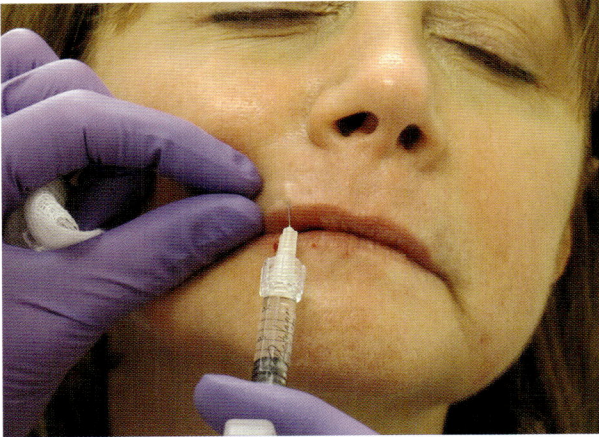

Fig. 16.5 Hyaluronic acid (HA) fillers can be used to correct perioral rhytids. The lines are first treated with superficial placement of the HA.

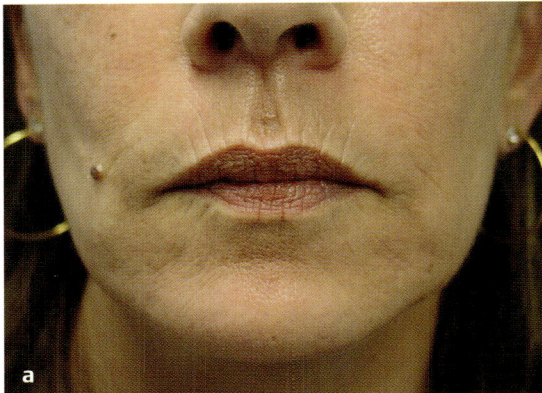

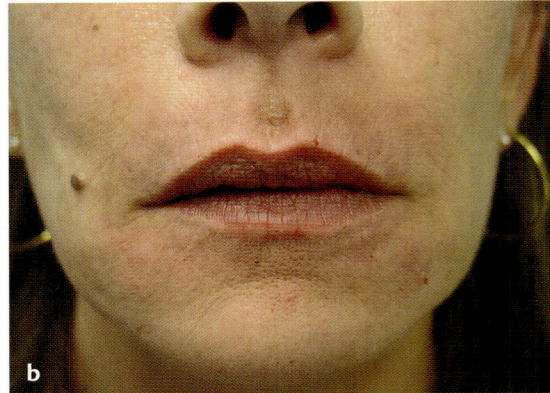

Fig. 16.6 Rhytid augmentation. **(a)** Patient prior to perioral rhytid augmentation with hyaluronic acid (HA) filler. **(b)** Patient post–perioral rhytid augmentation with HA filler showing dramatic improvement in the rhytids.

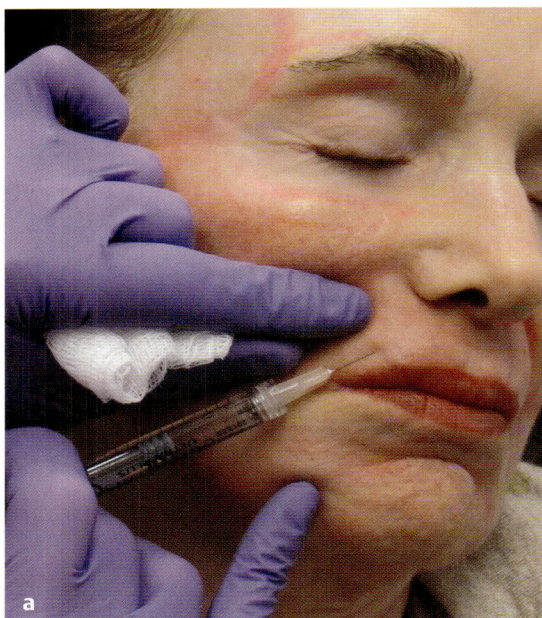

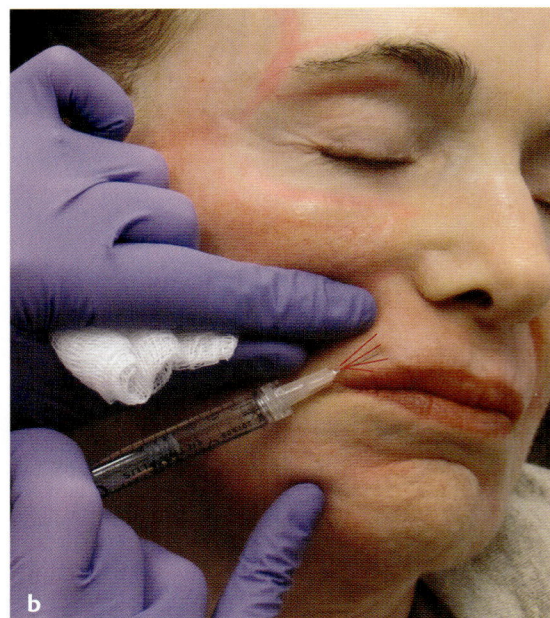

Fig. 16.7 The lateral cutaneous upper lip should be augmented with a fanning technique to optimize cosmesis **(a,b)**.

the orbicularis oris (pucker lines) or the depressor anguli oris (marionette folds).

HA fillers, such as Restylane or Juvederm Ultra Plus, are the agents of choice for lip augmentation. An additional benefit of Restylane is that it can easily flow through a 30-gauge needle that is bent at a 45-degree angle. This angle allows for easy placement of the filler in a more comfortable hand position for the physician. First, augmenting the vermilion–cutaneous border along its entirety adds definition.[22] This is followed by retrograde injections into the mucosal lip body to restore volume (**Fig. 16.8a,b**). Perioral rhytids are injected in a superficial fashion into the deficit and into two levels for the rhytids, as mentioned earlier. Neither PLLA nor CaHA is recommended for use in lip augmentation due to the risk of visible and palpable nodules.

Correction of Facial Scars and Soft Tissue Atrophy

Synthetic fillers and autologous fat transfer also have an important role in the correction of facial scars resulting from acne vulgaris, varicella, surgery, and other causes of soft tissue atrophy. When the defect is ad-

herent to the underlying fascia, filling techniques can often improve cosmesis by improving the contour. Soft tissue augmentation can be combined with additional treatment modalities, including subcision, punch grafting, and laser resurfacing, for optimal results.

Acne Scarring

Various synthetic fillers, including HA, CaHA, PMMA, PLLA, and silicone, have been reported to successfully treat cutaneous scarring from acne vulgaris. Fillers can be used for this purpose with two different objectives. Injecting HA fillers directly under the defect can result in immediate improvement of the scar appearance.[23] Alternatively, CaHA or PLLA can provide deep structural support that can also improve the appearance of acne scars.[23,24]

For immediate results in the treatment of valley, also known as rolling or saucerized, scars, the authors favor injection of an HA filler, such as Restylane, just below the deficit (**Fig. 16.9a,b**). The needle is then redirected with filling at a slightly deeper dermal level to yield structural support. Combining

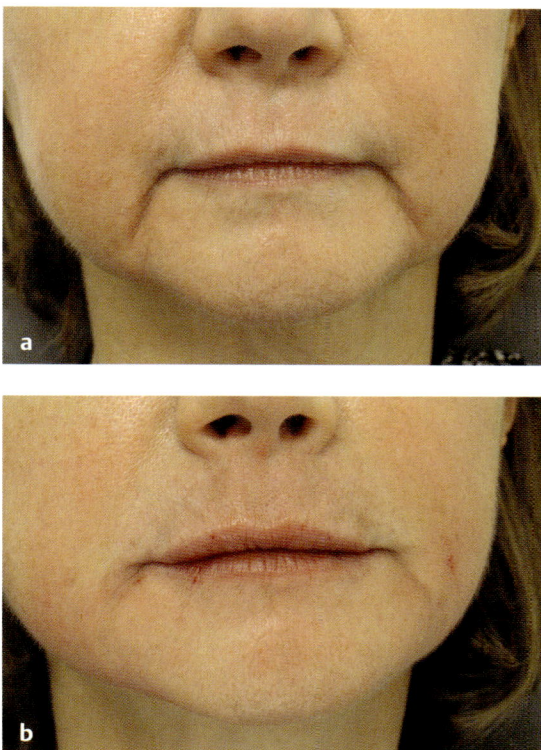

Fig. 16.8 Melomental fold and lip augmentation. **(a)** Patient prior to melomental fold and lip augmentation. **(b)** Patient post–melomental fold and lip augmentation displaying volume restoration.

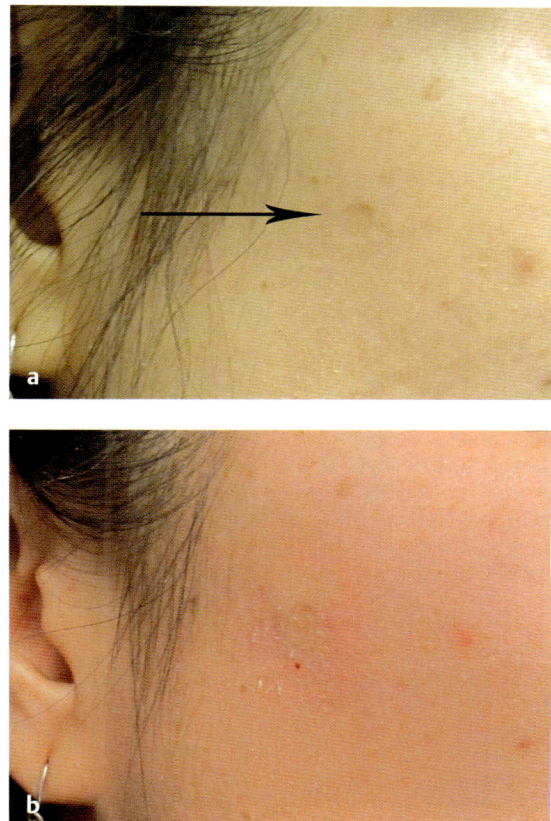

Fig. 16.9 **(a)** Patient with a boxcar scar of the right cheek prior to Restylane (Medicis Pharmaceutical) injection. **(b)** Patient immediately after Restylane (Medicis Pharmaceutical) injection beneath a valley scar of the right cheek.

soft tissue augmentation with a series of subcisions, or "subdermal incisionless undermining," may offer the patient more permanent results.[23] Subcision with a tribeveled 22-gauge needle attached to a 3 mL syringe will release the tethered scar from the dermis and can stimulate collagen deposition.[25] The suggested subcision end point is the ability to freely move the needle beneath the scar without resistance.[25] This technique is employed frequently by the authors for successful correction of acne scars.

CaHA has been reported to be effective in the treatment of saucerized acne scars but ineffective for ice-pick scarring.[24] Multiple sessions, injecting volumes of 0.1 to 0.3 mL per treatment, led to a 50 to 75% improvement in over half of the study participants.[24] The results typically last at least 1 year.

PLLA has been reported to improve scars from acne and varicella through direct stimulation of collagen production.[26] Beer described instilling PLLA into the atrophic scar with the end point being elevation of the scar to the level of surrounding skin.[26] After a series of treatments, a statistically significant reduction in scar size was achieved. Autologous fat transfer can also successfully treat acne and varicella scarring in a manner similar to that of PLLA.

Due to the temporary nature of other augmenting agents, permanent fillers such as PMMA and silicone have also been studied in the treatment of acne scars. PMMA, in combination with subcision, was reported to induce a noticeable improvement in atrophic facial acne scars in 96% of treated scars in a single-center, open-label pilot study.[27] Liquid silicone can result in correction of depressed, broad-based acne scars with a microdroplet, multiple injection technique.[28] Multiple sessions by a physician skilled in silicone injections are suggested to avoid overcorrection.

Correction of Soft Tissue Atrophy

Depressed scars from trauma or surgery, as well as facial hemiatrophy, can be treated with autologous fat transfer or various soft tissue fillers. HA fillers can be used to augment traumatic scars, and injection directly under the defect will result in immediate correction of the scar appearance. One vial of Restylane (Medicis Pharmaceutical) significantly improved cosmesis of the chin region in a patient status posttraumatic fall (**Fig. 16.10a,b**). Alternatively, dissection of fibrous scar attachments with a blunt cannula followed by autologous fat transfer has been well described in the correction of depressed scars adherent to underlying fascia.[29] Autologous fat transplantation in the treatment of progressive facial hemiatrophy or Parry-Romberg syndrome can lead to aesthetic improvement and patient satisfaction.[30] Patients without adequate fat reserves or history of weight fluctuations may be better candidates for atrophy correction with PLLA. One vial of PLLA was injected into the left buccal cheek in a linear and cross-hatching manner. This resulted in significant improvement in facial asymmetry in the patient shown (**Fig. 16.11a,b**).

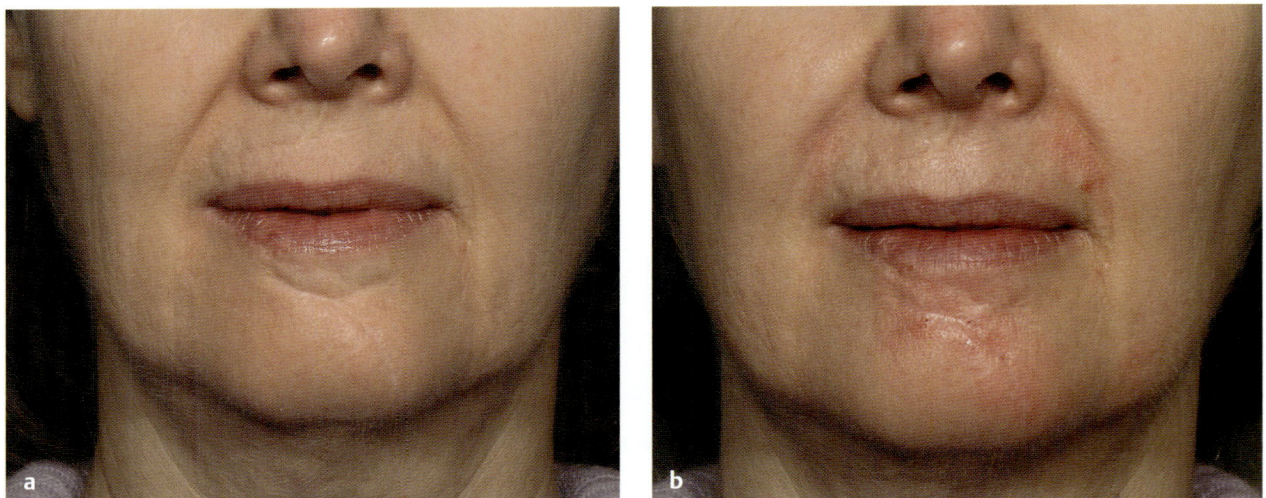

Fig. 16.10 **(a)** Patient with traumatic scar of the chin region. **(b)** Patient immediately after Juvederm (Allergan) injection to augment the traumatic chin scar.

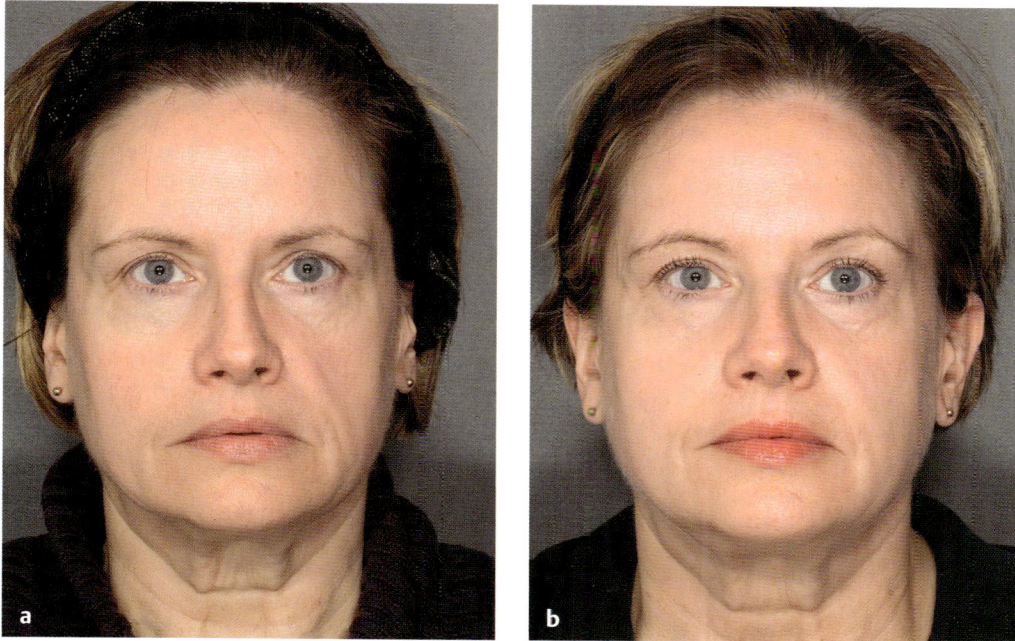

Fig. 16.11 **(a)** The patient suffered a fall with subsequent left buccal nerve weakness and facial hemiatrophy. **(b)** Five months after injection of one vial of poly-L-lactic acid showing correction of left buccal cheek soft tissue atrophy.

■ Complications and Their Management

Adverse reactions to soft tissue filling agents may include mild erythema (which fades within hours of the procedure), ecchymosis, transient palpable nodules, visible blue hue, cutaneous necrosis due to vascular compromise, and persistent inflammatory nodules. It is critical that the physician recognize an adverse event and initiate appropriate action immediately.

Tyndall Effect and Hyaluronic Acid Fillers

Filler placement at the correct level is critical in optimizing outcomes and minimizing side effects. Shortly after injection of the HA fillers, a palpable nodule can sometimes be felt by the patient if excess filler is deposited in a localized area. This is best treated with massage to the area starting 48 hours after treatment. HA fillers placed too superficially can result in a visible blue hue, known as the Tyndall effect (**Fig. 16.12**). If this occurs along a rhytid or a skin fold, it can be resolved by nicking the skin with a 22-gauge needle and expressing the material. If the collection is in the lower eyelid region, it may appear as a diffuse bluish discoloration. This will resolve with the injection of hyaluronidase into the area of concern.

Embolization

When injecting soft tissue fillers, it is essential to be aware of the potential for vascular compromise.[31] The risk is greatest when working medially on the face in areas such as the melolabial fold, the nasojugal crease, or the dorsum of the nose. The glabellar region has been described in the literature as the site most at risk for vas-

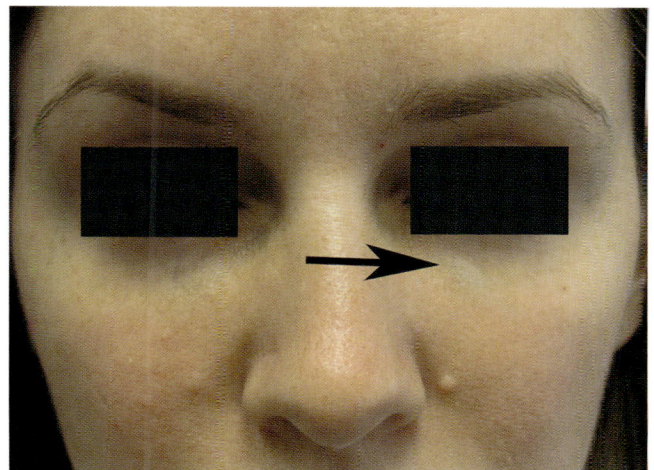

Fig. 16.12 Hyaluronic acid fillers placed too superficially can cause the Tyndall effect, or visible blue hue, as shown.

cular compromise and skin necrosis.[31,32] Embolization of fillers and fat can result in skin slough and scarring, vision loss,[33,34] and, in the most severe cases, stroke.[35]

In 2004, a case report of blindness with PMMA[34] was described, and more recently, the first documented case of visual loss following periorbital injection of PLLA was reported.[33] Inadvertent cannulation of an arterial lumen likely resulted in a bolus injection that progressed proximally. The authors hypothesized that the sequence of an inadvertent intra-arterial cannulation, retrograde flow of viscous product, and secondary embolization from a more proximal source, the ophthalmic artery, resulted in this devastating complication.[33] Another proposed risk factor in the case was prior rhinoplasty, which may have altered the normal vascular anastomoses.[33]

Early recognition of arterial or venous occlusion is critical. Although arterial compromise has been described as an immediate blanching and severe pain, venous occlusion may present with a delayed, dull pain and dark discoloration.[31] Immediate blanching should prompt the physician to aspirate, massage to disperse the agent, and apply warm compresses for induction of vasodilation.[31,32] If the filler contains anesthetic, the patient may not report immediate onset of pain, so one must look for skin blanching. Hyaluronidase should be injected diffusely into the area when using hyaluronic fillers to help relieve any pressure on the vasculature that may be contributing to the ischemia. Glaich et al advocate the application of nitroglycerin paste to the affected area. In addition to the previously mentioned steps, a low-molecular-weight heparin should be considered in the event of glabellar necrosis.[32] Large areas of skin necrosis or ischemia may improve with hyperbaric oxygen to speed wound healing. Additional measures include aspirin, low-level laser treatments (during wound healing), and diligent wound care to reduce the risk of secondary bacterial infection. Injection of limited volumes through the smallest-gauge needle possible, retrograde injection, and keeping the needle moving have been advocated to prevent this complication.

Nodules and Inflammatory Reactions

Patients may develop inflammatory skin nodules at any time after treatment with a soft tissue filler. However, it is most commonly seen with PLLA (**Fig. 16.13**). Inflammatory skin nodules post–soft tissue injection should be treated as infection until proven otherwise. Tissue culture for aerobic bacteria, anaerobic bacteria, and mycobacteria should be obtained.[31] Incision and drainage are recommended if the nodule is fluctuant.[36] Empirical antibiotics should be initiated with an oral macrolide or tetracycline derivative for a 4 to 6 week course[31,34] because it may take 4 to 6 weeks for the mycobacterial culture to complete. The authors favor the use of the macrolide clarithromycin after obtaining cultures. Intralesional corticoste-

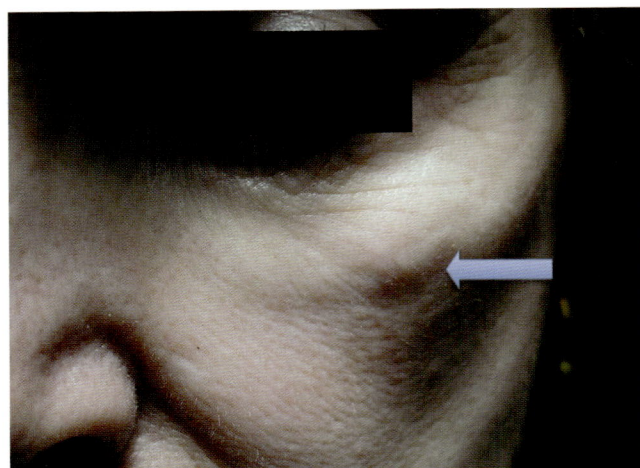

Fig. 16.13 Patient who developed a nodule months after injection of Sculptra (PLLA) (Sanofi-Aventis U.S.).

roid can improve the appearance of the nodules once infectious etiologies have been excluded.

Lip nodules have been reported with the injection of CaHA for lip augmentation.[6] Tear-trough fullness has also been reported after the injection of CaHA. This may be due to either lymphedema or overcorrection.[6] Less experienced practitioners should avoid the injection of this filler into the tear-trough regions. The treatment of these nodules is either firm massage, intralesional steroid, excision, or simply allowing the nodules to resolve spontaneously over time.

The most commonly reported side effect with PLLA (Sculptra, Sanofi-Aventis) is the formation of subcutaneous nodules.[10] The nodules typically appear with a mean latency of 6 months. Higher dilution volumes (5 mL or more) and a longer reconstitution period (about 7 days) have been proposed to help reduce the risk of nodules.[10,37]

The most frequently reported adverse events associated with PMMA from a case series on adverse events from fillers were erythema, swelling, and nodule formation.[36] The inflammatory nodules seen with this agent may have a longer interval from injection to reaction, with the mean time reported by Zielke et al being 37.1 ± 25.4 months and a maximum of 6.5 years.[38]

■ Conclusion

In conclusion, a comprehensive understanding of the properties of individual soft tissue fillers will guide the aesthetic physician in selecting the appropriate agent for a particular patient and location. Injecting at the appropriate depth, knowledge of facial anatomy, and patient variables are critical factors in optimizing outcomes. The authors' anatomical algorithm supports the use of a combination of fillers to achieve overall facial rejuvenation and to correct soft tissue atrophy.

References

1. Obagi S. Correction of surface deformities: Botox, soft-tissue fillers, lasers and intense pulsed light, and radiofrequency. Atlas Oral Maxillofac Surg Clin North Am 2004; 12(2):271–297

2. Carruthers J, Cohen SR, Joseph JH, Narins RS, Rubin M. The science and art of dermal fillers for soft-tissue augmentation. J Drugs Dermatol 2009;8(4):335–350

3. Monheit GD. Hylaform: a new hyaluronic acid filler. Facial Plast Surg 2004;20(2):153–155

4. Werschler WP, Weinkle S. Longevity of effects of injectable products for soft-tissue augmentation. J Drugs Dermatol 2005;4(1):20–27

5. Bergeret-Galley C. Comparison of resorbable soft tissue fillers. Aesthet Surg J 2004;24(1):33–46

6. Sklar JA, White SM. Radiance FN: a new soft tissue filler. Dermatol Surg 2004;30(5):764–768, discussion 768

7. Mayer R, Lightfoot M, Jung I. Preliminary evaluation of calcium hydroxylapatite as a transurethral bulking agent for stress urinary incontinence. Urology 2001;57(3): 434–438

8. Beasley K. Dermatol Surg 2010;36(4):524–526

9. Burgess CM, Quiroga RM. Assessment of the safety and efficacy of poly-L-lactic acid for the treatment of HIV-associated facial lipoatrophy. J Am Acad Dermatol 2005; 52(2):233–239

10. Rossner F, Rossner, Hartmann V, et al. Decrease of reported adverse events to injectible polylactic acid after recommending an increased dilution: 8-year results from the Injectible Filler Safety Study. J Cosmet Dermatol 2009;8(1):14–18

11. Woerle B, Hanke CW, Sattler G. Poly-L-lactic acid: a temporary filler for soft tissue augmentation. J Drugs Dermatol 2004;3(4):385–389

12. Sculptra prescribing information. www.sculptraaesthetic. com. Accessed October 17, 2011

13. Bauer U. Improvement of facial aesthetics at 40 months with injectable poly-L-lactic acid (PLLA). The 17th Congress of the International Society of Aesthetic Plastic Surgery; August 28–31, 2004; Houston, Texas. Abstract p164.

14. Cohen SR, Berner CF, Busso M, et al. Five-year safety and efficacy of a novel polymethylmethacrylate aesthetic soft tissue filler for the correction of nasolabial folds. Dermatol Surg 2007;33(Suppl 2):S222–S230

15. Coleman SR. Structural Fat Grafting. St. Louis, MO: Quality Medical Publishing; 2004

16. Obagi S. Autologous fat augmentation for addressing facial volume loss. Oral Maxillofac Surg Clin North Am 2005;17(1):99–109, vii

17. Pessa JE, Desvigne LD, Lambros VS, Nimerick J, Sugunan B, Zadoo VP. Changes in ocular globe-to-orbital rim position with age: implications for aesthetic blepharoplasty of the lower eyelids. Aesthetic Plast Surg 1999;23(5):337–342

18. Kranendonk SK, Obagi S. Autologous fat transfer for periorbital rejuvenation: indications, technique, and complications. Dermatol Surg 2007;33(5):572–578

19. Lambros V. Volumizing the brow with hyaluronic acid fillers. Aesthet Surg J 2009;29(3):174–179

20. Shaw RB Jr, Katzel EB, Koltz PF, Kahn DM, Girotto JA, Langstein HN. Aging of the mandible and its aesthetic implications. Plast Reconstr Surg 2010;125(1):332–342

21. Donofrio LM. Fat distribution: a morphologic study of the aging face. Dermatol Surg 2000;26(12):1107–1112

22. Sarroff DS, Saini R, Gotkin RH. Comparison of filling agents for lip augmentation. Aesthet Surg J 2008;28(5): 556–563

23. Fife D. Practical evaluation and management of atrophic acne scars: tips for the general dermatologist. J Clin Aesthet Dermatol 2011;4(8):50–57

24. Goldberg DJ, Amin S, Hussain M. Acne scar correction using calcium hydroxylapatite in a carrier-based gel. J Cosmet Laser Ther 2006;8(3):134–136

25. Fulchiero GJ Jr, Parham-Vetter PC, Obagi S. Subcision and 1320-nm Nd:YAG nonablative laser resurfacing for the treatment of acne scars: a simultaneous split-face single patient trial. Dermatol Surg 2004;30(10):1356–1359, discussion 1360

26. Beer K. A single-center, open-label study on the use of injectable poly-L-lactic acid for the treatment of moderate to severe scarring from acne or varicella. Dermatol Surg 2007;33(Suppl 2):S159–S167

27. Epstein RE, Spencer M. Correction of atrophic scars with Artefill: an open-label pilot study. J Drugs Dermatol 2010;9(9):1062–1064

28. Barnett JG, Barnett CR. Treatment of acne scars with liquid silicone injections: 30-year perspective. Dermatol Surg 2005;31(11 Pt 2):1542–1549

29. de Benito J, Fernández I, Nanda V. Treatment of depressed scars with a dissecting cannula and an autologous fat graft. Aesthetic Plast Surg 1999;23(5):367–370

30. Sterodimas A, Huanquipaco JC, de Souza Filho S, Bornia FA, Pitanguy I. Autologous fat transplantation for the treatment of Parry-Romberg syndrome. J Plast Reconstr Aesthet Surg 2009;62(11):e424–e426

31. Sclafani AP, Fagien S. Treatment of injectable soft tissue filler complications. Dermatol Surg 2009;35(Suppl 2): 1672–1680

32. Glaich AS, Cohen JL, Goldberg LH. Injection necrosis of the glabella: protocol for prevention and treatment after use of dermal fillers. Dermatol Surg 2006;32(2):276–281

33. Roberts SA, Arthurs BP. Severe visual loss and orbital infarction following periorbital aesthetic poly-L-lactic acid (PLLA) injection. Ophthal Plast Reconstr Surg 2012;28(3):e68–e70

34. Silva MT, Curi AL. Blindness and total ophthalmoplegia after aesthetic polymethylmethacrylate injection: case report. Arq Neuropsiquiatr 2004;62(3B):873–874

35. Gleeson CM, Lucas S, Langrish CJ, Barlow RJ. Acute fatal fat tissue embolism after autologous fat transfer in a patient with lupus profundus. Dermatol Surg 2011;37(1): 111–115

36. Lowe NJ, Maxwell CA, Patnaik R. Adverse reactions to dermal fillers: review. Dermatol Surg 2005;31(11 Pt 2): 1616–1625

37. Lam SM, Azizzadeh B, Graivier M. Injectable poly-L-lactic acid (Sculptra): technical considerations in soft-tissue contouring. Plast Reconstr Surg 2006;118(3, Suppl): 55S–63S

38. Zielke H, Wölber L, West L, Rzany B. Risk profiles of different injectable fillers: results from the Injectable Filler Safety Study (IFS Study). Dermatol Surg 2008;34(3): 326–335, discussion 335

17 Treatment of Nasal Defects and Acne Scars with Microdroplet Silicone

Jay G. Barnett and Channing R. Barnett

Key Concepts

- Injections of medical-grade liquid silicone can permanently improve nasal defects, acne scars, and other facial scars.

- The advantages of medical-grade liquid injectable silicone over other injectable filler substances are precision of placement and permanence.

- Although technique dependent, the utilization of medical-grade liquid silicone injections for appropriate indications is safe and provides natural-appearing results.

■ Introduction

This chapter discusses the use of injections of medical-grade liquid silicone to improve external nasal defects (the nonsurgical rhinoplasty) and to treat scars, including surgical, traumatic, and acne scars. Also, the recommended concepts and techniques involved in obtaining optimum results in these treatments are highlighted based on more than 40 years of experience with liquid silicone injections. Although silicone injection for facial defects is widely utilized, it must be stressed that this is an off-label use, and the patient should be informed of this prior to any procedure as part of the informed consent.

■ Background: Basic Science of Procedure

Soft tissue augmentation is sought to enhance various body contours and to restore soft tissue loss as-sociated with both normal aging and with diseases and trauma damaging to cutaneous structures. Many types of filler have been used for correction or restoration of facial contour deformities.[1]

Filler Material Requirements

For a filler material to be useful in correcting soft tissue abnormalities, it should be able to produce permanent, aesthetically pleasing cosmetic results with a minimum of undesirable reactions.[1] An ideal filler is autologous, easy for the physician to use with respect to material injectability and injection techniques, minimally painless on injection, and inexpensive. It is also preferred that such a filler be permanent while producing minimal side effects, such as bruising, bleeding, infection, migration, scarring, tissue loss, or reaction. In addition, physicians in the United States prefer the material to be approved by the U.S. Food and Drug Administration (FDA).

Significant factors associated with fillers and their uses include defect selection and injection technique (skill of administration).[1] Many types of filler have been used to correct postsurgical, posttraumatic, or inherited facial deformities and irregularities.[2–12] It should be noted that the only liquid filler substance that maintains precision and permanence in improving and correcting soft tissue defects is medical-grade liquid silicone, a silicone preparation purified and sterilized so that it can be used for medical and biological purposes.[6]

Silicone

Two liquid injectable silicone (LIS) products are currently approved by the FDA: Silikon 1000 (Alcon, Fort Worth, TX) and Adato Sil-ol 5000 (Bausch and Lomb, Rochester, NY). Although these products were approved for use in the eye as a tamponade for retinal detachments, they can be used off-label for correcting external nasal defects and treating scars. Physicians must keep in mind that commercial advertisement of off-label use of a product is not permitted under FDA guidelines. Silikon 1000 and Adato Sil-ol 5000 are forms of sterile purified polydimethylsiloxane of different viscosities. The viscosity of liquid silicone is expressed in centistoke (cs) units with one stoke (i.e., 100 cs) being the viscosity of water. Silikon 1000 has a viscosity of 1,000 cs and is less viscous than Adato Sil-ol 5000, which has a viscosity of 5,000 cs.

The higher the viscosity of the silicone, the larger the needle needed for its injection; the larger the needle, the more bruising, bleeding, and discomfort for the patient. Therefore, of the two available FDA-approved products, the less-viscous Silikon 1000, which can be injected with a 27-gauge half-inch needle, is preferred over the Adato Sil-ol 5000, which requires a 25-gauge 5/8 inch needle. Other syringe-needle configurations can be used based on individual physician preferences. Before these LIS products, another medical-grade liquid silicone product was available at 350 cs, which was even less viscous then Silikon 1000.

LIS fulfills most of the criteria for an ideal filling substance.[13–16] It is a clear, colorless, odorless, tasteless, and stable substance. It lacks mutagenic, carcinogenic, and teratogenic effects; no true allergies to silicone have been documented. The hypothesized mechanism of action is a combination of the displacement of the dermal connective tissue by silicone microdroplets, and the possible production of thin-walled collagen capsules that surround the silicone microdroplets.[17] LIS can be stored for long periods of time at room temperature and does not allow for the growth of microorganisms.[16] It does not soften or harden, remains unaltered within the range of human body temperature, and is chemically unaltered by exposure to sunlight, air, and most chemicals.[13] Although technique dependent, the advantages of LIS over other injectable filler substances are its precision and permanence. Zappi et al reported on the long-term histological host response to liquid silicone, demonstrating its permanence and inertness, reflected by the lack of any adverse reaction to its presence.[18]

The senior author (JGB) has used LIS for correcting nasal defects, acne scarring, and other scars for more than 40 years. He has reported on the use for treating acne scars for up to 30 years[13] and also for correcting nasal defects.[14] Many other authors have reported on the beneficial use of LIS for correcting facial defects.[6,19–24]

■ Pertinent Anatomy

External Nasal Defects

The nasal contour is a series of gentle curves and arches that allow the individual elements of the nose to blend seamlessly. The concavity of the nasal root should flow smoothly into the nasal dorsum, which, in turn, gently courses into the nasal tip. The nasal tip, alae, and columella consist of several interrelated curves. Distortion of any of these parts can adversely affect the appearance of the nose.

Subtle nasal defects can be seen in a variety of circumstances, including natural evolution, post-traumatic injury, postcosmetic surgical rhinoplasty, postnasal lesion removal, and after Mohs nasal reconstructive surgery. External nasal imperfections and deformities that are not expected to improve can be corrected without having to surgically manipulate the nose. In the absence of functional compromise, relatively more conservative approaches and problem-focused solutions are available.

The ability to readily improve or correct irregularities and asymmetries in the nose with an injectable material is very appealing because imperfections, especially after surgical treatment and rhinoplasty, are common. The use of a filler in correcting external nasal defects minimizes patient discomfort and financial expense, and it eliminates anesthetic risk and downtime, all usually associated with surgical intervention. Cutaneous fillers are less traumatic and more ideal for contour deformities than operative implants or incisions.

Efficacy means that the material fills the defect to create a natural appearance with a seamless transition from treated to untreated skin, maintaining the natural contours. Ideally, the filler should be permanent to avoid the need for retreatment after reaching the desired outcome. The use of LIS for the improvement or correction of nasal defects provides a simple minimally invasive, permanent solution in the form of a nonsurgical rhinoplasty.

Acne, Traumatic, and Surgical Scarring

Acne can produce many different types of skin defects, including inflammation and scarring. Acne scarring can be described as deep, shallow, wide (broad-based), pitted, ice-pick, depressed, hypo- and hypertrophic, keloidal, or hypo- and hyperpigmented. The choice of corrections, therefore, is dependent on the type of scar or acne defect. Several techniques for facial acne scar revision have been described. These include laser, dermabrasion, shave excision, punch elevation, punch excision with full-thickness graft replacement, silicone augmentation, electro-desiccation, and scar reduction with intralesional corticosteroids.[13,25,26]

Owing to the fibrous nature of both pitted and ice-pick scars, the benefit of treating these two types of scars by soft tissue augmentation is limited compared with the benefit obtained in treating depressed or broad-based scars. The use of augmentation in the treatment of broad-based depressed scars was first reported in 1983, and the two filler substances mentioned at that time were silicone and collagen.[25] The senior author has treated several thousand patients over the course of 40 years for different types of acne scars. Minor bleeding and bruising at the injection sites can occur with treatments, but persistent redness or swelling does not occur. Although no significant adverse reactions have occurred in any of these patients, fewer than 10 have had areas of minimal overcorrection, meaning that the scar was injected with slightly more silicone than was needed. Such overcorrections can be treated with minor surgical corrections, such as light electrosurgery, shave excision, or injections of small quantities of low-concentration triamcinolone acetonide.

In the case of traumatic or postsurgical scars, soft tissue augmentation can restore the appearance of the skin's surface. Silicone is an ideal filler for this type of scar revision because it is precise and permanent.

■ Technical Aspects of Procedure

Once the patient and physician have decided together on the treatment, the first step is to photograph the area(s) being treated. The photographs should be taken from the frontal view as well as from both the right and left sides. Additional photographs are recommended at follow-up treatments. The usefulness of these photographs cannot be overstated when physicians are confronted with patients' questions after treatment.

Betadine solution can be used as an antiseptic marker to highlight the areas being treated. Topical anesthetic ointment is not needed when injecting into external nasal defects and scars; most patients find the discomfort to be minimal.

The injection technique used with LIS when treating nasal defects and scarring is referred to as the micro-droplet, multiple injection approach. Each depressed scar or defect can be injected at different points in one treatment session. At each puncture point, minute amounts of LIS, ranging from 0.02 to 0.1 mL per puncture, are injected below the depressed defect at the level of the mid to deep dermis or superficial subcutaneous level. The injections are made using a 1 mL Luer Lock syringe with an appropriately sized needle, as discussed earlier. Silikon 1000 is the sili-

cone used for the correction of nasal defects, scars, and acne scars because it is less viscous and can be used with a smaller needle (27-gauge half-inch).[13]

As the LIS is injected, one can see the depressed defect rise. The size and nature of the defect will dictate the number of treatment sessions necessary, ranging from one in the case of very few small irregularities, to two to four for larger defects or greater involved areas. If multiple sessions are necessary, it is preferable that they be done in stages rather than at one time to prevent overcorrection as well as to minimize the amount of silicone used. Allowing at least a few weeks between treatment sessions enables the defect or scar to stretch, reconfigure, or accommodate the presence of the silicone.[13-15] The silicone stays permanently where it is placed, neither shifting nor drifting with time. Additionally, it does not prevent other treatments in the area, such as surgery, laser procedures, chemical peeling, or dermabrasion. However, if the area of the repaired scar is surgically moved or removed after silicone treatments, the silicone in the defect will go with it.

■ Postoperative Care

Following silicone injections, the treated areas are wiped clean with water. The patient is instructed to hold gauze with moderate pressure over the treated areas for 5 to 10 minutes to minimize any pinpoint bleeding, bruising, or swelling. Makeup can be applied immediately, and the patient can resume work and routine activities, including sports and air travel, as soon as the patient desires. There is no need for downtime following silicone injection.

■ Expected Results

The use of injections of silicone in the cases next described prevented the need for primary or secondary surgeries, many of which could not duplicate the degree of improvement achieved simply and easily by liquid silicone injections.

Correction of Nasal Defects (Nonsurgical Rhinoplasty)

The patients illustrated in **Figs. 17.1, 17.2, 17.3, 17.4, 17.5, 17.6,** and **17.7** are representative of the various nasal defects that can be corrected using medical-grade liquid silicone as already described.

Case 1 is a young woman with significant nasal deformities of long-standing duration; she is shown before treatment (**Fig. 17.1a**) and immediately (5 minutes) after treatment with 0.5 mL of LIS in one treatment session (**Fig. 17.1b**).

Case 2 is a 50-year-old woman with depressions on the dorsum of the nose. She had a rhinoplasty 25 years prior to being seen. Nasal defects before treatment (**Fig. 17.2a**) and immediately (5 minutes) after treatment with 0.4 mL of LIS in one treatment session (**Fig. 17.2b**).

Case 3 is a 40-year-old man with a history of two rhinoplasties 2 and 3 years prior to being seen. In addition, he had HA injected 1 year and then 6 months prior to being seen. He is shown before treatment (**Fig. 17.3a**) and immediately (5 minutes) after treatment with 0.05 mL of LIS in one treatment session (**Fig. 17.3b**).

Case 4 is a 25-year-old woman with depressions on the dorsum and right side of her nose before treatment (**Fig. 17.4**; **Fig. 17.5a**). Results are shown immediately (5 minutes) after treatment with 0.3 mL of LIS in one treatment session (**Fig. 17.4**; **Fig. 17.5b**).

Case 5 is a 43-year-old man with a depressed nasal tip scar resulting from an avascular necrosis secondary to collagen injections by another physician. The patient had rhinoplasties done 3 years and 2 years before the collagen injections (**Fig. 17.6a**). The patient had three treatments of 0.02 mL, 0.01 mL, and 0.01 mL of LIS at monthly intervals to allow the fibrous scar to stretch between treatments. The proximal raised fibrous edge of the scar was treated with light electrodesiccation. **Fig. 17.6b** shows him 6 years after LIS treatment.

Case 6 is a 61-year-old woman with a depressed, telangiectatic scar on the dorsum of the tip of her nose resulting from a graft used to repair the defect from a basal cell carcinoma treated 4 years before (**Fig. 17.7a**). The patient is shown (**Fig. 17.7b**) 2 years after three treatments of 0.1 mL, 0.1 mL, and 0.05 mL with 2 months between the first and second treatments and 18 months between the second and third treatments.

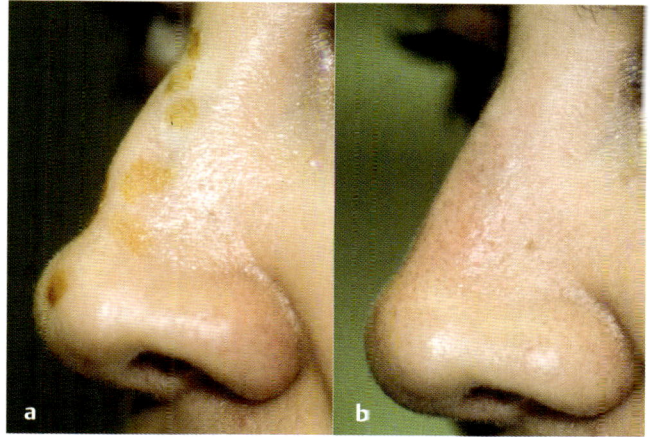

Fig. 17.1 Pretreatment (**a**) and 5 minutes after (**b**) one injection treatment for nasal deformity.

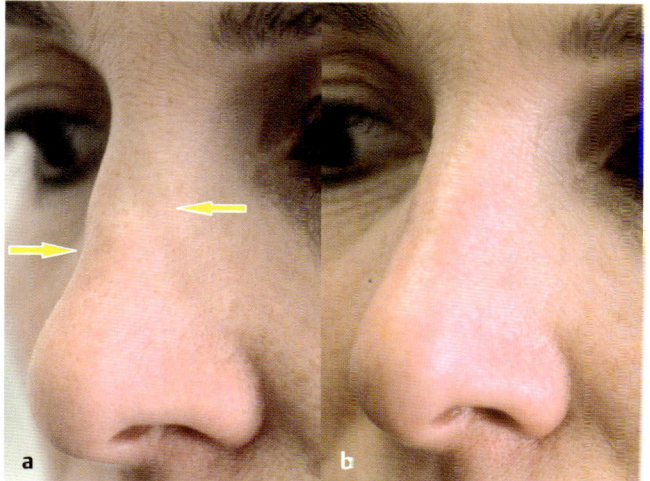

Fig. 17.2 Pretreatment (**a**) and 5 minutes after (**b**) one injection treatment for nasal deformity.

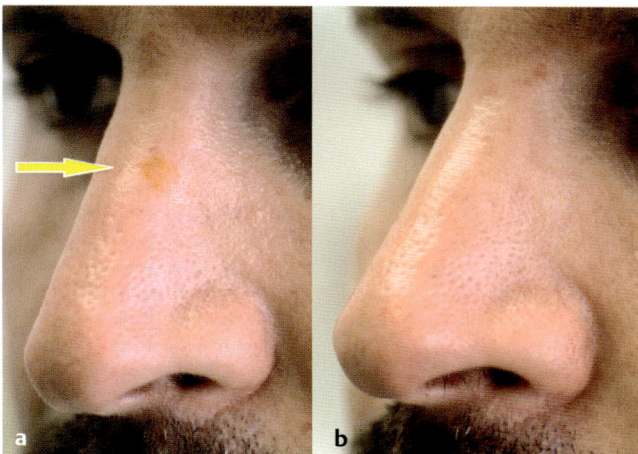

Fig. 17.3 Pretreatment (**a**) and 5 minutes after (**b**) one injection treatment for nasal deformity.

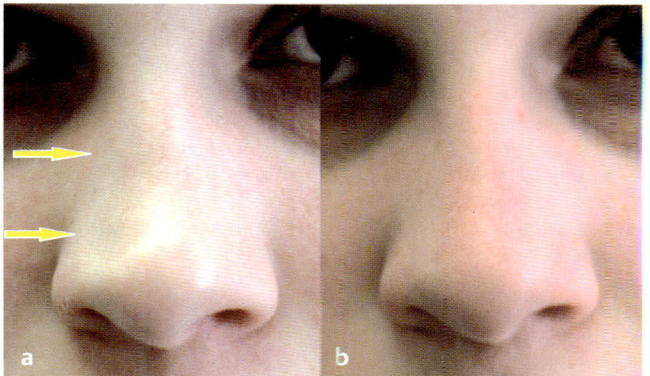

Fig. 17.4 Pretreatment (**a**) and 5 minutes after (**b**) one injection treatment for nasal deformity.

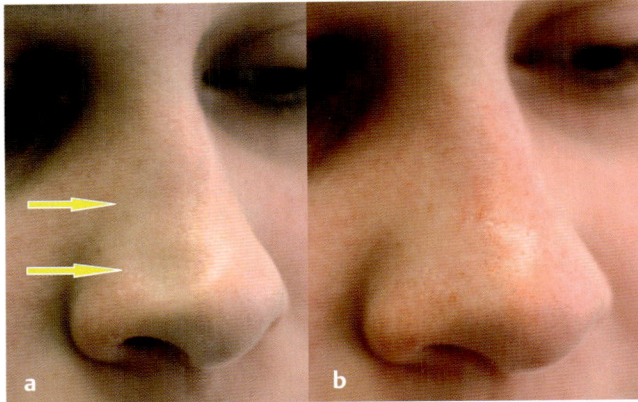

Fig. 17.5 Pretreatment **(a)** and 5 minutes after **(b)** one injection treatment for nasal deformity.

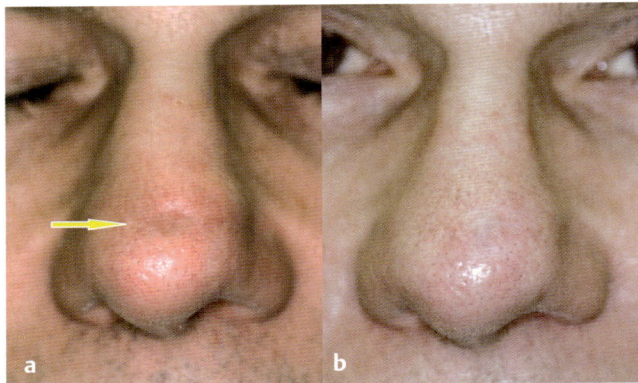

Fig. 17.6 Pretreatment **(a)** and 6 years after **(b)** three monthly injection treatments for nasal deformity.

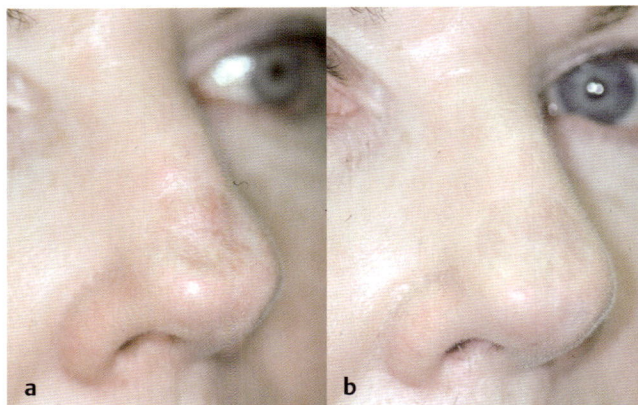

Fig. 17.7 Pretreatment **(a)** and 2 years after **(b)** three injection treatments for nasal deformity, with 2 months between the first and second and 18 months between the second and third treatments.

Correction of Acne Scarring

The patients illustrated in **Figs. 17.8, 17.9, 17.10, 17.11,** and **17.12** are representative of the immediate and long-term benefits of silicone injections in treating depressed, broad-based acne scars.

Case 1 is a 42-year-old woman with numerous depressed, soft, broad-based acne scars on her face, particularly on her temples. Over 20 years ago, she had a facial dermabrasion. At the initial treatment, the acne scars on her face were injected with a total dose of 0.8 mL of LIS. The pretreatment (**Fig. 17.8a**) and 5 minutes posttreatment (**Fig. 17.8b**) images reveal the immediate correction of her acne scars.

Case 2 is a 53-year-old man with extensive broad-based, depressed acne scars on his neck for over 30 years. At the initial treatment, these acne scars were injected with a total of 2.4 mL of LIS. Pretreatment (**Fig. 17.9a**) and 5 minutes immediately posttreatment (**Fig. 17.9b**) are shown.

Case 3 is a 20-year-old man who presented with numerous broad-based acne scars on his face of several years' duration. These acne scars were injected with LIS six times over 2 years with a total dose of 6.4 mL used. Pretreatment (**Fig. 17.10a**) and 6 years posttreatment (**Fig. 17.10b**) of the right side of his face, as well as pretreatment (**Fig. 17.11a**) and 6 years posttreatment (**Fig. 17.11b**) of the left side of his face are shown.

Case 4 is a 28-year-old man with depressed, broad-based acne scars of 10 years' duration on the right side of his chin. The acne scars were injected with LIS twice at monthly intervals. A total amount of 0.3 mL of LIS was used. The pretreatment (**Fig. 17.12a**) and 15-year post-treatment (**Fig. 17.12b**) images reveal the long-term permanent correction.

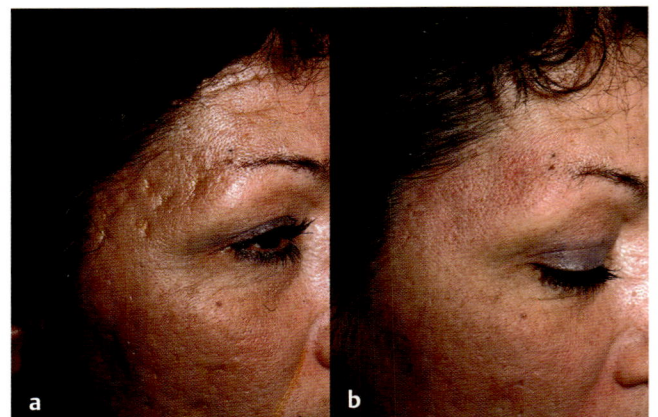

Fig. 17.8 Pretreatment **(a)** and 5 minutes after **(b)** one injection treatment for acne scarring.

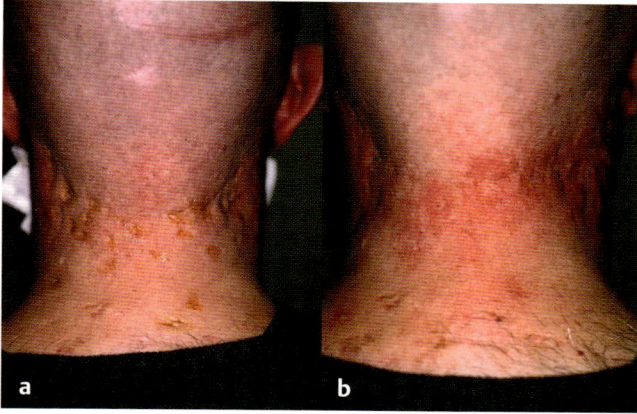

Fig. 17.9   Pretreatment **(a)** and 5 minutes after **(b)** one injection treatment for acne scarring.

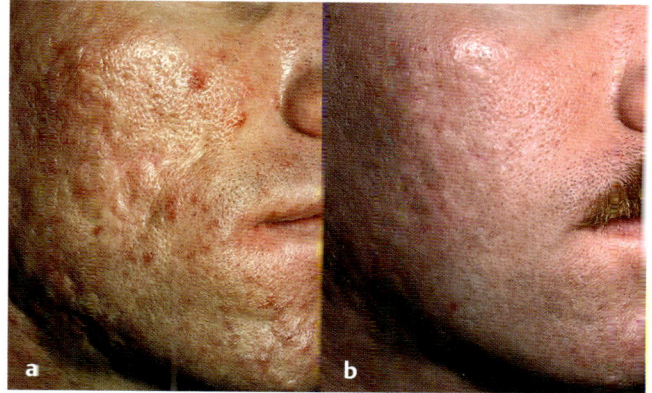

Fig. 17.10   Pretreatment **(a)** and 6 years after **(b)** six injection treatments over 2 years for acne scarring shown for the right side of the face.

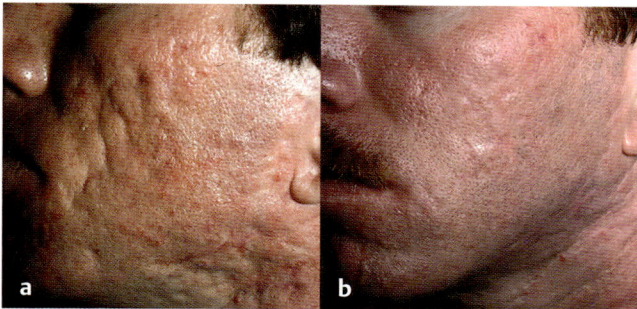

Fig. 17.11   Pretreatment **(a)** and 6 years after **(b)** six injection treatments over 2 years for acne scarring shown for the left side of the face.

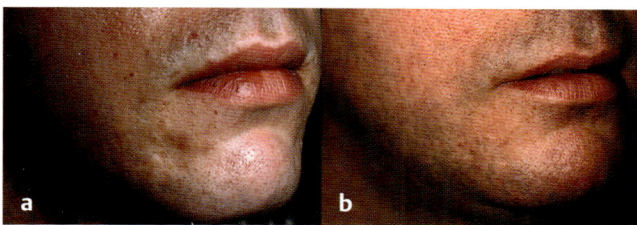

Fig. 17.12   Pretreatment **(a)** and 15 years after **(b)** two monthly injection treatments for acne scarring.

Correction of Surgical and Herpes Zoster Scarring

Case 1 is a 62-year-old man with a deeply depressed linear, postsurgical scar on the right side of his forehead resulting from the removal of a meningioma 4 years prior. The scar before treatment (**Fig. 17.13a**) and immediately after treatment with 3.2 mL of LIS in one treatment session (**Fig. 17.13b**).

Case 2 is a 24-year-old woman with depressed, fibrous-rimmed scars of the glabella and right side of her nose following a herpes zoster infection 6 months earlier. At 6 months, light electrodesiccation of the fibrous, raised scar edges was performed, and 3 months after that the patient had four treatments of injections over 8 months with a total amount of 2.6 mL of LIS injected. Pretreatment (**Fig. 17.14a**) and 1 year post–silicone injections are shown (**Fig. 17.14b**).

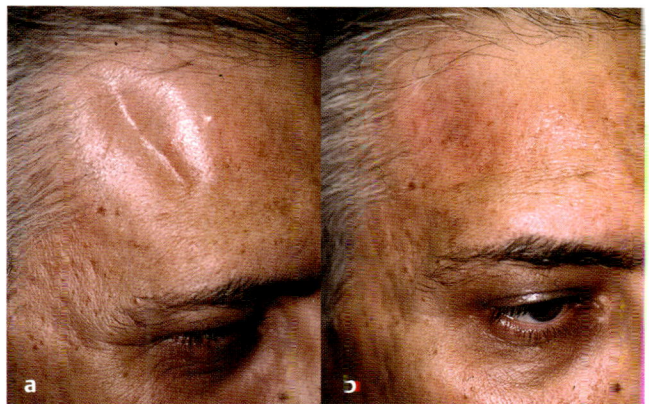

Fig. 17.13   Pretreatment **(a)** immediately after **(b)** one injection treatment for surgical scarring.

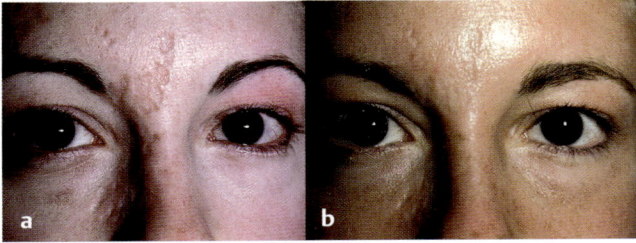

Fig. 17.14 Pretreatment **(a)** and 1 year after **(b)** four injection treatments over 8 months for herpes zoster scarring. Three months before silicone injection, the patient had also undergone light electrodesiccation of the raised scar edges.

■ Complications and Their Management

Numerous authors have raised concerns about LIS and its long-term safety and adverse tissue reactivity.[27–29] Silicone has been implicated in a variety of local and systemic adverse inflammatory reactions.[30] Treatment-site reactions, including pain, erythema, tissue induration, ecchymosis, pigmentation, excessive tissue elevation, and migration of the injected material to local and distant areas, have been reported. More severe complications, including granulomas, subcutaneous nodules, skin induration, cellulitis with nodule formation, local lymph node enlargement, and ulceration, have also been reported.[31] Following injections of large amounts of silicone, physicians have reported tissue destruction and scarring, granulomatous hepatitis, and acute pneumonitis.[32–35] None of the aforementioned reports have associated any such side effects or complications with the use of silicone for the treatment of acne scars, nasal defects, or other facial depressed scars in which only very small volumes of the material are employed.

Often, most granuloma-related reports are associated with impurities in the silicone and silicones associated with other substances. In the 1980s and 1990s, there was controversy regarding the relationship between silicone breast implants and the development of systemic disease.[36] However, in 1996, Hochberg and Perlmutter demonstrated that there is no evidence of a significant statistical association between the two.[37]

Despite these concerns, the long-term experience of physicians skilled in the administration of liquid injectable silicone has shown it to be safe and efficacious for soft tissue augmentation.[16,38] In the authors' experience, which includes 40 years of utilizing liquid silicone injections in many different situations, only occasional minor bruising and swelling have occurred. The rare case of overcorrection can be treated with minor surgical corrections, such as light electrosurgery, shave excision, or injections of small quantities of low-concentration triamcinolone acetonide.

■ Conclusion

As a precise and permanent filling substance used for soft tissue augmentation, silicone can improve or eliminate external nasal defects, surgical or traumatic scars, and acne scars using the microdroplet, multiple injection technique, in which very small amounts are used. In the opinion of the authors, injectable silicone is the filler of choice that should be used for the aforementioned conditions because it is precise and permanent, and it produces natural-appearing results. Let it also be noted that silicone can be used for cosmetic and reconstructive enhancement of lips; volume correction of facial hollows, grooves, and eyelid creases; as well as hand and earlobe restoration and rejuvenation.

References

1. Klein AW, Rish DC. Substances for soft tissue augmentation: collagen and silicone. J Dermatol Surg Oncol 1985;11(3):337–339
2. Klein AW, Rish DC. Injectable collagen update. J Dermatol Surg Oncol 1984;10(7):519–522
3. Castrow FF II, Krull EA. Injectable collagen implant—update. J Am Acad Dermatol 1983;9(6):889–893
4. Milojevic B. Complications after silicone injection therapy in aesthetic plastic surgery. Aesthetic Plast Surg 1982;6(4):203–206
5. Piechotta FU. Silicone fluid, attractive and dangerous. Aesthetic Plast Surg 1979;3:347–355
6. Selmanowitz VJ, Orentreich N. Medical-grade fluid silicone: a monographic review. J Dermatol Surg Oncol 1977;3(6):597–611
7. Watson W, Kaye RL, Klein A, Stegman S. Injectable collagen: a clinical overview. Cutis 1983;31(5):543–546
8. Goldberg DJ. Breakthroughs in US dermal fillers for facial soft-tissue augmentation. J Cosmet Laser Ther 2009;11(4):240–247
9. Humphrey CD, Arkins JP, Dayan SH. Soft tissue fillers in the nose. Aesthet Surg J 2009;29(6):477–484
10. Jones DH. Semipermanent and permanent injectable fillers. Dermatol Clin 2009;27(4):433–444, vi
11. Carruthers J, Cohen SR, Joseph JH, Narins RS, Rubin M. The science and art of dermal fillers for soft-tissue augmentation. J Drugs Dermatol 2009;8(4):335–350
12. Rivkin A, Soliemanzadeh P. Nonsurgical injection rhinoplasty with calcium hydroxylapatite in a carrier gel (Radiesse): a 4-year, retrospective, clinical review. Cosmet Dermatol 2009;22(12):619–624
13. Barnett JG, Barnett CR. Treatment of acne scars with liquid silicone injections: 30-year perspective. Dermatol Surg 2005;31(11 Pt 2):1542–1549
14. Sclafani AP, Romo T III, Barnett JG, Barnett CR. Adjustment of subtle post-operative nasal defects: managing the "near-miss" rhinoplasty. Facial Plast Surg 2003;19:349–361
15. Barnett JG, Barnett CR. Silicone augmentation of the lip. Facial Plast Surg Clin North Am 2007;15(4):501–512, vii–viii

16. Orentreich DS. Liquid injectable silicone: techniques for soft tissue augmentation. Clin Plast Surg 2000;27(4):595–612

17. Brown LH, Frank PJ. What's new in fillers? J Drugs Dermatol 2003;2(3):250–253

18. Zappi E, Barnett JG, Zappi ME, Barnett CR. The long-term host response to liquid silicone injected during soft tissue augmentation procedures: a microscopic appraisal. Dermatol Surg 2007;33(2, Suppl 2):S186–S192, discussion S192

19. Webster RC, Kattner MD, Smith RC. Injectable collagen for augmentation of facial areas. Arch Otolaryngol 1984;110(10):652–656

20. Aronsohn RB. A 22-year experience with the use of silicone injections. Am J Cosmet Surg 1984;1:21–28

21. Fulton JE. The elevation of acne scars with injectable silicone. Am J Cosmet Surg 1990;7:99–105

22. Orentreich DS, Orentreich N. Injectable fluid silicone. In: Roenigk R, Roenigk HH, eds. Dermatologic Surgery. New York, NY: Marcel Dekker; 1989:1349–1395

23. Duffy DM. Injectable liquid silicone; new perspectives. In: Klein AW, ed. Tissue Augmentation in Clinical Practice: Procedures and Techniques. New York, NY: Marcel Dekker; 1998:237–267

24. Prather CL, Jones DH. Liquid injectable silicone for soft tissue augmentation. Dermatol Ther 2006;19(3):159–168

25. Orentreich N, Durr NP. Rehabilitation of acne scarring. Dermatol Clin 1983;1:405–413

26. Orentreich D, Orentreich N. Acne scar revision update. Dermatol Clin 1987;5(2):359–368

27. Rapaport M. Silicone injections revisited. Dermatol Surg 2002;28(7):594–595

28. Wilkie TF. Late development of granuloma after liquid silicone injections. Plast Reconstr Surg 1977;60(2):179–188

29. Winer LH, Sternberg TH, Lehman R, Ashley FL. Tissue reactions to injected silicone liquids: a report of three cases. Arch Dermatol 1964;90 588–593

30. Clark DP, Hanke CW, Swanson NA. Dermal implants: safety of products injected for soft tissue augmentation. J Am Acad Dermatol 1989;21(5 Pt 1):992–998

31. Rapaport MJ, Vinnik CH, Zarem H. Injectable silicone cause of facial nodules cellulitis, ulceration, and migration. Aesthetic Plast Surg 1996;20(3):267–276

32. Mastruserio DN, Pesqueira MJ, Cobb MW. Severe granulomatous reaction and facial ulceration occurring after subcutaneous silicone injection. J Am Acad Dermatol 1996;34(5 Pt 1):849–852

33. Raszewski R, Guyuron B, Lash RH, McMahon JT, Tuthill R. A severe fibrotic reaction after cosmetic liquid silicone injection: a case report. J Craniomaxillofac Surg 1990;18(5):225–228

34. Ellenbogen R, Rubin L. Injectable fluid silicone therapy human morbidity and mortality. JAMA 1975;234(3 308–309

35. Chastre J, Basset F, Viau F, et al. Acute pneumonitis after subcutaneous injections of silicone in transsexual men. N Engl J Med 1983;308(13):764–767

36. Brozena SJ, Fenske NA, Cruse CW, et al. Human adjuvant disease following augmentation mammoplasty. Arch Dermatol 1988;124(9):1383–1386

37. Hochberg MC, Perlmutter DL. The association of augmentation mammoplasty with connective tissue disease, including systematic sclerosis (scleroderma): a meta-analysis. Curr Top Microbiol Immunol 1996;210:411–417

38. Webster RC, Fuleihan NS, Gaunz JM, et al. Injectable silicone for small augmentations: twenty-year experience in humans. Am J Cosmet Surg 1984;1:1–10

18 Soft Tissue Fillers for Facial Augmentation

Thomas L. Tzikas

Key Concepts

- Soft tissue facial fillers have developed into one of the most popular and widely used methods for facial rejuvenation.

- Cross-linked hyaluronic acid (HA) products are among the most studied and versatile products and are used more than all other fillers combined.

- The most common injection-site reactions are edema, erythema, tenderness, ecchymosis, and itching.

- Treatment of impending skin necrosis consists of warm compresses, oral steroids, nitroglycerin topical paste for vasodilation, topical antibiotic ointment, hyaluronidase if HA was injected, hyperbaric oxygen, and/or deep subcutaneous heparin injection.

Introduction

The last decade has seen a tremendous increase in minimally invasive cosmetic procedures, most notably injectable synthetic soft tissue facial fillers. A better understanding of facial aging as a result of soft tissue atrophy has fueled this dramatic rise. These office-based procedures are fairly straightforward to perform, have minimal downtime for the patient, and, when combined with neurotoxins and laser skin treatments, can result in impressive rejuvenative outcomes. Today there are a wide variety of short-duration, long-duration, and permanent fillers available for use in the United States. This chapter reviews many of these products, with special emphasis on techniques to optimize the result while limiting complications.

Background: Basic Science of Procedure

Soft tissue volume restoration has received a greater amount of emphasis in the treatment of the aging face during the past 15 years. The idea of vertical facial descent with loss of elasticity being the main cause of facial aging has been supplanted by the idea that volume depletion occurs at multiple tissue levels, including skeletal and subcutaneous tissue.[1–3] Facial beauty in a youthful face consists of fullness, softness, symmetry, and proper proportions. There is a smooth distribution and transition of skeletal and subcutaneous soft tissue between adjacent aesthetic zones of the face, with a resultant balance between volume and shape. Aging of the face involves tissue involution, with flattening and hollowing of facial features. Some of the earliest accounts of soft tissue augmentation utilized autologous fat over a century ago.[4] Other permanent products, such as paraffin, were used at the end of the 19th century but were discontinued due to severe granulomatous reactions. Silicone has been injected for well over 50 years but was banned by the U.S. Food and Drug Administration due to concerns about its safety.[5] Silicone is available today in 1,000 centistoke formulation for opthalmologic use and is utilized as an off-label cosmetic filler.[6]

The first widely used injectable fillers to be used in the United States were the bovine collagen products. They were introduced in the late 1970s and consisted of Zyderm and cross-linked Zyplast (Allergan, Irvine, CA) for the treatment of moderate fine lines and rhytids. The results were effective but short lived and resulted in about a 5% incidence of severe allergic reaction.[7,8] Therefore, skin testing was required, which delayed patient treatments. The limitations of collagen products led to the development of longer-lasting, nonallergic, and more versatile fillers. Today, the emphasis in facial volume enhancement has been transformed from simple wrinkles and filling of folds to regional and panfacial augmentation.

■ Patient Selection

The ideal patient for injectable fillers has relatively good skin elasticity and minimal skin laxity. Patients with thin skin and limited soft tissue have an increased risk of visible irregularity of the injected product. Patients with chronic disease, especially autoimmune disorders, and pregnant or lactating females are not appropriate candidates for treatment.

Discussion of patient expectations, including correction and longevity, is critical in obtaining satisfactory results, and an explanation of the various fillers with benefits and limitations must be provided prior to the treatment. A thorough comprehension by both the clinician and the patient of the potential reactions and complications is necessary. Preinjection standardized photographs are imperative because results with fillers can be less noticeable than with surgical intervention.

■ Technical Aspects of Procedure

Ideal filler substances have FDA approval and are nonallergenic, noncarcinogenic, nonmigratory, easy to store, cost-effective, reproducible, durable, and malleable enough to provide a "natural" look and feel. The injection procedure should be relatively simple to perform, with minimal discomfort and with few adverse sequelae. Each product has its unique characteristics and is used differently in each patient. It should be noted that, although many surgeons use some of these techniques and products in the manner described, there may be off-label uses of the fillers.

Products can be categorized by the duration of the effect. Hyaluronic acids (HAs) are temporary fillers that have a lasting effect of ~ 6 months. Intermediate or semipermanent fillers have durations of up to 18 months and are composed of calcium hydroxylapatite (CaHA, Radiesse, Merz Aesthetics, San Mateo, CA) and poly-L-lactic acid (PLLA, Sculptra, Sanofi-Aventis U.S., Bridgewater, NJ). Permanent filler products available consist of Silikon 1000 (Alcon, Fort Worth, TX, off-label use) and collagen with polymethyl methacrylate (PMMA, Artefill Suneva Medical, San Diego, CA). Products may be safely combined in the same patient during the same treatment session.

Techniques with previous fillers for simply filling lines on the face have been replaced with structural augmentation of deeper tissue levels with larger volumes of products. Evaluation of the face as a whole allows volume enhancement to be more comprehensive and to give a lifting effect to the face rather than treating only rhytids. A list of the facial regions with the author's preferred products is provided in Table 18.1. Product selection may vary with such factors as patient age, skin elasticity, and soft tissue thickness.

Table 18.1 Preferred product by region

Region	Primary filler choices	Secondary filler choices
Malar/submalar	CaHA, PLLA	Juvederm Ultra Plus,[b] Perlane[c]
Tear trough	Restylane[a]	Juvederm Ultra[d]
Nasolabial folds	HAs, CaHA	PLLA, PMMA, silicone
Marionette-prejowl sulcus	HAs, CaHA	PLLA, silicone, PMMA
Mandible	CaHA, PLLA	HAs
Lip augmentation	HAs, silicone	
Perioral rhytids	Silicone	HAs
Temple	PLLA, CaHA	HAs
Brow	CaHA	HAs, PLLA
Glabellar/forehead rhytids	HAs, CaHA	Silicone
Nose	HAs, CaHA	Silicone

Abbreviations: CaHA, calcium hydroxylapatite; HAs, hyaluronic acids; PLLA, poly-L-lactic acid; PMMA, polymethyl methacrylate.
[a]Medicis Pharmaceutical, Scottsdale, AZ.
[b]Allergan, Irvine, CA.
[c]Medicis Pharmaceutical, Scottsdale, AZ.
[d]Allergan, Irvine, CA.

Patients undergoing soft tissue facial filler injections should be instructed to refrain from taking blood thinners, such as aspirin (as long as it is not medically necessary), nonsteroidal anti-inflammatory drugs, many vitamin supplements (vitamin E, fish oils, ginger, Ginkgo biloba, ginseng, garlic), and alcohol, ideally for 2 weeks prior to the injection. The procedure is performed using strict aseptic technique (alcohol or chlorhexidine), making sure the skin is cleansed of all dirt and makeup. A compounded topical anesthetic cream (20% benzocaine, 6% lidocaine, 4% tetracaine, Pharmacy Creations, Randolph, NJ) is applied to the treatment area for at least 10 minutes, with local injectable anesthetics sometimes being used, especially in the perioral region (dental block). The incorporation of lidocaine within most of the current products has greatly reduced discomfort associated with the injection. Ice is applied to the face prior to, during, and after the injection.

Hyaluronic Acid (Restylane, Perlane, Juvederm)

Cross-linked HA products are among the most studied and versatile products, have become the standard in the United States, and are used more than all other fillers combined. HA is naturally occurring in the skin but it has a very short half-life due to its sensitivity to hyaluronidases and is therefore cross-linked in the manufacturing process to prevent degradation. HA is obtained through the fermentation of Streptococcus equi. HA fillers are biocompatible, stable in vivo, safe, effective, and well tolerated.[9]

The most popular HA products used in the United States today are Restylane, Perlane (Medicis Pharmaceutical, Scottsdale, AZ, Q-Med AB, Uppsala, Sweden), Juvederm Ultra XC, and Juvederm Ultra Plus XC (Allergan, Irvine, CA). They are all FDA approved for implantation into the mid-to-deep dermis for the correction of moderate to severe facial wrinkles and folds, such as nasolabial folds. The concentration of HA is 20 mg/mL for Restylane and Perlane and 24 mg/mL for Juvederm Ultra XC and Ultra Plus XC. Ideally, Juvederm Ultra XC and Restylane can be injected with either a 30-gauge half-inch or a 29-gauge half-inch needle. Juvederm Ultra Plus XC and Perlane are most commonly injected with a 27-gauge half-inch needle. All the foregoing products are cross-linked in a phosphate buffer with 0.3% lidocaine, which significantly reduces pain at the injection site.

Juvederm products are monophasic, where 100% of the HA molecule is cross-linked, and Restylane (smaller gel particle size) and Perlane (larger gel particle size) are biphasic products, where they contain both cross-linked and un-cross-linked HA. Juvederm has a higher degree of cross-linking between HA molecules (6 to 8%) and is supplied in 0.8 mL syringes versus 2% for Restylane, which is supplied in 1 mL syringes. The higher percentage of cross-linking between HA molecules increases the viscosity of the material (reduces the ability to flow) and theoretically lasts longer.

Injection techniques vary with the injector and may include serial puncture, linear threading, cross-hatching, or deep depot injections for regional augmentation. The filling effect of these products is a result of displacement of tissue and the hydrophilic properties, which attract water to the injection site. The author's preference is using Juvederm Ultra Plus XC and Perlane for deeper dermal or subcutaneous injections, such as the nasolabial folds, for supraperiosteal injections in areas such as the prejowl sulcus, and for volume restoration to the upper cheeks. Juvederm Ultra XC is a preferred product for lip augmentation because it results in a smoother and broader augmentation as compared with Restylane.

Restylane is the product of choice for tear-trough correction because it has a less characteristic hydrophilic effect and produces less edema ▶ Video 18.1. The technique involves using a minimal amount of local anesthetic to block the infraorbital nerve and to inject the filler using a 0.7 mm microcannula (Tulip, San Diego, CA). Other, newer, disposable, blunt-tipped cannulas are also available in 25 and 27 gauge by 1-, 1.5-, and 2-inch length (TSK Laboratory, Tochigi-Ken, Japan). The advantage of blunt-tip cannulas over standard needles is the ability to inject large volumes with less trauma, edema, and bruising and with a reduced risk of injecting into arteries or vessels. A sharp needle is used to make the entry site in the mid cheek, and the cannula is used to deposit small aliquots of material in the tear-trough deformity. It is imperative to inject at the level of the supraperiosteal tissue plane, to massage the material to the desired position, and not to overcorrect. Often, Restylane is diluted with 0.2 to 0.3 mL of 1% lidocaine, utilizing a transfer syringe, to reduce the hydrophilic effect of the material in this area of extremely thin skin. The hydrophilic effect of Juvederm is more pronounced and may result in visible accumulation of product in the tear trough or in the Tyndall effect. Therefore, if Juvederm is to be used in the tear trough, undercorrection is advised. HAs also have the added safety advantage of allowing one to correct excess fullness or superficial placement simply by injecting hyaluronidase. For these reasons, HAs have become the preferred fillers in the thin-skinned tear-trough region (Fig. 18.1a,b).

Other HA fillers available in the United States include Hydrelle (Anika Therapeutics, Bedford, MA), Prevelle Silk (Mentor, Santa Barbara, CA), and Puragen. Hydrelle (Anika Therapeutics), which has the highest concentration of HA per syringe at 28 mg/mL, was the first FDA-approved HA product to include lidocaine. Prevelle Silk also contains lidocaine and

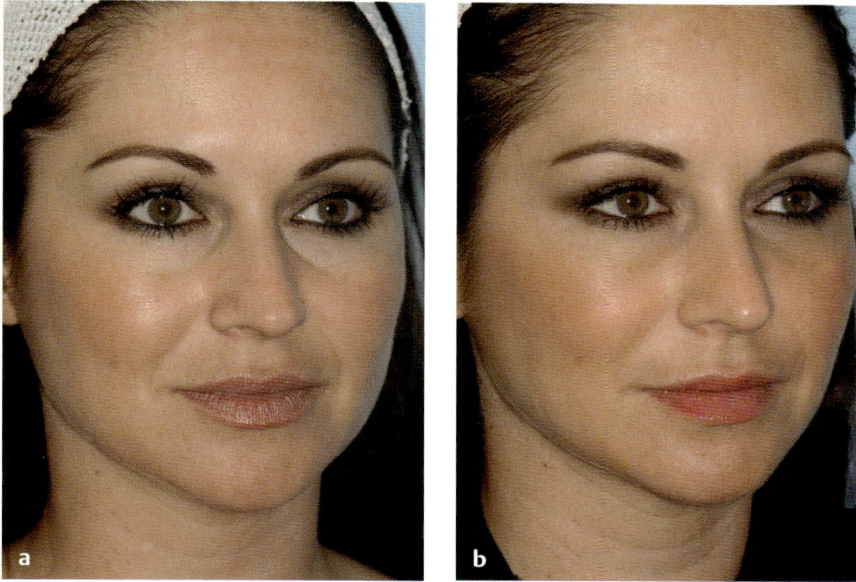

Fig. 18.1 (a) Before treatment of tear-trough depressions and nasolabial folds. (b) One month after Restylane (Medicis Pharmaceutical) cannula injection to the tear trough deformities bilaterally (1 mL total) and one vial (0.8 mL) Juvederm Ultra Plus XC (Allergan) to the nasolabial folds.

has an HA concentration of only 5.5 mg/mL, which provides a correction for 2 to 3 months. Puragen has a small particle size, improves flow characteristics, and reportedly can persist for 9 to 12 months.

Calcium Hydroxylapatite (Radiesse)

CaHA (Radiesse, Merz Aesthetics, San Mateo, CA) has a unique profile that makes it particularly well suited for facial augmentation. Radiesse (Merz Aesthetics) is a viscous filler composed of CaHA microspheres (25 to 45 μm) suspended in an aqueous carboxymethylcellulose gel carrier and is injected with a 28-gauge needle. When placed into soft tissue, CaHA provides immediate correction. As the gel carrier is absorbed, the CaHA particles act as a scaffold for new tissue formation and collagen deposition. Over time, the CaHA particles are broken down into calcium and phosphate ions and are slowly removed via the body's normal metabolic pathways. Radiesse is approved by the FDA for facial cosmetic applications, such as correction of moderate to severe wrinkles and folds, including nasolabial folds, and restoration or correction of signs of facial lipoatrophy in people with human immunodeficiency virus (HIV). Longevity of aesthetic correction in the face has been reported to range from 9 to 18 months with an average correction of 12 months.[10–12]

Radiesse is packaged in either 1.5, 0.8, or 0.3 mL syringes. An accessory kit is provided that contains a female-to-female Luer Lock connector and a 3 mL syringe that is used to mix the product with 0.3 mL of lidocaine. This mixture has significantly decreased the discomfort of injection but has not affected the durability or efficacy.

Radiesse is a thicker product than HAs and has the advantage of increased volume augmentation, especially in areas such as the cheeks, temples ▶ Video 18.2, pre-jowl sulcus, and deep nasolabial folds. It provides excellent volume restoration when injected in the supraperiosteal plane (Fig. 18.2a–c; Fig. 18.3a,b). Adverse events are similar to other fillers but CaHA has an increased incidence of nodule formation when injected into the lips and is therefore not generally indicated as an off-label filler for lip augmentation. The injection technique is similar to other products but is also used as a depot injection, especially for midface augmentation. Another unique method of midface injection is using an intraoral approach ▶ Video 18.3. Care must be taken to clean the intraoral mucosa usually with Betadine (Purdue Products, Stamford, CT), and to avoid injecting a patient with poor oral hygiene using this method. Another consideration is to be aware of the location of the infraorbital nerve and avoid its injury.

Poly-L-Lactic Acid (Sculptra)

Poly-L-lactic acid (PLLA, Sculptra, Sanofi-Aventis) is FDA approved for the treatment of HIV lipoatrophy and for the correction of shallow to deep nasolabial folds, contour deficiencies, and other facial wrinkles ▶ Video 18.4. Sculptra consists of microparticles of PLLA, sodium carboxymethylcellulose, and mannitol in a freeze-dried state, and is reconstituted with sterile water for injection. Generally, the product is reconstituted with 5 mL of sterile water, but reconstitution can also be done with sterile saline, bacteriostatic saline, and/or lidocaine. The author's preferred method is to reconstitute Sculptra 3 to 4

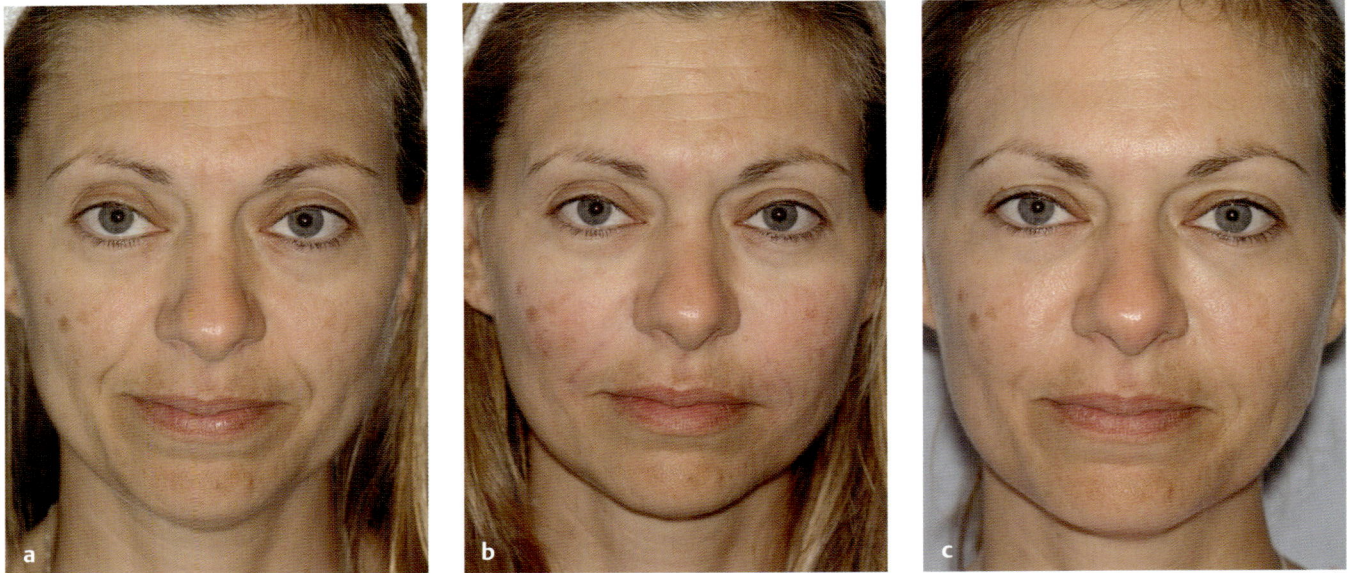

Fig. 18.2 **(a)** Before treatment with fillers and neurotoxin. **(b)** Immediately following Botox treatment to the upper face, Juvederm Ultra cannula injection to the infraorbital hollows (0.8 mL), and Radiesse 1.5 mL intraoral injection to the malar regions bilaterally, and Radiesse 1.5 mL injection to the nasolabial folds. **(c)** Two weeks following Botox treatment to the upper face, Juvederm Ultra cannula injection to the infraorbital hollows (0.8 mL) and Radiesse 1.5 mL intraoral injection to the malar regions bilaterally, and Radiesse 1.5 mL injection to the nasolabial folds.

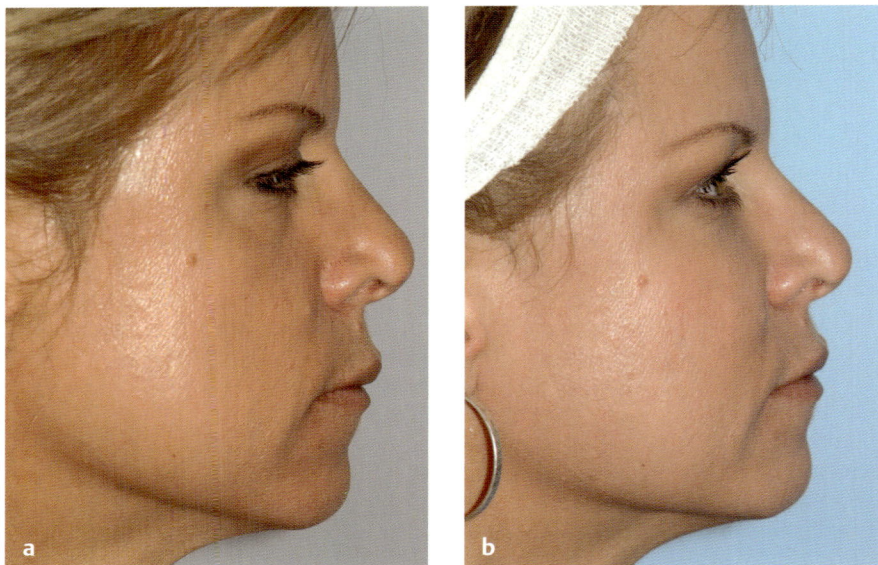

Fig. 18.3 **(a)** Before midface and infraorbital augmentation. **(b)** Two months after Radiesse intraoral injection 1.5 mL to the midface, Restylane 1 mL and Juvederm Ultra 0.8 mL cannula injection to the infraorbital region.

days prior to injection with 5 mL sterile water and then add 1 mL 1% lidocaine with 1:100,000 epinephrine immediately prior to the injection. PLLA is injected in a fanning retrograde fashion at or below the subdermal level using a 25-gauge needle. The product is massaged by the injector, and the patient is also instructed to massage the treated areas using a

topical moisturizer for 3 minutes, 3 times per day for 3 days. The reconstituted liquid is absorbed in 2 to 3 days, and PLLA is believed to elicit the stimulation of fibroblasts, which in turn produce collagen, adding volume to the treated area.[13]

Two to three sessions of one or two vials spaced 4 to 8 weeks apart are generally required to achieve the desired amount of augmentation, but this can vary with several factors, such as age, thickness of skin, and location of injection. The duration of the effect can be up to 18 to 24 months. Unlike most other facial fillers there is a gradual augmentation over time, with the aesthetic end point determined after approximately three treatment sessions by the patient and the clinician. The main adverse event with PLLA is subcutaneous nodule formation. The incidence of nodules can be reduced by using a greater dilution of the product and it should be administered by trained practitioners in the appropriate facial regions. PLLA is an excellent augmentation product, especially for the malar area and temples, but it should be avoided in the infraorbital and perioral regions because these areas result in a higher incidence of nodule formation (**Fig. 18.4a,b**).

Polymethyl Methacrylate (Artefill)

Polymethyl methacrylate (PMMA, Artefill, Suneva Medical, San Diego, CA) is the only permanent synthetic injectable soft tissue filler approved by the FDA for cosmetic use, having obtained approval for augmentation of the nasolabial folds in 2006. Artefill consists of 20% PMMA microspheres larger than 20 µm and 80% bovine collagen solution containing 3.5% bovine collagen, 2.7% phosphate buffer, 0.9% sodium chloride, 0.3% lidocaine hydrochloride, and 92.6% water for injection. The product can be stored for up to 18 months under refrigerated conditions. It has an opaque off-white appearance and is typically injected with a 26-gauge needle in the deep dermal or dermal–subcutaneous plane. Due to the presence of bovine collagen, an intradermal skin test is required 4 weeks prior to the injection to identify patients with a hypersensitivity reaction. Two to 3 months following the injection, the collagen vehicle is absorbed, leaving the PMMA microspheres, which are then encapsulated by the host collagen. Overcorrection should be avoided, and gradual volume enhancement is achieved over multiple staged injection sessions spaced several months apart. A recent 5 year safety and satisfaction study by Narins and Cohen found one granuloma out of 1,008 patients and an 80% satisfaction rate for the 18-month follow-up period.[14]

Silikon 1000

Although Silikon 1000 (Alcon, Fort Worth, TX) is not currently FDA approved for cosmetic indications, a thorough rendition of popularly used filler materials would not be complete without a description of its off-label use. For several decades, injectable liquid silicone oil has been one of the most controversial products used in the medical profession. Opponents cite that it should not be used in humans for injection because of long-term complications, such as granuloma formation ulceration, and migration. Proponents claim that it is a superior filler with predictable corrections and persistence of results, and they note that complications are a result of impurities in the product and injection of large volumes. Silikon 1000 (Alcon) is a highly purified 1,000 centistoke oil that was approved by the FDA in 1997 as an injectable intraocular tamponade to treat retinal detachment. It is therefore used off-label for cosmetic injection.

Early formulations of silicone, such as the Dow Corning 360 formula, were in many instances contaminated with heavy metals and other impurities and were used on thousands of patients for large-volume injection (750 to 2,000 mL) into breasts, faces, and buttocks. This use of an impure product officially ended with a judicial decree with Dow Corning in 1965.

Dermatologist Norman Orentreich developed and popularized the microdroplet technique using medical-grade silicone over several injection sessions. This technique resulted in a gradual correction

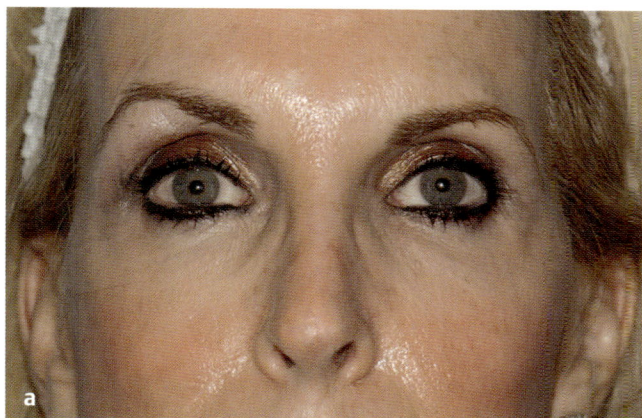

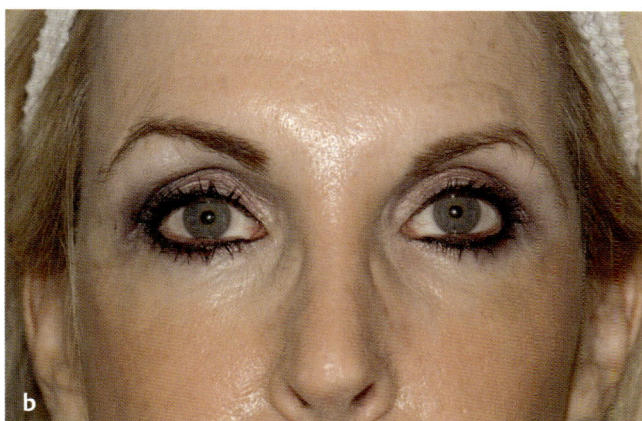

Fig. 18.4 **(a)** Before treatment of the temple hollows with filler. **(b)** Two months after injection of the temples using poly-L-lactic acid (PLLA) 1.5 mL on each side.

of the deformity and minimized the complications seen with large-volume injection. Silicone injections elicit a mild fibroblastic response, resulting in a slow increase in tissue volume over time. The amount of collagen production following the injection is equally as important as the volume of injected silicone. Therefore, waiting at least 1 month between injection sessions is important.

The author uses the following injection technique ▶ Video 18.5: (1) use a 1 mL syringe filled to 0.5 mL with silicone attached to a 27-gauge half-inch needle; (2) use topical and/or local anesthetic; (3) perform the injection as a microdroplet serial puncture (0.1 to 0.2 mL) in the subdermal plane at 2 to 3 mm intervals. Ice is applied during and after the injection. Ecchymosis is more common with silicone as compared with other fillers because of the injection technique. The patients require several treatment sessions, usually three to four, for correction of rhytids or lip augmentation, and treatments are spaced at least 4 to 6 weeks apart. The volume of silicone utilized is between 0.5 and 1.5 mL per treatment session and is dependent on the areas treated.

Silicone is an excellent filler for glabellar, nasolabial, and marionette folds as well as for facial acne scars, postrhinoplasty deformities, and HIV lipoatrophy (**Fig. 18.5a–c**; **Fig. 18.6a,b**). Injection into the tear trough should be completely avoided because of the increased risk of surface irregularity. Injection for patients who are pregnant, have chronic inflammatory disease, or are highly allergic should be avoided. Complications from Silikon 1000 injection are related to injection technique, such as beading, which results from injection into the superficial dermis. Excessive quantities injected into lips, especially by nonphysician injectors, can be successfully excised using a lip reduction technique (**Fig. 18.7a–c**). Granuloma formation is not unique to silicone and can occur with other injectable products. Treatment involves the use of antibiotics; topical, systemic, and intralesional steroids; and possibly surgical excision.[15]

■ Complications and Their Management

The most common injection-site reactions, which are self-limiting, are edema, erythema, tenderness, ecchymosis, and itching. Use of ice packs at home for several hours following the treatment and head elevation when sleeping will help reduce the amount of swelling. Ecchymosis may be immediate or delayed due to needle disruption of dermal veins. Resolution may be gradual over 3 to 10 days, and patients need to be made aware that this will not affect the final result. Oral and topical *Arnica montana* formulations have also been helpful in reducing the potential for ecchymosis. Camouflage makeup, especially with a green base, may help hide redness and bruising. Understanding facial vascular anatomy and utilizing bright lighting during the treatment session will decrease the likelihood of disrupting medium-caliber vessels.

Inappropriate superficial placement of the filler, resulting in visible lumps and bumps, can be treated with massage, aspiration, topical or intralesional steroid, incision and drainage, pulsed dye laser, or hyaluronidase for HA products.

Hypersensitivity can occur with any product, and as noted previously, collagen skin testing must be performed approximately 1 month prior to PMMA injection. A history of sulfa allergy must be ascertained prior to injection with Hydrelle because its preparation involves the incorporation of sodium metabisulfite as an antioxidant. Infection can result from inadequate cleansing of the skin with either alcohol or chlorhexidine solution. If an infection is suspected, appropriate cultures and sensitivities are obtained, and prompt antibiotic treatment is started. Antiviral prophylaxis may also be required to prevent herpetic viral outbreak, especially with lip augmentation.

Cannulation or occlusion of medium-sized vessels, usually with thicker, more viscous fillers, can result in skin necrosis. Symptoms can be instant or delayed by several hours or even longer than 1 to 2 days and can consist of pain, redness, breakdown of

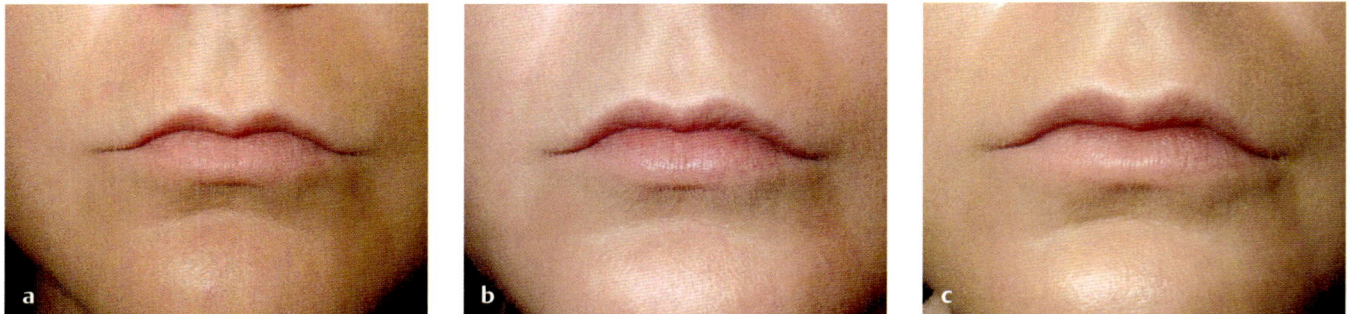

Fig. 18.5 (a) Before lip augmentation. (b) One month after 1 mL silicone injection to the upper and lower lips. (c) Three months after two treatments with 2 mL total silicone of lips.

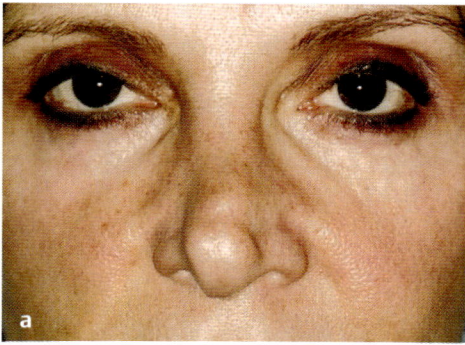

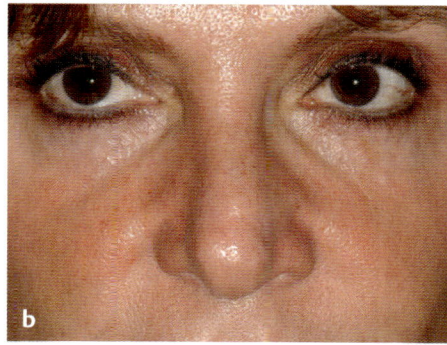

Fig. 18.6 (a) Several years following poor surgical result from rhinoplasty. (b) Six months following three treatments with silicone injection to nasal dorsum. A total of 1.2 mL silicone was used.

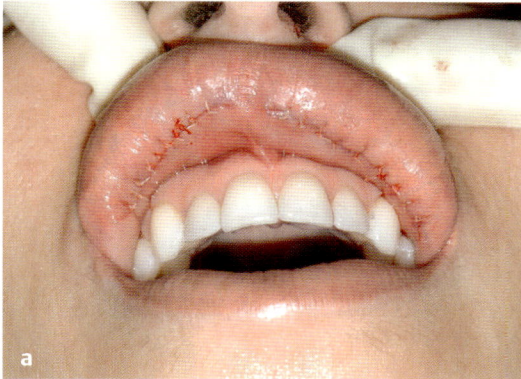

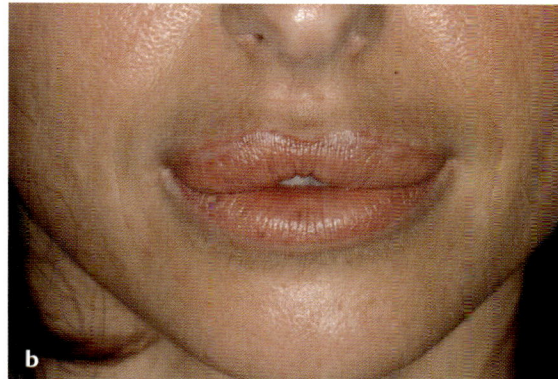

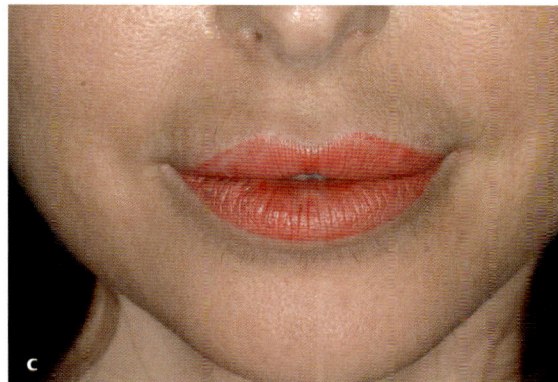

Fig. 18.7 (a) Lip reduction and excision of overinjected silicone of lips. (b) Before excision of silicone from lips. Note the excessive volume and unnatural appearance, especially of the upper lip. (c) Six months following excision of silicone from lips.

the skin, eschar formation, and serous and/or purulent discharge. The areas of the face most noted to develop skin necrosis are within the supratrochlear vasculature of the glabella and the angular vessels, resulting in lateral nasal skin necrosis. In the glabellar region, injection can compress or obstruct the supratrochlear vessels, which have minimal collateral circulation. Precautions that can be utilized to limit this complication are to inject more superficial and medial, aspirate prior to injection, use a low volume of product, and possibly treat the area in two separate sessions. Once recognized, treatment of impending skin necrosis consists of warm compresses, oral steroids, nitroglycerin topical paste for vasodilation, topical antibiotic ointment, hyaluronidase if HA was

injected, hyperbaric oxygen, and/or deep subcutaneous heparin injection.

The tear trough and infraorbital region have special considerations due to thin lower eyelid skin and the potential for malar edema. HAs (especially Juvederm) have hydrophilic effects, which can result in the Tyndall effect. This is a result of the effect of light scattering by colloidal particles in suspension, in which blue light is scattered more strongly than red. The cause of visible product in the infraorbital region is due to excessive superficial injection volume and can be avoided by undercorrection. Treatment consists of hyaluronidase injection. Viscous products, such as CaHA, FLLA, or FMMA, are to be avoided in this area because of the increased incidence of difficult-to-correct nodules.

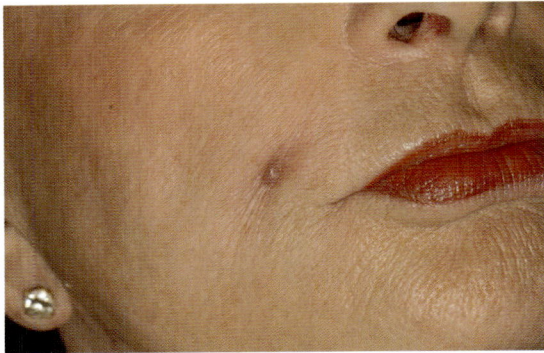

Fig. 18.8 Hypersensitivity reaction several months following Juvederm injection. It was treated with antibiotics and topical and oral steroids without improvement. Definitive treatment consisted of surgical excision.

Patients with preexisting malar edema should be injected with extreme caution in this area because filling at the level of the malar septum (a relatively impermeable membrane that allows tissue edema to accumulate superior to its cutaneous insertion) can result in decreased lymphatic drainage and worsening malar edema. This malar edema is very difficult to eradicate and may take longer than 1 year for resolution. Decreased dietary sodium intake, diuretics, head elevation, and warm compresses can all be helpful to expedite reduction of the visible tissue swelling.

Biofilm formation has been implicated in delayed hypersensitivity reactions with implants and long-term fillers (**Fig. 18.8**). A biofilm is defined as a structured community of microorganisms within a self-developed polymeric matrix irreversibly adherent to a living or inert surface. This can have up to 1,000-fold resistance to antibiotic penetration and can be very difficult to treat. Biofilms are difficult to diagnose because they are slow growing and often produce negative culture results. Steroids and non-steroidal anti-inflammatory drugs seem to aggravate and prolong the inflammation in a biofilm, and early treatment with antibiotics is recommended.[16]

Herpes outbreaks have been reported in some patients after facial injection with various fillers, compelling some practitioners to prescribe antiviral prophylaxis prior to lip injections. There are rare reports of serious or life-threatening complications after filler injection, including anaphylactic shock, sepsis, and blood clot in the retinal artery, leading to blindness, skin breakdown, and abscess needing drainage.

■ Conclusion

Soft tissue facial fillers have developed into one of the most popular and widely used methods for facial rejuvenation. Through extensive study, the products utilized by today's clinicians have a long, proven safety record with a large number of treatment applications. Results have been reproducible, more natural, and longer lasting, with more emphasis having been placed on overall facial volume augmentation. Patient outcomes have been enhanced by greater experience with these products, and complications have been limited.

References

1. Shaw RB Jr, Katzel EB, Koltz PF, et al. Aging of the facial skeleton: aesthetic implications and rejuvenation strategies. Plast Reconstr Surg 2011;127(1):374–383

2. Lambros VS. What age(s) for face lifts? Plast Reconstr Surg 1999;103(3):1076

3. Coleman SR. Facial recontouring with lipostructure. Clin Plast Surg 1997;24(2):347–367

4. Neuber F. Fat transplantation. Chir Kongr Verhandl Dtsch Gesellch Chir. 1893;22:66

5. Food and Drug Administration. Silicone gel-filled breast prostheses; silicone inflatable breast prostheses: patient risk information—FDA. Notice. Fed Regist 1991;56(187):49098–49099

6. Coleman SR. Injectable silicone returns to the United States. Aesthet Surg J 2001;21(6):576–578

7. Fagien S, Klein AW. A brief overview and history of temporary fillers: evolution, advantages, and limitations. Plast Reconstr Surg 2007;120(6, Suppl):8S–16S

8. Matarasso SL. Injectable collagens: lost but not forgotten—a review of products, indications, and injection techniques. Plast Reconstr Surg 2007;120(6, Suppl):17S–26S

9. Baumann LS, Shamban AT, Lupo MP, et al; JUVEDERM vs. ZYPLAST Nasolabial Fold Study Group. Comparison of smooth-gel hyaluronic acid dermal fillers with cross-linked bovine collagen: a multicenter, double-masked, randomized, within-subject study. Dermatol Surg 2007;33(Suppl 2):S128–S135

10. Tzikas TL. A 52-month summary of results using calcium hydroxylapatite for facial soft tissue augmentation. Dermatol Surg 2008;34(Suppl 1):S9–S15

11. Felderman LI. Radiesse for facial rejuvenation. Cosmet Dermatol 2005;18:823–826

12. Busso M, Karlsberg PL. Cheek augmentation and rejuvenation using injectable calcium hydroxylapatite (Radiesse). Cosmet Dermatol 2006;19:583–588

13. Lowe NJ, Maxwell CA, Lowe P, Shah A, Patnaik R. Injectable poly-L-lactic acid: 3 years of aesthetic experience. Dermatol Surg 2009;35(Suppl 1):344–349

14. Narins RS, Cohen SR. Novel polymethylmethacrylate soft tissue filler for the correction of nasolabial folds: interim results of a 5-year long-term safety and patient satisfaction study. Dermatol Surg 2010;36:766–774

15. Narins RS, Beer K. Liquid injectable silicone: a review of its history, immunology, technical considerations, complications, and potential. Plast Reconstr Surg 2006;118(3, Suppl):77S–84S

16. Dayan SH, Arkins JP, Brindise R. Soft tissue fillers and biofilms. Facial Plast Surg 2011;27(1):23–28

19 Facial Liposculpture and Fat Transfer

Stephen E. Metzinger, James N. Parrish Jr., and Aldo B. Guerra

Key Concepts

- Volume loss contributes significantly to the aged appearance of the face, and autogenous fat is an attractive option for volume replacement.

- Adipocyte-derived stem cells carried with the fat grafts seem to improve the quality and texture of the overlying skin.

- Atraumatic transfer of fat is critical for success. Use of gentle harvest techniques with low negative pressures and gentle handling, and transplant of small aliquots of adipose tissue ensure optimum survival of the graft.

- Use of small, blunt cannulas is essential to avoid embolization and arterial occlusion.

■ Introduction

Historically, it was believed that facial fat was a contiguous sheet of tissue and that facial aging was the result of the relentless downward pull on the facial skin and soft tissue. However, over the past 5 decades, several investigators have changed our understanding of facial aging. In 1965, Gonzalez-Ulloa and Flores proposed that facial aging involved changes in muscle and bone, as well as skin and fat.[1] Further, recent work has demonstrated that facial fat is not a continuous sheet of tissue but rather is compartmentalized throughout the face.[2] This discovery has allowed the evolution of improved techniques for facial rejuvenation.

For optimal results, the face should be considered in three dimensions, and the accepted surgical modalities of tightening and resurfacing of the skin are combined with the addition of volume. These principles should form the three limbs of the tripod for facial rejuvenation. Consideration of an individual's appearance based on systematic mapping and a three-dimensional evaluation of the four levels of facial structure (bone, muscle, fat, and skin) will help the clinician to choose the most appropriate modalities for facial rejuvenation.

Autologous fat transplantation can be used to address all four levels of volume deficiency in the face and can provide a stable and potentially long-lasting alternative to off-the-shelf fillers. Transplanted fat can survive well in the face with meticulous grafting technique, although more than one injection in some areas may be required to achieve optimal outcomes. Appropriate counseling, realistic expectations, and exacting technique make fat transfer an effective method of soft tissue augmentation.

■ Background: Basic Science of Procedure

Autologous fat has been used for aesthetic facial surgery for over 100 years.[3–6] In the 1950s, however, Peer demonstrated a graft survival rate of only 50% at 1 year.[7] Enthusiasm subsequently waned for the technique while dermal adipose grafts and artificial materials gained in popularity.[8] A new resurgence of interest occurred when Ellenbogen described free pearl fat grafts to the face.[9] The development of liposuction by Illouz then provided a large supply of autologous fat in an injectable form, which appeared to survive when reinjected.[10–12] This readily available material further bolstered the application of autologous fat transplantation for facial aesthetics. Refinements in technique have now produced more reliable results, and the concept of three-dimensional facial sculpting has led to the widespread application of autologous fat grafting to the face.[13–14]

Currently, there are two major theories describing the fate of grafted fat. Peer and Paddock proposed the host cell replacement theory, whereby host histiocytes phagocytize free fat and become adipocytes. The graft is thus replaced by host cells.[16]

This idea has been replaced by the cell survival theory.[7,17] In this paradigm, circulation is restored to the grafted fat cells in a manner similar to the revascularization of a skin graft. Up to postoperative day 4, host cells such as polymorphonuclear leukocytes and lymphocytes infiltrate the graft. Within the vessels of the graft, blood cells are clumped and the graft survives by plasma imbibition. On or about the fourth day, neovascularization becomes evident. Host histiocytes act to remove fat from nonsurviving cells, and these scavenged cells tend to be the more mature adipocytes.

Some researchers believe centrifugation removes some of the mature, or "weaker" adipocytes, leaving more preadipocytes and resulting in a fat graft far more likely to be revascularized.[18,19] Rigotti believes most mature fat cells are disrupted, and it is the adipose-derived stem cells carried with the graft that repopulate the recipient area. Removal of disrupted cells thus explains the loss of volume in the grafted areas.[20,21] Most likely, the combination of cell revascularization and some stem cell differentiation accounts for treatment successes, but more study is required for definitive answers.

■ Technical Aspects of Procedure

The technique for autologous fat transfer can be divided into three parts: harvesting the graft, processing the graft, and reintroduction of the graft. Each is equally important to the success of the procedure.

Harvesting

Donor Site

Different donor sites have been advocated for the harvest of autogenous fat.[22–26] We prefer the abdomen because it is easily accessible and stab incisions can be hidden within the umbilicus or in the hair-bearing skin of the pubic area. Most studies have failed to show an advantage of one donor site over another.[25–27] Other common donor sites include the lumbar and trochanteric areas, the thighs including the knees, the arms, and the para-axillary area.

Tumescent Solution

Sterile technique is employed for fat harvest and injection. We recommend prophylactic antibiotics. Local anesthesia is used to anesthetize the site for a small stab incision. Through this incision, tumescent fluid is introduced into the region. The same incision is used for harvesting.

The choice of tumescent fluid varies. Our solution consists of 1 mg of epinephrine, 200 mg of lidocaine, and 5 mEq of sodium bicarbonate in 1 L of normal saline. Dosages of lidocaine up to 35 mg/kg can be used, although usually less is required for fat harvesting. Recently, a study on the effects of local anesthetics on preadipocytes found the immediate viability and the ability to differentiate were affected, with lidocaine demonstrating one of the strongest effects.[28] One study noted that lidocaine potently inhibited glucose transport in adipocytes as well as their growth in culture. This effect, however, was only noted as long as the lidocaine was present. Adipocytes resumed normal metabolism and growth once they were washed.[29]

The β-adrenergic effects of catecholamines increase lipolysis in adipocytes, but it is unclear if there is a clinical effect of epinephrine in the tumescent solution used in fat transplantation.[30]

As an alternative, fat harvesting can be accomplished with minimal infiltration of lidocaine or "dry" without tumescent solution, thereby increasing the proportion of fat to residual fluid per harvested syringe.

Cannula and Negative Pressure

Atraumatic transfer of fat is a key principle for success. Trauma to fat in the process of harvesting or reintroduction affects the survival of the graft. Although a nonviable graft will initially appear to have corrected the problem, eventual resorption of the tissue negates the result.

Fat consists of adipose cells, which have thin cell membranes enmeshed in a fibrous network. Without the supporting fibers, the cells tend to collapse. An additional supporting network of connective tissue creates the lobules of fat, which can be observed grossly. Harvesting fat while retaining the supporting elements preserves the structural integrity of the tissue and helps the grafted fat survive in the transplanted site. The primary innovation of the Coleman technique was the use of a blunt-tipped cannula with dull distal openings, which harvests parcels of fat with intact architecture. These are small enough to pass through a 17-gauge injection cannula. The small parcels of fat placed in this manner allow maximal surface area contact with the recipient area.[31]

For harvesting, a 10 mL Luer Lock syringe is attached to the harvesting cannula, and the plunger is gently withdrawn to provide 1 to 2 mL of negative pressure. Larger cannulas combined with low aspiration pressure reduce trauma to the adipose tissue. Another commonly utilized technique designed to harvest the fat in parcels of readily transferable size uses the Lipivage system (Genesis Biosystems, Lew-

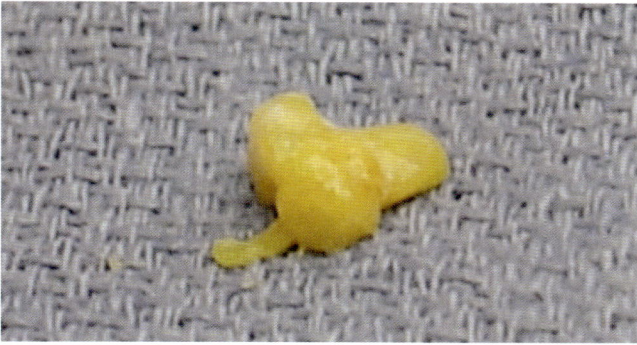

Fig. 19.1 The harvested fat is plump, young, viable, and selected for maximum survival.

isville, TX). The aspiration cannula is connected to a low-suction (< 15 mm Hg) aspiration system used to harvest the fat. Traditional vacuum or syringe aspiration may be used as long as low pressure and large cannulas (4 or 5 mm) are utilized. A gentle passing motion for aspiration further limits trauma to the adipocytes (**Fig. 19.1**) ▶ **Video 19.1**.

An alternative technique involves the use of a single-use disposable aspiration and injection kit, the Viafill System (Lipose, Maitland, FL). The kit includes a centrifuge, aspiration and injection syringes and cannulas, and centrifuge tubes. Fat aspiration is performed using a low negative pressure technique. The aspiration cannula has a diameter of 14 French and measures 12 cm in length. Centrifugation is performed at a low force of 50 g for a brief 2 minutes.

There is some controversy regarding the effect of negative pressure on the adipocyte.[32–37] Despite a wide range of results, the fact remains that many groups have demonstrated either structural or metabolic derangements of fat cells after harvest with high negative pressures.[32–34] Therefore, avoidance of trauma to the adipocytes is essential. The keys to atraumatic harvest are large cannulas, low negative pressures, and gentle passage of the cannula.

Processing

The goal of fat cell processing is to create the isolation and preparation of the best cells for reinjection while minimizing potential damage. The stromal vascular fraction remaining in the harvested fat can facilitate rapid degradation and must be removed. Strategies include systems such as Lipivage or Viafill, centrifuge, or gravity separation. There are advantages and disadvantages to all techniques. The Lipivage system is a closed filtration system, avoids

exposure to excessive g force and provides sterility and lack of exposure to air.

An alternative is the use of the centrifuge. Some investigators have demonstrated deleterious effects of a centrifuge on adipocytes, whereas others have had favorable results.[38,39] After centrifugation, those fat cells surviving the process tend to be younger and tougher and are found in the compacted region of viable adipocytes.[19,21,40] In addition, the layers of the compacted region differ with regard to the number of viable adipocytes. The bottom portion of the fat layer demonstrates 250% more viable cells when compared with the top layer and 140% more viable cells when compared with the middle layer.[40,4] Therefore, using the bottom layer of the centrifuged cells is recommended.

Gravity is also an alternative for separation and is used by some to produce the least trauma to the adipocyte. One disadvantage is the time required. Another is the possibility that some viable cells are not included in the fraction that is grafted.[39] Our technique utilizes both filtration and gravity separation. After the fat has been gently harvested and filtered by the Lipivage system, it is transferred to 30 or 60 mL syringes via a locking system and allowed to separate by gravity for 30 minutes (**Fig. 19.2**). The excess fluids, including the upper layer of oil from disrupted fat cells and the lower layer of blood and lidocaine are then removed and the fat transferred to 1 mL syringes for injection. The technique minimizes trauma and obtains a large number of viable cells. An alternative is the Viafill system using a sterile closed system and a low-g-force centrifuge ▶ **Video 19.1**.

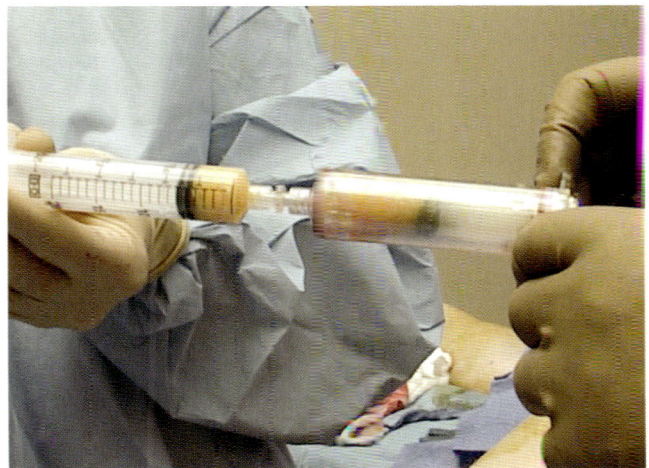

Fig. 19.2 Fat is transferred to a 30 mL syringe for gravity separation, never leaving the sterility of the operative field.

Grafting

The goal with any grafting procedure is to maximize graft survival by gentle reintroduction of fat cells into a well-vascularized bed. A Coleman Type II (Byron Medical, Tucson, AZ) 7 cm straight injecting cannula is inserted using a 2 mm stab incision made with an no. 11 blade knife and is used with the compacted fat cells in a 1 mL syringe. Small tunnels are created by advancing the cannula, and the fat is injected 0.1 to 0.2 mL at a time, only while withdrawing the injecting cannula. To reduce embolization, never inject with a sharp needle nor when advancing the injection cannula. The creation of small tunnels helps keep the grafted fat adherent to the recipient site, whereas independent tunnels prevent fat from leaking out. Care should be taken to avoid overfilling the tunnels because this can adversely affect graft survival. Do not use force; this creates an uncontrolled graft unlikely to survive. However, it is important to feel a small amount of resistance while injecting. If the injection goes too easily, it is likely that fat has already been placed in this location, and further injection will reduce graft survival.

Slight overcorrection is important to compensate for absorption of the liquid carrier. A general recommendation is for 30% overcorrection. After the fat is deposited, gentle digital pressure is used to check for placement and contour regularity. Additional facial surgical procedures can be completed at the time of lipoinjection if the procedures do not involve the graft recipient areas. Operating on a freshly injected area will disrupt the fat placement.

Patient Preparation

The face is divided into forehead, cheek, periorbital, nasal, perioral, and neck subunits (**Fig. 19.3**). Each subunit is examined for three-dimensional (3-D) volume loss and is then broken down into grafting units. Preoperative photographs are taken with and without a flash. Photographs taken without flash will often accentuate areas of volume loss not apparent in standard flash photos. It is helpful to compare preoperative photographs to pictures taken of patients in their early twenties, preferably full face, nonsmiling views to better appreciate the degree of volume loss present.

The patient is marked preoperatively sitting upright in an area with direct overhead lighting, often supplemented with side lighting as needed to identify the areas of volume deficiency to be grafted.

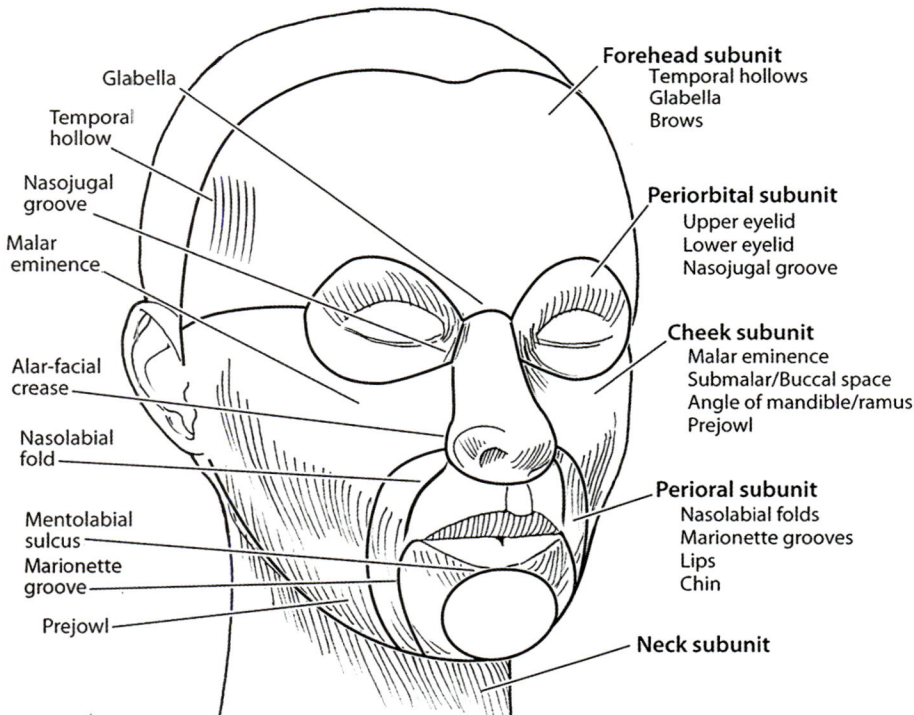

Fig. 19.3 Gonzales-Ulloa aesthetic subunits of the face.

Injection

By 3-D analysis of each subunit, an estimate of grafting volume as well as planes of injection can be formulated in a preoperative plan (**Table 19.1**).

The Forehead Subunit

Fat injections to the forehead should only be performed using a blunt injection cannula. Injections are only made parallel to the lines for wrinkles.

Temporal Hollows

The temporal hollows are marked pretreatment to accentuate the posterior aspect of the lateral orbital rim just above the zygomatic arch. This area is usually the deepest part of the hollow and is often asymmetric between sides. Access points are made at the temporal hairline and work best with two different vectors. Special care must be taken when injecting the temporal hollow to avoid injury to the frontal branch of the facial nerve.

Table 19.1 Pertinent anatomy and facial subunits

Units	Subunits
Forehead	Forehead
	Brows
	Glabella
	Temporal hollows
	Supraorbital units
Periorbital	Lower eyelids
	Upper eyelids
	Lateral orbital rim
	Nasojugal groove
Cheek	Malar eminence
	Submalar area
	Mandible angle
	Mandible ramus
	Prejowl area
Perioral	Nasolabial folds
	Lips
	Labiomental crease
	Marionette lines
	Chin
	Philtrum
Neck	Submentum
	Neck
	Suprahyoid
	Subjowl

The most visually important part of the temporal hollow is adjacent to the lateral orbit and the tail of the brow. The key to a good result is depth of injection, which should be in the plane immediately adjacent to the deep temporal fascia. This plane is deep to visible vessels and the frontal branch of the facial nerve. Injection should be performed while one is withdrawing the cannula, and care should be taken to avoid the sentinel vein.

The goal is expansion of the temporal hollow. Placement of 4 to 10 mL of fat in each hollow is done as evenly as possible, expecting ~ 30% resorption. Most of the fat should be placed anterorly. It is not unusual to have asymmetry between hollows, but care must be taken not to overfill because the goal is to level the temporal hollow, not make it convex. With the temporal hollow leveled, the tail of the brow rotates anteriorly, giving the impression of rising and lengthening.

Brows

Access to the brows is best via a lateral stab incision. The cannula is inserted lateral to medial below the brow in the muscle layer, and 1 mL of fat is placed on withdrawal using two vectors and two passes. The authors will add a second microaliquot placement in the subcutaneous plane more superficially but with only 0.5 to 1 mL of fat graft. This volume makes the brows look fuller and gives the illusion of autorotation and lift (**Fig. 19.4**). We prefer to use a Coleman Type I cannula (Byron Medical) to avoid damage to nerves and reduce the risk of vessel cannulation and embolization.

Glabella

Access to the glabella and radix is best through a medial brow stab incision ▶ Video 19.1. We prefer a plane below the muscle but supraperiosteal to avoid nerves and vessels in this region. Multiple passes and vectors are used for volume replacement with feathering onto the nasal dorsum and midforehead. Usually 1 to 2 mL are used and an additional 0.5 to 1 mL is placed in the subcutaneous plane if there are deep vertical rhytids. Gentle digital pressure is used to confirm volume placement, and care should be used at all times when one is working around the orbit ▶ Video 19.1.

The Periorbital Subunit

Great care must be observed when injecting into the periorbital subunit to avoid superficial injections and palpable lumps. Injections parallel and at crossing directions should be in the submuscular and subperiosteal planes.

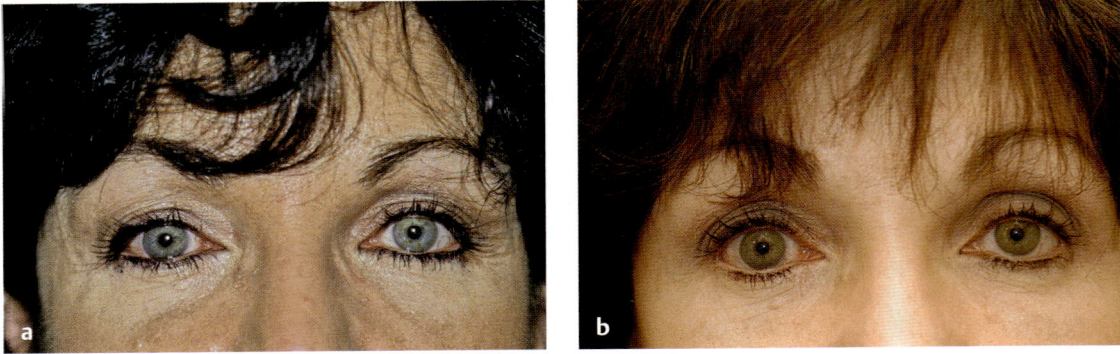

Fig. 19.4 Preoperative **(a)** and 3 year postoperative **(b)** fat injection to the lower eyelid/orbital rim, glabella, brow, infrabrow, and temple.

Upper Eyelids

This is really the area below the eyebrow but not into the glabella. The authors pre-tunnel this area to obtain the correct plane, which is subdermal and accessed via medial brow incisions. We will contour the left upper eyelid from the right medial brow and the right upper eyelid from the left medial brow. The lateral aspect can be volumized from the ipsilateral lateral brow incision. The vessels in this area tend to be very fragile, therefore we only use Coleman Type I (Byron Medical) cannulas in this region (very blunt). The volume used is 1.0 to 1.5 mL total for each lid. Anything more than this will look artificial and edematous. If more volume is needed, it should be done at a separate session.

Lower Eyelids

For the lower eyelids, we use two primary incisions on each side. The lateral brow gives excellent exposure to the lateral orbital rim and to the lateral lower eyelid. The lateral inferior temple at the level of the zygomatic arch usually in the hairline also gives great exposure to the lateral orbital rim and the crow's feet. This incision can be adjusted to the conditions at hand and moved more medial if necessary. The placement of fat is best in two planes: immediately subdermal (dermis–muscle interface) and in the orbicularis oculi muscle itself. Great care is taken not to perforate the orbital septum. In the lower eyelids superior to the infraorbital rim the goal is to remain superficial at all times. Small volumes of 0.25 to 1.0 mL seem to be adequate for the lower lid (**Fig. 19.4**). Great care is taken to avoid clumps. Lateral orbital rim volume is 1.0 to 5.0 mL and is best placed in the supraperiosteal and muscular planes.

Nasojugal Groove

For the nasojugal groove, a midcheek incision is best, with fat placed against the periosteum in the anterior malar fold (tear trough) if possible. The lower lid can

also be feathered with a vertical approach from this incision. No arcus marginalis release is needed because the motion of multiple passes creates an autorelease if the cannula is in the correct plane. Although some placement in the orbicularis oculi is desirable, a small feathering into the subdermal plane is needed for full correction. This maneuver can be quite tricky, and only small volumes must be used. Care should also be taken to prevent fenestration of the thin skin in this area. Remember, smaller volumes with multiple passes work best. Feathering toward the malar eminence in the muscle layer is needed for overall volume. About 2 mL total on each side are needed for the lower lids and nasojugal groove together; more volume in this thin skin will tend to create contour irregularities.

The Cheek Subunit

Malar Eminence/Submalar Space/Buccal Space

The malar eminence should be the most projecting point of the cheek, and it is important to correctly identify and accentuate this area in the volumizing process. Access to this area is from the lateral brow, midcheek, and lateral lip areas. Through these three ports, one can reach every area of the cheek and access the supraperiosteal, muscular, and subdermal planes with multiple vectors. Feathering into the lower eyelid, lateral orbital rim, and submalar areas is very important. Placement of 5 to 7 mL of grafted fat into these areas restores fullness and creates a more youthful look. It is sometimes necessary to add a second session if more volume is required. Filling of the malar eminence and the submalar and buccal space gives the illusion of cheek lift secondary to the increased volume (**Fig. 19.5**).

Angle of Mandible/Ramus/Prejowl

The angle of the mandible, mandibular ramus (**Fig. 19.6**) and prejowl area (**Fig. 19.5**) can be accessed from the posterior earlobe cleft. This is well hidden

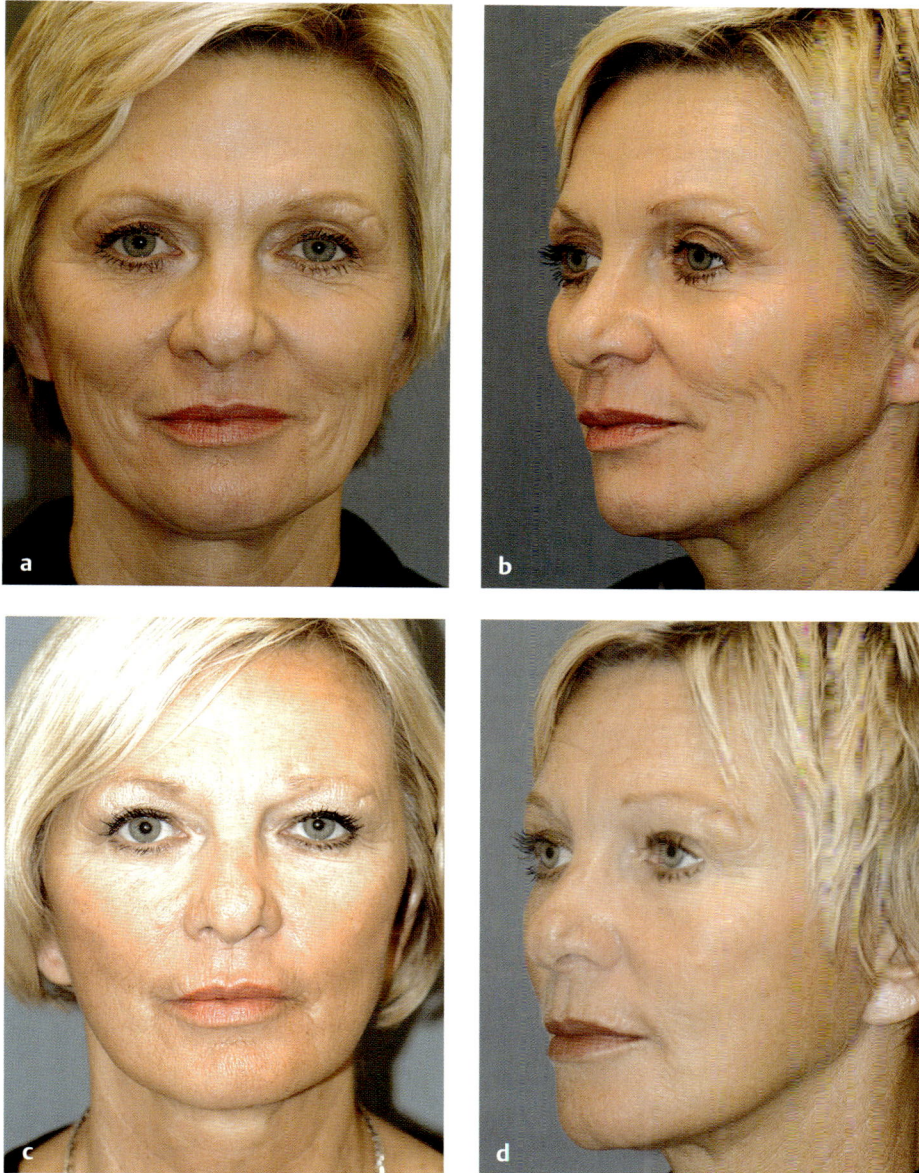

Fig. 19.5 Preoperative **(a,b)** and 3.5 year postoperative **(c,d)** facelift with concomitant fat injections to anterior cheek, lower eye lid/orbital rim, nasolabial fold (left 9 mL, right 7 mL); prejowl (3 mL left, 3 mL right); jawline (left 1 mL, right 1 mL); upper lip (1 mL) lower lip (1.5 mL); glabella, brow, infrabrow (6 mL); and temple (left 2 mL, right 2 mL).

and allows multiple vectors. Additional areas of access include the lateral lip, labiomental sulcus, and anterior mandible itself. The plane is subdermal and superficial to the platysma. In some deep grooves, a subperiosteal component may be attempted but will probably result in a supraperiosteal injection. Depending on volume demand, 4 to 5 mL are usually placed on the anterior mandibular border, and 7 to 10 mL are incorporated into the angle, ramus, and posterior mandibular border. Once again, feathering is important. Placement is critical if liposuction has been previously performed or is contemplated for the jowl.

If placement is too low or too much volume is used, it will make the jowl worse. It is better to undercorrect than to risk making the jowl more pronounced.

The Perioral Subunit

Nasolabial Folds

We prefer two access points and three different planes. The superior access point is via the alar-facial crease or the nasolabial isthmus ▶ **Video 19.**. This is based on surgeon preference and the condi-

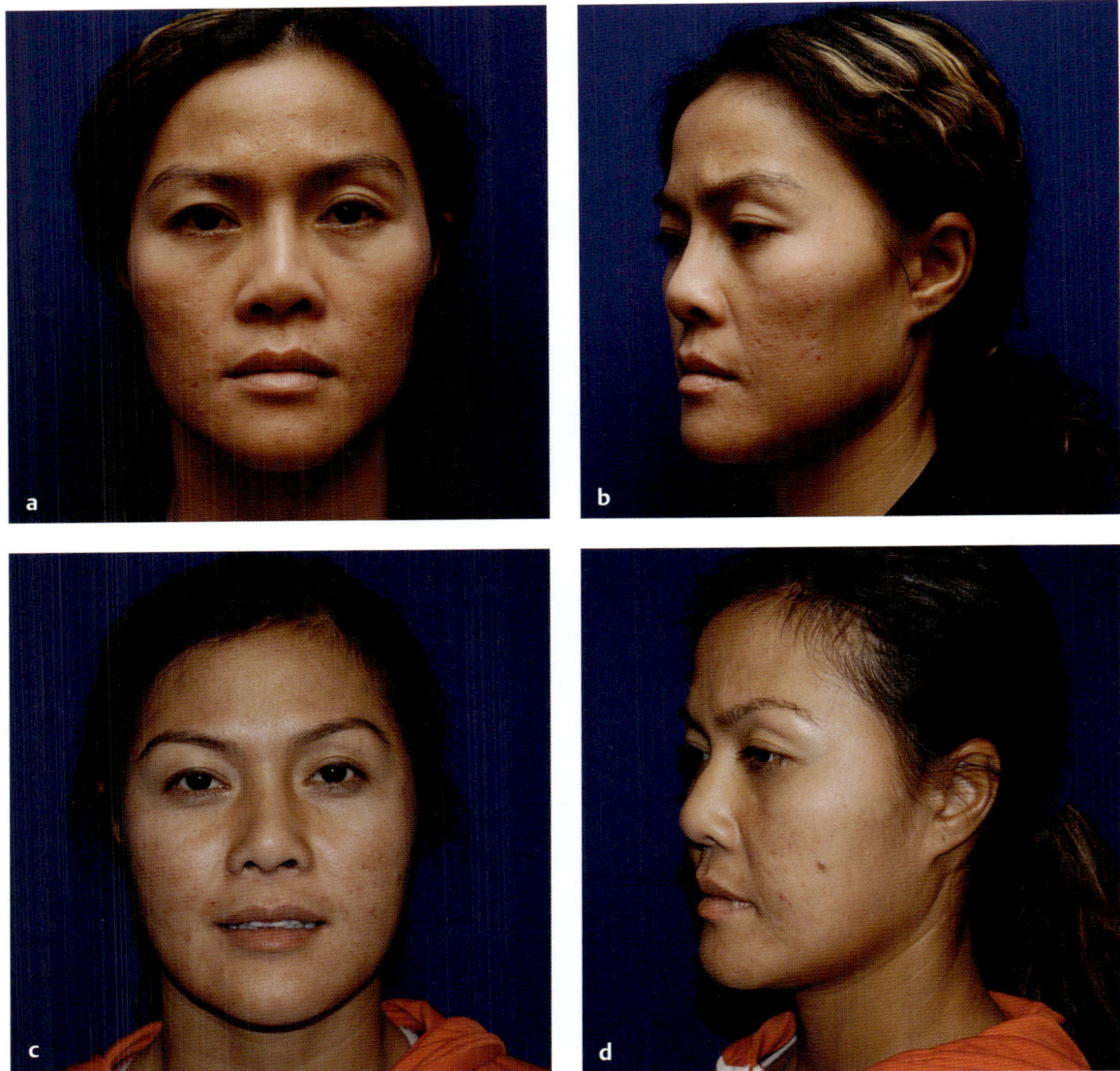

Fig. 19.6 Preoperative anteroposterior (AP) **(a)** and oblique views **(b)** prior to autologous fat grafting to the mandibular ramus, and angle and feathering fat grafting to the preparotid/submalar area and melolabial folds. Postoperative AP **(c)** and oblique views **(d)** after autologous fat grafting to the mandibular ramus and angle and feathering fat grafting to the preparotid/submalar area and melolabial folds. There was no reduction of the zygomatic malar eminence.

tions at hand. The superior passes are best in the supraperiosteal and muscular layers. The vectors are parallel to the fold but feather to the cheek and upper lip. The inferior access is at the modiolus, upper lip crease, or inferiormost aspect of the fold itself, whichever of these is least conspicuous and gives the best access (**Fig. 19.7**). The vector is again parallel to the fold and is muscular and subdermal in fat graft placement. Care is taken to avoid vessels in the area and to inject only on withdrawal of the cannula. Remember the key to good volume replacement is infiltration of the entire area, not just an individu-

al line or wrinkle. Feathering must be smooth and without clumps. It is also important to focus on adding support to the area and not just on eliminating the fold. Volume can range from as little as 2 mL to as much as 10 mL depending on premaxillary deficiency and the depth of the fold. Think in 3-D terms and try to replace volume in all levels from bone to the submucosa (**Fig. 19.8**). The Coleman Type I (Byron Medical) cannula works best in this area. If a horizontal component is needed to feather or access a difficult spot (scar), this can be approached from a midcheek access point.

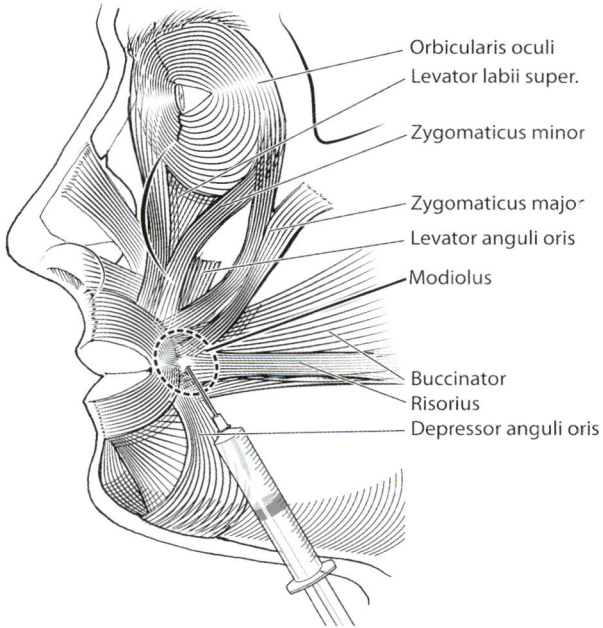

Fig. 19.7 Injection to the nasolabial fold via the modiolus.

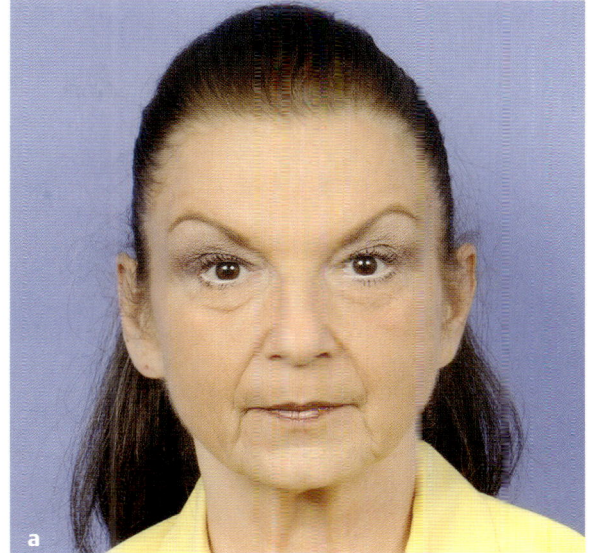

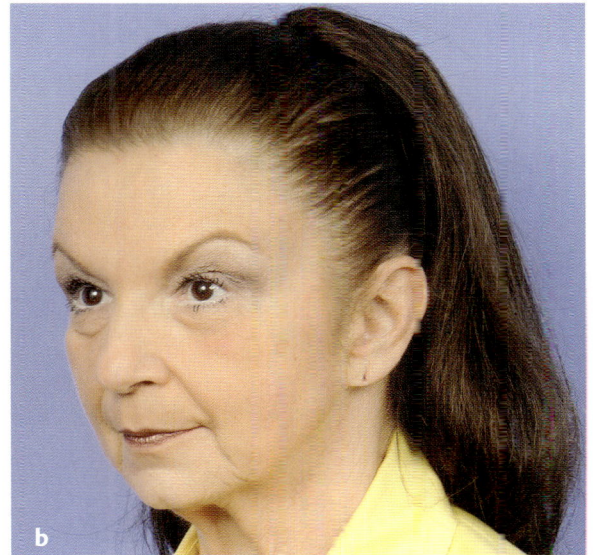

Fig. 19.8 Preoperative **(a,b)** and 1 year postoperative **(c,d)** views for autologous fat grafting to the nasolabial folds, marionette lines, and full rhytidectomy.

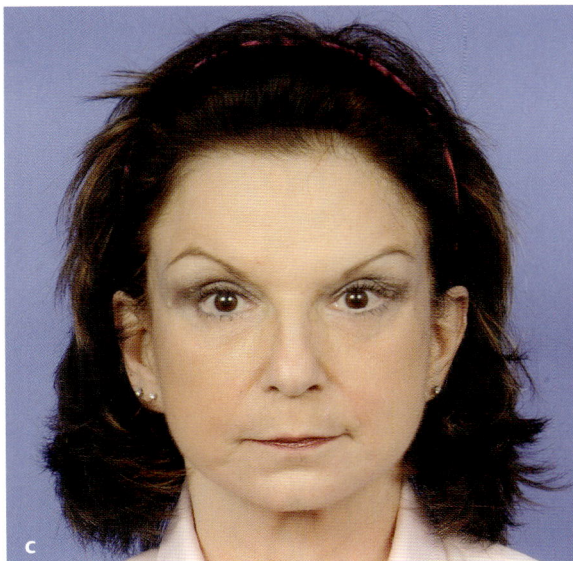

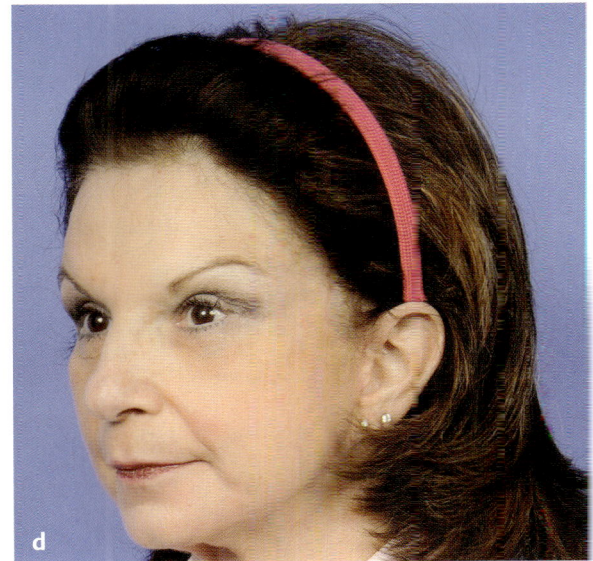

Marionette Grooves (Lines)

The marionette grooves (lines) can be approached from many directions. We prefer to use the inferior incision we used to infiltrate the nasolabial folds whether it is from the modiolus, inferior fold, or midcheek ▶ **Video 19.1** (**Fig. 19.9a–c**). The chin pad, lateral mental region, or oral commissure may also be used. This area requires a smaller volume, usually 1 to 3 mL. Once again, multiple passes with multiple vectors give the best results. The increase in volume to this area tends to lift the corners of the mouth and give a more youthful, rested appearance (**Fig. 19.8**). An additional benefit we have anecdotally noted is an improvement in the quality and the texture of the overlying skin. We attribute this beneficial effect to the action of adipose-derived stem cells.

Lips

The lips are a difficult area to treat. Placement of fat into different levels or parts of the lips leads to different results. Not all the changes have been favorable. The goal of lip augmentation is to project the vermilion of the lip to create an attractive full (pouty) lip with the smallest volume possible (**Fig. 19.10**). This is accomplished by horizontal passes in the submucosa and orbicularis oris muscle. Small microaliquots are necessary to prevent clumping. Remember the vermilion is key, and the lip is more forgiving with small clumps of fat than with large ones. Access is via the modiolus and is used for both upper and lower lips. Volume used in the white roll is 0.5 to 1.0 mL. Remember to approach from both sides. The body of the lip is usually 0.75 to 1.5 mL. More fat is usually

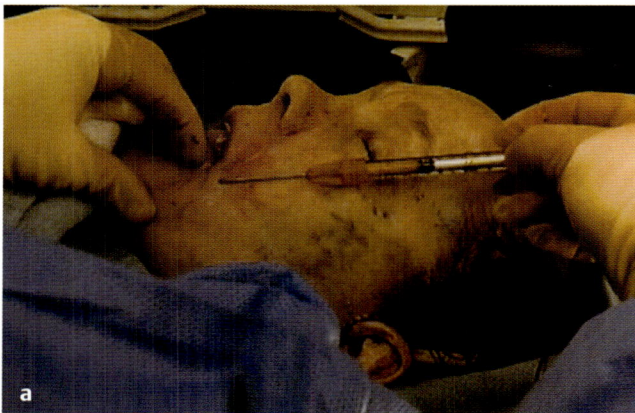

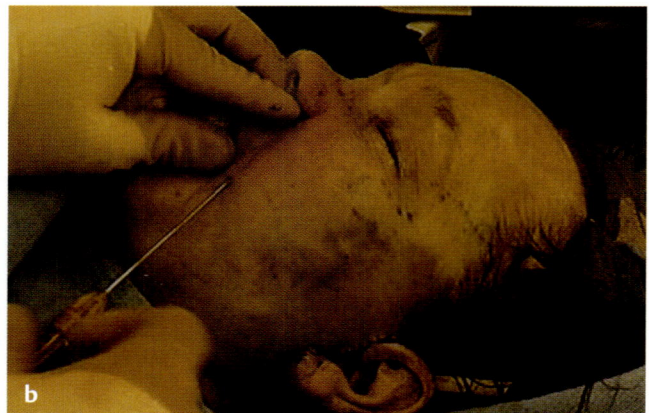

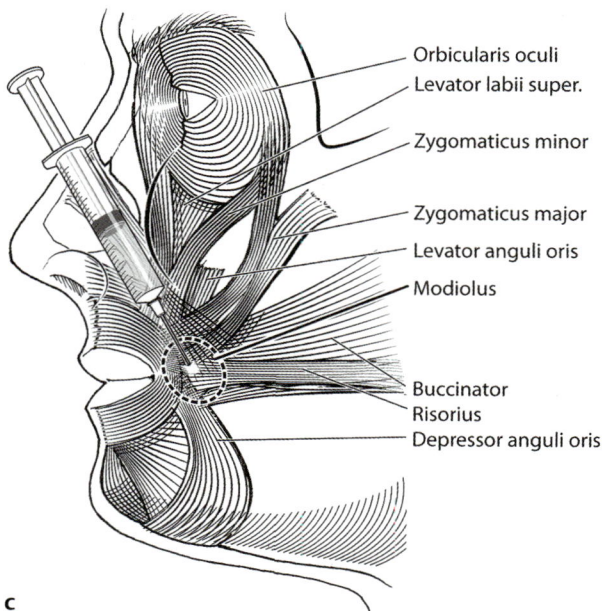

Orbicularis oculi
Levator labii super.

Zygomaticus minor

Zygomaticus major
Levator anguli oris
Modiolus

Buccinator
Risorius
Depressor anguli oris

Fig. 19.9 Injection to the marionette lines via the modiolus (a–c).

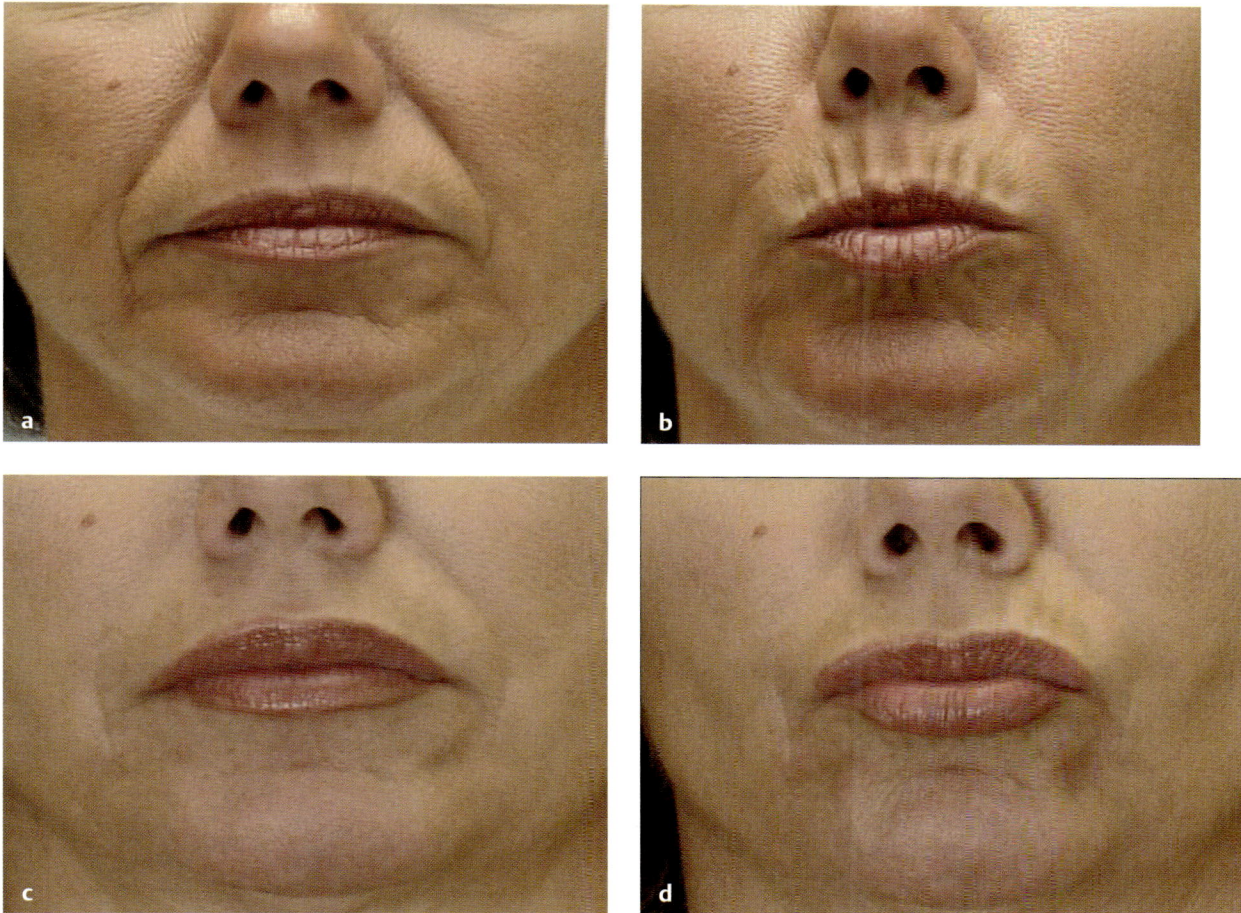

Fig. 19.10 Preoperative **(a,b)** and 6 month postoperative views **(c,d)** with autologous fat grafting to the lips and marionette lines.

placed in the body of the lower lip as opposed to the upper. The Coleman Type II cannula (Byron Medical) seems to work best unless there is previous scarring. In instances of revision or scar, the Coleman Type III cannula (Byron Medical) works best. Additional fat is placed at the tubercle and in the philtral columns to add volume and create a fuller look. Augmentation of the muscle will initially cause eversion of the vermilion and mucosa because of edema. As the edema subsides, so does the eversion. This area tends to lose volume the fastest and often requires multiple procedures to obtain the desired result. We attribute this to movement and traction injury to the grafted fat, but it may simply be the complexity of the vermilion and the body of the lip.

Chin

The chin is an ideal area for volume enhancement, either as a sole treatment (**Fig. 19.11**) or as an adjunct for prosthetic chin augmentation or sliding genioplasty. Additionally, feathering into the jawline enhances support to the prejowl area and creates a more youthful appearance.

The contour of a youthful chin is without ptosis and has two distinct lateral protuberances with a central flattening or midline cleft. Access to this area is via the midline cleft or submentum paired with the modiolus or midmandibular border. Two access points give more versatility and provide multiple vectors. Grafting should be in the supraperiosteal, muscular, and subdermal planes. Typically, 4 to 6 mL of volume are injected but can be more depending on the amount of feathering. If too much fat is placed, the chin can look amorphous.

The Neck Subunit

The neck is less commonly treated with autologous fat; however, rhytids along the neck and soft tissue deflation can be treated with fat injections at the subcutaneous and platysmal level. The cannula must be blunt, and care must be taken to avoid the superficial vessels of the neck. Subplatysmal injection is not recommended.

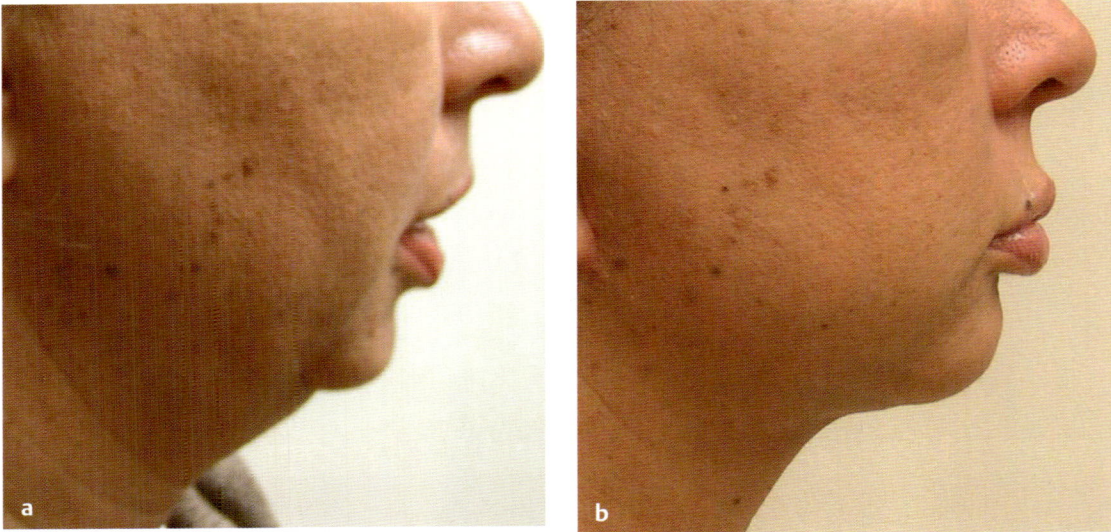

Fig. 19.11 Lateral view of chin preoperative **(a)** and 1 year postoperative **(b)**. Patient's lips were also augmented.

■ Postoperative Care

If the fat has been placed in an appropriate tunnel, the chance for migration is minimal. Massage and excessive facial animation are discouraged to prevent migration of fat away from the recipient sites. Compression dressings are in general ineffective; however, ice compresses can be applied for 24 to 48 hours to minimize inflammation.

■ Expected Results

Although autologous fat transplantation for nasolabial folds appears to be safe and effective, most authors have found the duration of correction can be variable. Serial injection may be performed at 3 month intervals. In our experience, three procedures should be anticipated, but this is not always necessary. Even distribution of the injection is crucial because excess bulk in a particular area may isolate the fat in the central region from the new blood supply. Even with multiple sessions, fat grafting to the lips has been suboptimal.

Retention varies in different parts of the face, and fat seems to "take" best in areas in which fat atrophy is the problem, such as the cheeks and the periorbital and mandibular subunits. When fat is being used to replace bony remodeling or mucosal atrophy (both occur in the perioral area), retention can be less predictable.

■ Complications and Their Management

Major concerns of fat grafting are undercorrection and overcorrection. Undercorrection can result from placement of less than the ideal volume of fat or from graft resorption. Although placing too little fat obviously fails to correct the defect, increasing the amount of injected fat does not always reduce problems. Graft migration can be caused by infiltrating too much fat into a particular site and forcing it into an undesirable area. Overfilling can increase graft necrosis, resulting in palpable irregularities and eventual resorption. As a rule, undercorrection is generally easier to treat than overcorrection, and additional fat may be grafted at a separate sitting to complete the correction.

When one is creating tunnels for fat graft placement, some resistance should be felt. If no resistance is encountered during placement of the cannula, a previously grafted area may have been entered and caution must be exercised to prevent overinjection. When one is grafting scarred areas, grafts tend to move to areas of least resistance and clumping may occur. If clumping is still present after 1 month, the patient can be instructed on doing self-massage at the site in question.

Removing excess graft is more difficult because the host tissue infiltrates into the graft. If overcorrection does occur, it is prudent to allow a period of time for edema to resolve and for some of the expected resorption of the graft. If the overcorrection persists, microliposuction can be performed.[42]

Edema is usually evident for 2 weeks after the procedure. However, as in any surgery, prolonged edema is possible and troubling to the patient. Bleeding complications are usually limited to transient mild ecchymosis that rapidly resolves. Small hematomas are more unusual and can sometimes be associated with the use of sharp needles for graft placement. Donor site scarring is also a potential concern. Contour irregularities can result from overly aggressive harvesting in a small area.

Although rare, infections can occur. The most common source of infection is the oral mucosa. There have also been reports of atypical mycobacterial infections after fat grafting.[42,43] Importantly, atypical mycobacterial infections have been associated with inadequately sterilized surgical instruments.[44-46] A disposable, single-use system should eliminate these risks. Severe systemic infections are rare with autologous fat grafting but have been reported with large-volume fat injections and can lead to life-threatening sepsis and residual deformity.[47] A sound understanding of the principles and techniques of surgical sterility with fat grafting is essential to avoid infectious complications.

Embolization and arterial occlusion can be reported after autologous fat injections. Tissue necrosis, blindness, and fatal stroke can result.[48-50] Blindness is caused by central retinal artery occlusion and has been reported with injection of the glabellar area,[48] the nasolabial folds,[51] and the lower lip.[52] Review of two cases of blindness revealed that sharp needles were used to inject relatively large volumes, presumably with increased pressure.[50] Central retinal artery occlusion is likely produced when a sharp needle cannulates a distal branch of the ophthalmic artery. High-pressure injection then propels a column of filler proximal to the origin of the central retinal artery where it then progresses distally to the eye.[50]

■ Conclusion

With increased recognition of the role of volume loss in the aged appearance of the face comes a need for readily available and inexpensive biocompatible filler. Autogenous fat meets these requirements. With gentle handling of the adipocytes and meticulous surgical technique, an excellent aesthetic result can be obtained.

Acknowledgment

Special thanks to Richard Zeph, MD, FACS, for his assistance with the text and photographs in this chapter.

References

1. Gonzalez-Ulloa M, Flores ES. Senility of the face—basic study to understand its causes and effects. Plast Reconstr Surg 1965;36:239–246

2. Rohrich RJ, Pessa JE. The fat compartments of the face: anatomy and clinical implications for cosmetic surgery. Plast Reconstr Surg 2007;119(7):2219–2227, discussion 2228–2231

3. Bruning P. The biographical history of fat transplant surgery. Am J Cosmet Surg 1987;4:35

4. Neuber F. Fat transplantation. Chir Kongr Verhandl Dsch Gesellch Chir 1893 20:66

5. Hollander E. Plastik und Medizin. Stuttgart: FerinandEnke; 1912

6. Miller CC. Cannula Implants and Review of Implantation Techniques in Esthetic Surgery. Chicago, IL: Oak Press; 1926

7. Peer LA. Loss of weight and volume in human fat grafts: with postulation of a "cell survival theory." Plast Reconstr Surg 1950;5:217

8. Zocchi ML, Zuliani F. Bicompartmental breast lipostructuring. Aesthetic Plast Surg 2008;32(2):313–328

9. Ellenbogen R. Free autogenous pearl fat grafts in the face—a preliminary report of a rediscovered technique. Ann Plast Surg 1986;16(3):179–194

10. Illouz YG. Communications at the Societe Francaise de Chirurgie Esthetique, June 1978 and 1979

11. Illouz YG. L'avnir de la reutilization de la graisse pares liposuccion (souite). Rev Chir Esthet Lang Franc 10, 1985

12. Illouz YG. The fat cell 'graft': a new technique to fill depressions. Plast Reconstr Surg 1986;78(1):122–123

13. Coleman SR. Long-term survival of fat transplants: controlled demonstrations. Aesthetic Plast Surg 1995;19(5):421–425

14. Ramirez OM. Full face rejuvenation in three dimensions: a "face-lifting" for the new millenium. Aesthetic Plast Surg 2001;25(3):152–164

15. Fournier PF. Facial recontouring with fat grafting. Dermatol Clin 1990;8(3):523–537

16. Peer LA, Paddock R. Histologic studies on the fate of deeply implanted dermal grafts: observations on secretions of implants buried from one week to one year. Arch Surg 1937;34:268

17. Billings E Jr, May JW Jr. Historical review and present status of free fat graft autotransplantation in plastic and reconstructive surgery. Plast Reconstr Surg 1989;83(2):368–381

18. Garson S. Lipomolding of the reconstructed breast. Presented at the First International Fat Grafting Forum; New Orleans, October 15–16, 2010

19. Lee HY. Fat cell survival and centrifugation. Presented at the First International Fat Grafting Forum; New Orleans October 15–16, 2010

20. Rigotti G, March A, Gaiè M, et al. Clinical treatment of radiotherapy tissue damage by lipoaspirate transplant: a healing process mediated by adipose-derived adult stem cells. Plast Reconstr Surg 2007;119(5):1409–1422, discussion 1423–1424

21. Rigotti G. Fat grafting after radiation therapy. Presented at the First International Fat Grafting Forum; New Orleans October 15–16, 2010

22. Fulton JE, Parastouk N. Fat grafting. Facial Plast Surg Clin North Am 2008;16(4):459–465, vii

23. Markey AC, Glogau RG. Autologous fat grafting: comparison of techniques. Dermatol Surg 2000;26(12):1135–1139

24. Hudson DA, Lambert EV, Bloch CE. Site selection for fat autotransplantation: some observations. Aesthetic Plast Surg 1990;14(3):195–197

25. Rohrich RJ, Sorokin ES, Brown SA. In search of improved fat transfer viability: a quantitative analysis of the role of centrifugation and harvest site. Plast Reconstr Surg 2004; 113(1):391–395, discussion 396–397

26. Ullmann Y, Shoshani O, Fodor A, et al. Searching for the favorable donor site for fat injection: in vivo study using the nude mice model. Dermatol Surg 2005;31(10):1304–1307

27. Chajchir A, Benzaquen I, Wexler E, Arellano AH. Fat injection. Aesthetic Plast Surg 1990;14(2):127–136

28. Keck M, Zeyda M, Gollinger K, et al. Local anesthetics have a major impact on viability of preadipocytes and their differentiation into adipocytes. Plast Reconstr Surg 2010; 126(5):1500–1505

29. Moore JH Jr, Kolaczynski JW, Morales LM, et al. Viability of fat obtained by syringe suction lipectomy: effects of local anesthesia with lidocaine. Aesthetic Plast Surg 1995; 19(4):335–339

30. Skouge JW. The biochemistry and development of adipose tissue and the pathophysiology of obesity as it relates to liposuction surgery. Dermatol Clin 1990;8(3):385–393

31. Coleman SR. Structural fat grafts: the ideal filler? Clin Plast Surg 2001;28(1):111–119

32. Nguyen A, Pasyk KA, Bouvier TN, Hassett CA, Argenta LC. Comparative study of survival of autologous adipose tissue taken and transplanted by different techniques. Plast Reconstr Surg 1990;85(3):378–386, discussion 387–389

33. Niechajev I, Sevčuk O. Long-term results of fat transplantation: clinical and histologic studies. Plast Reconstr Surg 1994;94(3):496–506

34. Pu LLQ, Cui X, Fink BF, Cibull ML, Gao D. The viability of fatty tissues within adipose aspirates after conventional liposuction: a comprehensive study. Ann Plast Surg 2005; 54(3):288–292, discussion 292

35. Smith P, Adams WP Jr, Lipschitz AH, et al. Autologous human fat grafting: effect of harvesting and preparation techniques on adipocyte graft survival. Plast Reconstr Surg 2006;117(6):1836–1844

36. Shiffman MA, Mirrafati S. Fat transfer techniques: the effect of harvest and transfer methods on adipocyte viability and review of the literature. Dermatol Surg 2001;27(9): 819–826

37. Rohrich RJ, Morales DE, Krueger JE, et al. Comparative lipoplasty analysis of in vivo-treated adipose tissue. Plast Reconstr Surg 2000;105(6):2152–2158, discussion 2159–2160

38. Chajchir A, Benzaquen I, Moretti E. Comparative experimental study of autologous adipose tissue processed by different techniques. Aesthetic Plast Surg 1993;17(2): 113–115

39. Piasecki JH, Gutowski KA, Lahvis GP, Moreno KI. An experimental model for improving fat graft viability and purity. Plast Reconstr Surg 2007;119(5):1571–1583

40. Boschert MT, Beckert BW, Puckett CL, Concannon MJ. Analysis of lipocyte viability after liposuction. Plast Reconstr Surg 2002;109(2):761–765, discussion 766–767

41. Crawford JL, Hubbard BA, Colbert SH, Puckett CL. Fine tuning lipoaspirate viability for fat grafting. Plast Reconstr Surg 2010;126(4):1342–1348

42. Glasgold RA, Glasgold MJ, Lam SM. Complications following fat transfer. Oral Maxillofac Surg Clin North Am 2009;21(1):53–58, vi

43. Dessy LA, Mazzocchi M, Fioramonti P, Scuderi N. Conservative management of local *Mycobacterium chelonae* infection after combined liposuction and lipofilling. Aesthetic Plast Surg 2006;30(6):717–722

44. Soto LE, Bobadilla M, Villalobos Y, et al. Post-surgical nasal cellulitis outbreak due to *Mycobacterium chelonae*. J Hosp Infect 1991;19(2):99–106

45. Centers for Disease Control and Prevention. Rapidly growing mycobacterial infection following liposuction and liposculpture—Caracas, Venezuela, 1996–1998. MMWR Morb Mortal Wkly Rep 1998 Dec 18;47(49):1065–1067

46. Vijayaraghavan R, Chandrashekhar R, Sujatha Y, Belagavi CS. Hospital outbreak of atypical mycobacterial infection of port sites after laparoscopic surgery. J Hosp Infect 2006;64(4):344–347

47. Talbot SG, Parrett BM, Yaremchuk MJ. Sepsis after autologous fat grafting. Plast Reconstr Surg 2010;126(4): 162e–164e

48. Teimourian B. Blindness following fat injections. Plast Reconstr Surg 1988;82(2):361

49. Yoon SS, Chang DI, Chung KC. Acute fatal stroke immediately following autologous fat injection into the face. Neurology 2003;61(8):1151–1152

50. Coleman SR. Avoidance of arterial occlusion from injection of soft tissue fillers. Aesthet Surg J 2002;22(6):555–557

51. Lee DH, Yang HN, Kim JC, Shyn KH. Sudden unilateral visual loss and brain infarction after autologous fat injection into nasolabial groove. Br J Ophthalmol 1996;80(11): 1026–1027

52. Feinendegen DL, Baumgartner RW, Schroth G, Mattle HP, Tschopp H. Middle cerebral artery occlusion and ocular fat embolism after autologous fat injection in the face. J Neurol 1998;245(1):53–54

20 Neuromodulators

Kartik Nettar, Jason P. Champagne, and Corey S. Maas

Key Concepts

- A thorough history and physical exam allow for appropriate selection of patients who will benefit from injection while avoiding those who will likely not respond well to treatment or be placed at greater risk.

- A comprehensive understanding of the relevant anatomy of the upper face and muscular interactions is imperative for proper injection technique and optimal outcomes.

- Injection over the glabella and at the level of the brow, while avoiding injection 1 to 2 cm above the brow, will provide optimal results and prevent medial brow ptosis, a common adverse effect.

- Small amounts of neuromodulator can be injected into the frontalis muscle to help smooth the forehead without risk of significant depression of the brow.

Introduction

Since its initial application in the treatment of strabismus in children in the 1970s and 1980s, botulinum toxin type A's usage has grown exponentially.[1] Botox (Allergan, Irvine, CA) has become a layperson's term, and the procedure, once reserved to subspecialized corners of medicine, today is performed by practitioners from many branches of medicine, for applications cosmetic and functional. Botulinum toxin's U.S. Food and Drug Administration (FDA) indications currently include blepharospasm, strabismus, and dynamic glabellar rhytids.[2] However, its multiple off-label uses include lateral orbital rhytids, dynamic forehead lines, peau d'orange of the chin, platysmal bands, hyperhidrosis, and migraine headaches, to name a few.[3]

Three botulinum neuromodulators are currently available, having obtained FDA approval for cosmetic use in July 2011: onabotulinumtoxinA (Botox Cosmetic, Allergan), abobotulinumtoxinA (Dysport, Medicis Aesthetics, Scottsdale, AZ), and incobotulinumtoxinA (Xeomin, Merz Pharmaceuticals, Frankfurt, Germany). Myobloc, a botulinum toxin type B, demonstrated encouraging results in the treatment of hyperfunctional frown lines but fell out of favor largely because of its short duration of action and the pain associated with its injection.[4,5]

Because of their ease of use, quick results, and long history of safety, botulinum neuromodulators have become nearly ubiquitous in aesthetic medicine. However, the astute clinician must possess a sound knowledge of neuromodulator physiology, relevant anatomy, and potential complications to successfully treat patients.

■ Background: Basic Science of Procedure

Botulinum neuromodulator exists as a two-chain polypeptide consisting of a 100 kD heavy chain and a 49 kD light chain joined by a disulfide bridge. The light chain functions as a protease, cleaving a critical protein in the fusion of acetylcholine vesicles in the presynaptic nerve terminal at the neuromuscular junction. Synaptosomal-associated protein 25 (SNAP-25) is the protein cleaved by the type A neuromodulator, whereas vesicle-associated membrane protein (VAMP), syntaxin and synaptobrevin are proteins cleaved by other neuromodulator serotypes (B through G). By preventing fusion of the acetylcholine vesicle with the presynaptic axon terminal membrane, acetylcholine is not released into the neuromuscular cleft. This causes the target muscle to be weakened reversibly until new presynaptic vesicles can be generated. This regeneration period varies, based on the target muscle, dosage, and neuromodulator, but it is thought to be 3 months.[6]

Botulinum neuromodulator is rapidly denatured at temperatures exceeding 60°C. Therefore, both onabotulinumtoxinA and abobotulinumtoxinA are to be stored at temperatures between 2 and 8°C, before and after reconstitution. One purported advantage of incobotulinumtoxinA is its lack of need for refrigeration in transport and prior to reconstitution. This occurs because incobotulinumtoxinA is manufactured as a 150 kD protein without the accessory proteins found in nature and other formulations. The accessory proteins serve to stabilize botulinum toxin but must be kept at low temperature to prevent denaturation. Without accessory proteins, incobotulinumtoxinA continues to demonstrate long-term stability and potency, thus allowing for unrefrigerated transport of vials.[7]

■ Pertinent Anatomy

The injecting clinician must possess a sound knowledge of facial anatomy before embarking on any treatment, surgical or otherwise. Because neuromodulators target facial muscles, particular attention must be paid to facial muscular anatomy. It should

be noted that anatomy can vary slightly between patients, genders, and races, but over all, it is fairly consistent (**Fig. 20.1**).

Brow

The paired corrugator supercilii and procerus muscles constitute brow musculature. However, the inferior frontalis and superior orbicularis oculi are also in the region and must be recognized with any brow intervention.

The procerus originates from the nasal bones and inserts into the subcutaneous tissues between the medial eyebrows as a flat, unpaired muscle in a vertical orientation. Procerus contraction produces characteristic transverse nasal lines at the nasion.

The corrugator supercilii is a thick, paired muscle originating at the procerus medially and inserting laterally into the orbicularis oculi at the lateral brow. Corrugator contraction produces glabellar frown lines in a vertical orientation medial to the medial clubhead of the eyebrow. Many textbooks erroneously depict the corrugator as a long, vertically oriented muscle extending well into the midforehead. While there is a small subset of patients in whom the

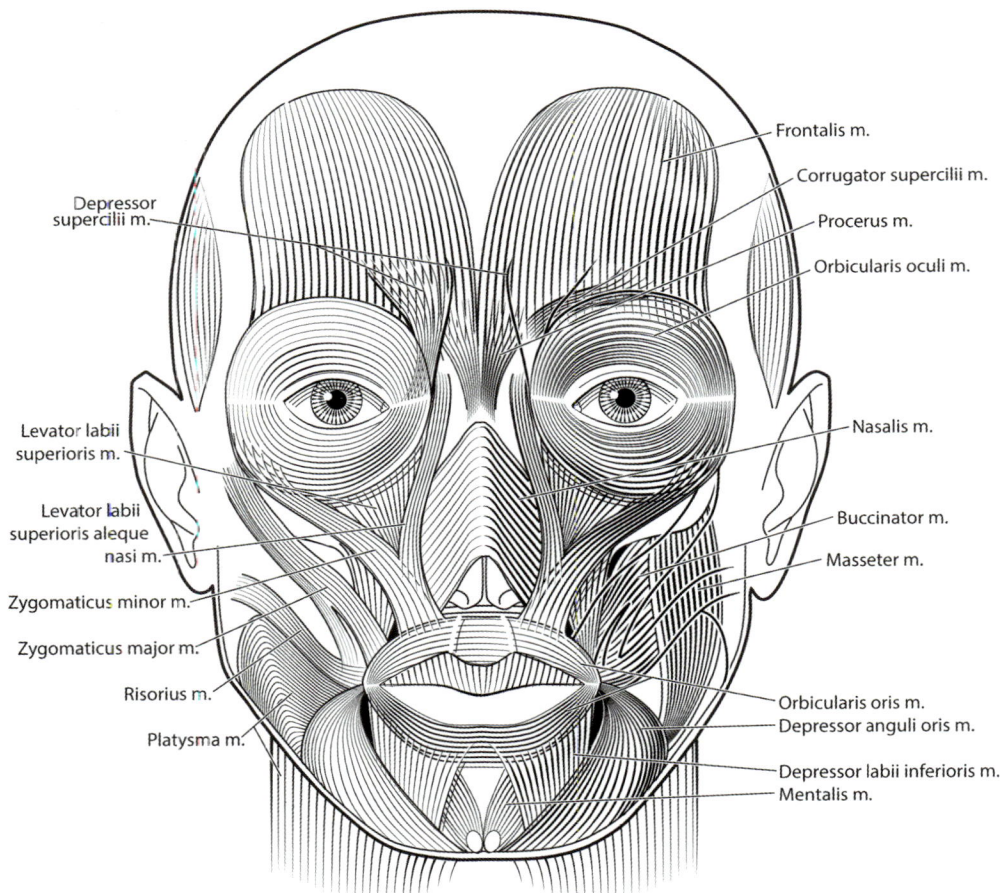

Fig. 20.1 Diagram of the facial muscles.

muscle takes an oblique course instead of paralleling the eyebrow, they exhibit more of an oblique rhytid and not the classic vertical line.

Forehead

The frontalis muscle is responsible for horizontal forehead lines, which trouble many patients. It originates in continuity from the galea aponeurotica superiorly and interdigitates with the procerus, corrugator supercilii, and orbicularis oculi muscle inferiorly. Most often, the muscle displays a midline dehiscence, creating two distinct bellies, rather than a single flat muscular sheet. Contraction of the frontalis causes elevation of the brow but also results in dynamic horizontal lines, which become curvilinear laterally.

Periocular Area

The orbicularis oculi encircles each eye as a wide, flat muscle. It extends out from the upper and lower eyelids and on to the brow and cheek. Medially, the muscle inserts into and around the medial canthal tendon and lacrimal sac, enabling a pumping action of the sac contents into the nasolacrimal ductal system. Laterally, a ligamentous contribution from the orbicularis oculi is dealt to the lateral canthal tendon, though this contribution is quite minor.

Contraction of the orbicularis oculi causes a sphincteric closure of the eyelids over the globe. As a result, lines tangent to the muscle project radially. In the lateral orbital area, these radial lines are better known as lateral orbital rhytids or crow's feet. It should be noted that in addition to its eye closure function, the orbicularis oculi is also the most powerful depressor of the brow.

Lower eyelid lines result from photoaging of eyelid skin. These lines may be accentuated by the underlying orbicularis oculi muscle. However, because the primary function of the orbicularis oculi in this area is closure of the lower eyelid, a fine balance exists between smoothing fine lines and causing ectropion. The muscles involved in facial expression are seen in relation to the overlying skin in **Fig. 20.2**.

Nose

Although nasal appearance is largely determined by bony and cartilaginous architecture, muscular anatomy can cause subtle aesthetic problems. A principal muscle on the nasal midvault is the paired, fan-shaped nasalis. Originating at the inferior nasal pyriform aperture, it travels transversely to insert into the aponeurosis of the contralateral muscle.[3] Contraction results in "bunny lines."

The depressor septi is an unpaired muscle at the base of the nose innervated by the buccal branch of the facial nerve. Arising from the incisive fossa

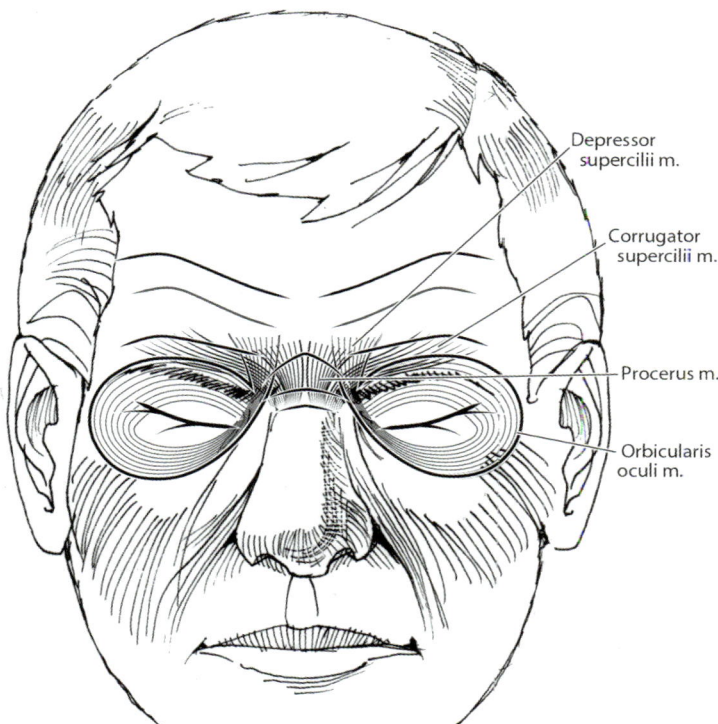

Fig. 20.2 Muscles of facial expression are seen in relation to the external landmarks.

of the maxilla, it inserts into the caudal septum. Its function is to constrict the nares. However, in doing this, the muscle also brings the nasal tip inferiorly (droopy nasal tip), particularly with a smile. As such, it has been postulated that its transection during rhinoplasty can help to alleviate the "smiling deformity."[8]

Perioral

Similar to the orbicularis oculi, the orbicularis oris functions as a sphincteric muscle encircling the mouth. Contraction of this muscle closes, protrudes, and purses the lips. The upper lip segment inserts into the maxilla just superior to the canine, and the lower lip segment originates on the mandible just lateral to the mentalis. Laterally, the orbicularis oris interdigitates with the depressor anguli oris (DAO) inferiorly and the risorius at the oral commissure.[9] Because of its sphincteric function, radial lip lines can result, often called smokers' lines, though most patients exhibiting them do not have a history of smoking. These lines can become particularly apparent in females as lipstick can bleed into the depths of the lip lines.

The DAO originates at the oblique line of the mandible and inserts at the modiolus of each oral commissure. The DAO's contraction pulls the oral commissures inferiorly and can cause a chronic downturned commissure resulting in a frowning appearance. Its opposing muscles are the risorius and zygomaticus major, which serve to elevate the oral commissure.

Chin

Medial to the DAO lies the mentalis. The mentalis originates at the incisor fossa of the mandible inferiorly and inserts into the skin of the lower lip superiorly. Contraction raises the chin to the lower lip and causes protrusion of the lower lip, thus deeming this the "pouting muscle." A deep transverse mental crease can result from hyperactivity of this muscle. Similarly, chin dimpling can become apparent, causing a peau d'orange (orange peel).

Masseter

The masseter is a short but strong muscle of mastication. It originates from the zygomatic arch and inserts into the lateral mandibular ramus. Innervated by the mandibular branch of the trigeminal nerve, it functions to elevate the mandible for chewing. Hypertrophy of this muscle can result in bulging of the cheeks and a widened facial contour.

Neck

Deep to the skin and within the superficial cervical fascia is the platysma. The platysma is a broad, flat, sheetlike muscle covering the entire neck. It originates from the superficial fascia of the pectoralis major and deltoid and ascends to insert into the orbicularis oris, DAO, risorius, mentalis, and the anterior third of the oblique lines of the mandibular ramus.[9] In the midline of the neck, the muscle dehisces, forming an inverted-v below the chin. Contraction of the muscle depresses the lower jaw and causes the lower lip and oral commissure to be drawn inferiorly.

Platysmal bands occur when skin overlying the muscle loses elasticity and are seen in aging. "Necklace lines" or transverse neck lines occur between the anterior borders of the sternocleidomastoid from a hyperfunctional platysma.

■ Patient Selection

Each patient should be treated with an individually tailored treatment plan. However, there are certain patient groups in which botulinum neuromodulators are contraindicated. These groups include those with a hypersensitivity to botulinum toxin and those with neuromuscular disorders, namely Lambert-Eaton syndrome, myasthenia gravis, and amyotrophic lateral sclerosis (ALS). In patients with inflamed or infected skin, deep dermal scarring, or dermatochalasia, caution and a thorough examination are required of the clinician. With any patient, it must be stressed that the goal of treatment is a natural, more refreshed appearance, as opposed to a drastic change.[10]

■ Technical Aspects of Procedure

Reconstitution of Neuromodulator

Protocol for reconstituting Botox and preparing prefilled syringes is as follows:

1. Remove Botox Cosmetic vial from freezer.
2. Apply gloves.
3. Attach a 19-gauge 1.5 inch needle to a 3 mL syringe.
4. Alcohol swab the stopper of preservative-free saline. Allow to dry.
5. Withdraw 2 mL of saline into the syringe.
6. Inject the preservative-free saline slowly into the stopper of the Botox vial. The handle of the 3 mL syringe may need to be held to stop rapid infusion of the saline.

7. Roll the vial gently and turn upside down once. *Do not shake.*
8. Remove the stopper of the vial. This will avoid dulling the needle.
9. Expel any air in the 0.5 mL insulin syringe and withdraw 0.4 mL of reconstituted Botox solution. This will yield 20 units of Botox in each syringe. Withdraw 0.2 mL of solution to yield 10 units of Botox. Repeat until all of the Botox solution has been withdrawn into the insulin syringes.

Protocol for reconstituting Dysport (Medicis Aesthetics) and preparing prefilled syringes is as follows:

1. Remove Dysport vial from freezer.
2. Apply gloves.
3. Attach a 19 gauge 1.5 inch needle to a 3 mL syringe.
4. Alcohol swab the stopper of preservative-free saline. Allow to dry.
5. Withdraw 1.5 mL of saline into the syringe.
6. Inject the preservative-free saline slowly into the stopper of the vial. The handle of the 3 mL syringe may need to be held to stop rapid infusion of saline.
7. Roll the vial gently and turn upside down once. *Do not shake.*
8. Remove the stopper of the vial. This will avoid dulling the needle.
9. Expel any air in the 0.3 mL insulin syringe and withdraw 0.3 mL of solution. This will yield 60 units of Dysport. Withdraw 0.15 of solution to yield 30 units of Dysport. Repeat until all of the solution has been withdrawn into the insulin syringes.

Injections

Brow

Correct placement of neuromodulator in the brow requires a proper understanding of the orientation of the corrugator supercilii muscle, as mentioned previously. As such, the neuromodulator should be injected in two positions for each brow. Approximately two thirds of the dose should be injected just at or slightly above the medial clubhead of the eyebrow. The remaining one third of the dose can then be injected 3 to 5 mm lateral to the first injection site, at approximately the mid eyebrow. In the senior author's (CSM) institution, the medial clubhead injection comprises 7.5 units of onabotulinumtoxinA or 23 units of abobotulinumtoxinA, whereas the more lateral injection consists of 2.5 units of onabotulinumtoxinA or 7 units of abobotulinumtoxinA.

When injecting, it is helpful to instruct the patient to frown to better visualize the bulk of the muscle. The muscle can then be grasped gently by the clinician with the thumb and forefinger of the noninjecting hand. The neuromodulator can then be injected at a 30 degree angle to the skin, entering from the contralateral direction. Care must be taken not to plunge the needle too deep (**Fig. 20.3a,b**).

Forehead

In treating the frontalis muscle, two points must be kept in mind. First, it is of paramount importance to avoid brow ptosis. It is therefore recommended that neuromodulator injections be placed at least 1.5 cm superior to the upper margin of the brows lateral to the midpupillary line. Moreover, in the pretreatment assessment, preexisting brow ptosis should be noted. In these patients, forehead treatment may be con-

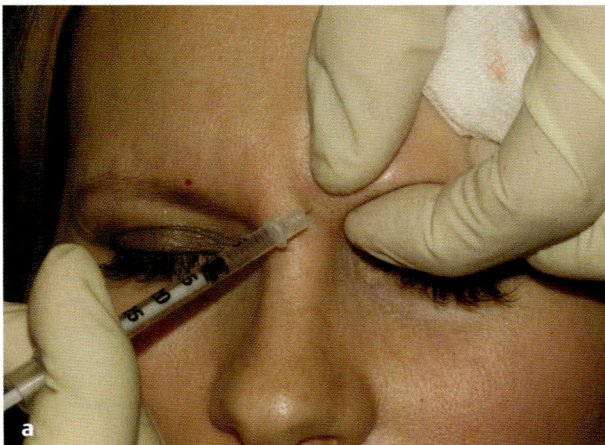

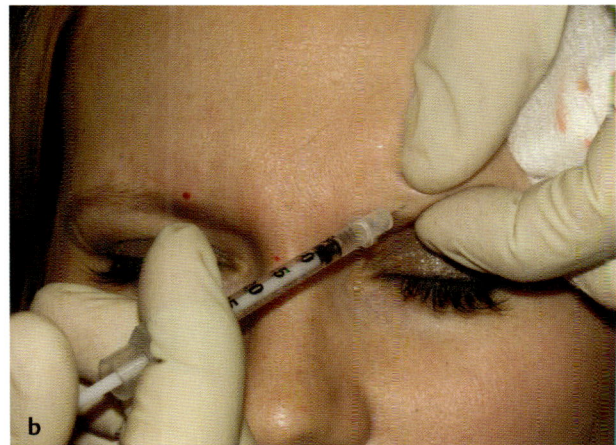

Fig. 20.3 Corrugator injections **(a,b)**. Typically, this injection is performed at least 1 cm above the orbital rim.

traindicated. It is important to educate the patient that forehead treatment attempts to strike a balance between frontalis muscle relaxation and adequate brow position.

When injecting the frontalis, one must inject immediately above the most inferior horizontal forehead crease. A total of 10 units of onabotulinumtoxinA or 30 units of abobotulinumtoxinA, divided into four equal aliquots, are then injected along the length of the forehead. Laterally, the point at which the forehead curves temporally is the lateralmost injection point. Medially, the medial canthus is the medialmost injection point. In patients with greater forehead height or numerous forehead lines, "extension therapy" can be added, consisting of three additional injections superiorly along the forehead. The first of this extension therapy is placed in the midline, whereas the other two are placed between the medial and lateral injection points bilaterally. Injections of the forehead can be made tangentially (**Fig. 20.4a,b**).

Lateral Orbit

Treatment of "crow's feet" is accomplished by injecting the lateral orbicularis oculi muscle ▶ **Video 20.1**. Injections should be placed at least 1 cm lateral to the lateral orbital rim to minimize intraorbital complications. A total of 10 units of onabotulinumtoxinA or 30 units of abobotulinumtoxinA, divided into four equal aliquots, are injected with the skin maximally spread apart in a craniocaudal direction to avoid traumatizing superficial blood vessels. Depending on the thickness of the patient's skin, the injection should be relatively superficial because of the thin height of the dermis in this area. Injections can be made tangential to the surface of the skin (**Fig. 20.5**).

Lower Eyelid

Lower eyelid lines can occur with photoaging and hyperkinetic orbicularis oculi muscle. To avoid posttreatment ectropion, a snap test must be performed to assess lower lid laxity. In patients with adequate recoil of the lower lid, a single small dose of neuromodulator (2 units onabotulinumtoxinA/6 units abobotulinumtoxinA) can be injected at a 30 degree angle to the skin and into the orbicularis oculi overlying the inferior orbital rim.

Nasalis Muscle

"Bunny lines" are best demonstrated and treated while the patient contracts their nasalis muscle, retracting the nose superiorly. A single superior midline injection point is utilized at the nasal dorsum immediately inferior to the procerus. A small dose (2 units onabotulinumtoxinA/6 units abobotulinumtoxinA) is utilized at this point.

Perioral Area

Radial lip lines, sometimes called lipstick lines, can occur along the upper lip, analogous to lateral orbital rhytids around the eye. Therefore, very small doses of neuromodulator (1 unit onabotulinumtoxinA/3 units abobotulinumtoxinA) can be injected evenly in four points just above the vermilion border. The lower lip should not be injected because of the risk of creating oral incompetence.

Downturned oral commissures, due to a tonic depressor anguli oris, can also be treated with small doses (2 units onabotulinumtoxinA/6 units abobotu-

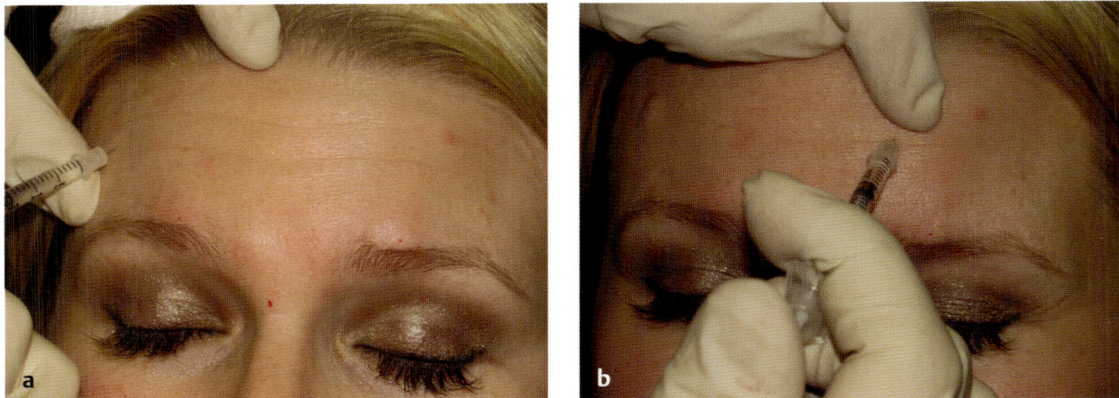

Fig. 20.4 Frontalis injections **(a,b)**.

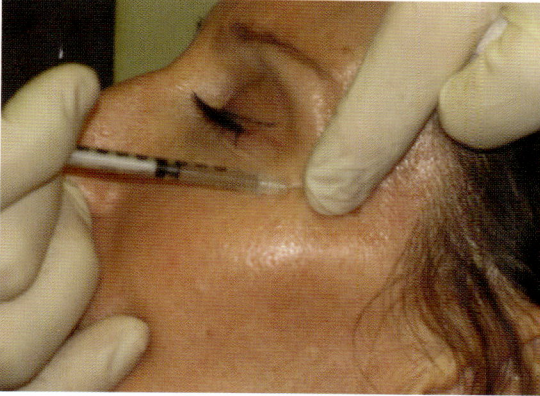

Fig. 20.5 Crow's feet or lateral canthus injection.

linumtoxinA) of neuromodulator injected immediately inferior and lateral to each oral commissure.

Chin

Peau d'orange or golf-ball dimpling can also be treated with neuromodulators. In this case, injections should be placed at the inferior aspect of the mentalis muscle to avoid injection into the orbicularis oris. Often, instructing patients to contract their mentalis and produce the undesirable dimpling assists in delineating the target muscle.

Masseter

While instructing the patient to bite down will better demonstrate the masseter, in patients seeking treatment, most often, this exercise is not necessary. Three separate injections of small doses of neuromodulator (2 units onabotulinumtoxinA/6 units abobotulinumtoxinA) into the body of the masseter can help in reducing its size while preserving its important function of mastication.

Neck

Treatment of platysmal bands can best be accomplished by grasping each band with the noninjecting thumb and forefinger while the patient is seated upright. Intramuscular injections are then delivered evenly in four aliquots (2 units onabotulinumtoxinA/ 6 units abobotulinumtoxinA) along the course of each band. One should not inject too deeply because severe complications may result, including dysphagia, dysphonia, and torticollis.

Transverse lines ("necklace lines") can similarly be treated with a neuromodulator in an evenly spaced distribution along the length of the rhytids. Smaller aliquots (1 unit onabotulinumtoxinA/2 units abobotulinumtoxinA) are injected tangentially into the rhytids, usually requiring two to three separate injections.

Postoperative Care

Minimal care is required after botulinum neuromodulator treatment. To assuage oozing from injection sites, firm pressure with cotton gauze can be applied by the clinician or patient for 5 minutes. Additionally, ice packs to the treatment area are advised to prevent bruising and edema. The vast majority of patients may resume their normal work and activities immediately after treatment.

Complications and Their Management

Due to their long history of safety and efficacy, botulinum neuromodulators are associated with few serious complications. Because the dosages used in aesthetic medicine, in particular, are small, serious adverse events are rare. Most adverse events are mild and temporary, including pain at injection sites, bruising, swelling, and flulike symptoms. To minimize bruising, clinicians may instruct patients to avoid aspirin, nonsteroidal anti-inflammatory agents, and vitamin E for up to 2 weeks prior to treatment. Additionally, the gentle application of ice packs, as mentioned previously, after injection aids in minimizing ecchymoses.

Most significant complications can occur when the clinician is unfamiliar with the relevant muscular anatomy. These result from diffusion of toxin into adjacent musculature which can lead to unexpected muscle weakening. Periorbital complications include an overtreated frontalis, brow ptosis, eyelid ptosis, asymmetry, cocked eyebrows, diplopia, ectropion, decreased strength of eye closure, and dry eyes. One should also carefully evaluate patients for any preexisting brow asymmetry or ptosis prior to treatment. Brow ptosis can generally be avoided by injecting no closer than 1 cm above the bony orbital rim in the midpupillary line and using lower doses in the frontalis.

Eyelid ptosis is one of the most commonly encountered complications. Though ptosis rates as high as 6.5% have been mentioned, clinical trial data suggest an approximate 3% rate with Botox Cosmetic and a 2% rate with Dysport. The etiology of eyelid ptosis is diffusion of the toxin into the levator palpebrae muscle. Further, some believe that older patients or those with loose skin or a weak orbital septum are more susceptible to ptosis. In certain cases, ptosis can be due to a weakened frontalis from botulinum neuromodulator that is compensating for a preexisting mild degree of eyelid ptosis. Although many believe that ptosis occurs because of diffusion of neuromodulator through the orbital septum to the levator palpebrae muscle, it is the senior author's assertion that hydrostatic pressure related to the injection can cause the neuromodulator to traverse the supraorbital or supratrochlear foramina and the superior orbital fissure. Thus, by minimizing the volume injected and increasing the concentration of botulinum neuromodulator per aliquot, as well as applying low plunger pressure during injection, ptosis can be avoided. In addition, one should avoid applying firm direct pressure at glabellar injection sites.

Eyelid ptosis can occur as early as 48 hours after treatment to as late as 14 days posttreatment and results after treatment of the glabellar complex. Duration rarely lasts more than 3 to 4 weeks but can be particularly aggravating to patients.

Diplopia and dry eyes are also well-described adverse effects of botulinum neuromodulator treatment when it is used for blepharospasm, facial spasm, or synkinesis and essential hyperlacrimation; these are extremely rare complications in cosmetic applications. Possible explanations for diplopia include incorrect placement of injections, larger volumes that lead to greater toxin diffusion/migration, or a defective orbital septum that allows the toxin to exert an effect on the extraocular muscles.[12] Dry eyes can result from diffusion of toxin into the lacrimal gland or paralytic lagophthalmos leading to reduced blink strength. One case report attributed this complication to an injection site 0.5 cm from the superior orbital rim.[13]

■ Conclusion

The advent of neuromodulators has afforded aesthetic clinicians another tool to rejuvenate the aging face. As newer neuromodulators become commercially available, demand for such treatments and their subsequent use will continue to grow. A strong grasp of facial muscular anatomy coupled with precise injectable technique will afford clinicians an opportunity to effect successful outcomes, in turn creating happy and satisfied patients.

References

1. Scott AB. Botulinum toxin injection into extraocular muscles as an alternative to strabismus surgery. J Pediatr Ophthalmol Strabismus 1980;17(1):21–25
2. Carruthers J, Carruthers A. Botulinum toxin (Botox) chemodenervation for facial rejuvenation. Facial Plast Surg Clin North Am 2001;9(2):197–204, vii
3. Loos BM, Maas CS. Relevant anatomy for botulinum toxin facial rejuvenation. Facial Plast Surg Clin North Am 2003;11(4):439–443
4. Ramirez AL, Reeck J, Maas CS. Preliminary experience with botulinum toxin type B in hyperkinetic facial lines. Plast Reconstr Surg 2002;109(6):2154–2155
5. Ramirez AL, Reeck J, Maas CS. Botulinum toxin type B (MyoBloc) in the management of hyperkinetic facial lines. Otolaryngol Head Neck Surg 2002;126(5):459–467
6. Schantz EJ, Johnson EA. Botulinum toxin: the story of its development for the treatment of human disease. Biol Med 1997;40(3):317–327
7. Grein S, Mander GJ, Taylor HV. Xeomin is stable without refrigeration: complexing proteins are not required for stability of botulinum neurotoxin type A preparations. Toxicon 2008;51(Suppl 1):13
8. Benlier E, Top H, Aygit AC. A new approach to smiling deformity: cutting of the superior part of the orbicularis oris. Aesthetic Plast Surg 2005;29(5):373–377, discussion 378
9. Petrus GM, Lewis D, Maas CS. Anatomic considerations for treatment with botulinum toxin. Facial Plast Surg Clin North Am 2007;15(1):1–9, v
10. Carruthers J, Fagien S, Matarasso SL; Botox Consensus Group. Consensus recommendations on the use of botulinum toxin type A in facial aesthetics. Plast Reconstr Surg 2004;114(6, Suppl):1S–22S
11. Alam M, Dover JS, Klein AW, Arndt KA. Botulinum A exotoxin for hyperfunctional facial lines: where not to inject. Arch Dermatol 2002;138(9):1180–1185
12. Aristodemou P, Watt L, Baldwin C, Hugkulstone C. Diplopia associated with the cosmetic use of botulinum toxin A for facial rejuvenation. Ophthal Plast Reconstr Surg 2006;22(2):134–136
13. Northington ME, Huang CC. Dry eyes and superficial punctate keratitis: a complication of treatment of glabellar dynamic rhytides with botulinum exotoxin A. Dermatol Surg 2004;30(12 Pt 2):1515–1517

21 Endonasal Rhinoplasty

Paul J. Carniol, Dhave Setabutr, and Fred G. Fedok

Key Concepts

- The endonasal approach to rhinoplasty allows the surgeon to perform many of the same maneuvers as the open rhinoplasty approach.

- Excellent visualization of the nasal tip structures can be achieved with the cartilage delivery technique.

- Because there is no columellar incision, there is no risk of problems with the healing of the columellar incision or columellar scarring.

- Because there is less dissection with the endonasal approach, there may be less swelling.

■ Introduction

During the past decade, the external approach to rhinoplasty has been widely popularized. As is well documented in the literature, this is a useful approach for the procedure and offers distinct visualization advantages for teaching the procedure to residents.

Yet the endonasal approach to rhinoplasty also has some distinct advantages, including less surgical dissection, potentially more rapid execution, and the lack of a visible incision. Furthermore, the endonasal approach avoids the risk of a columellar scar or columellar healing problems, which can uncommonly include partial loss of the columella, requiring secondary reconstruction. Healing time may be reduced because there is less dissection and, in the authors' experience, frequently less swelling.

To perform an endonasal approach, it is important for the surgeon to have a thorough understanding of the underlying anatomy. Some surgeons will mark the underlying anatomy on the skin surface. As for all rhinoplasty approaches, it is important to have a diagnosis of the underlying issues before starting the surgical procedure. It is also important to have a complete procedural plan before making any incisions. However, one must be prepared to amend the initial plan depending on the findings at surgery.

■ Background: Basic Science of Procedure

Sushruta Ayuveda was the first known person to describe external nasal surgery for reconstruction around 600 BC in India. Rhinoplasty was described in the nineteenth century by Orlando Roe[1] and Franz Joseph. Subsequently, rhinoplasty techniques were further refined and popularized by physicians such as Aufricht, Fomon, and Goldman.[2,3] The endonasal approach, with the use of transfixion incisions, became the primary approach through most of the 1960s and 1970s. More recently, external rhinoplasty has become more popular than endonasal rhinoplasty. Despite this, many surgeons advocate for the use of the endonasal approach. For many patients the benefits of the endonasal approach are clear.

With both primary and revision cases, those that offer limited challenges are sometimes the most appropriate to address endonasally.[4] Before performing a rhinoplasty procedure, it is important to have an understanding of nasal anatomy that includes osseous, cartilaginous, and ligamentous structures. Endonasal rhinoplasty can be used to improve the nasal tip, dorsum, or both. Incising, suturing, or excising portions of the tip cartilages can be used to alter the shape, projection, and rotation of the tip. Struts, tip grafts, and alar batten grafts can also be employed.

■ Pertinent Anatomy

An understanding of the anatomy of the nose is crucial when one is evaluating the rhinoplasty patient. The paired nasal bones provide the bony framework of the upper nose.[5] Their attachments to the frontal bone and nasal processes of the maxillary bone complete the bony vault. The paired upper lateral cartilages and lower lateral cartilages, with their fibrocartilaginous support, provide the framework of the middle third of the nose, in addition to the septum and nasal bones. Specifically, the lower lateral cartilages form a fibrocartilaginous arch supporting the nasal lobule and nostrils.[5] The nasal septum supports the nose along its entire length. It supplies the dorsal profile between the nasal bones and nasal tip.[5] The caudal septum influences the appearance of the columella. To describe the dynamics of the tip, Anderson analogized nasal tip support to a tripod, with the lateral crura representing two legs and the conjoined medial crura the third leg.[5] Other authors have likened tip dynamics to a cantilevered spring model.[6]

Tip support is dependent upon the relationship of the lower lateral cartilages to the soft tissue and their intrinsic strengths. Male and female noses differ with respect to nasolabial angles and the incidence of dorsal humps. The ideal nasolabial angle ranges from 90 to 115 degrees.[7] In general, the angle is more acute in men and more obtuse in females.

Aesthetically, the nose should be symmetrical, proportioned, and balanced. The well-balanced nose is in harmony with the surrounding structures of the face. On analysis, one should be able to divide the face into equal horizontal thirds and vertical facial proportions equal to five eye widths across when viewed frontally.[7]

■ Patient Selection

Appropriate patient selection is critical for successful outcomes in endonasal rhinoplasty. Depending on the surgeon's level of expertise, the endonasal approach can be used for both primary and revision rhinoplasty procedures. Patients with excessive asymmetry or scarring due to multiple prior procedures may benefit more from an open approach. Ideal candidates for an endonasal approach are those that may be more symmetrical, have less challenging goals for correction, and have limited diagnostic uncertainties. In contrast, even complex patients whose goals are met with limited resection or grafting might be best benefited by an endonasal approach.

It is important to obtain preoperative photographs. These should include at least frontal, lateral, base, and oblique views. Lateral photos with and without smiling are at times important to analyze possible changes in the nasal tip with smiling and should be taken so that the patient's face is positioned in line in the Frankfort horizontal plane. Frontal, base, and oblique views provide the best way to assess side-to-side symmetry and reflect the views most seen by others in the day-to-day life of a patient.[4]

■ Technical Aspects of Procedure

Endonasal rhinoplasty can be used to address aesthetic issues in all aspects of the nose. Using the cartilage delivery technique, there is excellent visualization of the alar cartilages. Several types of maneuvers can be performed on the cartilages when exposed via delivery or closed technique. Portions of the lateral crura can be conservatively removed, incised, or reshaped with sutures. Tip grafts and struts can be placed and stabilized with absorbable sutures as needed. The nasal dorsum can also be managed through the same intercartilaginous incisions that are used in cartilage delivery.[8,9]

These and other maneuvers can be used to alter the nasal tip, including reshaping, narrowing, rotating, augmenting, and altering projection.

Surgical Instruments

A basic rhinoplasty set includes a sharp no. 15 blade scalpel, a no. 11 blade, nasal speculum, double ball retractors, single-prong hook, double-prong skin hooks, elevators, rasps, osteotomes, morselizer, crusher, Aufricht retractor, Fomon scissors, Stevens tenotomy scissors, Cottle-Neivert retractor(s), and sponges (**Fig. 21.1**).

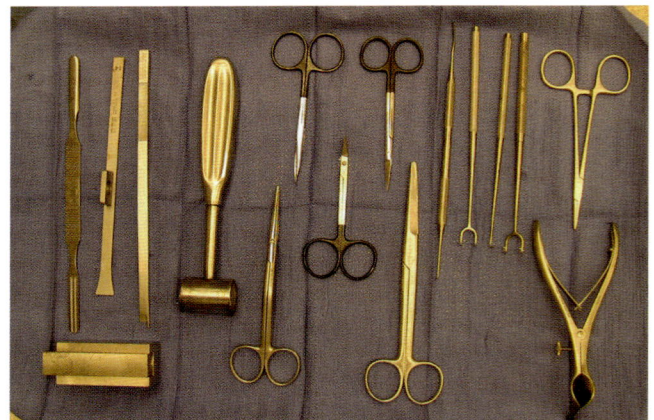

Fig. 21.1 Typical instruments used in endonasal rhinoplasty.

Patient Preparation

Patient preparation for the procedure starts with a prior discussion about the procedure, potential results, limitations and variations, risks, and the typical recovery course. Patients should also be instructed to avoid any medications or supplements that can predispose them to bleeding for the 2 weeks leading up to the procedure.

Endonasal rhinoplasty can be performed with general anesthesia, local anesthesia with intravenous sedation, or local anesthesia with oral sedation. Epinephrine within the local facilitates hemostasis. It is prudent for the physician to select the optimal anesthesia agents for the individual patient. Skin and intranasal markings should be completed before local anesthesia is injected.

Nasal Anesthesia

If the procedure is performed with oral sedation, it is particularly important to achieve adequate anesthesia by local infiltration or local blocks or both. The authors' preference for local anesthesia is 1% lidocaine with 1:100,000 epinephrine. When injecting local anesthesia, it is important to avoid distorting key structures, as well as not to exceed a safe total dose of local anesthesia. Overinjection of local anesthesia can also distort the patient's nasal anatomy or create avoidable swelling.

Surgical Approach

The incisions used to approach an endonasal rhinoplasty are varied, but the ones to be covered in this chapter will equip the surgeon for adequate management of the anatomy ▶ Video 21.1. Endonasal rhinoplasty is started by approaching either the nasal dorsum or the nasal tip. The marginal and intercartilaginous incisions are made adjacent to the endonasal proximal and distal edges of the lateral crura of the lower lateral cartilages. The marginal incision, combined with an intercartilaginous (IC) incision, provides delivery of the tip cartilage into the surgical field. The retrograde IC and cartilage-splitting approaches are nondelivery techniques.[2] The IC incision is useful for trimming relatively small cephalic portions of the lobular cartilage,[2] whereas the cartilage-splitting incision is used when there are more changes needed in tip rotation and supratip definition. Preservation of alar support, with integrity of the caudal lateral crus, is possible with both.[10]

The Marginal Incision

The marginal incision is made in the vestibular skin along the caudal margin of the lower lateral cartilage with a no. 15 blade scalpel (**Fig. 21.2a–f**). When making this incision, it is important to have a finger on the external skin so the depth of the scalpel can be palpated.

The Intercartilaginous Incision

The IC incision is performed under direct visualization with the use of a retractor or nasal speculum. The incision is made with a no. 15 blade scalpel positioned between the upper lateral cartilage and the lateral crus of the lower lateral cartilages. Care should be taken to avoid placing the incision along the free edge of the upper lateral cartilage to avoid scarring (**Fig. 21.3a–d**). While one is making this incision, it is best to have at least one finger palpating the external skin. This enables the surgeon to determine the depth of the incision and avoid injury to the overlying skin. The IC incision is usually made in conjunction with a marginal incision for the purposes of alar cartilage delivery and the excision of limited portions of the lower lateral cartilage.[11] The most cephalic part of the lateral crus to be resected can be marked with methylene blue or a fine marking pen. The amount of cartilage to be resected can be measured with a caliper or ruler. The relative positions of these incisions are shown in **Fig. 21.4**.

Alternative Alar Cartilage-Splitting Incision

The cartilage-splitting incision will accomplish two things. It will allow access to the nasal dorsum over the upper lateral cartilages as well as the completion or execution of a complete strip procedure with reduction of the superior aspect of the lateral crus of the lower lateral cartilage. To accomplish this incision, the surgeon must anticipate the amount and location of cartilage from the lower lateral cartilage that needs to be removed. Some surgeons will facilitate the position of the excision by placing a 25-gauge needle through the nasal ala and/or marking it with methylene blue. The incision is placed through the adherent vestibular lining on the underside of the lower-lateral cartilage and then extended through the cartilage itself (**Fig. 21.5a,b**). Once again, while one is making this incision, it is best to have at least one finger palpating the external skin. This enables the surgeon to determine the depth of the incision and avoid injury to the overlying skin.

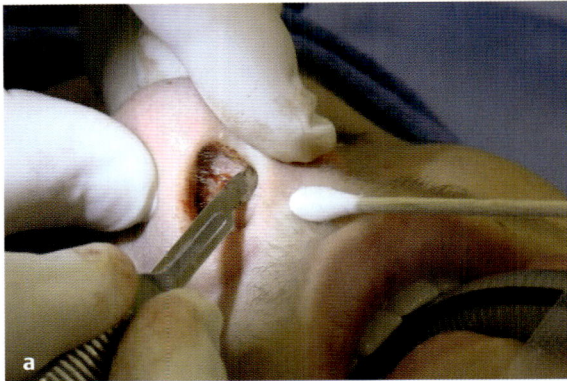

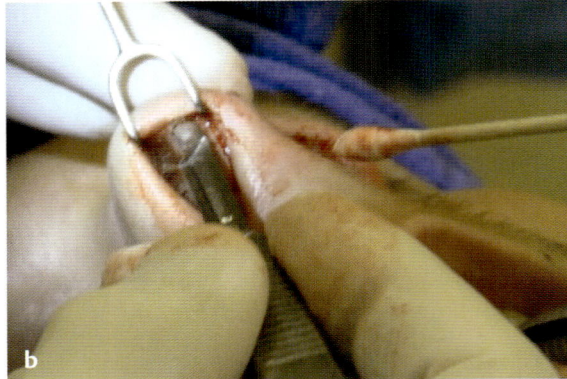

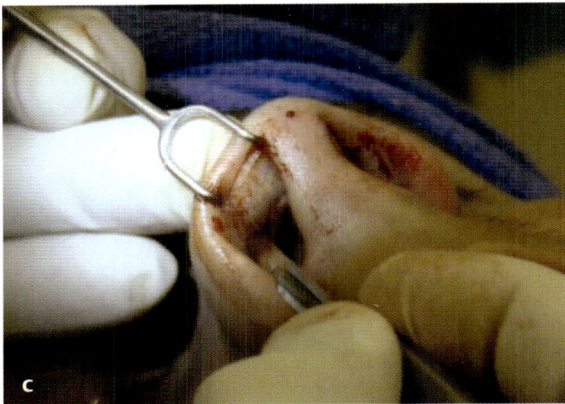

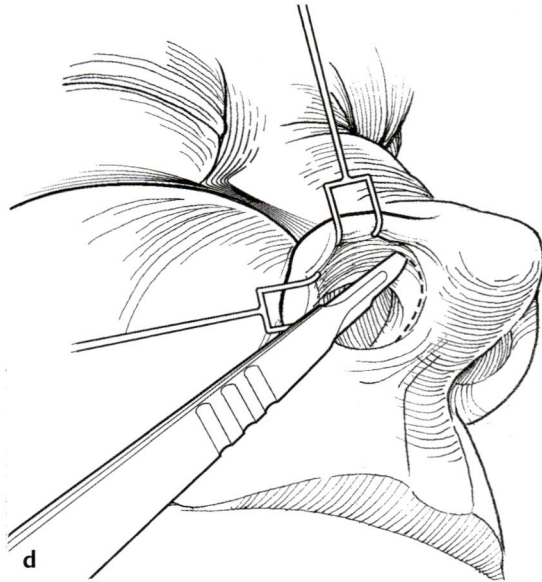

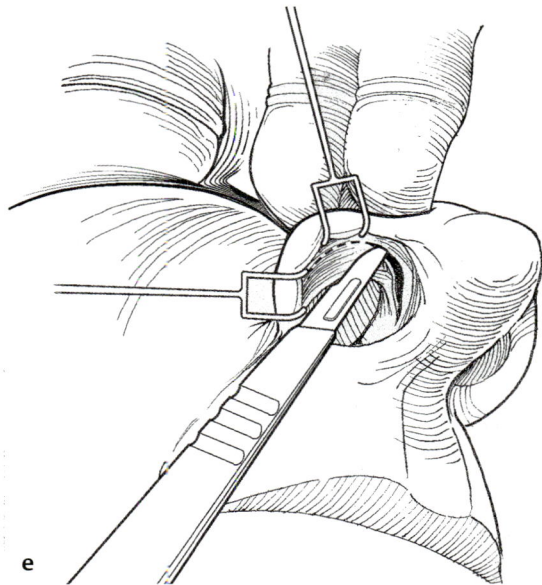

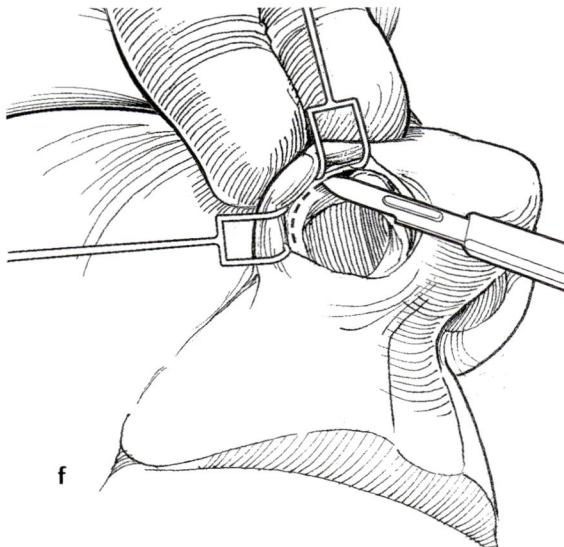

Fig. 21.2 Intraoperative photographs showing technique for a marginal incision **(a–c)**. Diagrams showing incision at the caudal end **(d–f)**. It is important to continually palpate the external skin while making these incisions to monitor the location of the scalpel blade.

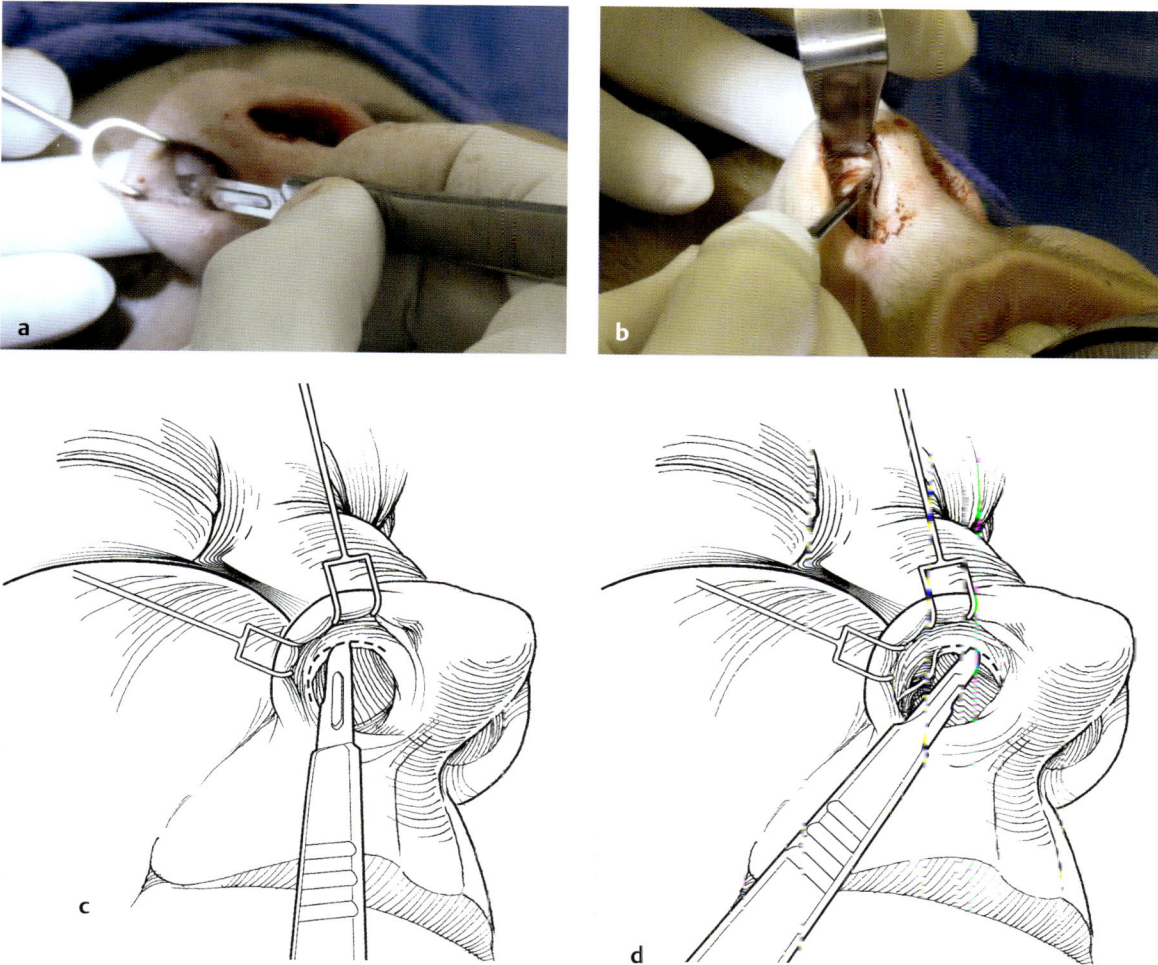

Fig. 21.3 Intraoperative photographs showing technique for an intercartilaginous incision **(a,b)**. The incision is made between the upper and lateral cartilages **(c,d)**.

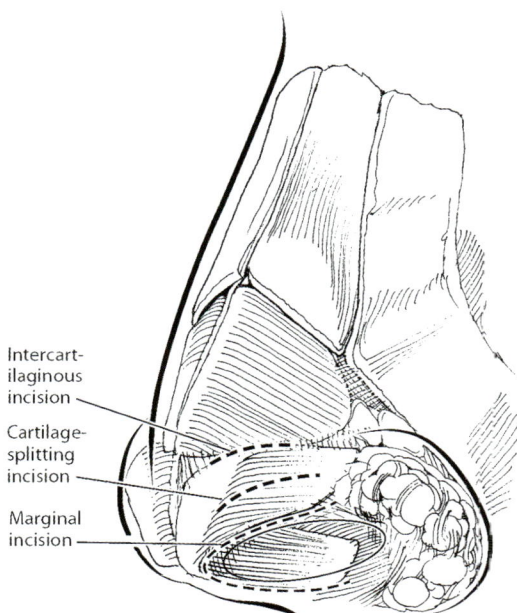

Intercart-
ilaginous
incision

Cartilage-
splitting
incision

Marginal
incision

Fig. 21.4 Drawing depicting relative positions of intercartilaginous, carti-lage-splitting, and marginal incisions.

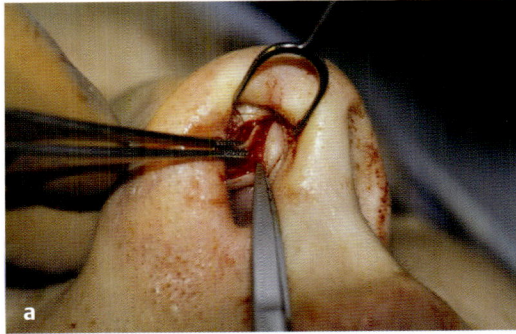

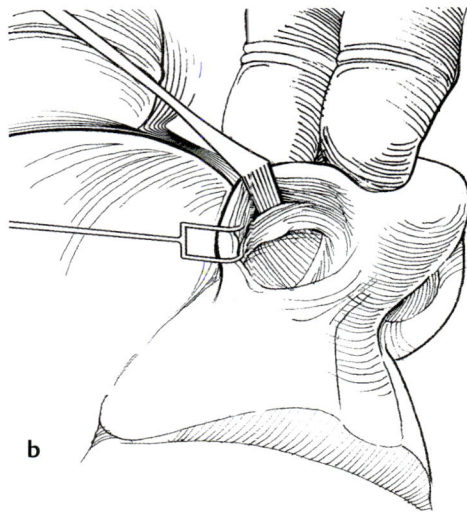

Fig. 21.5 Cartilage-splitting incision. (a) Intraoperative photograph showing technique for a cartilage-splitting incision. In the photo, the forceps is grasping the superior aspect of the lateral crus of the alar cartilage, which will be excised. (b) Drawing depicting cartilage-splitting incision.

The Retrograde Approach to the Tip

The retrograde approach will accomplish two things. It will allow access to the nasal dorsum over the upper lateral cartilages. It will also allow the completion or execution of a complete strip procedure with reduction of the superior aspect of the lateral crus of the lower lateral cartilage. Furthermore, with this approach, the soft tissue triangles of the nasal tip are not violated. The retrograde approach involves completing an IC incision and dissecting the vestibular lining retrograde over the underside of the lateral crus of the lower lateral cartilage. Then, under direct vision, a complete strip excision can be accomplished. Other surgical maneuvers can also be performed via this approach (e.g., various excisions and divisions) (**Fig. 21.6**).

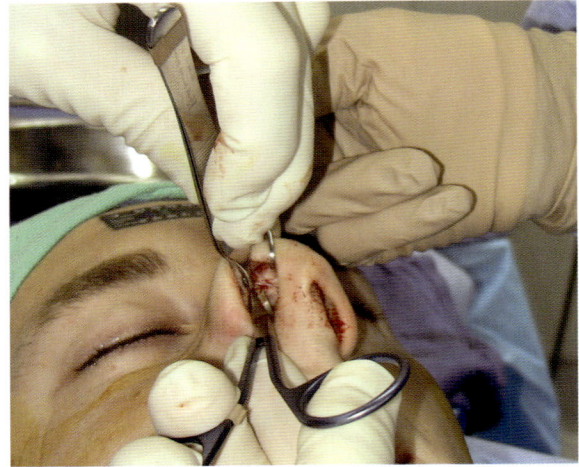

Fig. 21.6 Intraoperative photograph showing technique for a retrograde approach. When using a retrograde approach, it is important to preserve the vestibular lining and remove only a portion of the ala cartilage.

Alar Cartilage Delivery

Alar cartilage delivery spans the differences between an endonasal approach and an open approach to rhinoplasty and is the most common approach used for endonasal rhinoplasty. Through this technique, the surgeon is afforded complete visualization and access to the medial and lateral crura of the lower lateral cartilages. Therefore, multiple maneuvers can be performed on these cartilages to change the shape of the nose, and multiple types of grafts can also be placed.

To accomplish this technique, the surgeon completes an IC incision that is then brought down as a partial transfixion incision in front of the anterior superior septal angle. It can also be extended into a complete transfixion incision; it is important for this extension of the incision to be close to the caudal septal margin. A second incision is then made at the caudal margin of the lower lateral cartilages and not at the nostril margin. This incision is brought along the caudal edge of the lower lateral cartilage and under the soft triangle to a position at the caudal aspect of the medial crus of the lower lateral cartilage. Through blunt dissection, the cartilages are dissected away from the overlying skin. This creates a bipedicle flap of cartilage and underlying vestibular lining. Different surgeons have different preferences for the timing of the cartilage delivery. Some surgeons prefer to perform this prior to approaching the dorsum, whereas others perform this after approaching the dorsum. In patients who require dorsum reduction with planned use of significant cartilage struts or grafts in the nasal tip, it may be preferable to place these after the dorsum has been addressed (**Fig. 21.7a–d**). This is important because nasal dorsal maneuvers can dislodge tip grafts or struts.

The Approach to the Dorsum

The dorsum is typically approached through the IC incision by placing one's fingers on the external nasal skin to palpate throughout the dissection, or by placing traction against the overlying skin with a converse or similar retractor. The soft tissues can then be elevated off the middle vault of the nose using a no. 15 blade scalpel. Alternatively, this dissection can be performed using curved blunt-tip scissors, such as baby Metzenbaum or tenotomy type of scissors.

Soft tissues are elevated over the cartilaginous portions of the nasal dorsum above the plane of the perichondrium and below the periosteum, over the osseous portions. In thin-skinned noses, it is particularly important to elevate the periosteum prior to performing dorsum reduction. When performing this skin and soft tissue elevation, it is important to maintain attachment to the nasal bones laterally to minimize the risk of destabilizing the nasal bones when performing osteotomies (**Fig. 21.8a–c**).

Osteotomies

Osteotomies are easily employed during endonasal rhinoplasty. They can be performed to narrow the nose, straighten the nose, or reduce an open roof def-

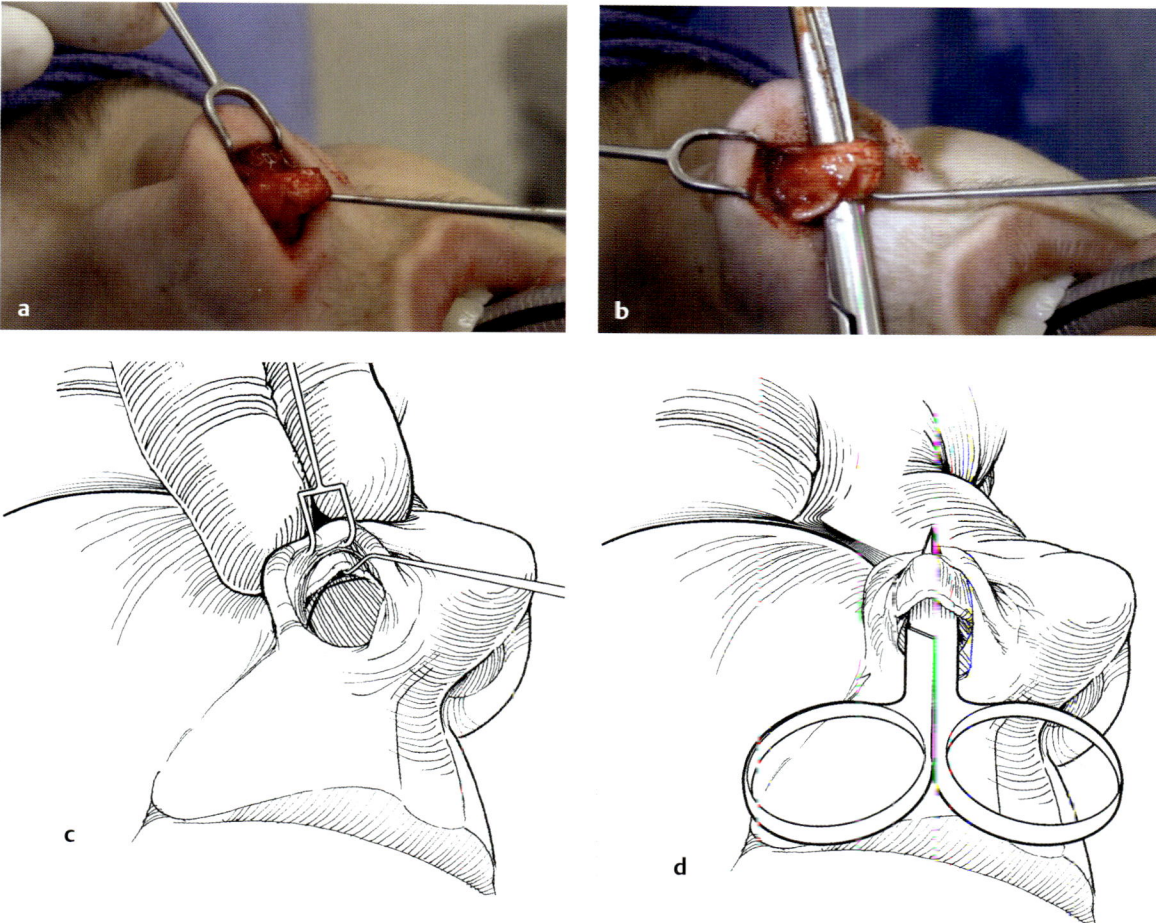

Fig. 21.7 Intraoperative photographs showing cartilage delivery technique **(a,b)**. Illustration shows the lower lateral cartilage being retracted with a single-pronged hook **(c)**. Further development of cartilage delivery with scissors being placed under the lower lateral cartilage **(d)**.

ter dorsal hump reduction. Osteotomies can be performed during endonasal rhinoplasty in a manner similar to that for the open approach. The osteotome is inserted low in the pyriform aperture, following the nasofacial groove. Depending on individual preference, this can be performed with 3 or 4 mm osteotomes or curved, guarded osteotomes. When performing osteotomies, it is important to be aware of the location of the tip of the osteotome at all times.

Reduction and Augmentation of the Nasal Dorsum

Reduction of the nasal dorsum can be performed using rasps or an osteotome. When using rasps, it is important to avoid separating the upper lateral cartilage from the nasal bones. For this reason, some surgeons prefer upbiting rasps to downbiting rasps; other surgeons prefer using graduated downbiting rasps.

The cartilaginous dorsum can be reduced with rasps designed for cartilage, a scalpel, or Fomon type scissors. It is important to perform adequate, but not excessive, reduction of the cartilaginous septum. This can be done under direct visualization or guided by external visualization.

Placement and Fixation of Grafts

Augmentation of the nasal dorsum begins with identification of the deficiency. A limited "pocket" is created over the area to be augmented, and a well-contoured autologous graft is placed in the precisely shaped area of exposure. Precise pockets typically require no suturing. However, if wide exposure has been created, the augmentation graft should be stabilized. Intranasal anchoring sutures can be placed.[4] Occasionally, sutures can be brought out through the skin to stabilize dorsal nasal grafts. If this is performed, the sutures must be loose and tied loosely over a soft bolster to avoid trauma to the skin and potential scarring. These tie-over sutures may be removed in 2 to 3 days. Nasal tip grafts can be stabilized by placement into pockets or intranasal suturing to other tip structures. Nasal struts are frequently held in place by adjacent structures after placement and do not require suturing.

The authors prefer autologous grafts. Septal cartilage is usually the first choice for grafts because it is the strongest and least pliable. Auricular cartilage has an elastic component, making it the second choice. When larger volumes of grafting material are necessary, costal cartilage can be used.

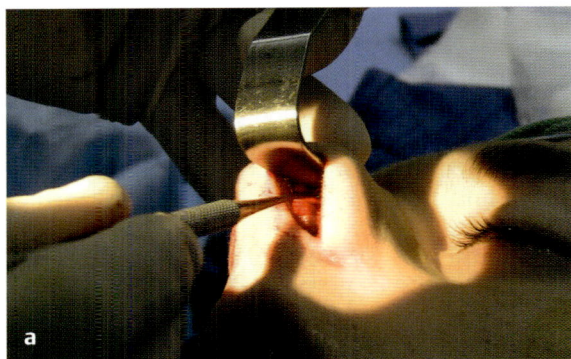

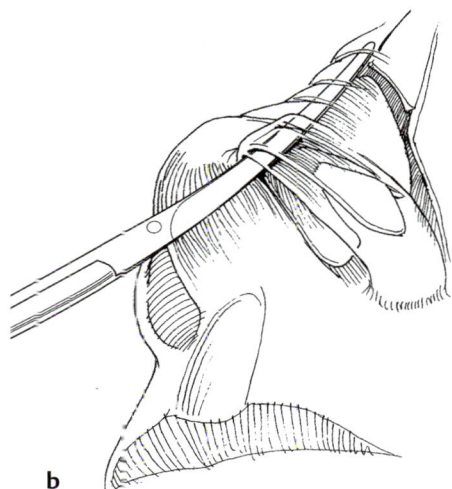

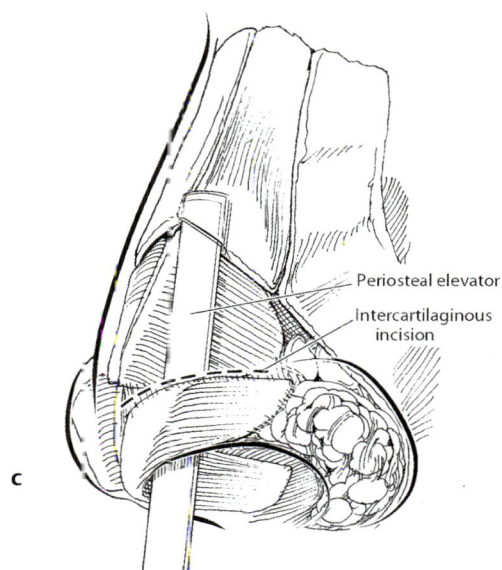

Fig. 21.8 **(a)** Intraoperative photograph showing the dorsal exposure possible through the intercartilaginous incision with the aid of an appropriate retractor. **(b,c)** Through the intercartilaginous incision the dorsum is approached and limited elevation of the dorsal skin and soft tissue is performed. Limited elevation of the dorsal skin and soft tissue is performed. Over the osseous nasal dorsum, periosteum of the nasal bones can be elevated with the skin and soft tissues.

At the end of the procedure, it is important to accurately close the intranasal incisions to avoid any tension, which can alter the appearance of the nose. Most of the intranasal wounds are closed with absorbable sutures.

Directed Techniques for the Office Setting

Resection of excess of the caudal septum can address alar–columellar disproportion. Alar rim or contour grafts, lateral crural strut grafts, and alar batten grafts to the lower lateral cartilages can also be placed under local anesthesia to correct various distortions of the nasal base and treat alar retraction.[4]

Dressings and Splints

The majority of patients will have minimal bleeding after this procedure and will not require intranasal packing. The use of internal splints and external dressings is dependent on both the procedure and the preference of the surgeon. Some surgeons place a small amount of oxidized regenerated cellulose over the incisions. There are several materials available for nasal splints. Those that involve heated splint material or plaster require attention to avoid burning the nasal skin because there may be increased sensitivity to thermal injury.

■ Postoperative Care

Patients are instructed not to perform any vigorous physical activity for several weeks and to avoid any activity that could cause nasal trauma for several months. They are asked to avoid any antiplatelet medications. Patients are advised to sleep on two to three pillows, sneeze with their mouth open, and avoid blowing their nose. The use of intranasal sprays and ointments varies depending on surgeon preference.

■ Expected Results

The usual results are improvements of the aesthetics and function of the nose. Realistic expectations should be established during the preoperative period via discussions between the patient and the surgeon. There may be swelling that resolves over a greater length of time than the patient initially anticipates. Ideally, the patient has been educated that the final result will not be realized until the first year has passed postprocedure. Meanwhile, there should be an absence of infection. Discomfort usually resolves over the first few days after the procedure. Examples of the varied challenges that can be managed endonasally are shown (**Fig. 21.9a–f**; **Fig. 21.10a–f**).

■ Complications and Their Management

Although uncommon, complications can occur in endonasal rhinoplasty. These include healing problems, bleeding, infection, septal perforations, nasal airway narrowing, inadequate preoperative evaluation, undesired results, and, rarely, cerebrospinal fluid leaks. If alloplastic implants are used, there are the additional risks of extrusion and fragmentation.

To reduce the risk of bleeding, it is important to review the patient's coagulation history and address any concerns. Preoperative instructions should include the avoidance of any preoperative medications or supplements that can decrease platelet adhesiveness.

Infection after rhinoplasty is uncommon, and there is some controversy about whether prophylactic antibiotics reduce the incidence of infection after rhinoplasty. However, many surgeons use prophylactic antibiotics due to concerns about the potential deleterious effects that infection can have on the aesthetic outcome.

With all rhinoplasty procedures, there is the potential for multiple types of undesired results. These include, but are not limited to, tip asymmetry, inadequate tip projection, nasal bossae, overly voluminous or deficient tips, inadequate or excessive tip rotation, dorsal asymmetry, open roof, asymmetrically depressed nasal bones, polly beak, and alar–columellar mismatches. Among the most common issues are small dorsal irregularities. Many revisions can be performed with an endonasal approach. The revision technique will vary depending on the issue that is being revised.

■ Conclusion

The endonasal approach to rhinoplasty should be part of each surgeon's available techniques for rhinoplasty. Many of the standard rhinoplasty maneuvers can be performed through this approach. Additionally, recovery may be more rapid with this approach than with external rhinoplasty.

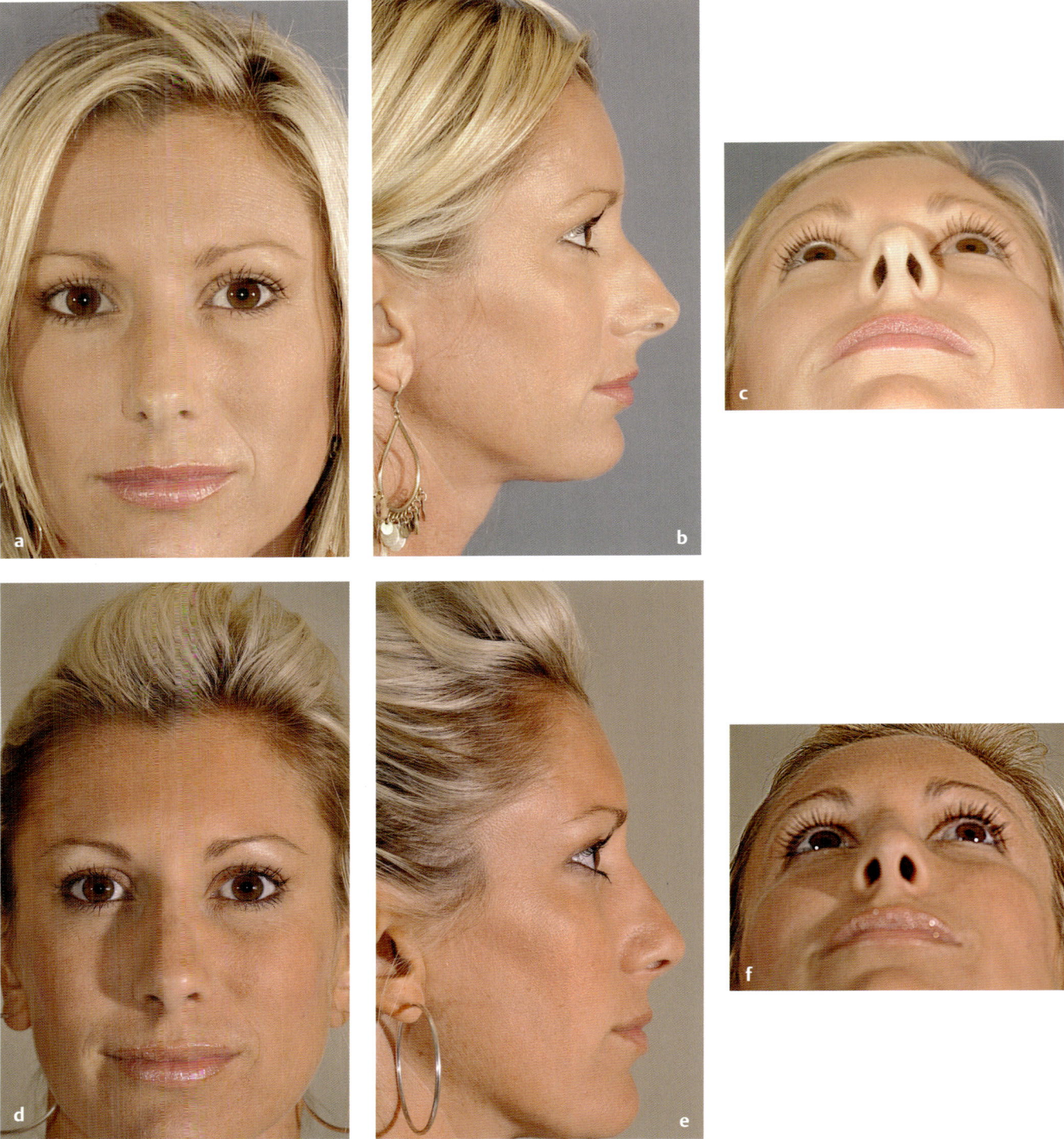

Fig. 21.9 Endonasal rhinoplasty preoperative photographs **(a–c)**; postoperative photographs **(d–f)**.

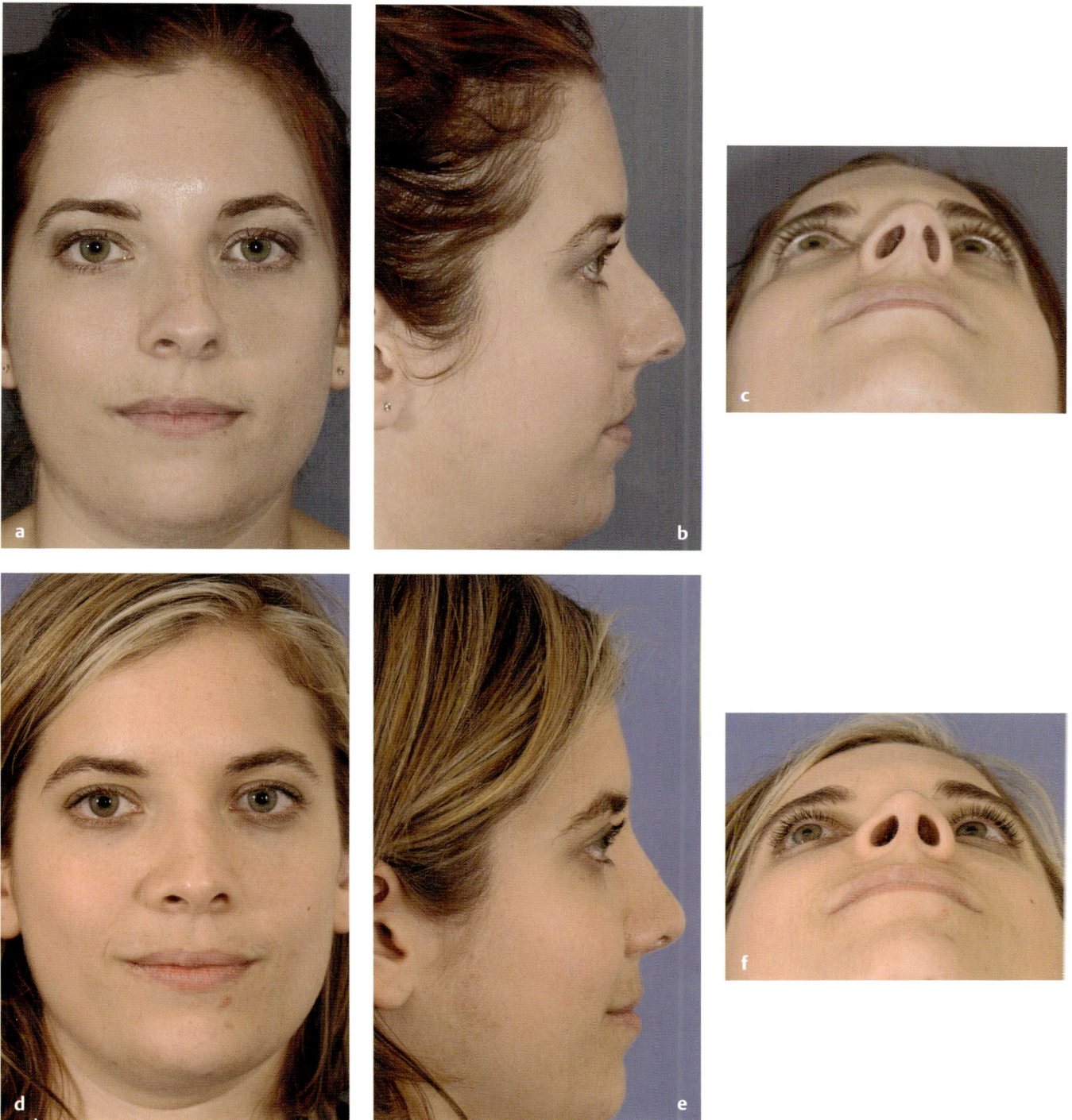

Fig. 21.10   Endonasal rhinoplasty preoperative photographs **(a–c)**; postoperative photographs **(d–f)**.

References

1. The deformity termed "pug nose" and its correction, by a simple operation: John O. Roe, M.D., Rochester, N.Y. (Reprinted from The Medical Record, June 4, 1887). Plast Reconstr Surg 1970;45(1):78–83

2. Kamer FM, Pieper PG. Nasal tip surgery: a 30-year experience. Facial Plast Surg Clin North Am 2004;12(1):81–92

3. Fomon S, Goldman IB, Neivert H, Schattner A. Management of deformities of the lower cartilaginous vault. AMA Arch Otolaryngol 1951;54(5):467–472

4. Fedok FG. Revision rhinoplasty using the endonasal approach. Facial Plast Surg 2008;24(3):293–309

5. Larrabee WF, Cupp C. Advanced nasal anatomy. Facial Plast Surg Clin North Am 1994;2:393–416

6. Westreich RW, Lawson W. The tripod theory of nasal tip support revisited: the cantilevered spring model. Arch Facial Plast Surg 2008;10(3):170–179

7. Larrabee WF Jr, Makielski KH. Surgical Anatomy of the Face. New York, NY: Raven; 1993:154–155

8. Anderson JR. A reasoned approach to nasal base surgery. Arch Otolaryngol 1984;110(6):349–358

9. Adamson PA, Galli SK. Rhinoplasty approaches: current state of the art. Arch Facial Plast Surg 2005;7(1):32–37

10. Tasman AJ, Palma P. The infracartilaginous approach revisited. Arch Facial Plast Surg 2008;10(6):370–375

11. McCollough EG, Mangat D. Systematic approach to correction of the nasal tip in rhinoplasty. Arch Otolaryngol 1981;107(1):12–16

22 Office Rhinoplasty Techniques

Ira D. Papel and Theda C. Kontis

Key Concepts

- Office-based rhinoplasty techniques can be used to address postoperative minor rhinoplasty revision issues.

- There are many less extensive nasal procedures that can be performed with simple local anesthesia in an office setting.

- Soft tissue fillers have provided another means for correcting subtle contour irregularities.

■ Introduction

The majority of rhinoplasty procedures will continue to be done in operating rooms, utilizing either general or monitored anesthesia techniques. Patients demand this for comfort and reduction of anxiety. Surgeons prefer anesthesia for rhinoplasty because it often creates a more comfortable surgical environment. Patient safety with airway safeguards is also emphasized in accredited surgical centers. This description applies to most primary and many revision rhinoplasty operations. On the other hand, there are many less extensive nasal procedures that can be performed with simple local anesthesia in an office setting. These techniques typically address postoperative rhinoplasty patients who need a minor revision or management of common postrhinoplasty healing patterns. If it can be done with local anesthesia in an office or exam room environment, it fits the scope of this chapter. All procedures described in this chapter are designed so that the patient can be discharged immediately to home, without complex postoperative care.

■ Technical Aspects of Procedures

Early Postoperative Procedures

The healing process in rhinoplasty is slow and frequently tests the patience of both surgeon and patient. Soft tissue edema, in addition to gradual scar contraction around the skeletal framework, may take years to finalize. Certain postoperative therapies and maneuvers can impact healing as this process unfolds.

One area that is frequently a problem is the supratip. In patients with marginal tip projection and thicker skin, this may show up early in the postoperative period. The mainstay of early treatment for this problem is prolonged taping and subcutaneous steroid injection. In our practice, it is not unusual to initiate steroid injections 1 week after surgery if the surgeon feels that it will help reduce supratip edema and prevent a deformity down the road. The initial treatment involves injection of 0.1 mL triamcinolone 10 mg/mL into the subcutaneous space just above the tip. It is important to avoid an intradermal injection because this may cause dermal atrophy and a significant contour defect. Over time, these defects may improve, but prevention is the best policy (**Fig. 22.1**).[1]

Taping of the nose after surgery is one of the mainstays of postoperative treatment. The purposes of taping are generally acknowledged to be stabilization, elimination of a potential space, and containment of edema in key areas. The supratip is probably the area where taping is most effective. After the initial dressing is removed at 1 week after surgery, retaping the nose is an option. Combined with steroid injection, taping for an additional 1 to 2 weeks can be quite effective in the treatment of early supratip edema.

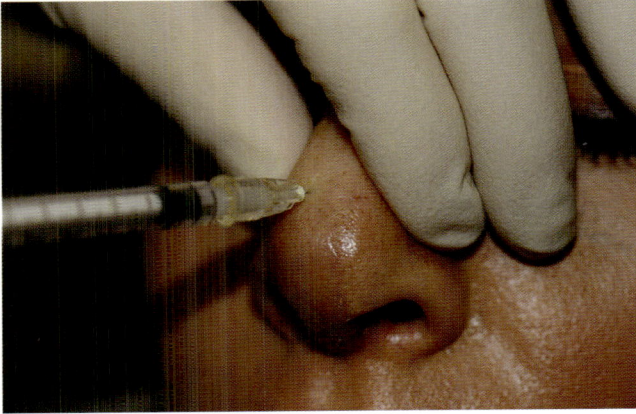

Fig. 22.1   Injection of triamcinolone 10 mg/mL into supratip subcutaneous space.

When rhinoplasty surgery involves osteotomies, malposition may occur early in the postoperative period. At the first visit after surgery, the surgeon can use digital pressure to realign the bones, usually after topical and regional local anesthetic is employed. Even with the local anesthetic, this can be uncomfortable for the patient. If the bones are too medial in position, intranasal pressure with a blunt instrument can be utilized to lateralize the bones, with reapplication of tape and splint for 1 more week.

Having the patient apply digital pressure on a regular basis can also treat subtle deviations of the bony structures. We routinely ask all rhinoplasty patients to apply bilateral pressure every 2 hours during the day for a period of 4 weeks. This must be demonstrated at the first postoperative visit to ensure the pressure is applied correctly (**Fig. 22.2a,b**).

Late Postoperative Procedures (> 6 Months)

Telangiectasias

Increased vascularization of the nasal dorsum soft tissue can occur after rhinoplasty, regardless of the surgical approach used (**Fig. 22.3**). This redness can be exacerbated by certain skin care products, sun exposure, hot flashes, and hot beverages or alcohol. Patients who find these telangiectasias troublesome often use cosmetics to camouflage the redness. If isolated telangiectasias occur, simple cauterization of the vessel(s) can be performed. The Hyfrecator unipolar cautery can be fitted with a 30-gauge metal hub needle by adding a small adapter to the handpiece. This allows direct cauterization of the targeted vessels without the need for topical or local anesthesia and does not injure the surrounding tissue.

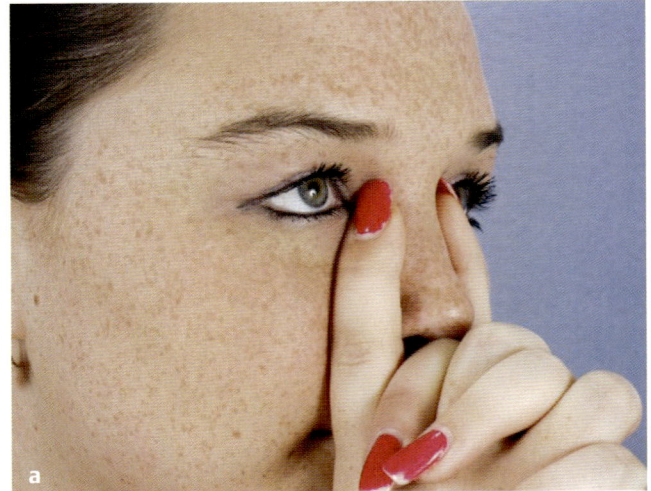

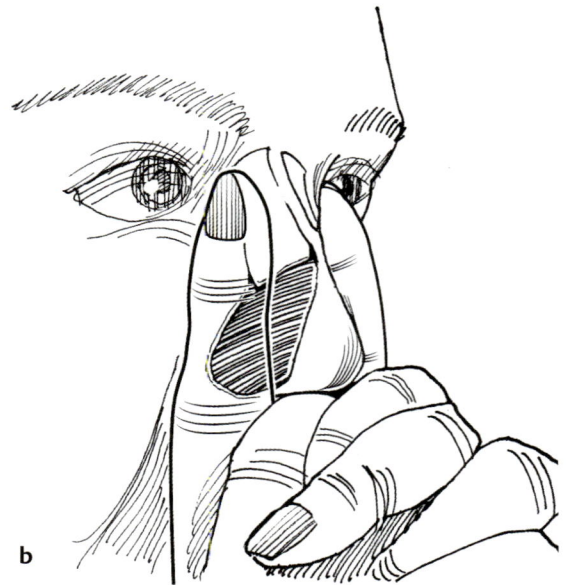

Fig. 22.2   **(a)** Digital pressure and finger alignment to help align nasal bones. **(b)** Finger placement in relation to underlying nasal bones.

Laser treatment is required when the telangiectasias are more diffuse. The flashlamp pulsed dye laser and the V Beam lasers (Syneron, Inc., Irvine, CA) are ideal for this situation. In addition, an yttrium-aluminum-garnet (YAG) laser can be used to treat this condition with excellent results, although more than one treatment may be necessary.

Cartilage Irregularities

As the soft tissue envelope thins over time, cartilage irregularities can become evident, especially in thin-skinned individuals. Both the dorsum and the nasal

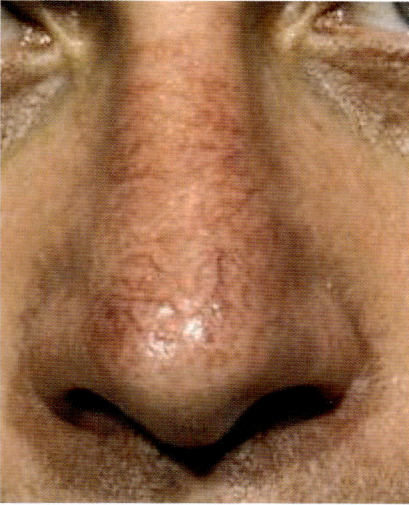

Fig. 22.3 Telangiectasia of nasal dorsum.

tip can have cartilaginous abnormalities that become noticeable in the late postoperative period. Most cartilaginous irregularities can be treated in the office in the minor procedure room under local anesthesia. Very small nodular irregularities can be treated using the needle shaving technique ▶Video 22.1. The cartilaginous lump is marked with a surgical marker, and local anesthesia is infiltrated. A 20-gauge needle is inserted into the skin, and the bevel of the needle is used to shave off the prominent cartilage (**Fig. 22.4a,b**).

Larger cartilaginous irregularities require an open procedure, usually performed in the minor procedure room. The irregularity is marked prior to injection. After local anesthesia is infiltrated, an intercartilagenous incision is performed, unilateral or bilateral, depending on the exposure needed. The nasal dorsum tissue is undermined, and the cartilaginous irregularity is excised and the fragment removed. The incisions are closed with 4–0 chromic suture. This procedure is tolerated well with either local anesthesia or with the addition of oral lorazepam preoperatively.

The nasal tip skin is the last area of the nose to regain its definition as the edema subsides. Occasionally, tip irregularities can become manifest late in the healing process. A nasal tip revision can also be performed in the local room with or without preoperative premedication with lorazepam. Surgical access can range from reopening the nose through the transcolumellar incision to delivering the tip for better visualization.

Camouflage of cartilaginous irregularities of the nasal tip can be achieved with the use of fascia or allograft. Fascia can be harvested from the temporalis muscle or from conchal perichondrium. Several types of allograft are also available for use. The fas-

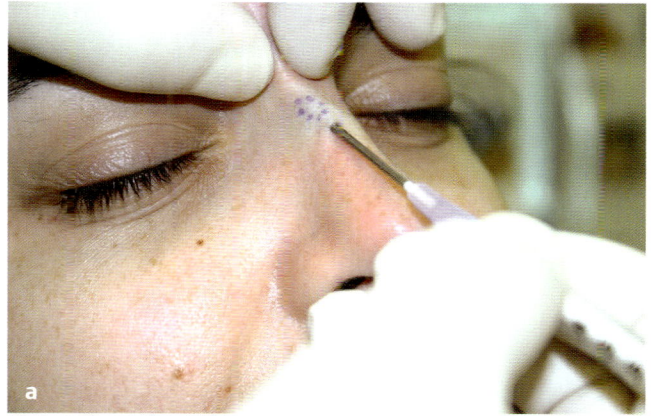

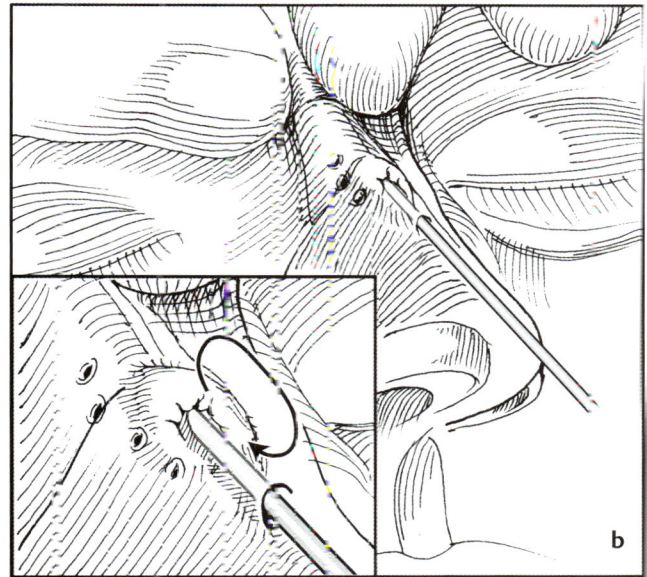

Fig. 22.4 (a) Demonstration of needle shave technique. **(b)** Shaving of dorsal irregularity using needle.

cia or allograft can be placed into a pocket dissected over the nasal tip cartilage, but care must be taken to ensure smooth, unfolded placement. More accurate placement can be achieved if the cartilages are better exposed by the open or delivery techniques, whereby the graft can be sewn into place over the nasal tip cartilages (**Fig. 22.5a–d**).[2]

Septal Shortening for Columellar Show

Increased columellar show can be an early or late complication of rhinoplasty. This can be treated under local anesthesia as a minor procedure. A hemitransfixion incision is made after infiltration of local anesthesia. The caudal aspect of the septum is isolated and trimmed conservatively. If necessary, a full transfixion

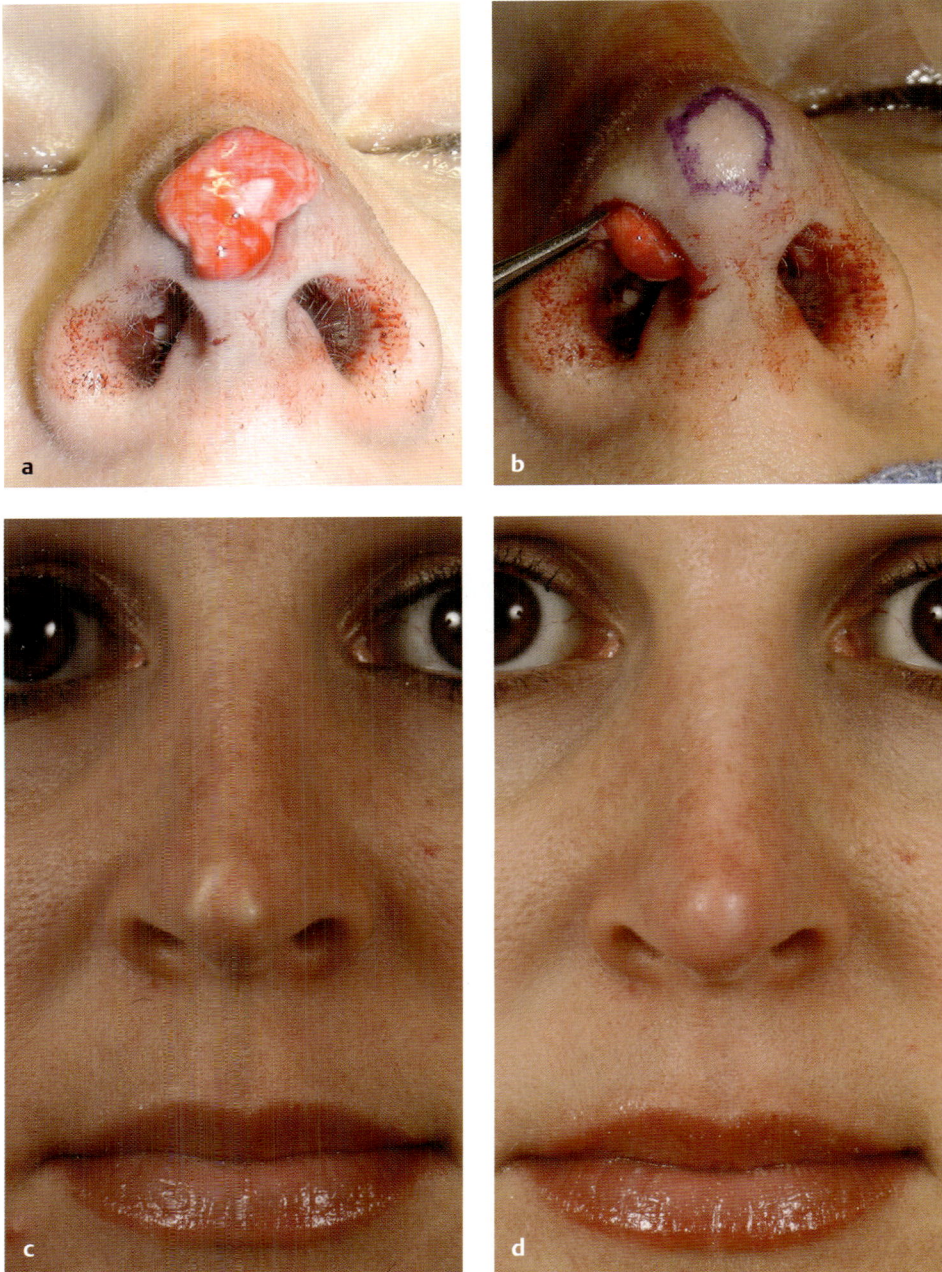

Fig. 22.5   Use of fascia to camouflage cartilage under thin skin. **(a)** Fascia in planned location. **(b)** Placement via marginal incision. **(c)** Preoperative view. **(d)** One year postoperative.

incision can be made and a small strip of vestibular mucosa excised. Care must be taken to avoid excision of excess nasal skin of the vestibule, which can result in chronic rhinorrhea or a "wet nose." The incisions are closed with 4–0 chromic sutures (**Fig. 22.6a,b**).

Scar Management: Dermabrasion

If not reapproximated exactly, the columellar incision used for the open rhinoplasty technique can result in an unacceptable scar. An inverted v or stair-step incision is usually made, and over time, the incision is usually barely visible. On occasion, the skin edges are not perfectly approximated, and an unacceptable transcolumellar scar can occur. In these cases, dermabrasion can be used to improve the minor scarring. Dermabrasion is performed in the minor procedure room under local anesthesia. This procedure will serve to improve uneven tissue edges.

Fillers in Rhinoplasty

The recent boom in noninvasive techniques has provided more tools for the cosmetic surgeon. Al-

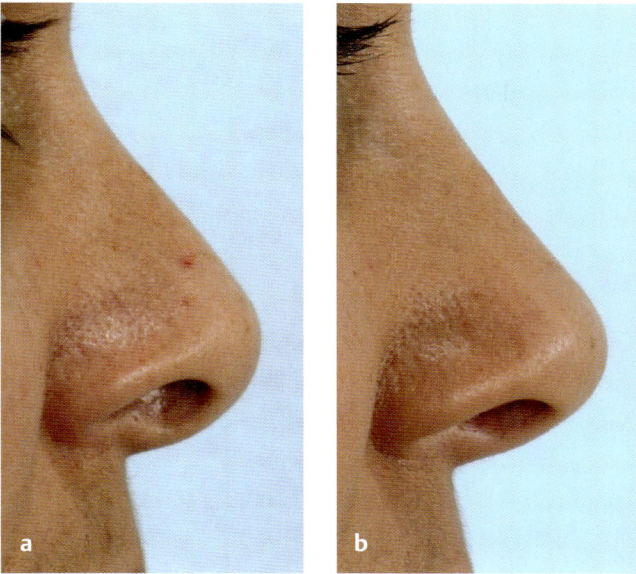

Fig. 22.6 Shortening the caudal septum can correct excessive columellar show. **(a)** Preoperative. **(b)** One year postoperative.

though off-label, some injectors are using fillers to improve nasal appearance, either as a primary treatment or postoperatively to correct contour irregularities.

The fillers most commonly used for nasal augmentation are the hyaluronic acids and calcium hydrox-

ylapatite. These fillers can be used cosmetically to augment the dorsum,[3] fill in dorsal depressions, and increase tip projection (nonsurgical rhinoplasty). They can also be used to straighten a crooked nose by filling in the depressed side. In addition, functional improvements can be made by using the filler to stiffen a weak ala to improve external valve collapse, or intranasally to improve a narrow internal nasal valve.

Injection for dorsal irregularities is performed in the office under topical anesthesia, if necessary. The injection is placed conservatively in the subcutaneous plane, and after a small injection, the product is molded into place. Small amounts of filler are sequentially placed until the desired improvement is realized. Patients are usually pleased to see their nasal deformity disappear in a few seconds (**Fig. 22.7a,b**). Similarly, injections can be placed in the dorsum to give the appearance of a straighter nose by filling in the concave side.

We prefer to use calcium hydroxylapatite when nasal valve issues are treated. For the patient with collapse of the external valve with deep inspiration, using filler to stiffen the ala will immediately improve external valve collapse by strengthening the ala. Internal valve collapse can also be corrected by injecting filler on the lateral aspect of the internal valve, through an intranasal injection (**Fig. 22.8a,b**). In one visit, small amounts of product are injected until the patient notes significant improvement in nasal airflow.

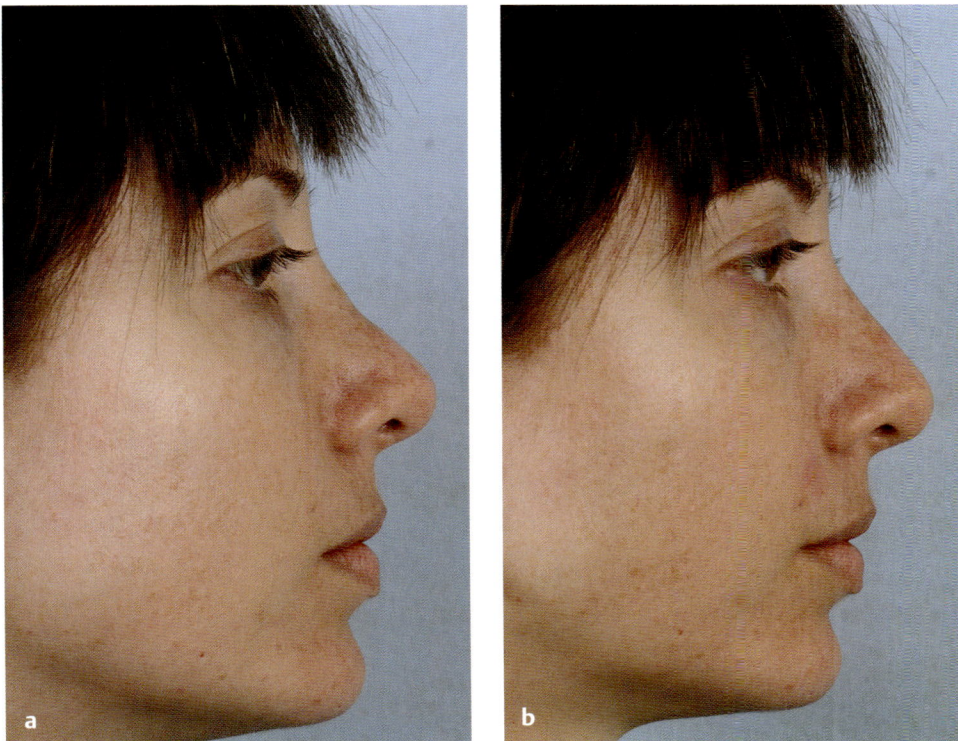

Fig. 22.7 Pre- **(a)** and postfiller **(b)** for dorsal correction.

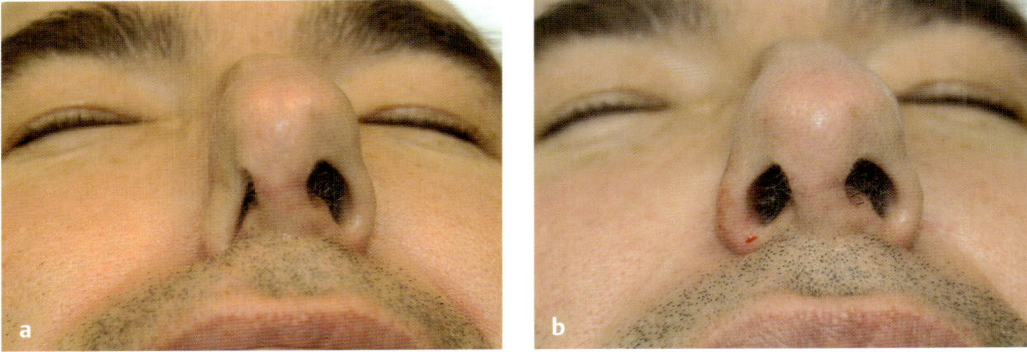

Fig. 22.8 **(a)** Collapse of external nasal valve with deep inspiration. **(b)** Lateral ala stiffened with Radiesse (Merz Aesthetics, San Mateo, CA). No collapse seen with deep inspiration.

In our practice, we prefer to begin injections of the nose with hyaluronic acids because the results can be reversed with hyaluronidase if necessary. Reflux of the syringe is required in this area to prevent vascular occlusion by the filler material. It is also advisable to have nitropaste on hand on the chance that vascular occlusion occurs (**Fig. 22.9**).

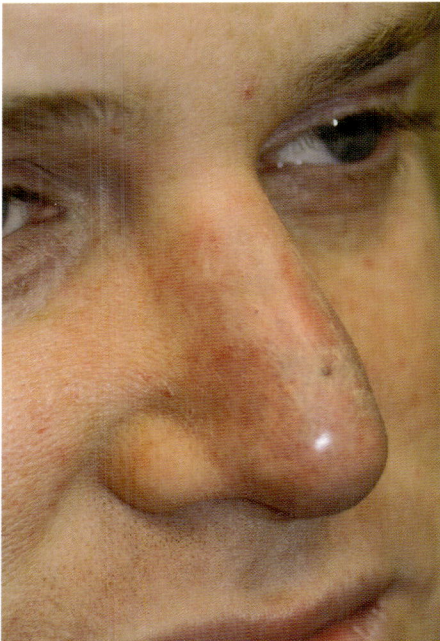

Fig. 22.9 Nasal vascular compromise after injection of Radiesse (Merz Aesthetics) for dorsal augmentation. It completely resolved with no sequelae.

■ Complications and Their Management

The Skin

Rhinoplasty surgery can affect the condition of nasal and facial skin. The application of substances like benzoin or Mastisol (Ferndale Laboratories, Ferndale, MI), in addition to occlusive tape, is irritating and can cause blockage of pores with inflammation or even infection. When the tape is removed, it is common to see pustules in the lower third of the nose. In most cases, this clears quickly with cleansing and removal of the adhesive. When inflammation persists, oral and/or topical antibiotics may be necessary. Topical retinoids are also helpful in refractory cases.

On rare occasions, a patient may incur a severe allergic reaction to the adhesive or tape (**Fig. 22.10**). This may become an emergency situation, leading to severe skin damage and potential scarring. Excessive itching and purulence oozing from the edges of the bandage are clues to the problem. Quick removal of the splints, tape, and adhesive is mandatory. Aggressive treatment with oral and topical steroids, antibiotics, and careful debridement will usually lead to a good outcome.[4]

Scarring

Any skin incision can create a problematic scar, and the nose is no exception. The most common areas used for rhinoplasty cutaneous incisions are the columella (**Fig. 22.11**), lateral alar creases, and percutaneous osteotomies. Patients with thick sebaceous

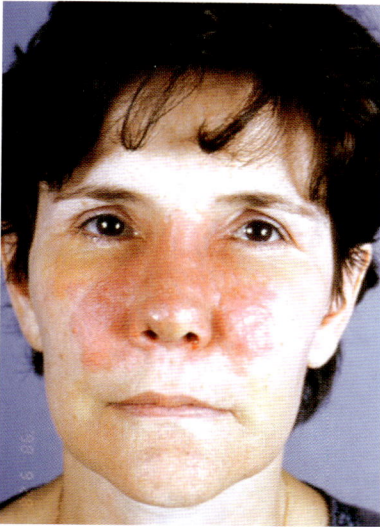

Fig. 22.10 Severe allergic reaction to Mastisol skin adhesive 1 week postoperative.

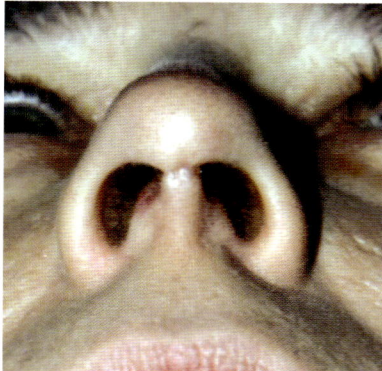

Fig. 22.11 Unacceptable columellar scar.

skin will typically display slower resolution of scars and more permanent deformities. The key to prevention of noticeable scars is proper placement and execution and meticulous closure with minimal tension. When incisions are not healing well, scar management techniques may be utilized.

Surgical scar revisions are rarely indicated after rhinoplasty. Hypertrophic and keloid scars are rare on the nose. Early intervention with either or both topical silicone ointment and sheeting may be helpful and can be prescribed for several months. Frequent massage with moisturizers or other scar management preparations can be helpful over time. In some patients with lighter skin pigmentation dermabrasion can be helpful. Dermabrasion can be accomplished with topical or local regional anesthetic injection. The proper time for dermabrasion is usually between 6 and 12 weeks in the early postoperative period, or any time after 1 year, if indicated.

■ Conclusion

Rhinoplasty is challenging surgery, even for experienced nasal surgeons. As the nose heals, telangiectasias, cartilaginous irregularities, and scars can become manifest. Although some post rhinoplasty complications require a return to the operating room, we have found that many small irregularities can be addressed under local anesthesia. Soft tissue fillers have also provided the means for correcting subtle contour irregularities, either on a postoperative nose or as a primary nonsurgical rhinoplasty procedure.

References

1. Hanasono MM, Kridel RW, Pastorek NJ, Glasgold MJ, Koch RJ. Correction of the soft tissue pollybeak using triamcinolone injection. Arch Facial Plast Surg 2002;4(1):26–30, discussion 31

2. Baker TM, Courtiss EH. Temporalis fascia grafts in open secondary rhinoplasty. Plast Reconstr Surg 1994;93(4): 802–810

3. Redaelli A. Medical rhinoplasty with hyaluronic acid and botulinum toxin A: a very simple and quite effective technique. J Cosmet Dermato 2008;7(3):210–220

4. Cohen DE, Kaufmann JM. Hypersensitivity reactions to products and devices in plastic surgery. Facial Plast Surg Clin North Am 2003;11(2):253–265

23 Brow Rejuvenation

Donn R. Chatham

Key Concepts

- The goal is a stable, natural, and, ideally, long-lasting improvement and/or elevation when necessary.

- Strict adherence to a single procedure, especially if arbitrary, cannot best serve all patients.

- Before selecting a brow-improvement procedure, the correct diagnosis should be made.

- Most patients requiring brow elevation nevertheless still require upper eyelid blepharoplasty.

- All brow lifts fall over time.

- In females, one goal is to raise the lateral brow above the orbit but allow the medial brow to remain at or slightly below the orbital rim (i.e., where it began).

- According to a quote by Val Lambros: "[. . .] brow lifts by whatever ilk have proved to be maddeningly inflexible, imprecise, and uncontrollable in the very patients who need the most care in the degree and location of elevation . . . good outcomes are usually from good preoperative configurations"

- Most of the literature has historically focused on lifting the brows. Contemporary procedures will focus equally on issues like positioning, shaping, brow and infrabrow fullness, and tissue integrity.

■ Introduction

The brow–lid complex is the key component in aesthetic facial appearance, and facial improvement must begin with this area in mind. As part of the periorbital region, the brows define the superior boundaries of the upper eyelid (the two function as a unit),[1] touch both the temple and the glabella, and serve as part of the "frame" that defines the eye. Let us explore the (sometimes misunderstood) region of the brow and how, as surgeons, we can help our patients in its analysis and rejuvenation. We focus on the brow and periorbit but not on upper or lower eyelid issues, which are covered in the next three chapters.

■ Background: Basic Science of Procedure

Lying in the inferior forehead, forming the superior-most frame of the eye, brows are the central focus for facial expression. Even a minor change in brow position alters the expression and perceived emotions of a person's face. Forehead height is typically one third of the face: longer foreheads connote aging and shorter ones connote youth.

Ideally, the periorbit resembles an oval with an open lateral end and a closed nasal line medially blending into a smooth and full glabella. The brow must either be above, at, or below the orbital rim, and in fact may do all three at once. An attractive and youthful brow–lid junction ("infrabrow") is convex, full, and smooth (**Fig. 23.1**).

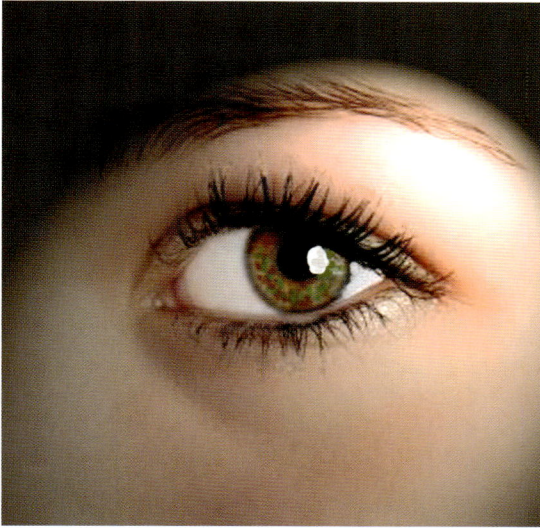

Fig. 23.1 Attractive and youthful brow lid junction (infrabrow).

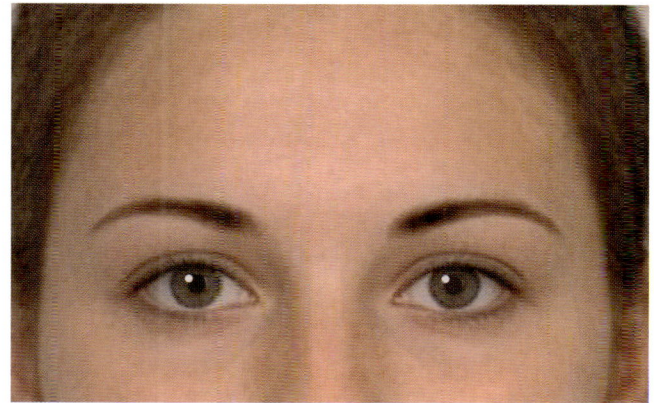

Fig. 23.2 Female brows.

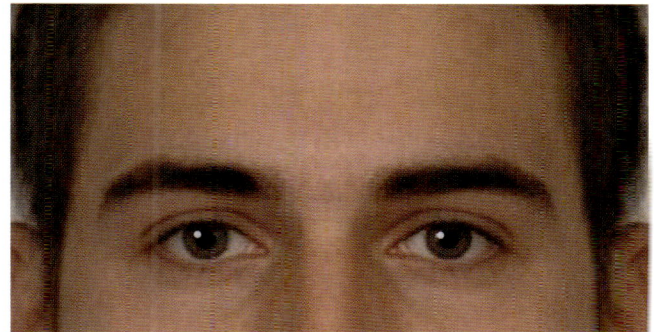

Fig. 23.3 Male brows.

Eyebrow shape is generally, but not always, considered more attractive if it takes a gentle arc, compared with a straight line. The shape of the brow is more important than the actual position of the brow and in part depends on the adjacent anatomy (balance) to look good. Additionally, brows that seem attractive on one face may not look good on another. Thus there is no one "perfect brow."

■ Pertinent Anatomy

What Is the Standard of Attractiveness?

One study asked participants to position brows where they liked them best. The preferred female brow began medially below the orbital rim and gently arched as it became lateral and above the orbital rim to a peak of 13 mm. For men, the preferred position was a lower, flatter brow just above or at the rim, with less of a tail. Both sexes peak the brow at the lateral canthus (**Figs. 23.2** and **23.3**).[2] Other studies support similar findings.[3]

In women, the peak of the ideal brow should be 0.5 to 1 cm above the supraorbital rim.[4] Westmore described the ideal brow: (1) the medial brow begins at the plane of the lateral ala/inner canthus, (2) the lateral brow ends from the oblique ala to the lateral canthus, (3) the medial and lateral brows lie at about the same plane, and (4) the apex lies on the vertical at the lateral limbus (**Fig. 23.4**).[5]

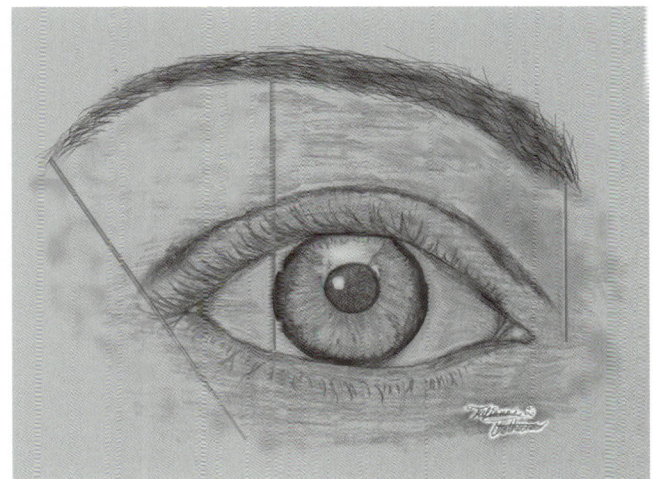

Fig. 23.4 Ideal vertical relationships between brow and eye: medial brow begins at medial canthus, brow peaks at lateral limbus, lateral brow ends at nasal ala-lateral lid oblique line.

However, mathematical and linear measurements should serve as a guide and not as an absolute goal. Each patient's anatomy is unique. Proper proportion and balance are more important. The "Golden Proportion," for example, is considered both mathematically and aesthetically vital based on the ratio of 1:1.6 comparing the brow height to the eyelid aperture of females and males, respectively (**Fig. 23.5**). In males, brows positioned above the rim give a feminizing appearance. Heavy, bushy brows are generally not considered a feminine attribute.

Culture, ethnic background, gender, and age, as well as current fashion trends, influence what is considered most attractive. African Americans, in general, have higher brows than Caucasians, according to one study.[6] Note that the shape of the brows of fashion models is often more dramatic than what is seen in typical society.[6]

Why Are Some Brows Unattractive?

Although the diversity of facial features makes humans more interesting, certain characteristics are generally considered unattractive. Brows might just represent the ultimate in "body language." Disharmony of the brows may convey an appearance or emotion discordant with how that person really feels ("I am told I look angry but I am not").[7]

By shape and position, the brow can indicate a range of emotions. For example, if brows are angled with the medial portion lowered in a scowl (overactive corruga-tor combined with procerus activity), this can convey an angry or hostile demeanor. Brows that encroach upon the upper lid convey a tired appearance, whereas brows that are excessively low laterally with an elevated medial position signify a sad look or fatigue.

Higher brows convey more alertness to a degree, but if taken even higher, then a surprised or goosed or unintelligent appearance results. Asymmetries in elevated position create an inquisitive look. An elevated brow in the deep-set eye patient may unmask the orbit, creating an emaciated look. Ideally, brow aesthetic surgery creates a more youthful, peaceful, relaxed face. But it can inadvertently create a surprised or bizarre look, too. Thus brow position can either positively or negatively affect how others perceive us and react to us (**Fig. 23.6a–d**).

Aging

How do brows age (**Fig. 23.7**)? Often the lateral brows descend, and with soft tissue thinning, this produces a more angular superior brow edge. Forehead creases develop, and with medial brow movement, the thicker brow skin moves the thinner glabellar skin, shifting it more medially and producing a crease, which over time changes from a dynamic crease to a passive crease. Upper lid ptosis, independent of eyelid and brow changes, can also occur.

Why do brows descend? (1) Tissue lateral to the temporal fusion line has no frontalis muscle to pull superiorly, (2) active orbicularis oculi and corrugator

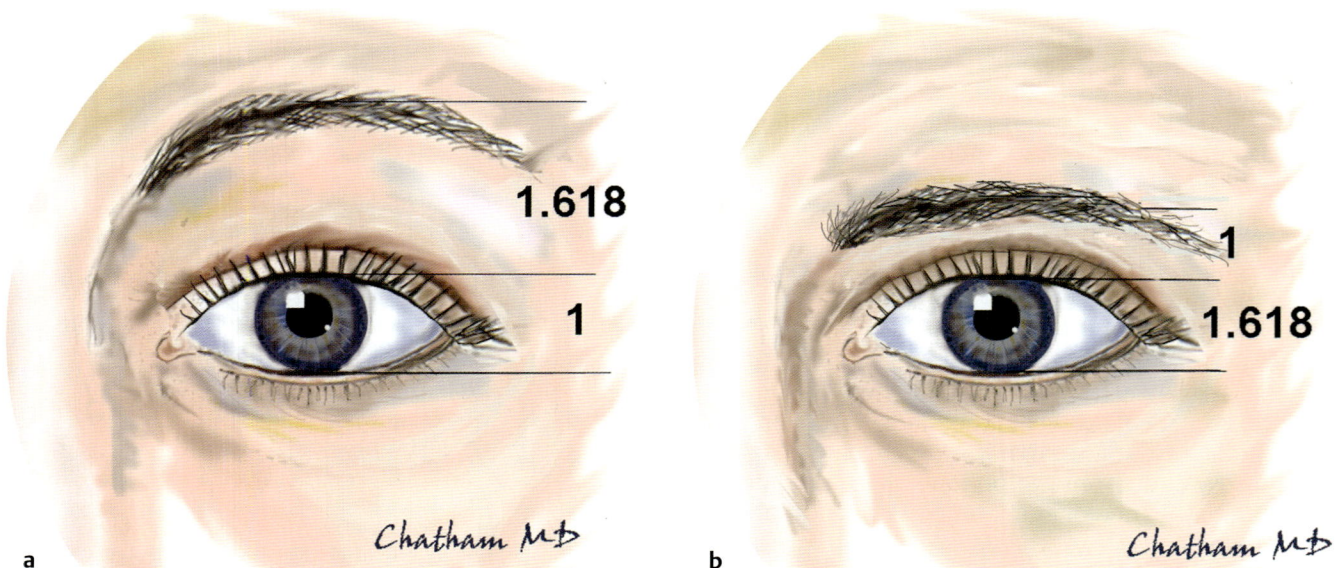

Fig. 23.5 (a) Ideal height of female brow: golden ratio. (b) Typical height of male brow: golden ratio reverse of female brow.

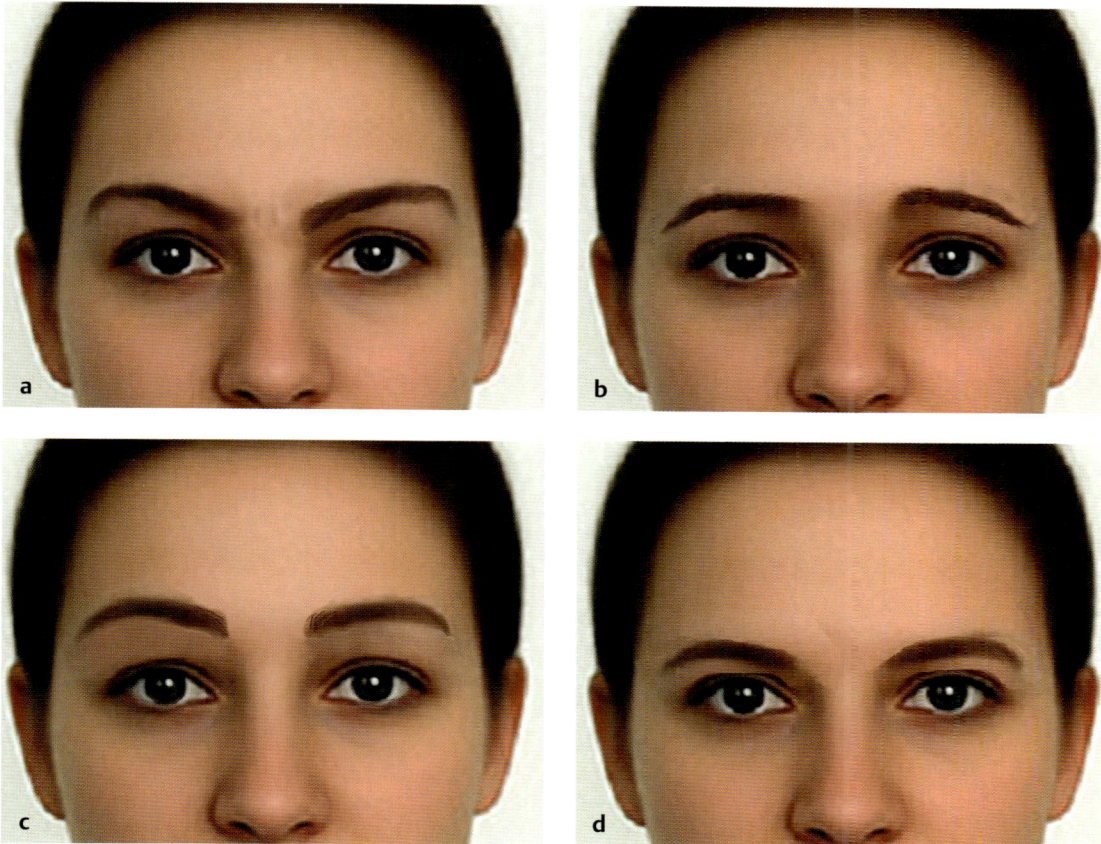

Fig. 23.6 Perceived emotions through brow positioning. **(a)** Angry. **(b)** Sad. **(c)** Surprised. **(d)** Tired.

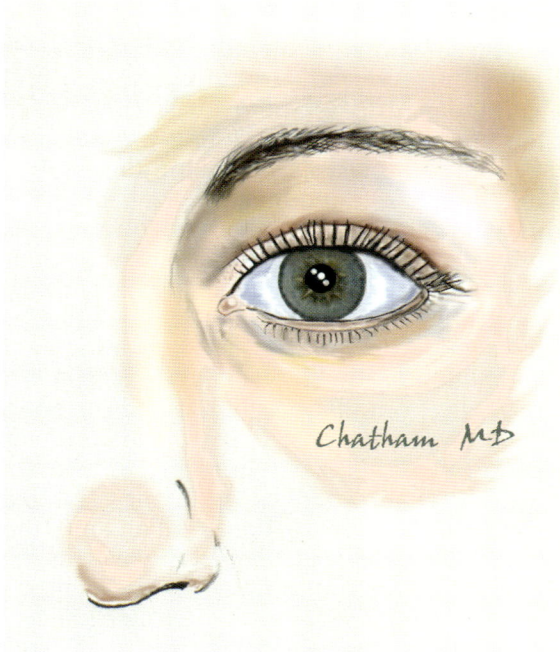

Fig. 23.7 Youthful brow with ideal attractive brow height, arch, and length.

supercilii muscles pull inferiorly, (3) the lateral orbital ligament inserts from the periosteum to the superficial temporal fascia but does not connect to the dermis, and (4) gravity (**Fig. 23.8**). But movement is not always in the inferior position. Van den Bosch et al noted that the midbrow elevates with advancing age in large numbers of women and in some men (**Fig. 23.9**).[8] Lambros studied a series of women over several years (an average 25 year span), and using digital analysis concluded that brows descended in 29% of women, remained stable in 41%, but actually elevated in 28%.[9]

Other studies demonstrated an elevation of the brows in aging women as well.[10] One compared two cohorts of women 20 to 30 years old with a second cohort age 50 to 60 years and measured three heights: medial brow, midbrow, and lateral brow positions. The 20- to 30-year-old group had average measurements as follows: medial 15.7 mm, middle 19.8 mm, and lateral 21.3 mm. The older 50- to 60-year-old group had average measurements as follows: medial 19.1 mm, middle 22.4 mm, and lateral 22.4 mm. All distances rose (medial 3.4, mid 2.6, lateral 1.1 mm) as aging progressed

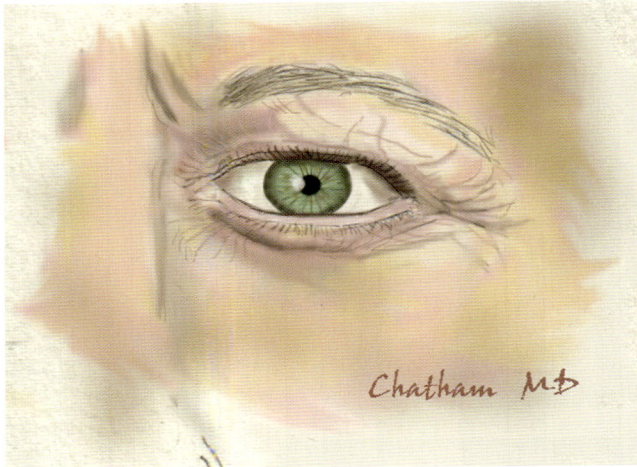

Fig. 23.8 Aging periorbit showing brow ptosis and dermatochalasis of lid.

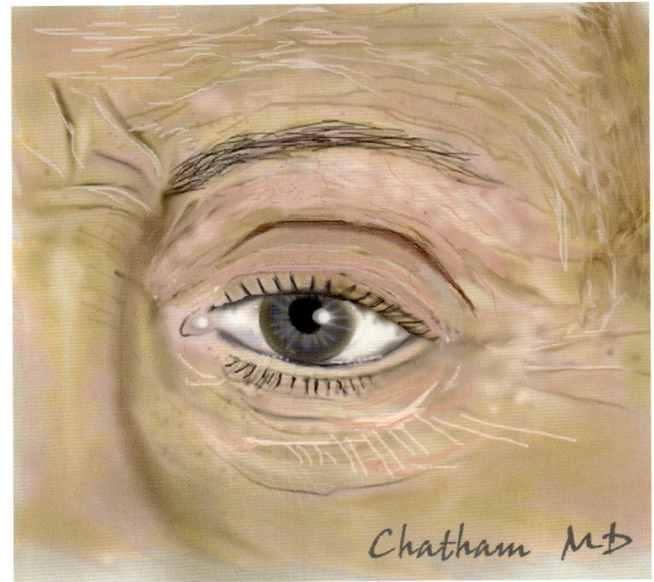

Fig. 23.9 Aging periorbit showing elevated brow with hollowing of upper lid.

In patients whose brows elevate, what is the reason? Some postulate it is overactivity of the frontalis, which compensates for gradual levator weakness.[11] One does see compensatory unilateral brow elevation when ptosis of the upper lid is present, and contracting the frontalis to lift the brows can improve vision. If, after blepharoplasty, the stimulus to elevate the brows is gone, the brows may indeed lower, in some cases diminishing the surgical results.[12]

But We Help Patients Look Better, Don't We?

A study surveyed a group of plastic surgeons and aestheticians and asked them what shape and position of brows they believe most attractive. Reviewing photos from 16 frequently cited medical articles, they also evaluated 100 preop photos to compare with 100 postop photos. Patients were from three different ethnic groups and had undergone brow surgery. Not surprisingly, both surgeons and aestheticians preferred the medial brow at the orbital rim and with an apex lateral slant. However, the surgical results, as judged by photographs, did not seem to produce the desired result, with brows either placed too high or the shape changed from a lateral slant to a less desirable flat or medial slant. The article said, "We conclude that the brow lift procedure, as documented in the plastic surgical literature, does not reliably achieve the most desirable aesthetic results for eyebrow height and shape."[13]

Other studies have opined that some popular surgical procedures create a result that is not attractive, including the tendency of some procedures to overelevate the brows, which created a surprised look in spite of our knowledge about what constitutes an attractive brow.[14] The fact that some patients who have undergone forehead lift procedures seek surgical reversal of their results suggests that sometimes a given procedure can be anatomically "too successful."[15]

■ Patient Selection

Patients often consult with surgeons when they desire a fresher, more rested, attractive, and youthful look. It is important to ask them what they notice about their brows. Sometimes patients are not even aware of the role brows play, thinking the issue is only related to upper lid redundancy. For example, if a woman wears bangs, she may have little awareness of her forehead and brows. When describing their eyelids, patients may use their fingertips to actually elevate their lateral brow, thinking they are addressing the lids only (Flowers sign). When horizontal creases are evident in the forehead, the surgeon can assume that the frontalis muscle has been used to elevate the brows to (unconsciously) compensate for a low position. Vertical (frown) lines suggest overactivity of the corrugator muscles. An upper lateral lid skin fold that extends beyond the eyelid and into the lateral periorbital tissues, or even to the level of the lateral lower lid, defines forehead ptosis and suggests a brow procedure may be indicated (Connell's sign).

Symmetry should be mentioned given that postprocedure the brow appearance will be scrutinized. But because human faces are inherently asymmetric, good proportion, balance, and brow shape are more important considerations. Prior to a procedure, pertinent questions include the following:

1. What does the patient request?
2. Is there a problem with brow descent?
3. Where were the brows during the twenties and thirties?
4. Is there adequate inflation (fullness) of the periorbital soft tissue?
5. Do the brows crowd the upper lid region?
6. Is there significant asymmetry?
7. Is there functional, including visual, disturbance?
8. Will the patient's hair pattern or style influence where possible incisions are made?
9. What are the shape and height of the forehead?
10. Is upper lid blepharoplasty necessary and can it be performed simultaneously?

■ Technical Aspects of Procedures

The prepared facial plastic surgeon has several options to offer patients, and a combination of techniques will serve the surgeon and patient well ▶ Video 23.1. A description of procedures follows, and while subdivided, naturally there is some overlap of techniques. At times it is advantageous to combine parts of "separate procedures" for the benefit of one patient.[16] Surgical procedures designed to improve brow aesthetics can be categorized as follows: (1) traditional versus nontraditional, (2) using general or sedation anesthesia versus local anesthesia, and (3) performed in a surgical suite versus an office setting.

Open Foreheadplasty

• Traditional, general or sedation anesthesia, surgical suite

It has been said that "open foreheadplasty techniques remain the standard against which other procedures are measured."[17] Utilizing an incision posterior to the anterior hairline (coronal) or just at the hairline (trichophytic or pretrichial) and extending bilaterally toward the superior auricles, the open foreheadplasty has been the mainstay in brow elevation for many years (**Fig. 23.10**). A large flap is created either in the subgaleal, subperiosteal, or subcutaneous plane. Once soft tissue release is accomplished in the superior orbital level, the entire forehead can be elevated and skin excised. Medial muscles can be divided or resected, and frontalis muscles may be partially scored under direct vision, if necessary.[17–19]

Dissection of the lateral scalp is taken deep to the temporoparietal fascia, just superficial to the deep temporal fascia, upon which dissection can be advanced inferiorly and medially. Subperiosteal dissection in the region of the superior lateral orbit requires that the ligaments and adhesions be adequately released to achieve lateral elevation. This includes the lateral brow thickening of the periorbital septum and temporal ligamentous adhesions and has been referred to as the orbital ligament (confluence of the anterior leaf of the deep galea and superficial temporalis fascia. Knize refers to the superior temporal septum (temporal crest, conjoint tendon) as the "zone of fixation."[20]

When dissecting in the temporal region, careful attention is paid to the position of the frontal branch of the facial nerve, which is just deep to the temporoparietal fascia lateral to the brow. It has been described as running halfway between the tragus and the lateral canthus and in close proximity to the sentinel vein[21] and 0.9 to 1.4 cm posterior to the lateral orbital rim.[22] And surgeons should remember it is not one ramus but several rami that cross the zygomatic arch, approximately half of which may be covered with from two to four rami.[23]

Likewise, understanding the position of the supraorbital and supratrochlear nerves (2.7 and 1.7 cm from midline, respectively) is vital to avoid sensory deficits due to unnecessary trauma to these nerves.

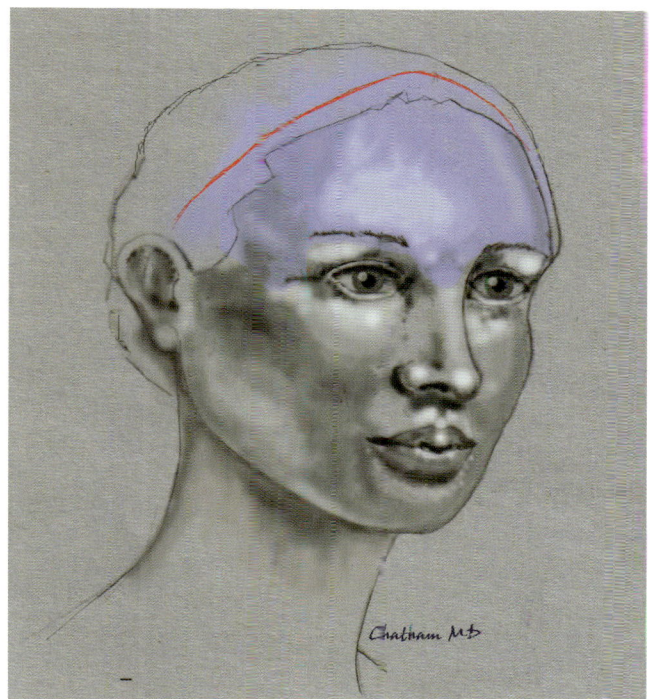

Fig. 23.10 Open foreheadplasty, coronal incision.

Manipulating the medial muscles (corrugator and procerus) allows the medial brow to elevate if desired. At the skin incision, one may need to resect approximately twice the skin at open incision in relation to amount of brow actually elevated (2:1), and this will lengthen the forehead unless a trichophytic incision is used.[24] Here the incision may be straight or irregularly shaped, beveling away from the hair follicles to encourage hair growth through the resultant scar. Here a subcutaneous or subgaleal or subperiosteal plane can be used (**Fig. 23.11**).

The pretrichial approach does shorten the forehead but does not necessarily lower the hairline unless the posterior scalp is mobilized and advanced, which usually requires a galeotomy.[25] Good candidates for hairline lowering include those with a high hairline, good scalp mobility, good hair, and no prior scalp surgery. Poorer candidates include those with a rigid scalp, thin or fragile hair, and previous transplants, as well as heavy smokers.

Pros: Works in an open access, and excessive skin is not just repositioned but removed. Results are believed by many to be longer lasting. The pretrichial scar can be camouflaged and is a good choice for heavily wrinkled forehead skin, which can be tightened well. When subcutaneous, there may be less postop itching and dysesthesias because the plane of dissection is superficial to the sensory nerves.

Cons: Produces a larger scar, and some hair loss (risky choice in males whose genetic hair pattern is still evolving). Sensory dysesthesias and paresthesias are frequent. Subcutaneous dissection requires meticulous attention to blood vessels and the position of the frontal branch of cranial nerve VII. Use caution in smokers.

Endoscopically Assisted Foreheadplasty

• *Traditional, general or sedation anesthesia, surgical suite*

In recent years, the endoscopically assisted forehead lift has been popular (**Fig. 23.12**). Via limited paramedian and lateral incisions (four or five), this procedure combines manual dissection with use of an endoscopic camera attached to a video monitor. Again, success in advancement of the forehead requires complete release of the arcus marginalis and temporal crest (conjoint tendon), as well as dissection caveats as previously discussed in the coronal approach section. The plane of dissection is typically subperiosteal or subgaleal,[26] and some techniques sometimes add a limited subcutaneous portion.[27]

A variety of centrally placed techniques can be utilized for fixation and include the Endotine and Ultratine devices (Microaire, Charlottesville, VA),[28] bone

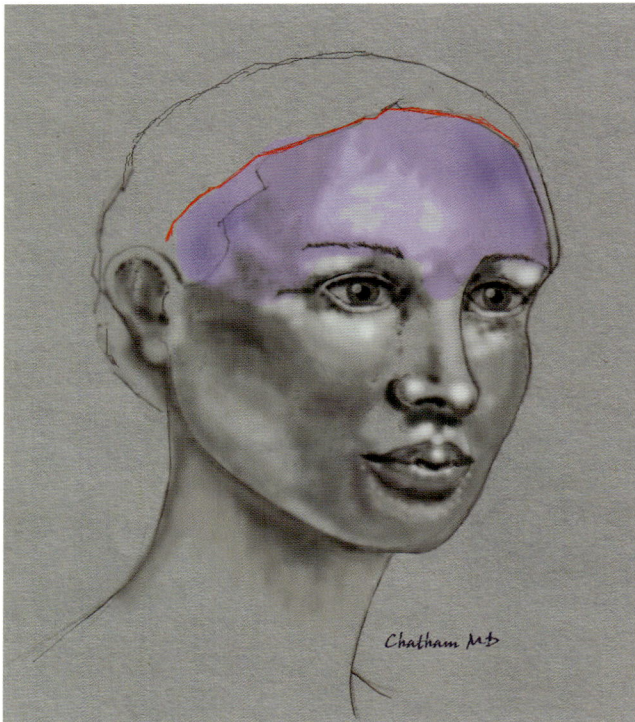

Fig. 23.11 Open foreheadplasty, trichophytic/pretrichial incision.

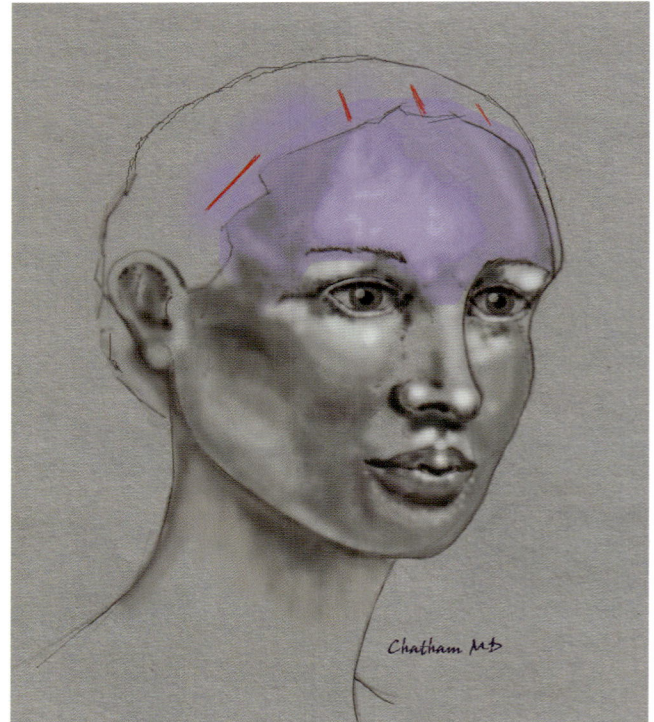

Fig. 23.12 Incisions, endoscopically assisted foreheadplasty.

tunnel,[29] subcutaneous suspension sutures,[30] and external and internal screws, plates, and tacks (Mitek Quickanchor screw, DePuy Mitek, Norwood, MA).

Application of tissue adhesives has also been employed. Lateral fixation via deep temporal fascia sutures is usually adequate for suspension and fixation. This not only may involve fixation for the temporoparietal fascia to the deep temporal fascia with strong sutures but also can include a window of resected temporalis fascia to promote additional scar tissue stabilization.[31] Laterally based suspension ribbons have also been employed.[32]

Note that when a drill is used in the anterior table of the skull, safety is paramount (i.e., avoidance of cerebrospinal fluid leak). Thickness is increased medially and posteriorly with thicker bone posterior to the coronal sutures. Drilling in the midline (sagittal sinus) and lateral to the temporal crest (thin temporal bone) is not recommended. In one study, cortical tunnels at 45 degrees never penetrated the inner table nor did Mitek screws, although one Endotine post did on one of 14 cadaver skulls.[33]

Although generally described as minimally invasive, there is considerable dissection involved, often subperiosteal. Only the incisions are minimally invasive. Of interest is a study by Chiu and Baker of 21 surgeons showing that the number of endoscopically assisted forehead procedures was dramatically reduced between 1997 and 2001, in part because several surgeons were not pleased with the results.[34]

Pros: Best for younger patients with low or low normal hairline with minimal wrinkles or muscle problems. Smaller incisions can lead to faster recovery, fewer sensory disturbances (usually), and less alopecia. There is no scalp resection.

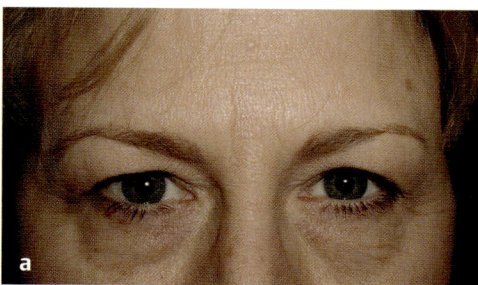

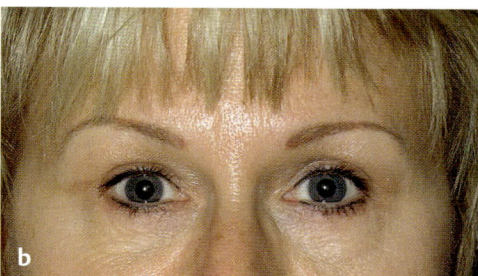

Cons: Less useful in older patients, high hairlines, thin-skinned men, extremely thick sebaceous skin, and very heavy, low brows. Curved foreheads can be problematic ("double convexity") because most equipment is straight. Resection of corrugators can be very time consuming. Specialized equipment and a fixation method are required. Some controversy about longevity exists, and **Fig. 23.13a,b** demonstrates a 1 year surgical result.

Direct Brow Lift

- *Traditional, general sedation or local anesthesia, surgical suite or office*

This procedure places the point of incision the closest to the brows, with the forehead incisions just above or slightly higher than the brows (**Fig. 23.14**). Dissection identifies the superior orbicularis muscle, into which are placed sutures that elevate the deep tissues. This can be unilateral and if significant asymmetry exists, skin excision can be tailored.

Pros: Placing the incision and lift in close proximity to the brow results in most elevation efficiency. This can easily be performed under local anesthesia and is best suited for older patients with rhytids, and where a scar is not a significant issue. There is excellent long-term durability.[35]

Cons: The visible scar limits patient suitability.

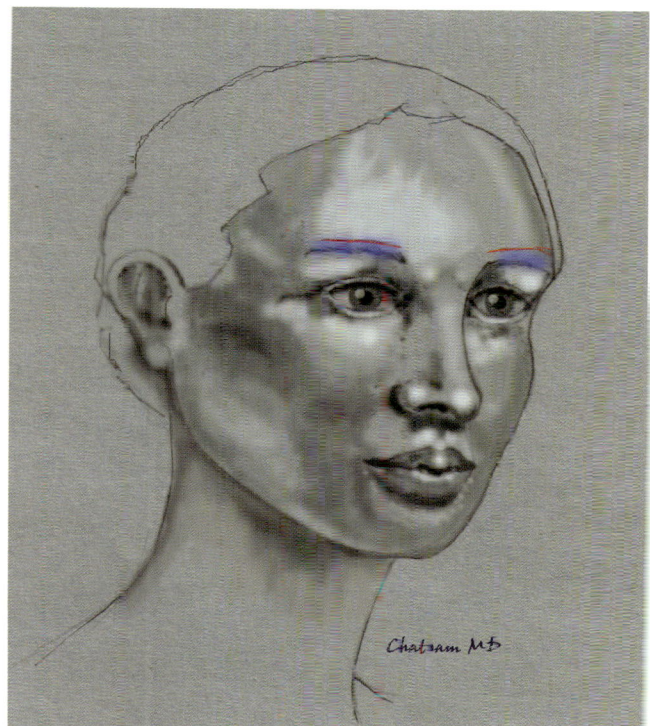

Fig. 23.13 Endoscopically assisted foreheadplasty. (a) Preoperative. (b) 1 year postoperative.

Fig. 23.14 Incisions, direct brow lift.

Subcutaneous Forehead Lift

• *Nontraditional, general sedation or local anesthesia, surgical suite or office*

A variation of the deeper dissections is the use of the subcutaneous lift. Here the dissection plane is superficial to the frontalis muscle and is based on nondisturbance of deep division of the supraorbital nerve branches and meticulous hemostasis. Indications may include a wrinkled forehead with brow ptosis, a secondary forehead lift, a short forehead with a desire to raise the forehead, or a long forehead and desire to shorten and advance. This can be performed under direct visualization without endoscopic equipment.[36,37]

Length and site of access incisions can vary from rather long pretrichial incisions to limited ones 4 or 5 cm long. An example of the latter is a short incision vertical to the lateral brow and extending from the velus hairs at the anterior lateral hairline into the temporal scalp (**Fig. 23.15a**) with digital dissection made inferiorly to ~ 2 cm above the brow. The undermined skin is now advanced superiorly, excess skin is removed, and careful suturing is performed at the incision. Additional dissection can be extended medially depending upon the forehead laxity of the patient (**Fig. 23.15b**). This can also be combined with additional approaches to the medial brow (i.e., transblepharoplasty access).[38]

Pros: Extended incision and dissection can place the brow where you want it. Pretrichial incision will not elevate the hairline and can lower it some. No specialized equipment is needed. Dissection is superficial to motor and sensory nerves (because the galea is not transected).

Cons: May take longer due to vascularity. Incisions and scars are longer than those of endoforehead. This cannot safely be combined with simultaneous, aggressive skin resurfacing.[39]

Midforehead Lift

• *Traditional, general sedation or local anesthesia, surgical suite or office*

This approach typically utilizes two fusiform incisions (which can be at uneven levels), placed in the midforehead near an existing crease (**Fig. 23.16**). One longer incision is occasionally used. Subcutaneous supramuscular skin undermining is performed to the brow, the skin is advanced, excess skin is excised, and deep tissues are secured to the periosteum with strong sutures. It is possible to engage the medial depressor muscles (corrugator and procerus) as well.

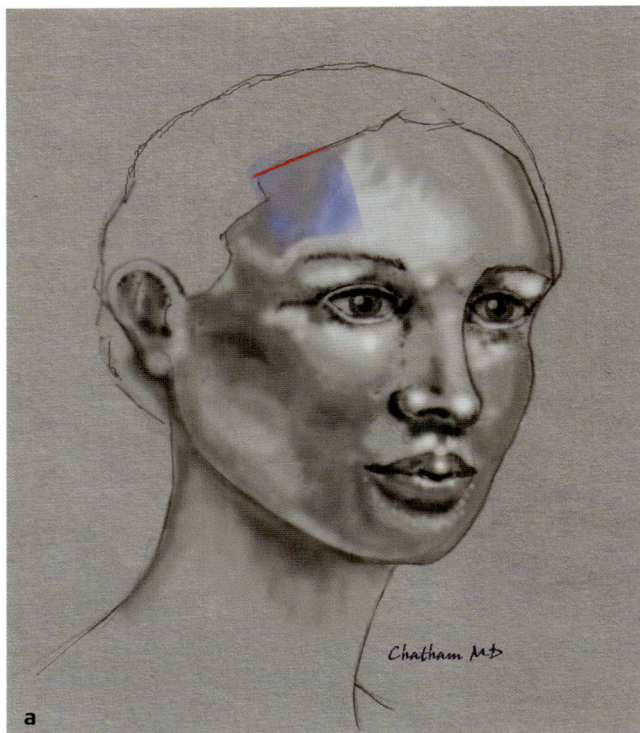

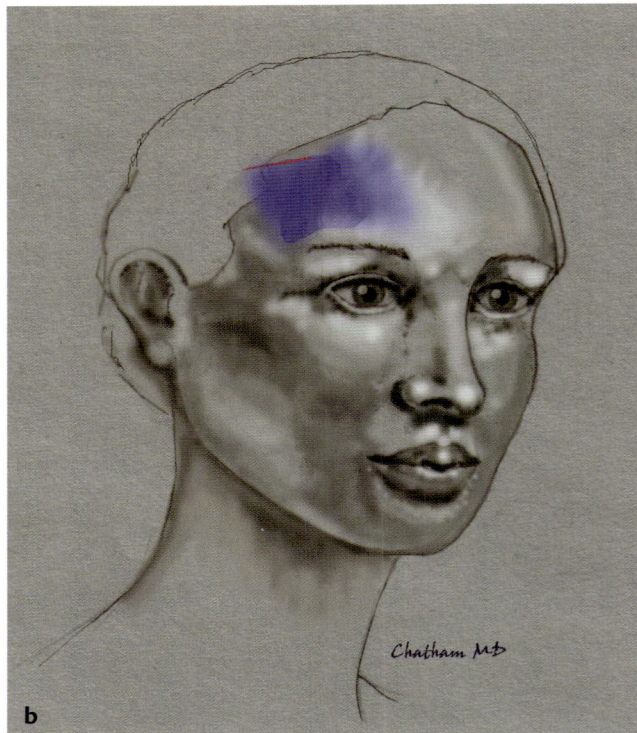

Fig. 23.15 Subcutaneous forehead lift. **(a)** Limited lateral incision. **(b)** Extended dissection.

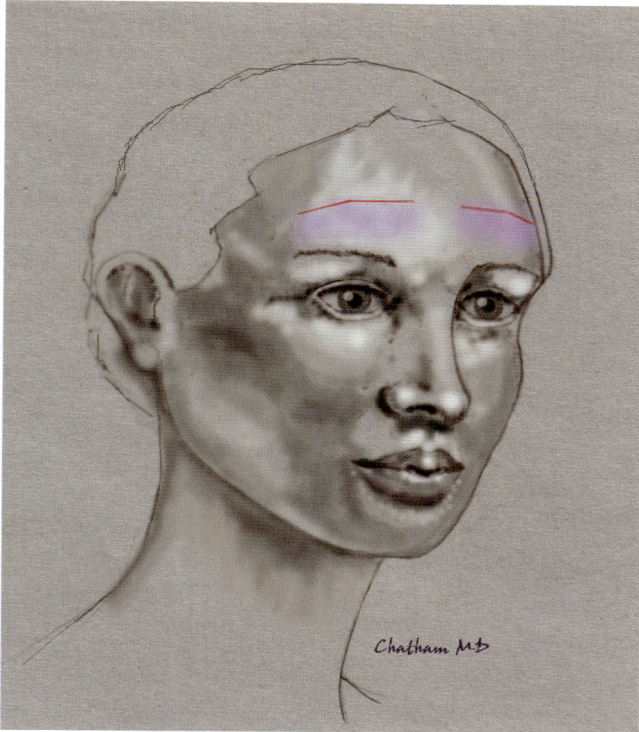

Fig. 23.16   Midforehead lift incisions.

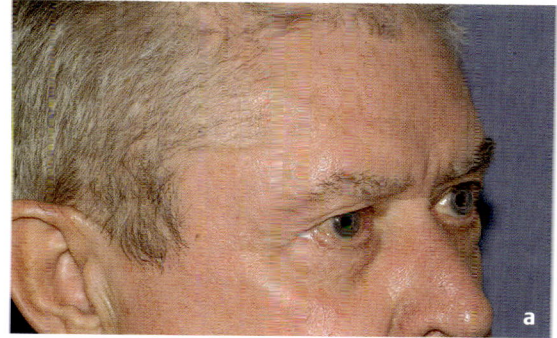

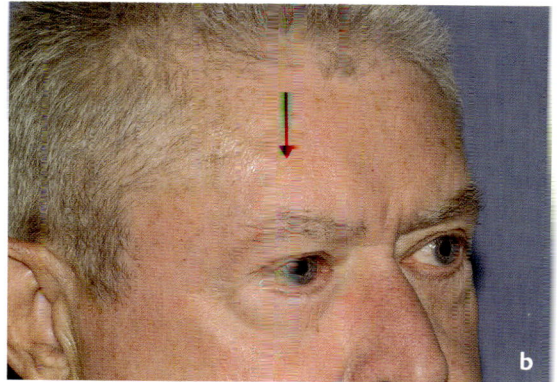

Fig. 23.17   Midforehead lift. (a) Preoperative. (b) Postoperative; note scar.

Pros: Incisions closer to the brows are useful in paralytic foreheads and ones with deep rhytids. This can produce excellent symmetry and longevity and only requires use of local anesthesia.

Cons: The visible scar requires properly selected patients (**Fig. 23.17a,b**).[40]

Transblepharoplasty Approach

- *Nontraditional, sedation or general anesthesia, surgical suite*

This procedure is usually simultaneously performed with an upper eyelid blepharoplasty (**Fig. 23.18**). Access to the supraorbital area is by dissection through the upper orbicularis muscle to gain access to the supra brow skull and lateral and medial musculature. Medially, depressor muscles may be modified or resected. The plane of dissection is typically subgaleal (supraperiosteal).[41,42]

The lateral approach (lateral to the supraorbital nerve) gains access to the lateral orbicularis and offers the option to suspend the lateral brow to the supraorbital tissues.[43,44] Laterally, sutures as well as absorbable fixation devices (Endotine Transbleph Implant, Coapt Systems, Palo Alto, CA), have been used to help

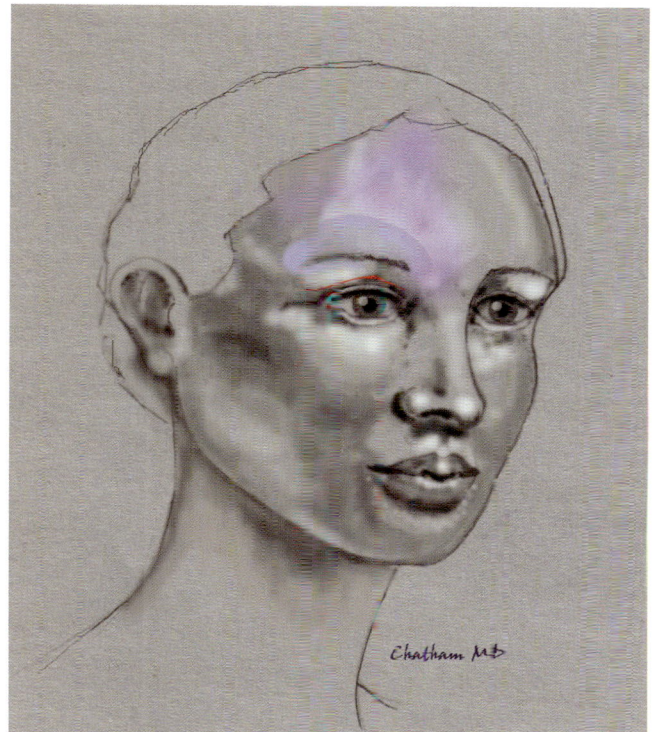

Fig. 23.18   Incisions, transblepharoplasty approach.

stabilize the brow.[45] Dissection may be extended superiorly to the hairline.[46] Note that laterally, periosteal fixation can result in restricted brow movement and dimpling. Some surgeons[47] utilize no periosteal fixation and achieve lateral lift via partial orbicularis muscle division (weakening the depressors) and by orbital ligament transection, galea release, and fat sculpting.

Pros: The incision is the one used for blepharoplasty, and there is no forehead scarring. Medial muscles can be addressed close to the incision. Lateral sculpting of heavy brow fat pads is possible. Balding men make good candidates. No special equipment is necessary.

Cons: Brow elevation is more subtle in comparison. Forehead hypesthesia may result from transection of the superficialmost branches of the supratrochlear, supraorbital, and lacrimal nerves. Most of the edema is concentrated postoperatively. Limits exist on affecting forehead rhytids or elevating skin. Lateral fixation may create more fullness above and lateral to the brow (masculinizing), as well as temporary puckering. Suturing to periosteum is tenuous.

Lateral Brow Lift

- *Nontraditional, general sedation or local anesthesia, surgical suite or office*

When modest isolated lateral brow elevation is desired, the lateral brow lift may be the choice (**Fig. 23.19**). The usual plane of dissection is just superficial to the deep temporal fascia and will require release of the temporal ligaments.[48]

This can also be performed subcutaneously, with care not to traumatize the frontal branch of the facial nerve, which lies just deep to this dissection. Access can be either from a more superior vector near the frontal hairline using approximately a 5 cm horizontal incision that is extended inferiorly, and even medially, to include most of the forehead, if desired. Alternatively, access may be more laterally from the temple (closer to the tail of the lateral brow) when more of a lateral vector is desired.[36,49,50] **Fig. 23.20a,b** shows pre- and postoperative views from a subcutaneous lateral brow lift.

Pros: Efficient and deals directly with the lateral brow containing skin. Wrinkling can be partially improved, and there is no need to release the orbital ligament bands.

Cons: There is somewhat limited access, especially to the medial brow, unless an additional incision is made. Delicate dissection in the area of the frontal branch of cranial nerve VII is required.

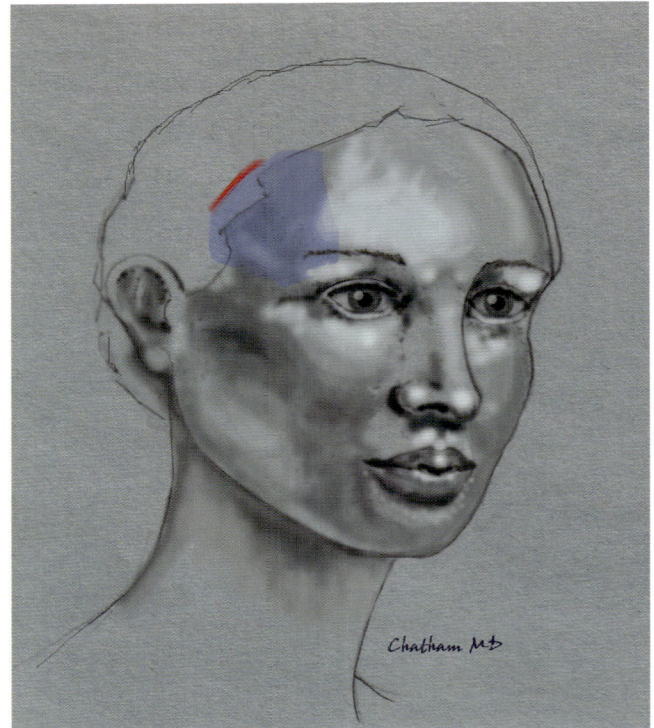

Fig. 23.19 Incisions, lateral brow lift.

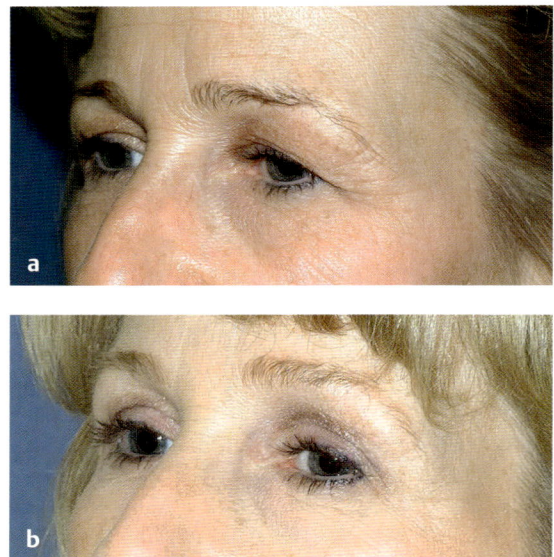

Fig. 23.20 Subcutaneous lateral brow lift. **(a)** Preoperative. **(b)** Postoperative.

Chemodenervation (Botulinum Toxin)

- *Nontraditional, no anesthesia, office*

Remembering that the brows are affected by muscles including the frontalis (elevator) and the corrugator supercilii and orbicularis oculi (depressors), by weakening one vector the other receives a competitive advantage (**Figs. 23.21**). Carefully placed botulinum, when properly administered, can create 2 to 4 mm of brow elevation, as well as soften glabellar frown lines, and is very useful for the patient not desirous of surgery.[51,52] The commercial botulinum products most widely used in the United States at the time of this writing are Botox (onabotulinumtoxin A, Allergan, Irvine, CA), Dysport (abobotulinumtoxin A, Medicis Aesthetics, Scottsdale, AZ), and Xeomin (incobotulinumtoxin A) (Merz Aesthetics, San Mateo, CA). All are effective and provide good results when proper dosing and technique are utilized. In females, corrugators can be longer than in males, whose corrugators are usually thicker. Some muscles require more botulinum toxin, and men usually require a larger dose than women (**Fig. 23.22a,b**).[53]

Dysport doses are sometimes calibrated in relation to existing Botox doses, and may be two to three times the appropriate Botox dosage. Xeomin doses are equivalent to those of Botox. Dose ranges for the medial (corrugator) muscles are 5 to 15 units in each muscle for Botox and 15 to 25 units for Dysport, but this can vary. Each corrugator is approached with one or two injection sites. Doses placed laterally under the tail of the brow may range from 3 to 6 units of Botox and 6 to 12 units of Dysport. This is exclusive of the dosage used for the treatment of "crow's feet," which may involve 7 to 15 units per each side, depending on the size and strength of that orbicularis. In addition, several units may also be used to calm the procerus, when it is active.

A 30-gauge needle works well, but so do 29- to 32-gauge needles. Preinjection chilling of the skin with a refrigerated cold pack seems to reduce discomfort; some have used a topical spray or even topical anesthetic cream. In our experience, reassurance coupled with a few seconds of cold pack is all that most patients require. Angling the needle at ~ 45 degrees toward the temple, and ~ 45 degrees entry (not directly perpendicular), and using one or two injection sites per each brow, 0.5 cm above the medial rim and 1 to 1.5 cm above the central brow, works well (**Fig. 23.23a,b**).

Asking the patient to frown often allows further visualization and palpation of the subcutaneous muscle, so the injection can be most precise. Some practitioners stabilize the head of the corrugator in the non-syringe-holding hand, and others simply

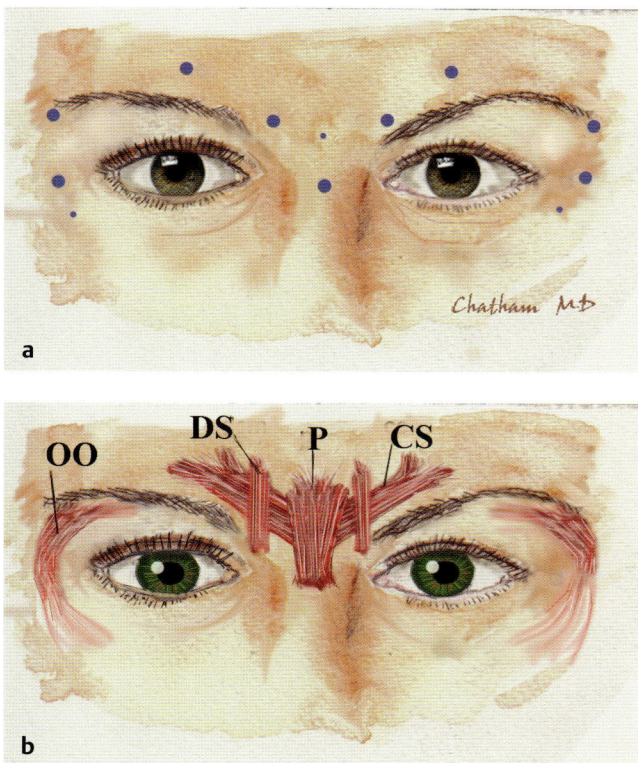

Fig. 23.21 **(a)** Skin injection points for neurotoxin therapy. **(b)** Diagrams of periorbital muscles. OO, orbicularis oculi; DS, depressor supercilii; P, procerus; CS, corrugator supercilii

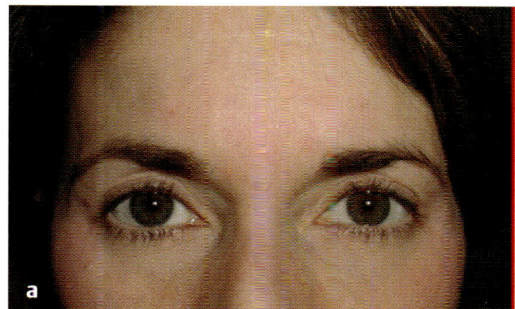

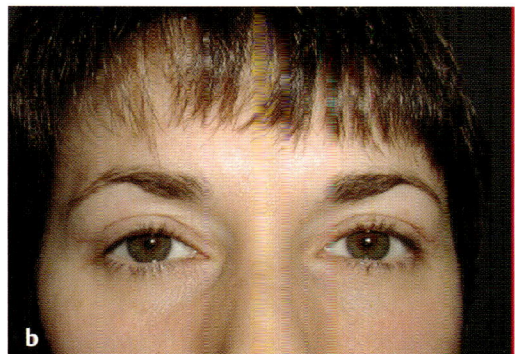

Fig. 23.22 Chemodenervation with Botox (Allergan). **(a)** Preoperative. **(b)** Postoperative.

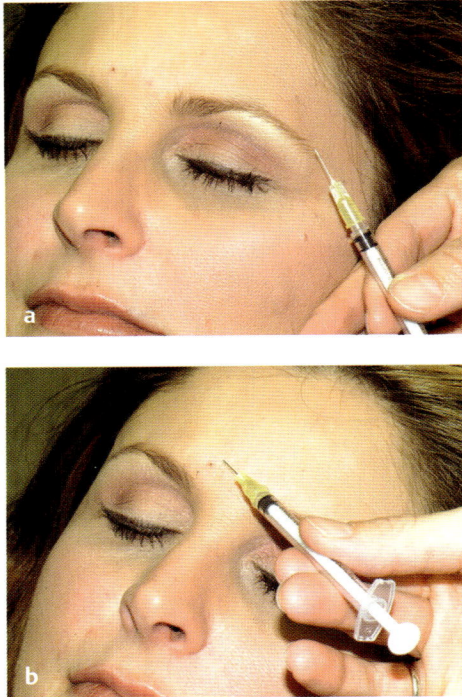

Fig. 23.23 Chemodenervation. (a) Lateral brow site. (b) Medial brow site.

inject the stationary suprabrow tissues. In thicker skin, the needle should be slightly deeper to engage the muscle. When the frontalis is also injected, some early techniques advocated a v-shaped forehead pattern, but this sometimes created a Spock-like or quizzical appearance when the lateral frontalis muscle would create a profound lateral arch.

Pros: Treatment is quick, low risk, and non-surgical.

Cons: Treatment lasts only 3 to 4 months, and an occasional delayed levator ptosis can be seen (3.2% reported from one study, and the effect is transient). Because it is classified as a pregnancy category C drug, botulinum should be avoided by pregnant or breastfeeding women. Contraindications may include disorders of the neuromuscular junction and some autoimmune diseases.[54]

Soft Tissue Fillers

• *Nontraditional, no anesthesia, office*

One of the desired goals of treatment is a smooth supraorbital (infrabrow) convexity (**Fig. 23.1**). This is more easily attainable with younger, more elastic skin. When performing upper lid blepharoplasty, leaving the orbicularis intact can help provide subcutaneous fullness, especially in the lateral one third of the upper infrabrow area. With older, nonelastic

skin, if one tries to achieve smoothness with brow elevation, the height must be to ridiculous dimensions.

Not all brows have a full infrabrow fullness, and even ones that do can deflate with time. The galea fat pad is a transverse band of fibroadipose tissue extending for ~ 2 cm above the orbital rims deep to the inferior frontalis muscle. Being mobile, with time it descends laterally and may seem confluent with the preseptal fat pad deep to the orbicularis oculi.[55] The presence of lateral orbital fat is significant because, with fat atrophy, overlying soft tissue becomes deflated. Dealing with "reinflation" in rejuvenation procedures should not be forgotten (**Fig. 23.24**).

Because one attribute of a youthful brow is a full convex infrabrow, techniques that "refill" the brow and infrabrow will help create a youthful contour along with an inflation, and thus slight "lift" of the lateral brow. **Fig. 23.25a–c** demonstrates an anterior view following lateral infrabrow volumization. **Fig. 23.26a,b** demonstrates placement of fat in the infrabrow to achieve rejuvenation plus slight lifting.

In addition to the lateral infrabrow area, at times the superior orbit will skeletonize and accentuate a deeply set or hollowed eye. Careful placement of an appropriate filler deep to the orbicularis along the inferior orbit just posterior to the rim can help soften this edge and decrease (fill) the perceived lid–brow distance. **Fig. 23.27a,b** demonstrates hyaluronic acid (HA) placed at the superior rim above the sulcus to soften orbital hollowing.

Fillers approved by the U.S. Food and Drug Administration (FDA) are most appropriate.[56] In addition to the collagen-injectible products (Zyderm, Allergan, Irvine, CA; Evolence, Johnson & Johnson, Brunswick, NJ), a newer generation of soft tissue fillers available in the United States includes HA, fat, calcium hydroxylapatite, and poly-L-lactic acid (PLLA). Autologous fat is also successfully used.[57] The HA fillers include Restylane and Perlane (Medicis); Hylaform, Captique, and Juvederm (Allergan), Prevelle (Genzyme, Mentor,

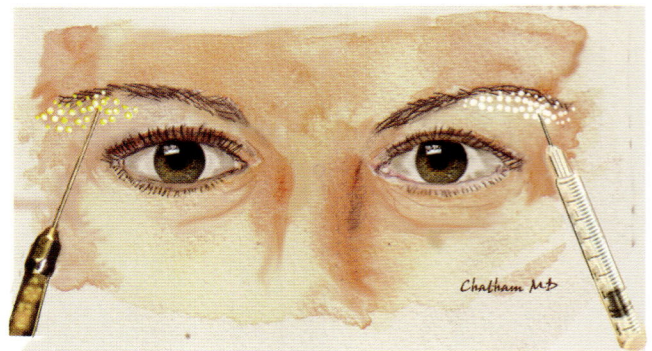

Fig. 23.24 Augmenting the infrabrow with autologous fat or fillers.

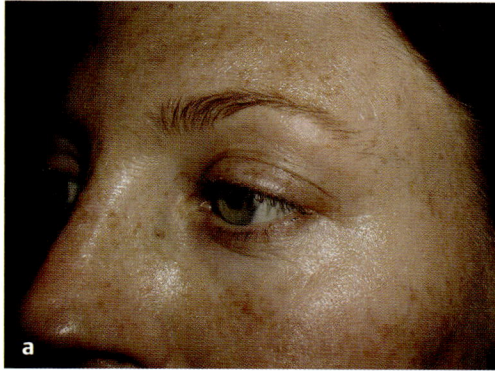

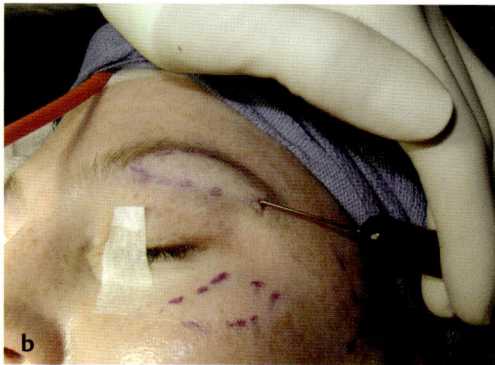

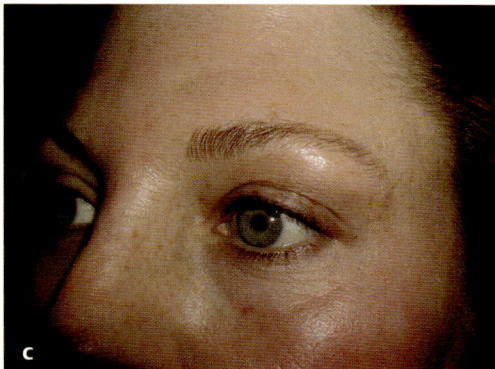

Fig. 23.25 Fat placement for lateral infrabrow volumization. **(a)** Preoperative. **(b)** Perioperative. **(c)** Postoperative.

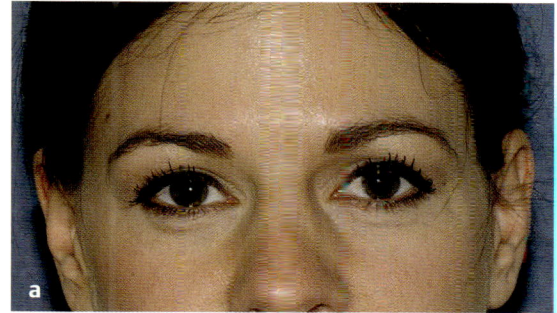

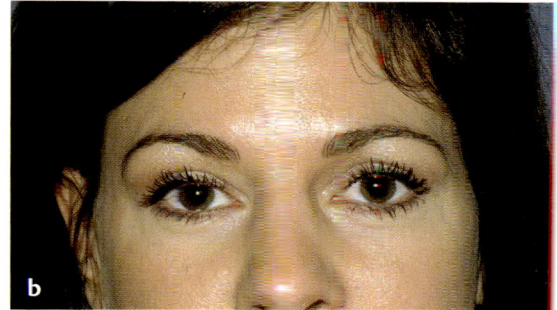

Fig. 23.26 Fat placement in the infrabrow. **(a)** Preoperative. **(b)** Postoperative.

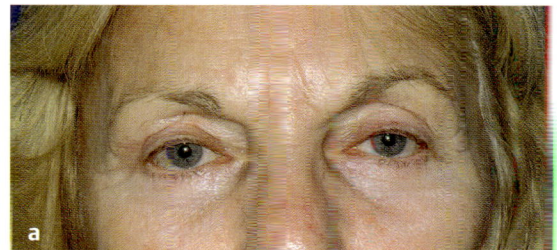

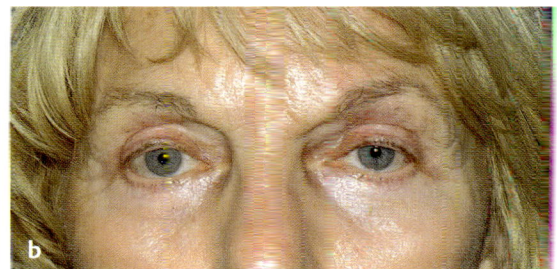

Fig. 23.27 Hyaluronic acid (HA) placement at the superior rim above the sulcus to soften orbital hollowing **(a)** Preoperative. **(b)** Postoperative.

Santa Barbara, CA), and Elevess (Anika Therapeutics, Bedford, MA).[58] Calcium hydroxylapatite is known as Radiesse (Merz Aesthetics, San Mateo, CA). PLLA is marketed as Sculptra (Sanofi-Aventis, Bridgewater, NJ). All have been successfully utilized in restoring facial volume and may be carefully employed.[59,60] It should be noted that, although many surgeons may use these products, some of these uses may be off-label applications.

Autologous fat is another option that skilled physicians have used in the face, including the periorbital[61] region.[62,63] Caution should be used in the eyelid region because the very thin skin and absence of

subcutaneous fat allow very little margin of error for improper or excessive placement of product. Use of Sculptra near the lids is ill-advised, and when using Sculptra, a greater dilution (i.e., 10 mL of diluent per vial) is associated with fewer nodular events. Although the use of fat or HA products to fill a hollow upper orbital sulcus has been successfully employed, it is very technique dependent, and visible and palpable nodules can occur. Sculptra and other fillers have been successfully used in improving the hollowing of the temporal fossa that is secondary to temporal fat wasting. When one is injecting subdermally/subcutaneously, careful technique is mandatory, which includes slow injection made upon withdrawal when possible. Aspiration of the syringe to detect any inadvertent intravascular entry avoids potential embolization, as does an appreciation for the location of usually subcutaneous vascular routes.

When HA has been injected suboptimally and needs removal, injection of the enzyme hyaluronidase in small aliquots can be used to dissipate it.

Pros: These are office procedures with ease of use and reasonable duration (6 to 12 months for HAs, 9 to 18 months for calcium hydroxylapatite, 18 to 24 months for PLLA, though this varies). Good lateral brow structure can be achieved.

Cons: One must avoid placement that is too superficial. There is the potential for vascular injection, and rarely, granulomatous reaction.[64] Imprecise placement along the upper lid can result in lumps, and the longevity of fat may vary.

Cable Suture Suspension

- *Nontraditional, general sedation or local anesthesia, surgical suite or office*

Various forms of subcutaneous/percutaneous suspension sutures and threads have been employed to suspend and fixate the brows to a more superior site in the forehead. Suspension sutures and threads create a linear stress on each suture.[65–68]

Pros: Relatively noninvasive, and the position of brows can be evaluated with each suture.

Cons: Pulling hard dimples the skin. Long-term reliability is questionable.

■ Postoperative Care

Following injectibles, patients are advised to refrain from strenuous physical activity for several hours. This may reduce the risk of delayed bruising and additional swelling. In the case of the neuromodulators, it seems wise to discourage massage or tissue manipulation, which may serve to "squeegee" the drug toward the upper lid levators. Immediately postinjection, we apply a very thin layer of antibiotic ointment to the puncture sites. We do encourage massage of the deposits of fillers, especially if the patient feels nodules in the first few days. Massage of PLLA is most important, and the "5-5-5 rule" (firm massage 5 minutes daily 5 times a day for 5 days)

helps distribute these particles to avoid clumping and unwanted nodules.

Postoperative care following incisional procedures will follow standard wound care instructions. Attention to cleanliness and topical antimicrobials help with healing. Avoidance of strenuous behavior for a week or two, depending on the extent of dissection, seems to help postoperative edema resolve more quickly. Perioperative broad-spectrum antibiotics, adequate analgesia, and anti-inflammatory medicines containing arnica and bromelain seem to have additive value. And, although "old-fashioned," we suggest liberal use of topical ice compresses in any area that is healing, both for comfort and for swelling reduction. Postsurgical patients are given detailed instructions and are encouraged to call the surgeon for any signs of problems.

■ Complications and Their Management

Complications can occur even in the best-planned and executed procedures, and sometimes lie distal rather than proximal to the surgical instrument. Although avoidance of problems always remains the gold standard, management is vital as well. Smaller procedures carry less risk. For example, the possible untoward effects of levator ptosis or brow ptosis secondary to neuromodulators are temporary and are best managed by empathetic patient support and encouragement. Using ophthalmic drops containing an adrenergic stimulator of Müller's muscle when levator ptosis is present may see some improvement with Iopidine ophthalmic drops (Alcon, Fort Worth, TX) (apraclonidine 0.5%). When using HA fillers around the orbit, if excessive volume is used and results in visible lumps or unattractive mounds, this can be reduced with small aliquots of hyaluronidase injected into the HA filler (Amphadase, Amphastar Pharmaceuticals, Cucamonga, CA; and Vitrase, Bausch & Lomb, Rochester, NY). Nodules of calcium hydroxylapatite and PLLA are more difficult to soften and may require excision if too prominent, although resolution is expected with time. Intravessel embolization must be avoided, and avoidance of injecting with excessive pressure, use of blunt-tipped microcannulas, adhering to gentle unhurried technique, and avoiding vascular areas will reduce this risk. Topical use of nitroglycerin paste, heat, and massage may help improve skin vascular perfusion when impending vascular compromise to skin is suspected.

Surgical procedures involve different potential risks and complications. Less than ideal scarring may be treated with routine modalities. When scars are thicker or potentially hypertrophic, use of topical creams or gels containing steroids may help, and intralesional injection of triamcinolone (Kenalog, Bristol Meyers Squibb, New York, NY) may be necessary. When sensory nerve endings are divided, the patient will experience sensory compromise, with paresthesias, dysesthesias, and/or anesthesias. These generally improve with time and healing, but in the case of a prolonged or focal area of pain, then a neuroma associated with collagen (scar) deposition may be an issue. If injectable steroid does not help, and an injectable trial of a local anesthetic temporarily improves the pain, then consideration might be given to a local resection of the offending scar.

■ Conclusion

To achieve the aesthetic goal of an attractive brow and periorbital complex, the facial surgeon needs a clear understanding of what constitutes the pleasing brow. Anatomy varies from patient to patient; therefore, a creative approach to each individual patient is essential. The next step is to assist patients in best understanding their most valuable options. When surgical elevation is required, the most favorable incisions for the patient may be selected, apprising the patient of the pros and cons. When additional volume is needed, either autologous or "off-the-shelf" fillers can be utilized. Neuromodulators may also temporarily enhance results. Some patients may need a comprehensive combination of techniques, whereas others may need very little at all. One size does not fit all patients, and the well-trained and creative surgeon will try to recommend options best suited for the anatomy, age, and tolerance of each individual patient.

References

1. McCord CD. Eyelid Surgery: Principles and Techniques. Philadelphia, PA: Lippincott-Raven; 1995

2. Sclafani AP, Jung M. Desired position, shape, and dynamic range of the normal adult eyebrow. Arch Facial Plast Surg 2010;12(2):123–127

3. Schreiber JE, Singh NK, Klatsky SA. Beauty lies in the "eyebrow" of the beholder: a public survey of eyebrow aesthetics. Aesthet Surg J 2005;25(4):348–352

4. Codner MA, Kikkawa DO, Korn BS, Pacella SJ. Blepharoplasty and brow lift. Plast Reconstr Surg 2010;126(1): 1e–17e

5. Westmore, MG. Facial Cosmetics in Conjunction with Surgery. Course at Aesthetics Plastic Surgery Society; May 1974; Vancouver, BC

6. Price KM, Gupta PK, Woodward JA, Stinnett SS, Murchison AP. Eyebrow and eyelid dimensions: an anthropometric analysis of African Americans and Caucasians. Plast Reconstr Surg 2009;124(2):615–623

7. Pastorek NJ, White WM. The angry face syndrome. Arch Facial Plast Surg 2011;13(2):131–133

8. van den Bosch WA, Leenders I Mulder P. Topographic anatomy of the eyelids, and the effects of sex and age. Br J Ophthalmol 1999;83(3):347–352

9. Lambros V. Observations on periorbital and midface aging. Plast Reconstr Surg 2007;120(5):1367–1376, discussion 1377

10. Matros E, Garcia JA, Yaremchuk MJ. Changes in eyebrow position and shape with aging. Plast Reconstr Surg 2009;124(4):1296–1301

11. Troilius C. Subperiosteal brow lifts without fixation. Plast Reconstr Surg 2004;114(6):1595–1603, discussion 1604–1605

12. van den Bosch WA, Leenders I Mulder P. Topographic anatomy of the eyelids, and the effects of sex and age. Br J Ophthalmol 1999;83(3):347–352

13. Freund RM, Nolan WB III. Correlation between brow lift outcomes and aesthetic ideals for eyebrow height and shape in females. Plast Reconstr Surg 1996;97(7):1343–1348

14. Gunter JP, Antrobus SD. Aesthetic analysis of the eyebrows. Plast Reconstr Surg 1997;99(7):1808–1816

15. Yaremchuk MJ, O'Sullivan N, Benslimane F. Reversing brow lifts. Aesthet Surg J 2007;27(4):367–375

16. Carniol PJ, Baker S. Combining techniques to optimize upper facial rejuvenation. Facial Plast Surg Clin North Am 2006;14(3):247–251

17. Marten T. Open forehead plasty. In: Knize D, ed. The Forehead and Temporal Fossa. Philadelphia, PA: Lippincott Williams & Wilkins; 2001:154–187

18. Ortiz-Monasterio F, Barrera G, Olmedo A. The coronal incision in rhytidectomy—the brow lift. Clin Plast Surg 1978;5(1):167–179

19. Flowers RS, Ceydeli A. The open coronal approach to forehead rejuvenation. Clin Plast Surg 2008;35(3):331–351, discussion 329

20. Knize DA. The forehead and temporal fossa. In: Knize D, ed. The Forehead and Temporal Fossa. Philadelphia, PA: Lippincott Williams & Wilkins; 2001:55

21. Quatela VC, Graham HD, Sabini P. Rejuvenation of the brow and midface. In: Papel I, ed. Facial Plastic and Reconstructive Surgery. 2nd ed. New York, NY: Thieme; 2002:171–185

22. Agarwal CA, Mendenhall SD III, Foreman KB, Owsley JQ. The course of the frontal branch of the facial nerve in relation to fascial planes: an anatomic study. Plast Reconstr Surg 2010;125(2):532–537

23. Gosain AK, Sewall SR, Yousif NJ. The temporal branch of the facial nerve: how reliably can we predict its path? Plast Reconstr Surg 1997;99(5):1224–1233, discussion 1234–1236

24. Marten T. Open forehead plasty. In: Knize D, ed. The Forehead and Temporal Fossa. Philadelphia, PA: Lippincott Williams & Wilkins; 2001:154–187

25. Guyuron B, Rowe DJ. How to make a long forehead more aesthetic. Aesthet Surg J 2008;28(1):46–50

26. Horn CE, Thomas JR. Subgaleal endoscopic browlift with absorbable fixation. Facial Plast Surg Clin North Am 2006;14(3):175–184

27. Ramirez OM. Endoscopically assisted biplanar forehead lift. Plast Reconstr Surg 1995;96(2):323–333

28. Stevens WG, Apfelberg DB, Stoker DA, Schantz SA. The Endotine: a new biodegradable fixation device for endoscopic forehead lifts. Aesthet Surg J 2003;23(2):103–107

29. Malata CM, Abood A. Experience with cortical tunnel fixation in endoscopic brow lift: the "bevel and slide" modification. Int J Surg 2009;7(6):510–515

30. Foustanos A, Zavrides H. An alternative fixation technique for the endoscopic brow lift. Ann Plast Surg 2006; 56(6):599–604

31. Hönig JF, Frank MH, Knutti D, de La Fuente A. Video endoscopic-assisted brow lift: comparison of the eyebrow position after Endotine tissue fixation versus suture fixation. J Craniofac Surg 2008;19(4):1140–1147

32. Pascali M, Gualdi A, Bottini DJ, Botti C, Botti G, Cervelli V. An original application of the Endotine ribbon device for brow lift. Plast Reconstr Surg 2009;124(5):1652–1661

33. Walden JL, Orseck MJ, Aston SJ. Current methods for brow fixation: are they safe? Aesthetic Plast Surg 2006;30(5): 541–548

34. Chiu ES, Baker DC. Endoscopic forehead rejuvenation, I: Limitations, flaws, and rewards. Plast Reconstr Surg 2007;119(3):1115–1116, author reply 1116–1119

35. Castañares S. Forehead wrinkles, glabellar frown and ptosis of the eyebrows. Plast Reconstr Surg 1964;34:406–413

36. Wolfe SA, Baird WL. The subcutaneous forehead lift. Plast Reconstr Surg 1989;83(2):251–256

37. Guyuron B. Subcutaneous approach to forehead, brow, and modified temple incision. Clin Plast Surg 1992;19(2): 461–476

38. Miller TA, Rudkin G, Honig M, Elahi M, Adams J. Lateral subcutaneous brow lift and interbrow muscle resection: clinical experience and anatomic studies. Plast Reconstr Surg 2000;105(3):1120–1127, discussion 1128

39. Niamtu J III. The subcutaneous brow- and forehead-lift: a face-lift for the forehead and brow. Dermatol Surg 2008;34(10):1350–1361, discussion 1362

40. McKinney P, Mossie RD, Zukowski ML. Criteria for the forehead lift. Aesthetic Plast Surg 1991;15(2):141–147

41. Knize DM. Transpalpebral approach to the corrugator supercilii and procerus muscles. Plast Reconstr Surg 1995;95(1):52–60, discussion 61–62

42. Guyuron B, Michelow BJ, Thomas T. Corrugator supercilii muscle resection through blepharoplasty incision. Plast Reconstr Surg 1995;95(4):691–696

43. Sokol AB, Sokol TP. Transblepharoplasty brow suspension. Plast Reconstr Surg 1982;69(6):940–944

44. McCord CD, Doxanas MT. Browplasty and browpexy: an adjunct to blepharoplasty. Plast Reconstr Surg 1990;86(2): 248–254

45. Sclafani AP. Comprehensive periorbital rejuvenation with resorbable Endotine implants for trans-lid brow and midface elevation. Facial Plast Surg Clin North Am 2007;15(2):255–264, viii

46. Langsdon PR, Metzinger SE, Glickstein JS, Armstrong DL. Transblepharoplasty brow suspension: an expanded role. Ann Plast Surg 2008;60(1):2–5

47. Burroughs JR, Bearden WH, Anderson RL, McCann JD. Internal brow elevation at blepharoplasty. Arch Facial Plast Surg 2006;8(1):36–41

48. Knize DM. Limited-incision forehead lift for eyebrow elevation to enhance upper blepharoplasty. Plast Reconstr Surg 1996;97(7):1334–1342

49. Miller TA, Rudkin G, Honig M, Elahi M, Adams J. Lateral subcutaneous brow lift and interbrow muscle resection: clinical experience and anatomic studies. Plast Reconstr Surg 2000;105(3):1120–1127, discussion 1128

50. Bernard RW, Greenwald JA, Beran SJ, Morello DC. Enhancing upper lid aesthetics with the lateral subcutaneous brow lift. Aesthet Surg J 2006;26(1):19–23

51. Dyer WK, Jung RT. Botulinum assisted brow lift. Facial Plast Surg Clin North Am 2000;8(3):343–354

52. Carruthers J, Carruthers AC. The use of botulinum toxin type A in the upper face. Facial Plast Surg Clin North Am 2006;14(3):253–260

53. Kane MA, Brandt F, Rohrich RJ, Narins RS, Monheit GD, Huber MB; Reloxin Investigational Group. Evaluation of variable-dose treatment with a new U.S. botulinum toxin type A (Dysport) for correction of moderate to severe glabellar lines: results from a phase III, randomized, double-blind, placebo-controlled study. Plast Reconstr Surg 2009;124(5):1619–1629

54. Carruthers A, Carruthers J, Lowe NJ, et al. One year randomized multicenter two period study of the safety and efficacy of repeated treatments with botulinum toxin type A in the treatment of glabellar lines. J Clin Res 2004;7:1–20

55. Knize DM. Reassessment of the coronal incision and subgaleal dissection for foreheadplasty. Plast Reconstr Surg 1998;102(2):478–489, discussion 490–492

56. Baumann L, Blyumin ML. Update on dermal filling agents: the University of Miami Department of Dermatology's Cosmetic Center perspective. Review. Cosmet Dermatol 2008;21(6):268–274

57. Coleman SR. Concepts of aging: rethinking the obvious. In: Coleman S, ed. Structural Fat Grafting. St Louis, MO: Quality Medical Publishing; 2004

58. Klienerman R, Emanuel P, Goldernberg G. Treatment with hyaluronic acid fillers. Cosmet Dermatol 2010;23(9): 405–409

59. Carruthers JD, Carruthers A. Facial sculpting and tissue augmentation. Dermatol Surg 2005;31(11 Pt 2):1604–1612

60. Tzikas TL. Autologous fat grafting for midface rejuvenation. Facial Plast Surg Clin North Am 2006;14(3):229–240

61. Berman M. Rejuvenation of the upper eyelid complex with autologous fat transplantation. Dermatol Surg 2000; 26(12):1113–1116

62. Obagi S. Autologous fat augmentation: a perfect fit in new and emerging technologies. Facial Plast Surg Clin North Am 2007;15(2):221–228, vii

63. Lam SM, Glasgold MJ, Glasgold RA. Complementary Fat Grafting. Philadelphia, PA: Lippincott Williams and Wilkins; 2006

64. Chabra I, Obagi S. Severe site reaction after injecting hyaluronic acid-based soft tissue filler. Cosmet Dermatol 2011;24(1):14–21

65. Sulamanidze MA, Paikidze TG, Sulamanidze GM, Neigel JM. Facial lifting with "APTOS" threads: featherlift. Otolaryngol Clin North Am 2005;38(5):1109–1117

66. Mutaf M. Mesh lift: a new procedure for long-lasting results in brow lift surgery. Plast Reconstr Surg 2005;116(5):1490–1499, discussion 1500–1501

67. Ellis DA. Thread-lift techniques. In: Truswell WH, ed. Surgical Facial Rejuvenation. New York, NY: Thieme; 2011

68. Matros E, Garcia JA, Yaremchuk MJ. Changes in eyebrow position and shape with aging. Plast Reconstr Surg 2009;124(4):1296–1301

24 Upper Eyelid Blepharoplasty

Fred G. Fedok and Paul J. Carniol

Key Concepts

- The overall goal of surgery is to create a natural, nonoperated appearance.

- For patients with visual field loss due to blepharochalasis and upper eyelid skin redundancy, an additional goal is to alleviate visual field obstruction.

- The emphases in technique have shifted to skin removal with conservation of fat and the avoidance of eyelids with an overoperated appearance.

- If a browlift and upper eyelid blepharoplasty are performed together, care must be taken to avoid excessive excision of upper eyelid skin to avoid lagophthalmos.

■ Introduction

The eyes are the windows. . . . Most adults of the Western world can finish this common expression, and in many ways, the expression is true. Given their central location, the eyelids' contours and movements account for a large part of the expressiveness of the face and convey much of a person's nuances of communication. These factors have motivated both men and women to seek to maintain a healthy, youthful appearance and expressiveness through eyelid enhancement surgery.

■ Background: Basic Science of Procedure

The term *blepharoplasty* was coined by Von Graefe in 1817 to describe a reconstructive technique. In the late 1920s, French surgeons, such as Bourget, advocated removal of herniated orbital fat for cosmetic reasons. In 1951, Castenares described the fat compartments of the upper and lower eyelids. Until recently, fat removal had remained an integral part of blepharoplasty. During the last decade, the emphases in technique have shifted to skin removal with conservation of fat and the avoidance of eyelids with an overoperated appearance.[1,2]

Upper eyelid blepharoplasty is usually performed for cosmetic concerns, functional impairment of vision, or both. Each situation is frequently accompanied by an excess or prominence of eyelid skin, fat, or orbicularis muscle. This tissue redundancy is caused by the aging process or secondary to a familial propensity. Lid malposition and ptosis may also be concerns. In most situations, management of the excessive tissues of the upper eyelid includes some consideration of brow position; to ignore the close anatomical relationship between the brow and the upper eyelids in performing surgery of the region potentially jeopardizes the final aesthetic and functional outcomes. The goal is to achieve facial harmony and optimal function while maintaining latitude for individual variation.[3–5]

■ Pertinent Anatomy

That the face on frontal projection can be divided into vertically oriented thirds is a well-recognized concept (**Fig. 24.1**). In this model, the upper facial

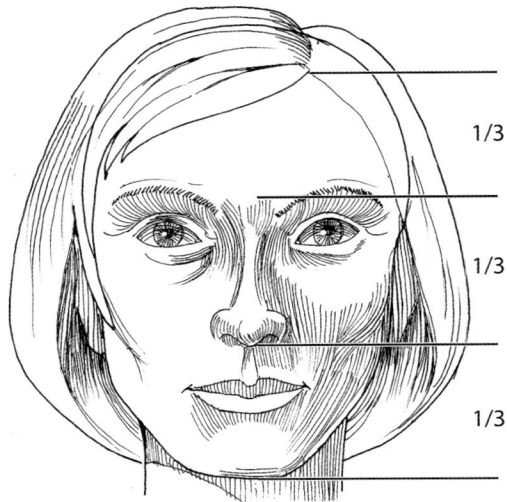

Fig. 24.1 Facial thirds.

third is bordered by the anterior hairline above and the glabella below.[6] Definitions and boundaries of the facial thirds are somewhat inconsistent from author to author, but in general, the brows and the upper eyelids are included in the upper third of the face and should be considered as a unit. More specifically, the position of the brow and its symmetry should be assessed whenever considering alteration of the upper eyelid. If a browlift and upper eyelid blepharoplasty are performed together, care must be taken to avoid excessive excision of upper eyelid skin, because the patient can develop lagophthalmos.

Eyebrow ptosis and asymmetry are frequent contributing factors to undesirable features of the upper eyelid. In general, it is considered acceptable for the male brow to be at the level of, or just superior to, the orbital rim. The male brow is usually more horizontally oriented and straighter, thicker, less defined, less refined, and without the curved elegance of the female brow. In females, it is considered more aesthetically pleasing if the brow is positioned higher than the orbital rim, with an arching elevation at either the lateral level of the lateral canthus or the limbus. Most of these gender-based differences should be preserved when one is performing surgical correction[7] to avoid an undesirable feminizing or masculinizing effect (**Fig. 24.2a,b**).

The upper eyelid, as is the lower eyelid, is a trilamellar structure. The anterior lamella is composed of skin and the orbicularis muscle. The middle lamella of the eyelid is the orbital septum, which fuses with the posterior lamella as it attaches to the tarsal plate. The posterior lamella is composed of the levator aponeurosis, Müller's muscle, and the conjunctiva.[8] The inferior portion of the posterior lamella is the tarsal plate, measuring 10 to 11 mm wide. The levator aponeurosis of the upper eyelid fuses to the orbital

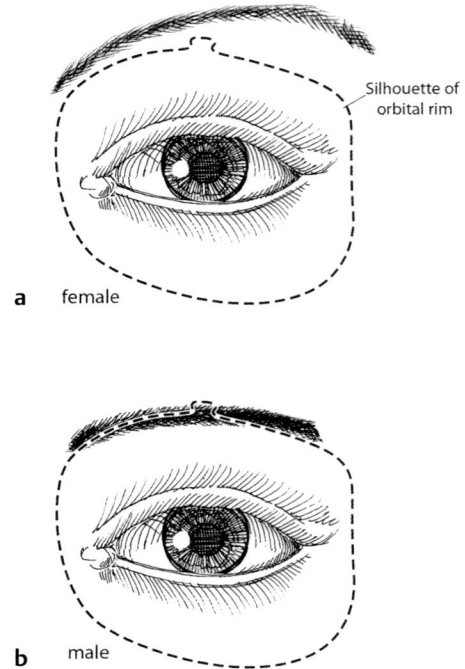

Fig. 24.2 Ideal brow and eyelid characteristics. **(a)** Female patient. **(b)** Male patient.

septum ~ 2 to 3 mm above the superior margin of the tarsus. This fascial structure is in continuity with the conjunctiva at the fornix, and, in combination with Müller's muscle, retracts the conjunctiva and the tarsus on upward gaze (**Fig. 24.3**).[9]

The visible external anatomical landmarks of the upper eyelid include the ciliary margin, the supratarsal crease, and the superior palpebral sulcus. In occidental patients, the mid–upper border of the tarsal plate is marked by the presence of the supratarsal crease. In the adult male, the supratarsal crease lies 8 to 10 mm superior to the lid margin and can be less

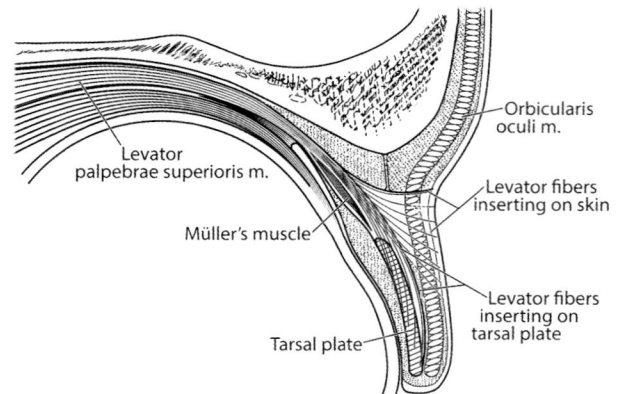

Fig. 24.3 The upper eyelid on cross-section.

defined than in females, where the distance is 10 to 12 mm (**Fig. 24.4**).[10]

The upper eyelid skin is the thinnest skin on the body. There is usually an absence of subcutaneous fat and only limited skin adnexal structures. The dermis is thin, and at times the skin is almost translucent. These qualities of the skin predispose it to laxity and redundancy with aging. Alternatively, some of these same structural features make the eyelids particularly good surgical sites, and incisions generally heal very well.

The orbicularis muscle lies immediately under the dermis, with only a loose layer of connective tissue separating the two. It is innervated by the temporal, buccal, and zygomatic branches of the facial nerve. The muscle is commonly described as consisting of three parts: the orbital part, the preseptal aspect, and the pretarsal part. The pretarsal orbicularis is contiguous with the medial and lateral canthal ligaments (**Fig. 24.5**).

Management of bulging orbital fat is central to the topic of blepharoplasty. On a familial or involutional basis, a laxity of support structures occurs, thus allowing a bulging or prominence of orbital fat to occur. Clinically, this produces varying bulging of the orbit-al fat that is seen as baggy or swollen eyelids. This is commonly referred to as orbital fat pseudoherniation because the fat remains behind the orbital septum; no true hernia occurs. The orbital fat is semicompartmentalized. Although the orbital fat shares a common space posterior to the globe, in the context of blepharoplasty this fat is clinically described as occupying distinct compartments in the anterior orbit. There are two upper eyelid fat compartments and three lower eyelid compartments (**Fig. 24.6**). In the upper eyelic, the compartments are the nasal and the central or middle compartments. The lacrimal gland occupies the lateral aspect of the superior orbit. In the course of performing upper eyelid blepharoplasties with the removal of pseudoherniated fat, the anterior eyelid skin, the orbicularis muscle, and the medial orbital septum are entered.

■ Patient Selection

Motivation

Because this is elective surgery, it is extremely important that patients are proper candidates for surgery. The patients' motivations must be sound, they have to be willing to accept imperfection, they have to possess realistic goals, and they have to be willing to accept the prospect of additional surgery. The management of patients with cosmetic eyelid concerns is guided by the careful assessment of the patient, the establishment of a "diagnosis" based on anatomical and aesthetic parameters, and an approach based on sound surgical principles. A thorough evaluation of the patient is therefore necessary, as it would be in any other aspect of medicine and surgery. Both psychological and medical issues should be explored.

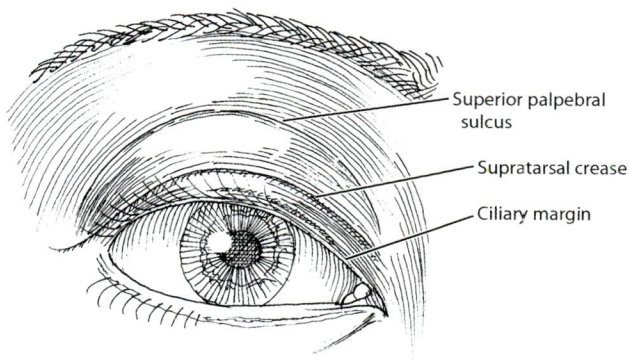

Fig. 24.4 Pertinent external landmarks of the upper eyelid.

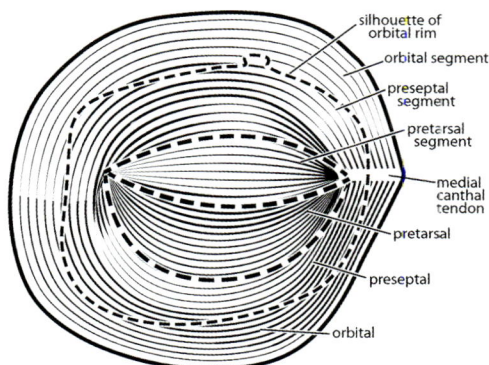

Fig. 24.5 The orbicularis muscle.

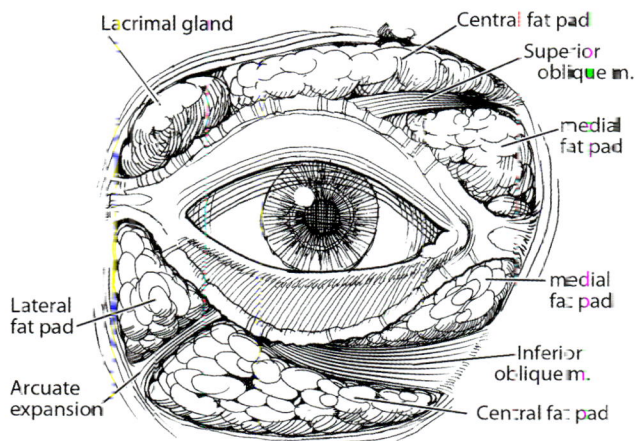

Fig. 24.6 The fat compartments of the upper and lower eyelid.

The overall goal of surgery is to create a natural, nonoperated appearance. For patients with visual field loss due to the blepharochalasis and upper eyelid skin redundancy, the other goal is to alleviate the visual field obstruction.[11–13] Problems that can be addressed at the time of upper blepharoplasty routinely include brow malposition and asymmetry, excess skin, and pseudoherniation of orbital fat. Problems that cannot be addressed through blepharoplasty alone include rhytids, pigmentation abnormalities, malar bags, and ptosis. Other features of the patient's eyelid and adjacent structures or surgery that should be noted and discussed with the patient include skin lesions, lacrimal gland ptosis, prominent orbital rims, edema, or any other abnormality or asymmetry. These associated conditions and their adjunctive treatments should be discussed with the patient before undergoing blepharoplasty (**Fig. 24.7a,b**; **Fig. 24.8a,b**; **Figs. 24.9** and **24.10**).

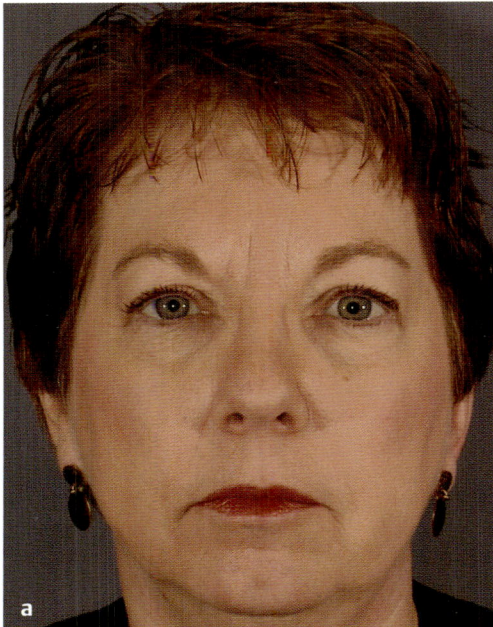

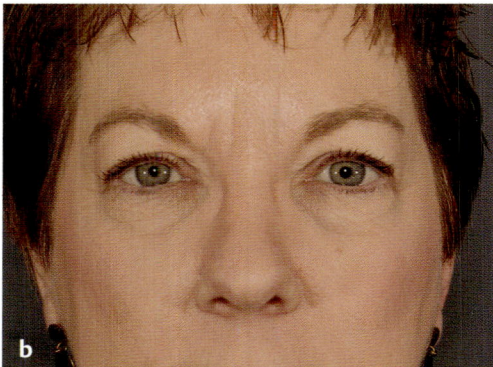

Fig. 24.8 **(a,b)** A patient who is a less favorable candidate for simple upper eyelid blepharoplasty. She has left upper eyelid ptosis with encroachment of the pupil and probable levator dehiscence.

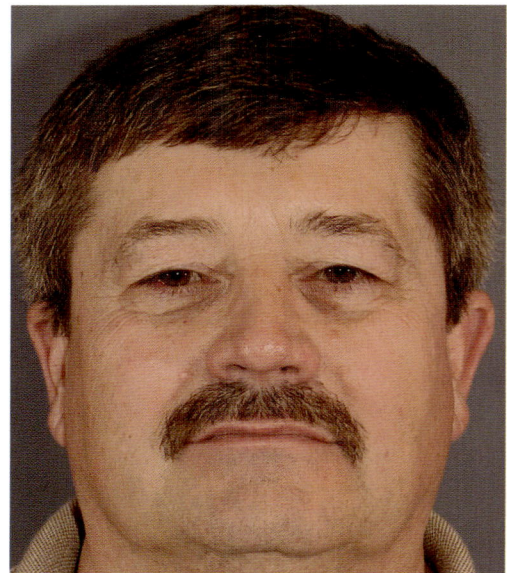

Fig. 24.7 **(a,b)** A favorable candidate for upper eyelid blepharoplasty with acceptable brow position, excessive eyelid skin, and good position of upper eyelid margin.

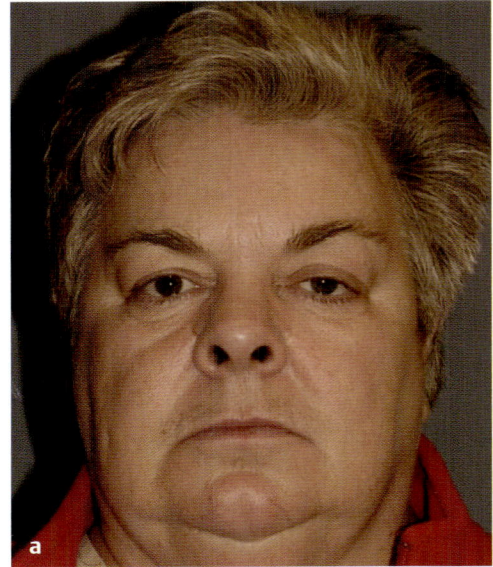

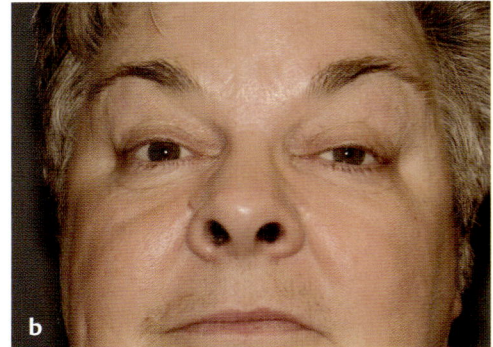

Fig. 24.9 Mild brow asymmetry.

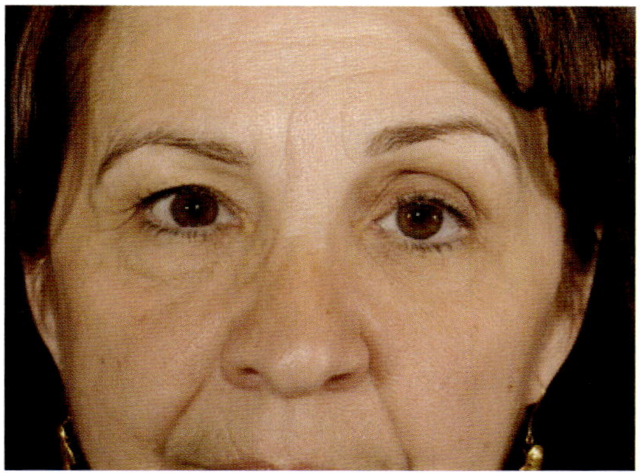

Fig. 24.10 Severe brow asymmetry and deepening of left superior orbital sulcus possibly suggestive of levator dehiscence.

Preoperative Evaluation

A set of standardized clinical photographs should be taken to document aesthetic and functional features of the patient's periorbital areas and face.

In evaluating the patient for eyelid blepharoplasty, several parameters should be assessed. The patient must be in good general health and able to withstand the modest rigors of blepharoplasty surgery. This procedure can be performed under local anesthesia, local anesthesia with conscious sedation, or brief general anesthesia.

The physician should obtain a detailed ophthalmological history, including at least dry eyes, epiphora, previous surgery, visual acuity, and diplopia. The history should focus on eye-related symptoms, medical conditions that might affect the eyes or soft tissues of the face, the patient's candidacy for surgery, and whether surgery is contraindicated.

All patients are assessed for visual acuity, lacrimal function, eyelid function, presence of ptosis and lagophthalmos, tone and position of the lower eyelid, presence of excess and laxity of eyelid skin, pseudoherniation of orbital fat, and rhytids. Many practitioners perform a Schirmer's test on all patients; some perform the test only if there is a history of dry eyes or epiphora.

Formal visual field testing may be necessary if the patient has a complaint or physical findings suggesting a peripheral visual deficit. Formal ophthalmological consultation or optometric consultation may be obtained based on the results of history or examination, or as a screening for disorders that might affect the patient's candidacy for surgery. Some practitioners do this only if there appears to be an ophthalmological abnormality based on their evaluation.

Palpebral fissure length, shape, and size should be assessed. Eyelid position and symmetry should be noted, in regard to both the upper and lower eyelids. The upper eyelid margin should lie between the superior limbus and the pupil. The pupil should not be encroached by the eyelid margin or ptosis is present. Ideally, the upper eyelid should fuse laterally with the lower eyelid at a sharp lateral canthal angle with the lower eyelid central margin position abutting the iris with an absence of scleral show. The patient's eye opening and closure should be observed for the presence of lagophthalmos and asymmetries. The eyelids should be observed for the presence of rhytids, laxity, and redundancy of skin.[14-16]

Many patients are noted to have a tendency to "rounding" or lateral inferior rotation of their lower eyelid. This may be secondary to involutional laxity of the lower eyelid, or it may be an individual characteristic of the eyelid without any inherent laxity. In either case, because this is generally thought of as an unfavorable characteristic, it should be pointed out to the patient before surgery.

When the skin of the eyelids is assessed, redundancy can be evaluated visually and demonstrated by grasping the redundancy between the thumb and index finger. This will give an indication of thin, draping excess characteristic of the effects of aging in dermatochalasis, or instead, the thickened redundancy of a familiar disorder, blepharochalasis.

The presence of fat pseudoherniation should be evaluated with the patient in neutral gaze and with them gazing upward, downward, to the left and right. The presence of fat pseudoherniation and asymmetry should be noted in all the potential locations in the upper and lower eyelids along with the location and relative amounts of fat (**Fig. 24.11a,b**).

A regional examination of the face is undertaken to assess both medical and aesthetic concerns. Patients should be examined in the upright position and while they are looking at themselves in a mirror, as well as without the mirror. The examiner will notice that some patients involuntarily raise their brow and open their eyes as soon as they see themselves in a mirror. If that behavior is demonstrated, it should be pointed out to the patient. It may be necessary to demonstrate to the patient this automatic tendency to elevate the brows by comparison of their photographs.

The assessment of various other factors is necessary. The patient's brow position should be at acceptable aesthetic levels (i.e., above the orbital rim) and symmetrical. The position and symmetry of the brow are examined in repose and in animation. Brow position will usually be a major consideration regarding upper eyelid skin redundancy. In front of a mirror, the examiner should demonstrate for the patient the effect of manual placement of the brow in a more acceptable position on upper eyelid skin redundancy. The presence of furrows should be noted, as well as the presence of hyperactive corrugator and procerus muscles.

Other features of the patient's eyelid and adjacent structures or surgery that should be noted and discussed with the patient include proptosis, skin lesions,

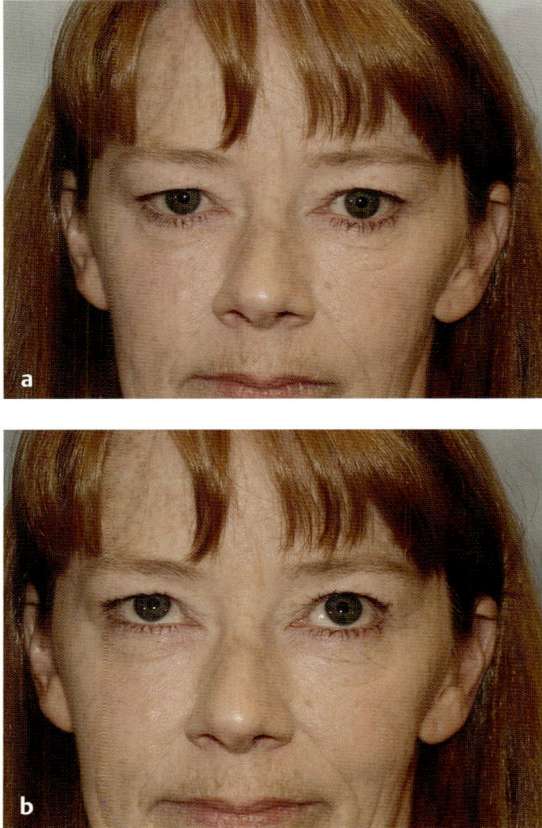

Fig. 24.11 Evidence of excessive or pseudoherniated orbital fat in the nasal fat compartments of the upper eyelids. **(a)** Neutral gaze; **(b)** upward gaze.

abnormal pigmentation, rhytids, malar bags, lacrimal gland ptosis, prominent orbital rims, edema, or any other abnormality or asymmetry. Although some of these issues can be addressed at the time of surgery, some cannot, and it is often beneficial to have all concerns discussed before the time of the procedure.

The consultation is ideally ended with a discussion of diagnoses, surgery or alternative management options, the goals of the management, and the risks of therapy versus no therapy. Further testing, consultations, design of incisions, redundant fat, eyelid position, rhytids, and correction of ptosis should be outlined.

■ Technical Aspects of Procedure

The goals of surgery should again be reviewed with the patient on the day of surgery. There should again be a brief discussion of the diagnoses and corrective plan, and any final concerns of the patient should be addressed. It is usually our preference to address the brow first when the decision has been made to change the position of the brow in conjunction with blepharoplasty. A variety of approaches and techniques are available

for brow correction, each with advantages and disadvantages ▶ **Video 24.1**. The decision to use a particular technique depends on the clinical situation, but further discussion of this topic is beyond the scope of this chapter (**Fig. 24.12**).

Skin Marking

Preoperatively, the amount of excess skin to be excised is determined by examining the patient in the upright position before the eyelids have been injected with any local anesthetic. Planning markings are made with a surgical marking pen. The inferior aspect of the proposed eyelid incisions is marked first. At the central portion of the eyelid, this marking and the subsequent incision are usually placed at, or just inferior to, the supratarsal crease, or 10 mm from the ciliary margin. Medially, this incision is carried to the level of the puncta but no further medially to avoid webbing of the incision. Laterally, in females, the incision is usually carried to approximately 1 cm over the orbital rim and is usually placed in a lateral eyelid crease. In males, the lateral extent of the incision is planned to terminate with only a minimal crossing onto the lateral orbital rim.

In marking the skin, one must verify that eye closure will be complete with the amount of skin excised, and hence, there should be a certain conservatism during the planned marking of the skin (**Fig. 24.13**). The forceps are used to determine the vertical height of the skin to be excised (so-called pinch test). This is done by grasping the skin with a smooth forceps. The tines of the forceps are adjusted to approximate the amount of skin to be removed while maintaining the

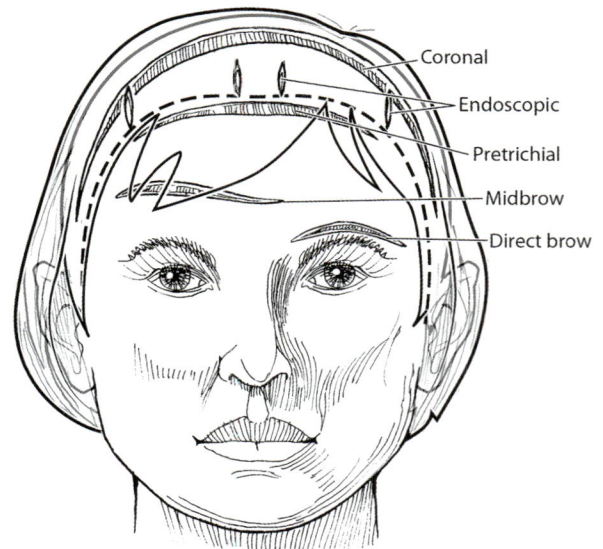

Fig. 24.12 Options for brow lifting. Graphic depicts the position of incisions depending on the technique.

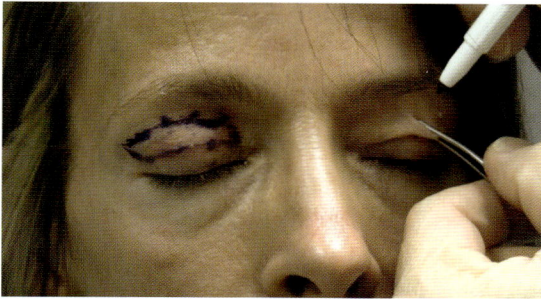

Fig. 24.13 Skin marking of a patient in the upright position prior to blepharoplasty.

lower tine of the forceps on the planned inferior incision and gently pinching the skin. This is repeated at several positions along the eyelid to determine some of the points for the placement of the upper eyelid incision. While the skin is pinched together, the patient's closed eyelid is observed. While the excess skin is held between the tines of the forceps, the eye should be observed to determine whether it can still be closed. The incisions should be limited to the thinner upper eyelid skin and should not extend into the thicker infrabrow skin. Often the thinner eyelid skin that can be removed has a different color and texture than the surrounding skin. The position of the brow should also be noted and should not be disturbed by this process. The amount of skin between the superior and inferior incisions varies between patients. Even in the same patient it can vary between the left and right eyes. It is important to avoid excess skin excision, which can cause lagophthalmos and problems with dryness (**Fig. 24.14a,b**).

Anesthesia

In the authors' practices, simple upper blepharoplasty is commonly performed under local anesthesia with or without oral sedation. Hemostasis and local anesthesia of the eyelids and brow is accomplished through the injection of a solution of 1 to 2% Lidocaine with 1:100,000 epinephrine. Hyaluronidase may be added to the solution to aid the dispersion of the local anesthetic solution in the tissues.

The Incision

The incision is made in the upper eyelid skin with a no. 15 scalpel. Because the skin is very thin, this should be performed with extreme care. The lower incision should be performed first. The lower incision usually cannot be adjusted because it is in the supratarsal crease. The superior limb can be adjusted and hence is performed next.

Removal of the Skin

In the authors' techniques, the skin is removed by blunt dissection using bibeveled scissors. After the section of skin is bluntly undermined, the incision

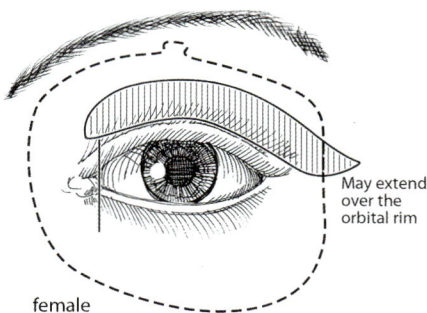

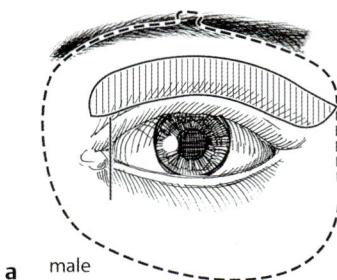

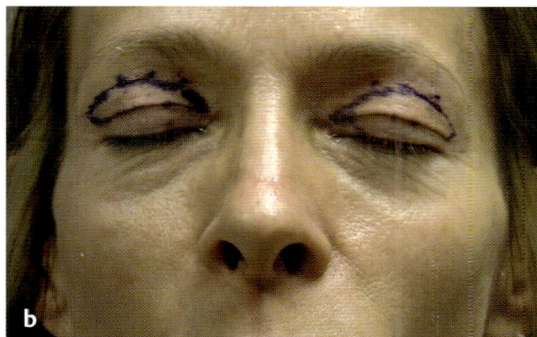

Fig. 24.14 Typical planning for skin excision in male and female patients **(a)** and a patient with completed skin marking prior to blepharoplasty, with slight variability of right and left markings **(b)**.

is completed with the scissors, and the skin is removed. When the removal of the skin is optimally performed, the orbicularis remains intact and can be variably removed as a separate step (**Fig. 24.15a–d**).

Removal of a Strip of Orbicularis

In the course of upper eyelid blepharoplasty, the orbicularis muscle has to be incised to access the orbital fat pads. Some authors will remove a strip of orbicularis at this time to accentuate the superior palpebral sulcus. In accessing the fat pads and during closure, the surgeon has to avoid injury or tethering of the levator apparatus.

In contrast, in certain techniques, such as westernization of the Asian eyelid, it may be necessary to "anchor" the lower incision to the levator aponeurosis during closure to create a supratarsal crease. It should be emphasized that this procedure should not be used for Asians who want to maintain an ethnic appearance.

Opening of the Orbital Septum and Delivery of Excess Fat

Prior to performing surgery, fat protruding from the upper eyelid compartments should be assessed. At surgery, after a strip of orbicularis muscle has been removed, an opening is made in the septum overlying any compartments in which the fat appears to be protruding or in which there was found to be protruding fat on the preoperative evaluation. This can be performed with the same type of small scissors used for the skin elevation and should be performed with meticulous hemostasis. The septum is opened as wide as is necessary using scissors, and the fat pads are sought in the expected locations. The fat is delivered into the wound by applying gentle pressure on the globe, rather than by pulling the fat pad into the wound, which increases the risk for retrobulbar hemorrhage or an undesirable skeletonized appearance. Although some surgeons will perform a gentle dissection with a fine instrument to deliver the excess fat, it is important not to place any traction on the protruding fat.

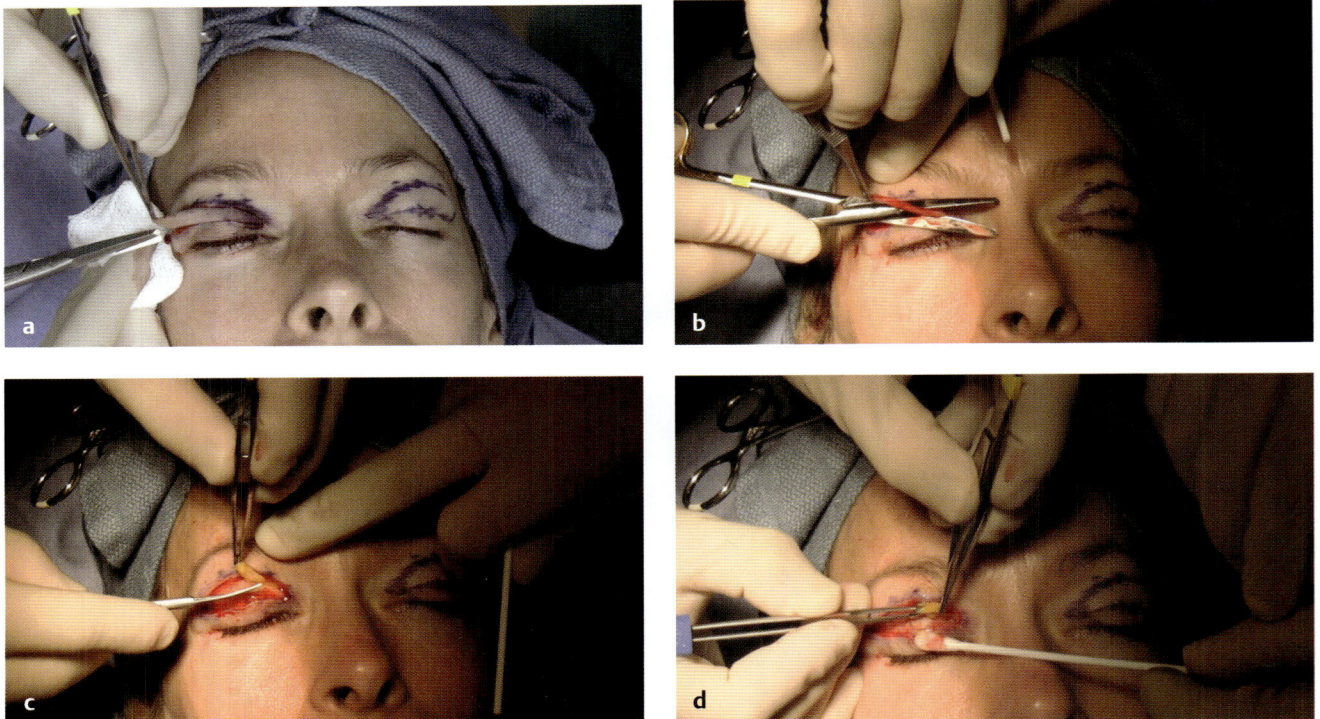

Fig. 24.15 Removal of skin during blepharoplasty after incision and undermining of skin with beveled scissors **(a)**. Removal of thin strip of orbicularis muscle **(b)**. Delivery of a portion of the central fat pad into the surgical field **(c)**. Bipolar cautery of the base of the portion of the fat pad prior to excision **(d)**.

Fat Removal

The protruding fat is teased away from the orbital septum. Lidocaine (1%) without epinephrine can be injected into the extension of the protruding fat outside of the orbital septum because the orbital septum will have provided an effective barrier to the initial local anesthetic injection. The protruding fat is cauterized with bipolar or battery-powered cautery and then cut and removed above the level of cautery with fine scissors.

Hemostasis

Meticulous hemostasis is obtained using bipolar or battery cautery.

Wound Closure

Because the upper eyelid skin is quite thin, the authors do not recommend closure with deep absorbable or permanent suture. External incisions can be closed with absorbable or permanent suture. It is most important that the sutures be removed as soon as the wound is stable to avoid suture marks and milia. The authors prefer the use of a running subcuticular 5 or 6–0 monofilament suture (**Fig. 24.16**).

■ Postoperative Care

Postoperative care is initially very similar to that for other facial surgeries. Conscientious use of iced compresses immediately postoperative and for up to

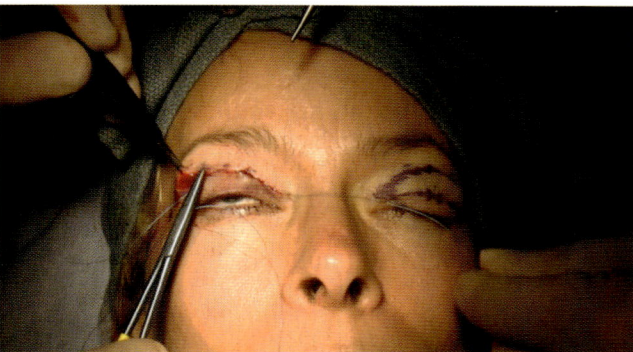

Fig. 24.16 Typical closure of a right upper blepharoplasty incision using monofilament subcuticular suture.

24 to 72 hours thereafter will significantly diminish bruising. Wounds are cared for four to six times a day with swab-applied H_2O_2 and a bland eye ointment. Sutures should be taken out in 5 to 7 days depending on healing and the patient's age. If completely epithelialized, patients can begin to wear makeup after 7 to 14 days. If there is a need to camouflage bruising because of social or job-related commitments, even the most reluctant male patient may be willing to use professional camouflage instruction from a skilled aesthetician or cosmetologist.

■ Expected Results

Attractive, functional eyelids are the goal of blepharoplasty. The eyelids must look natural, attractive, and gender appropriate without the use of makeup or other enhancements. The brows should be symmetrical and positioned at the level of the orbital rim or slightly above. Representative patient preoperative and postoperative photographs demonstrate the favorable results (**Fig. 24.17a–h**; **Fig. 24.18a–h**; **Fig. 24.19a–f**; **Fig. 24.20a–h**; **Fig. 24.21a,b**).

■ Complications and Their Management

All patients undergoing blepharoplasty should be informed of the functional and cosmetic risks. These include scarring, asymmetry, over-/underresection of fat, over-/underresection of skin, drug reactions, contact dermatitis, ecchymosis, hematoma, blindness, lagophthalmos, entropion, eyelid retraction, dry eyes, epiphora, unsightly scars, and milia.

Retrobulbar orbital hematoma is a true, sight-threatening medical emergency. Significant hematoma is usually heralded by the patient's experience of pain, which is not typical after blepharoplasty. In its pronounced and dangerous presentation, the patient will be proptotic. Palpation of the globe will reveal a tense resistance, which is indicative of increased orbital pressures. Emergency management includes some or all of the following interventions, depending on the clinical situation: lateral canthotomy and canthclysis, opening the eyelid wound, intravenous steroids, measurement of intraocular pressures, visual assessment, emergency ophthalmology consultation, and formal bony orbital decompression.

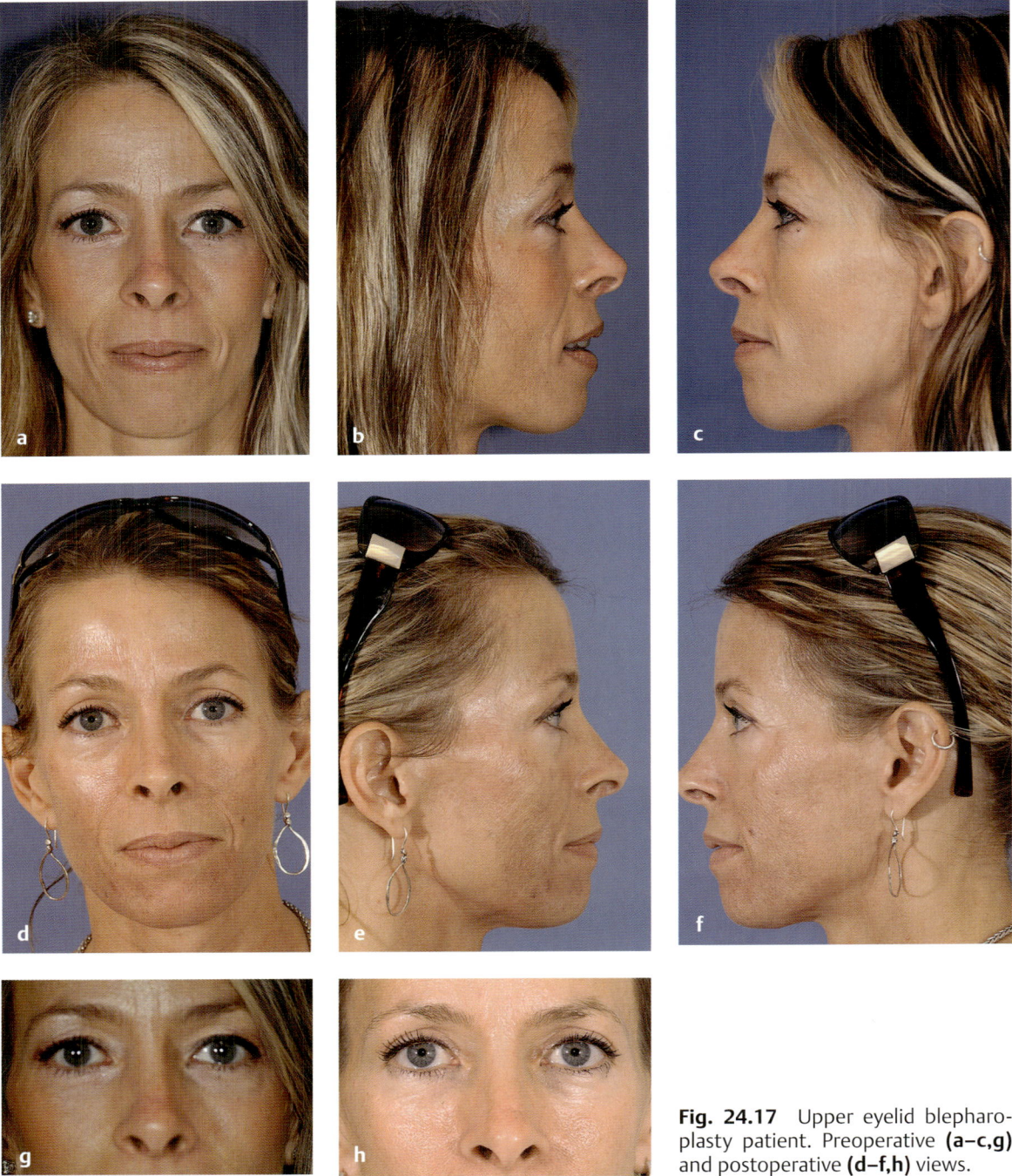

Fig. 24.17 Upper eyelid blepharoplasty patient. Preoperative **(a–c,g)** and postoperative **(d–f,h)** views.

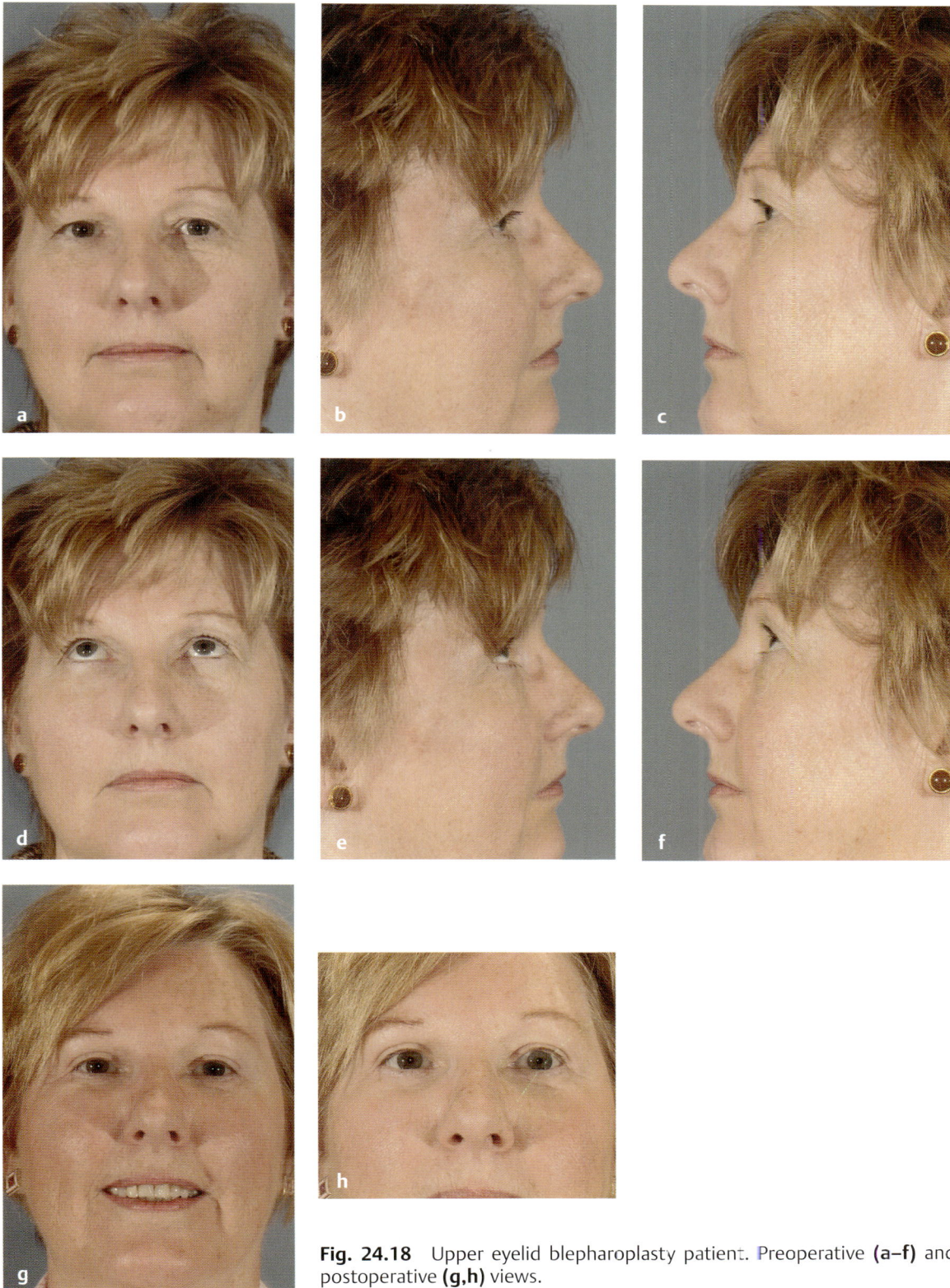

Fig. 24.18 Upper eyelid blepharoplasty patient. Preoperative **(a–f)** and postoperative **(g,h)** views.

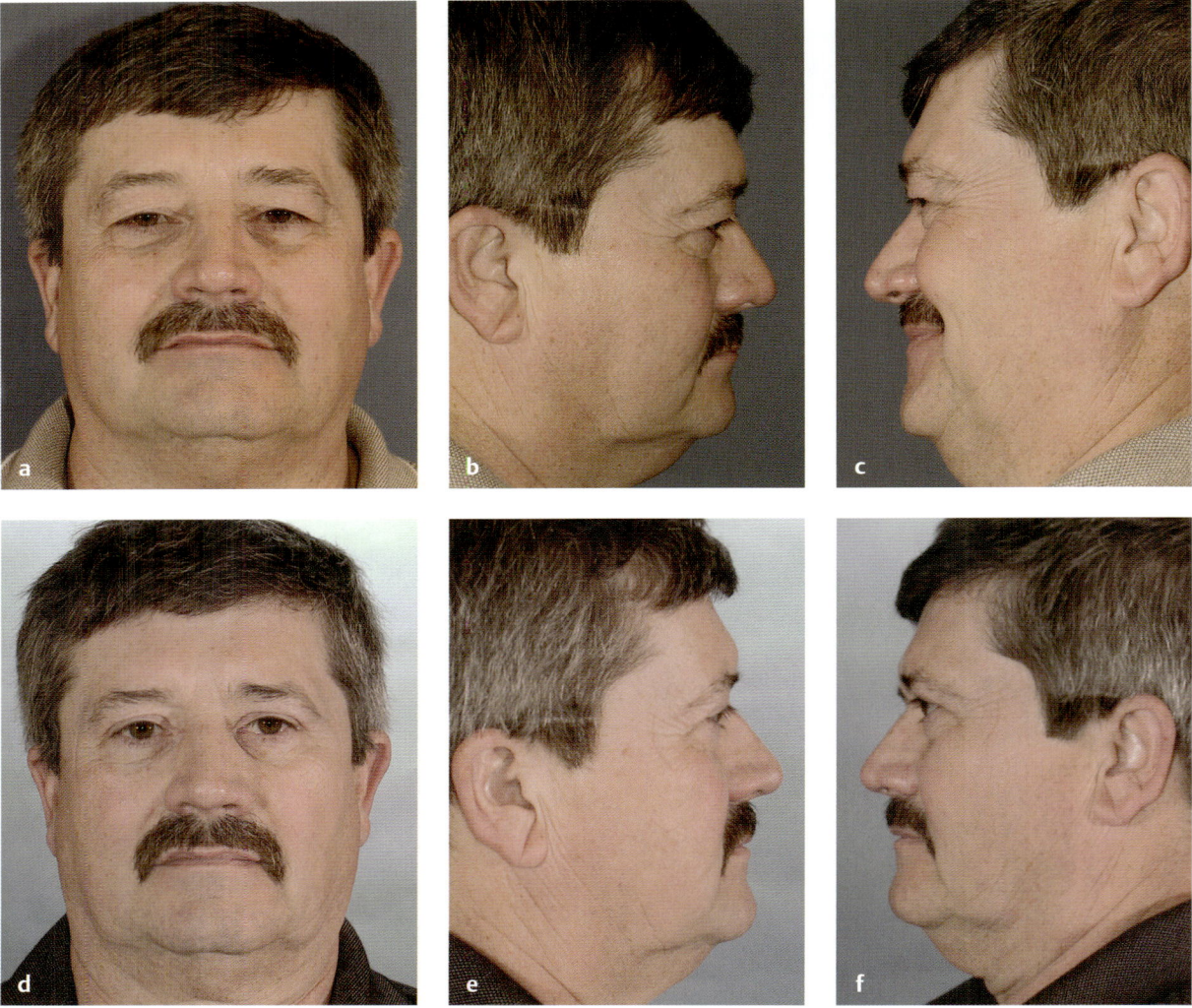

Fig. 24.19 Upper eyelid blepharoplasty patient. Preoperative **(a–c)** and postoperative **(d–f)** views.

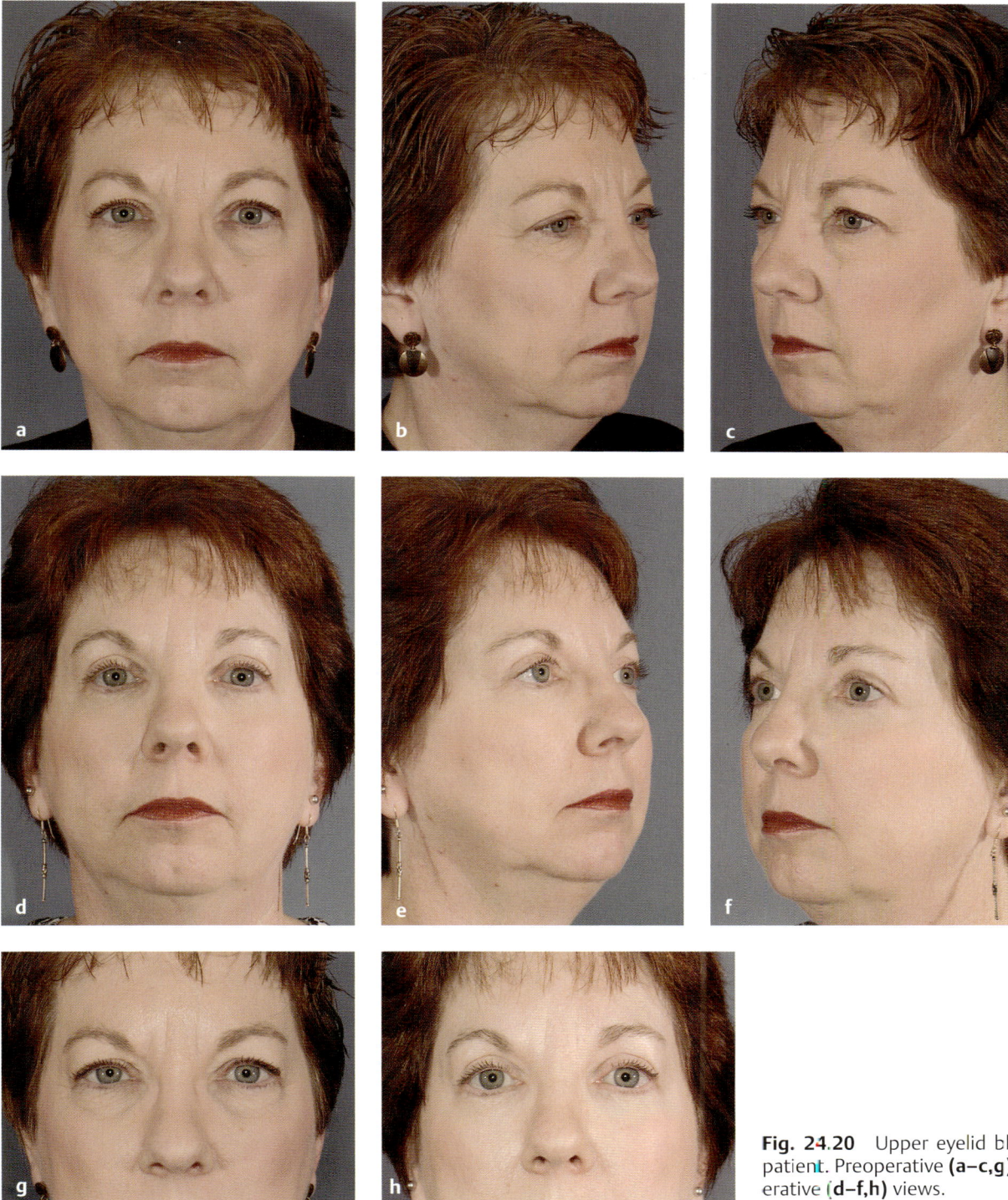

Fig. 24.20   Upper eyelid blepharoplasty patient. Preoperative (a–c,g) and postoperative (d–f,h) views.

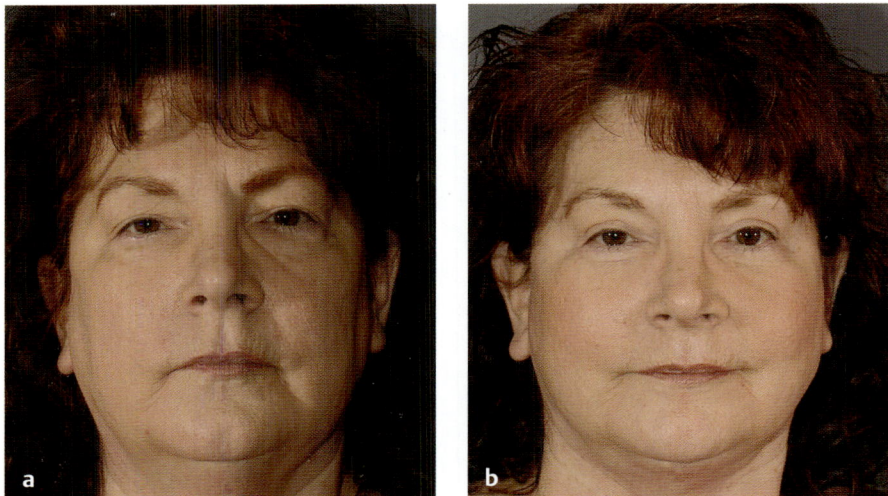

Fig. 24.21 Upper eyelid blepharoplasty patient. Preoperative **(a)** and postoperative **(b)** view.

■ Conclusion

Cosmetic and functional upper blepharoplasty is a rewarding and challenging discipline. Optimal patient selection and application of technique are dependent on a thorough appreciation of the aesthetic and surgical principles of the area. When performed in this fashion the results of upper blepharoplasty surgery are rewarding, and the relative benefits to the patient are enormous. The procedure is among the group of aesthetic procedures that can be safely and expertly performed in the office setting under minimal anesthesia.

References

1. Gentile RD. Upper lid blepharoplasty. Facial Plast Surg Clin North Am 2005;13(4):511–524, v–vi
2. Katzen LB. The history of cosmetic blepharoplasty. Adv Ophthalmic Plast Reconstr Surg 1986;5:89–96
3. Baylis HI, Goldberg RA, Kerivan KM, Jacobs JL. Blepharoplasty and periorbital surgery. Dermatol Clin 1997;15(4):635–647
4. Keller GS. Blepharoplasty and brow lifting. Facial Plast Surg 2010 26(3):175
5. Perkins SW, Prischmann J. The art of blepharoplasty. Facial Plast Surg 2011;27(1):58–66
6. Kerth JD, Toriumi DM. Management of the aging forehead. Arch Otolaryngol Head Neck Surg 1990;116(10):1137–1142
7. Fedok FG. Blepharoplasty in the male patient, male aesthetic surgery. Facial Plast Surg Clin North Am 1999;7(4):442–446
8. Zide BM, Jelks GW. Surgical Anatomy of the Orbit. New York, NY: Raven Press; 1985
9. Most SP, Mobley SR, Larrabee WF Jr. Anatomy of the eyelids. Facial Plast Surg Clin North Am 2005;13(4):487–492, v
10. Ridgway JM, Larrabee WF. Anatomy for blepharoplasty and brow-lift. Facial Plast Surg 2010;26(3):177–185
11. Pastorek NJ. Blepharoplasty update. Facial Plast Surg Clin North Am 2002;10(1):23–27, vii
12. Pastorek N. Upper-lid blepharoplasty. Facial Plast Surg 1996;12(2):157–169
13. McCollough EG, English JL. Blepharoplasty: avoiding plastic eyelids. Arch Otolaryngol Head Neck Surg 1988;114(6):645–648
14. Rohrich RJ, Coberly DM, Fagien S, Stuzin JM. Current concepts in aesthetic upper blepharoplasty. Plast Reconstr Surg 2004;113(3):32e–42e
15. Jelks GW, Jelks EB. Preoperative evaluation of the blepharoplasty patient: bypassing the pitfalls. Clin Plast Surg 1993;20(2):213–223, discussion 224
16. Zukowskl ML. Clinical evaluation of the blepharoplasty patient with brow ptosis. Aesthet Surg J 1998;18(1):51–52

25 Lower Blepharoplasty and Midface Rejuvenation

Christina K. Magill and Jonathan M. Sykes

Key Concepts

- The procedure chosen to rejuvenate the lower eyelid and midface depends on the comfort level of the surgeon and the individual needs of the patient.

- The lower eyelid and midface should be viewed as a single complex.

- Procedures to rejuvenate the lower eyelid–midface complex can be minimally invasive or surgical.

- Correctly diagnosing pathology in the lower eyelid and midface is critical; the surgeon must determine if there is a skin problem, horizontal lower eyelid laxity, excess periorbital fat in relation to the cheek, tear-trough deformity, malar fat pad descent, or a bony problem, such as a negative vector.

- Three-dimensional volume restoration is the aesthetic goal in treating the lower eyelid and midface complex.

◼ Introduction

A vast number of procedures exist to rejuvenate the lower eyelid and the midface. These include minimally invasive techniques, such as injectables and fillers, in addition to a wide array of surgical options. The technique ultimately chosen will depend on the needs of the individual and the preference of the surgeon.

The use of injectables and fillers can provide satisfactory lower eyelid and midface rejuvenation in selected patients. Botulinum toxin can address periocular rhytids when injected laterally. Soft tissue deficiency of the eyelid–cheek junction, often termed tear-trough deformity, can be carefully corrected with fillers. The use of injectables avoids the cost and recovery time of surgery and is a minimally invasive technique for lower eyelid and midface rejuvenation.

In patients with more significant midfacial aging, surgical procedures on the lower eyelid and midface are indicated. A transblepharoplasty, preauricular, or transtemporal approach can be used to access and rejuvenate the midface. The midface can be approached through the lower eyelid in several ways. The transblepharoplasty approach allows for lower eyelid fat removal and fat repositioning. Transblepharoplasty midfacial lifting can be done through a transcutaneous or a transconjunctival incision. Lower eyelid fat repositioning with skin removal and canthal repositioning are also possible through a transblepharoplasty approach. The preauricular and transtemporal approaches allow for a wide vector of tissue suspension and good scar camouflage.

The procedure chosen for lower eyelid and midface rejuvenation should consider the surgeon's comfort level, patient desires and expectations, and the required downtime. In choosing between the available options, the surgeon should assess anatomical and aesthetic needs, and patients should assess cost and their willingness to undergo the procedure(s). This chapter outlines the background of lower eyelid and midface treatment, pertinent anatomy, patient selection, technical aspects of the selected procedure, postoperative care, expected results, and complications.

◼ Background: Basic Science of Procedure

The facial plastic surgery literature describes a variety of strategies for treating the lower eyelid and midface complex.[1] Early literature of midface rejuvenative procedures describes skin-lift-only techniques, usually utilizing a lateral preauricular approach. Surgical techniques to address aging of the lower eyelid and midface have evolved to incorporate dissection and repositioning of the deeper tissues, including a combination of subperiosteal, sub–superficial musculoaponeurotic system (sub-SMAS), and deep plane techniques.[1] In synthesizing the vast options available, the early view of skin excision and tightening has shifted to a modern aim to support, fill, and suspend.[2]

The most important philosophical change in treating the lower eyelid and midface has resulted from the strategy of restoring three-dimensional volume where it has been lost or shifted.[3] Volume restoration can be accomplished surgically with autologous fat or with injectable fillers. The trend of combining surgical lifting with volume restoration has maximized midface rejuvenation while emphasizing natural-appearing results.

■ Pertinent Anatomy

The anatomy of the midface has not changed over time. However, the surgeon's understanding of what anatomical components contribute to midfacial volume has evolved. The lower eyelid and midface are now viewed as a single complex (**Fig. 25.1**). To be successful, the surgeon must understand the anatomical relationships and tissue layers of the midface and lower eyelid, including the aesthetics of the area that change with aging. The six prominent features in midfacial aging include (1) descent of the lower eyelid–cheek junction, leading to a hollowed appearance and attenuation of the infraorbital rim, (2) ptosis of the malar fat pad with loss or change of midfacial projection, (3) exposure and deepening of the tear trough, (4) prominence of the nasolabial fold, (5) midfacial skeletal bone loss, and (6) increase of bony orbit volume.[4,5] Treatment of these changes is based on the underlying anatomical structures involved.

The region of the lower eyelid–cheek complex begins at the lower eyelid margin superiorly and extends to the melolabial fold inferomedially. The medial boundary extends to the cheek–nose junction and is ill-defined. The most lateral aspect of the cheek ends conceptually along the anterior line of the masseter muscle and the frontal projection of the zygoma.

The tissue layers of the lower eyelid and midface guide procedural interventions in the area. In the lower eyelid, the most superficial layer is the skin, followed by the orbicularis oculi muscle (**Fig. 25.2**).[6] Together, the skin and orbicularis oculi muscle compose the anterior lamella of the lower eyelid. The fibrous orbital septum composes the middle lamella and contains the medial, central, and lateral fat pads of the lower eyelid (**Fig. 25.3**).[6] The posterior lamella of the lower eyelid consists of the tarsus, the lower eyelid retractors, and the conjunctiva.

The demarcation of the lower eyelid from the midface can be ill-defined and is created by the cutaneous attachments of the orbitomalar ligament, which is an extension of the infraorbital rim periosteum (**Fig. 25.4**).[6] The orbitomalar ligament forms a horizontal division between the fat pads of the orbit and the suborbicularis oculi fat pad (SOOF) of the upper midface, both of which are deep to the orbicularis oculi muscle. The inferior border of the orbicularis oculi muscle is continuous with the SMAS of the facial musculature. The midface SMAS envelopes the levator labii superioris alaeque nasi, levator anguli oris, and zygomaticus major and minor muscles. Overlying the SMAS in the inferior midface is the triangular malar fat pad. There is also a separate, fixed preperiosteal fat pad beneath the lip elevator musculature.[7]

The relationships between skin, fat compartments, suspensory ligaments, muscle, and bone can lead to aesthetic aging changes in the lower eyelid

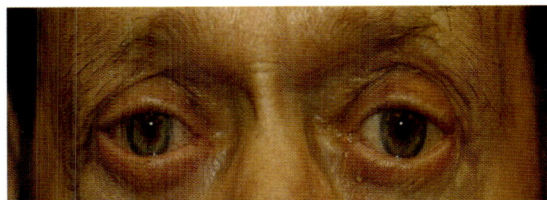

Fig. 25.1 A frontal photograph of a patient with volume deficiency of the midface. He has undergone upper and lower eyelid blepharoplasties in addition to canthal tightening. Tightening or lifting the lower eyelid without addressing the midface can lead to a suboptimal result in patients who need midfacial volume.

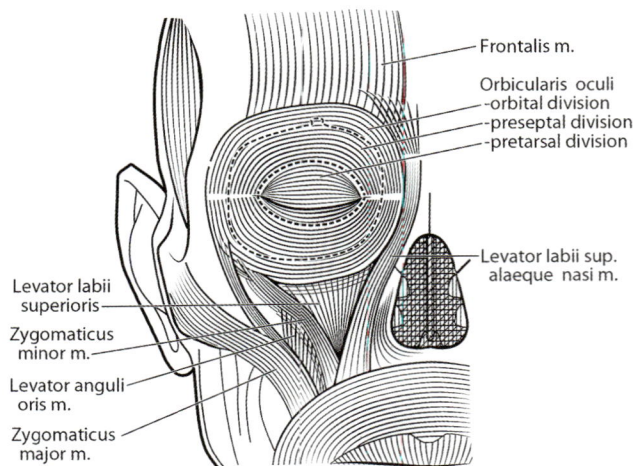

Fig. 25.2 The periocular musculature is shown. The orbicularis oculi has three named parts in surgical nomenclature that are not true anatomical separations: the orbital orbicularis, the preseptal orbicularis, and the pretarsal orbicularis.

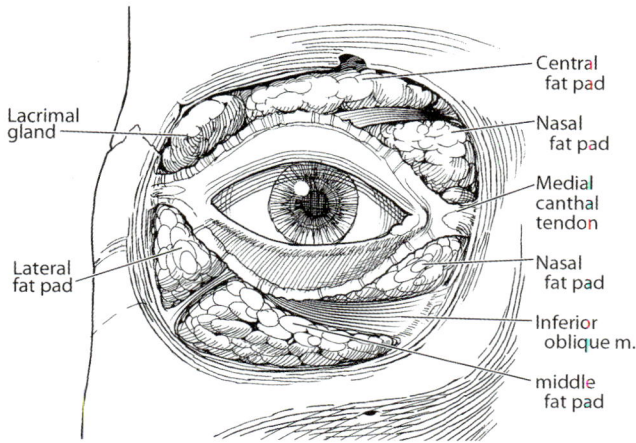

Fig. 25.3 The postseptal compartments of the upper and lower eyelids are shown. The lower eyelid has three fat pads that lie beneath the orbital septum. The nasal fat pad and the central fat pad are separated by the inferior oblique muscle.

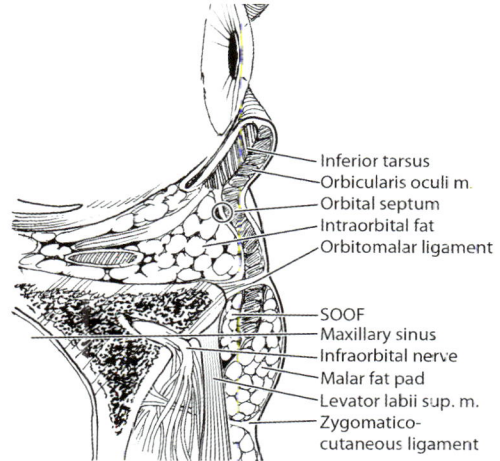

Fig. 25.4 A sagittal section through the lower eyelid and upper midface demonstrates the boundary created by the orbitomalar ligament between the lower eyelid fat pads and the suborbicularis oculi fat pad.

and midface. Correctly diagnosing the underlying anatomical etiology of changes in the lower eyelid–midface complex is critical. Problems that can be addressed include aging or redundancy of the lower eyelid skin (**Fig. 25.5**), horizontal lower eyelid laxity, inferior orbital fat prolapse or pseudoprolapse, the tear-trough deformity[6] (**Fig. 25.6a,b**), midface descent, and the presence of a skeletal negative vector (**Fig. 25.7**). **Table 25.1** provides a brief overview of these common problems, their etiology, and treatments.

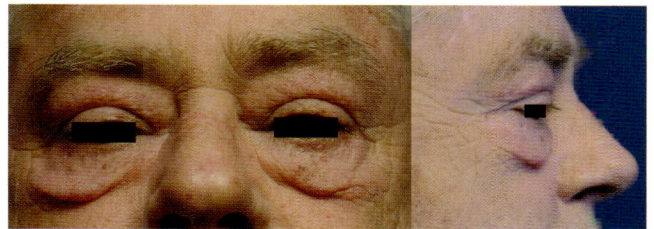

Fig. 25.5 The patient shown has excessive lower eyelid skin that creates prominent lower eyelid "bags." Removal of fat alone would not address the primary pathology of excess lower eyelid skin.

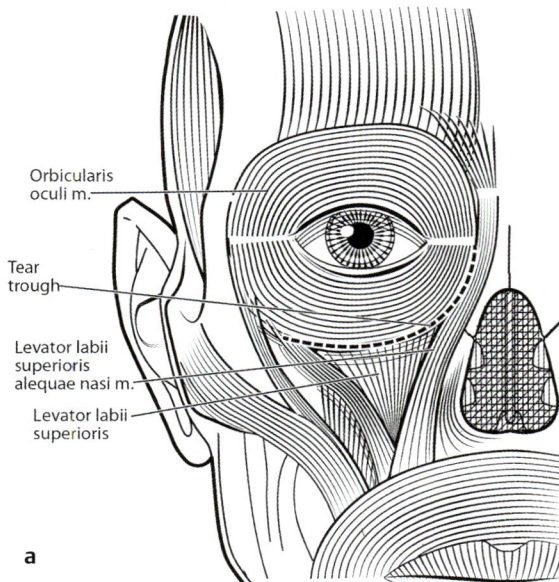

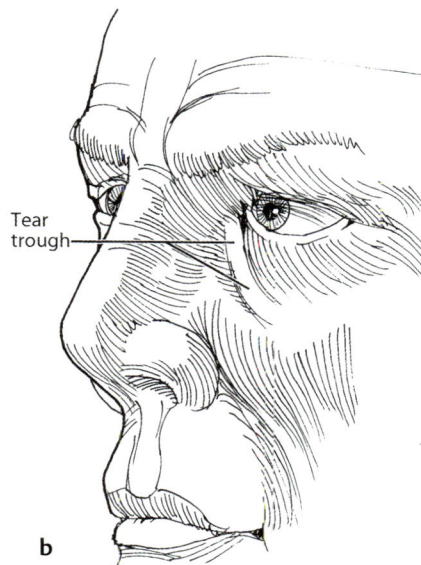

Fig. 25.6 The medial orbicularis oculi muscle and the superior levator labii superioris oblique nasi muscle define the tear trough (a). The tear trough is an area of the medial lower eyelid and midface junction that can become prominent with aging (b).

Table 25.1 Common problems causing aesthetic changes in the lower eyelid–midface complex

Lower eyelid–midface problem	Etiology	Treatment
Skin rhytids	Chronological aging and sun exposure can lead to periorbital fine lines and wrinkles	Skin resurfacing with CO_2 laser or trichloracetic acid peel, botulinum toxin to lateral periocular rhytids
Horizontal laxity	Involutional changes in the tarsus and/or shortening of the anterior lamella	Lateral tarsal strip or canthopexy; midface lift to recruit and support anterior lamellar tissue of the lower eyelid
Inferior orbital fat prolapse	Relaxation of the fibrous orbital septum	Inferior eyelid blepharoplasty (transconjunctival or transcutaneous)
Pseudo–fat prolapse	Edema of the lower eyelid gives the appearance of fat prolapse; pressure to fat pads in the upward gaze does not resolve fullness (as it would in true fat prolapse)	Address underlying cause of edema; possible restoration of midface volume with fillers, fat augmentation, or midface lift to balance inferior eyelid–midface complex
Tear-trough deformity	The groove between the levator labii superioris and levator alaeque nasi muscles can deepen with the herniation of postseptal fat over the orbitomalar ligament, and the descent of prezygomatic fat	Careful injection with hyaluronic acid–based fillers, or fat augmentation
Midface descent	Descent of the buccal fat pad	If hollowed appearance, filler or fat augmentation; possible midface lift
Negative vector	The inferior orbital rim falls posterior to the anterior convexity of the cornea (**Fig. 25.7**)	Cautious and conservative lower eyelid blepharoplasty, fat repositioning, restoration of midface volume to balance negative vector

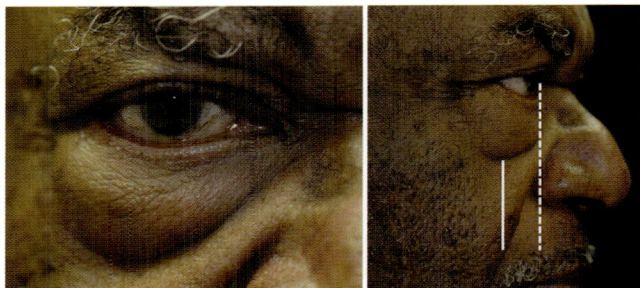

Fig. 25.7 A frontal and lateral view of a patient with ectropion, epiphora, and a prominent negative vector are shown. In the lateral view, the inferior orbital rim (*solid line*) falls posterior to the anterior convexity of the cornea (*dashed line*), thus creating a negative vector.

■ Patient Selection

Successful rejuvenation of the lower eyelid and midface hinges on a correct diagnosis by the surgeon and management of patient expectations. Patients should be made aware of the factors contributing to their aging and the options available to address them. The procedure chosen will depend on the motives of the patient and the comfort level of the surgeon.

Some patients desire a minimal approach, such as an injectable filler for the tear-trough depression or augmentation for generalized malar or inframalar volume loss. Fat augmentation is also an option in these areas. Injection of fillers or fat can be done as an isolated procedure or in combination with other procedures. A minimally invasive approach is excellent for patients who need mild-to-moderate aesthetic correction, desire minimal downtime, and have limited financial resources. Any of these factors may preclude a more involved surgical procedure.

Patients who are amenable to a midface lift need to be informed of the possible approaches, including a transtemporal or blepharoplasty approach. The benefits and risks of each approach and procedure should be discussed. Patients should also be made aware of the specific complications related to each approach so that they can make an informed decision.

Surgery of the lower eyelid can include fat removal, fat transposition, and possible tightening of the lower eyelid if lid laxity is present. The selection of patients for lower eyelid blepharoplasty is dependent on the underlying cause of their aesthetic problem. Taking a thorough ocular history and diagnosing preexisting ocular impairment usually improves outcomes and minimizes complications.

■ Technical Aspects of Procedure

The decision to perform a more invasive surgery versus an injectable procedure is based on a variety of parameters. These include the patient's expectations, the patient's tolerance of undergoing a procedure and have surgical downtime, economic considerations, and the surgeon's preferences and experiences with given procedures and techniques. The ultimate choice in what is selected to rejuvenate the midface should be a synthesis of these important factors. This section will outline the technical aspects of performing lower eyelid blepharoplasty, midface lifting, filler injection, fat augmentation, and botulinum toxin injection.

Lower Blepharoplasty

The prolapse of fat, in addition to lid laxity, can be addressed with a lower eyelid blepharoplasty (**Fig. 25.8**). A blepharoplasty approach can also be used to elevate the soft tissues of the midface. Incisions can be made through the conjunctiva or through the skin. Local anesthetic with intravenous sedation or general anesthetic can be used for the procedure, depending on the extent of work to be done and the comfort level of the patient and surgeon.

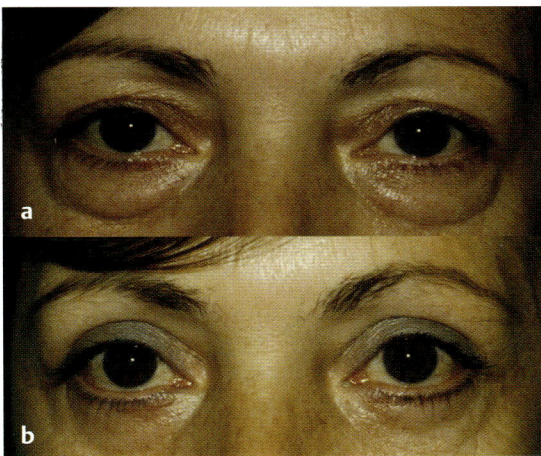

Fig. 25.8 Patient with lower eyelid fat herniation. Preoperative photograph (**a**). Postoperative photograph is shown after the patient has undergone a transconjunctival blepharoplasty with supratarsal fixation (**b**).

Transconjunctival Approach

A transconjunctival approach is the best option for younger patients who have no excess muscle or skin to be excised. Surgical steps include injection of local anesthesia, conjunctival incision, preseptal dissection, orbital fat exposure, fat excision, meticulous hemostasis, and conjunctival closure.

The procedure begins with noting the fat pads to be excised. Topical anesthetic is then placed in the conjunctival cul de sac, and a corneal shield is placed. A 1 mL syringe with a 30-gauge needle is used to gently inject the conjunctiva with Xylocaine 1% (AstraZeneca, Wilmington, DE) with 1:100,000 epinephrine. The injections should be placed in aliquots at the inferior tarsal border. A separate injection is done just beneath the lower eyelid skin. The incision of the conjunctiva at the inferior edge of the tarsal border is done with a no. 15 blade or a protected needle-tipped monopolar cautery on a low setting. Care is taken to avoid extending the incision past the medial aspect of the lower eyelid punctum. A 4–0 nylon or silk horizontal mattress suture is placed in the superior conjunctival edge to retract it superiorly for traction and corneal protection. A preseptal skin and muscle flap is then dissected anteriorly. The orbicularis oculi muscle is separated from the underlying orbital septum and retracted inferiorly with a Desmarres lid retractor. This maneuver helps to expose the orbital septum and underlying lower eyelid fat. The orbital septum is then incised with Westcott scissors just over the bulging fat. The fat pads are gently dissected from their fibrous attachments, and the base of the fat to be removed is cauterized. This maneuver avoids any bleeding and decreases the incidence of hematoma formation. It is advisable to conservatively excise fat to prevent a hollowed out or sunken appearance. Care must also be taken to avoid injury to the superficially located inferior oblique muscle, which lies between the medial and central fat pads. In general, the medial and central fat pads are easy to locate, but the lateral fat pad can be more challenging to identify.

In certain cases, the lower eyelid fat pads can be repositioned rather than removed. This technique diminishes the convexity produced by the herniated fat and augments the hollow, or concave, appearance immediately inferior to the convexity. The transposed fat is secured to the orbital rim or skin–muscle flap to alter the lower eyelid contour. After all aspects of lower eyelid blepharoplasty are performed and adequate hemostasis has been obtained, the conjunctival incision is closed with a medial, central, and lateral interrupted 6–0 fast gut suture.

Transcutaneous Approach

A transcutaneous approach is the best option for patients who have excess muscle or skin, or if eyelid positioning is to be performed. Surgical steps include injection of local anesthesia, subciliary incision, skin–muscle flap with preservation of the pretarsal orbicularis oculi muscle, preseptal dissection, orbital fat exposure, fat excision, meticulous hemostasis, and closure. It is also important to perform a lateral tarsal trip or canthopexy in patients who have lower eyelid laxity.

Before injecting local anesthetic, the position and prominence of the lower eyelid fat pads are assessed. A 1 mL syringe with a 30-gauge needle is used to inject the inferior eyelid skin along the subciliary line with Xylocaine 1% with 1:100,000 epinephrine. Further injection of local anesthetic is performed in the inferior eyelid skin and in any fat pads to be excised. The subciliary incision is made with a scalpel, and a skin-alone or skin/muscle flap can be raised, depending on the goals of the procedure. To remove fat, the orbicularis muscle is raised off the underlying orbital septum. After incising the orbital septum, the fat is then excised or transposed in a manner similar to that previously described in the tranconjunctival approach. After all aspects of fat removal or repositioning have been done, the flap is very conservatively trimmed if any skin excess is present. Great caution is necessary when excising skin to avoid postoperative ectropion. If lid laxity is present, a lateral tarsal strip or canthopexy can be performed. This involves suture fixation of the lateral canthal tendon to the orbital periosteum with a no. 5–0 monofilament long-lasting absorbable suture. The skin incision is then closed with interrupted 6–0 fast gut suture.

Midface Lifting

Transblepharoplasty Approach

The SOOF can be localized and lifted through a transconjunctival or transcutaneous blepharoplasty approach (**Fig. 25.9**) ▶ Video 25.1. After a preseptal dissection is performed to the level of the orbital rim, the SOOF can be accessed and lifted. The SOOF is located directly beneath the orbicularis oculi and inferior to the orbitomalar ligament. The SOOF can be vertically lifted through a preperiosteal or subperiosteal plane. In the preperiosteal plane, the SOOF layer is bluntly dissected and mobilized with a Freer elevator up to 2 to 3 cm below the inferior orbital rim. The mobilized SOOF can then be secured to the periosteum of the lateral orbital rim with an interrupted 4–0 braided or monofilament absorbable suture.

In the subperiosteal plane, the midface is dissected medially and laterally to the level of the infraorbital

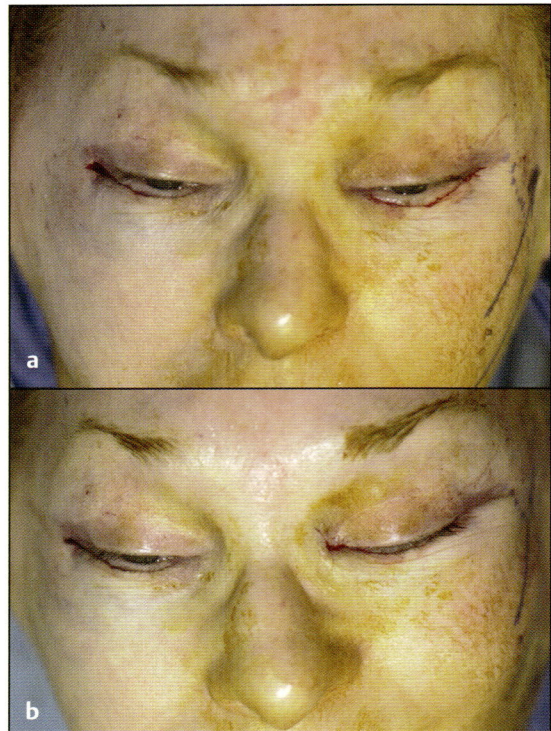

Fig. 25.9 Bilateral transcutaneous lower eyelid blepharoplasties. Intraoperative photograph of bilateral transcutaneous lower eyelid blepharoplasties **(a)**. A left-sided midface lift has been performed through a transconjunctival approach **(b)**.

nerve. A 2 to 3 mm strip of periosteum is left intact at the level of the rim. The dissection is performed inferiorly to the level of the gingival sulcus, at which point the periosteum is stretched or incised to provide any needed release. The superior edge of the dissected periosteal flap is anchored to the rim of intact periosteum using interrupted 4–0. After all aspects of the midface lift have been completed, the incisions made for this approach are closed in a similar manner to that described in the lower eyelid blepharoplasty section of this chapter (**Fig. 25.10a,b**).

Transtemporal Approach

The SOOF and midface can also be accessed from a lateral approach by making an incision behind the temporal hairline, in front of the temporal hairline with a pretrichial incision, or in a preauricular location. The advantage of a transtemporal approach to the midface is that the vector of lift can be both vertical and horizontal, depending on the goal of the surgeon and how suspensory sutures are placed. The surgical steps include injection of local anesthesia, placement of temporal or preauricular incision, dissection along the superficial layer of the deep tem-

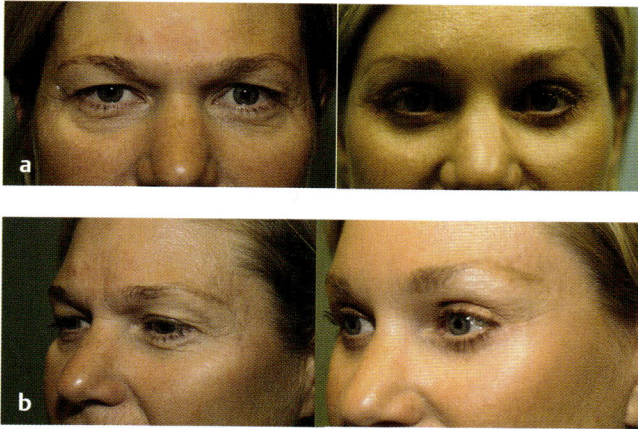

Fig. 25.10 The patient has undergone a brow lift, upper and lower eyelid blepharoplasties, and a transbelpharoplasty midface lift. **(a)** Frontal preoperative and postoperative photographs. **(b)** Oblique preoperative and postoperative photographs.

poralis fascia, blunt dissection over the zygoma deep to the temporoparietal fascia to avoid laceration or sharp injury to the temporal branch of the facial nerve, dissection deep to the orbicularis oculi to access the SOOF, and placement of suspension sutures. The transtemporal approach to the midface can be done as a single procedure, or in combination with a browlift, facelift, or neck lift. The operation may be performed with a patient under conscious sedation or general anesthesia, depending on the extent of the procedure and the comfort of the patient and surgeon.

The design and location of the incision for the transtemporal approach to the midface will depend on the location of the hairline and if any additional procedures are being performed in conjunction with midface lifting. For patients with a lower hairline, the incision can be placed 1.5 cm posterior to the temporal hairline or just in front of the hairline, with care to bevel the incision parallel to the hair follicles to help avoid postoperative alopecia at the location of the incision. For patients with a high hairline or with temporal hair loss, the incision can be placed in a preauricular or pretrichial location.

The transtemporal approach begins with identifying the superficial layer of the deep temporal fascia, which is a thick, shiny white layer of tissue immediately superficial to the temporalis muscle. Dissecting directly onto this layer allows the temporal branch of the facial nerve to be reflected superficially within the temporoparietal fascia and protected. Dissection along the superficial layer of the deep temporal fascia extends to the orbital rim medially and over

the zygoma inferiorly. As the dissection proceeds inferomedially, a plane transition is made to a level beneath the orbicularis oculi muscle. For any dissection over the zygoma, blunt techniques are best employed to help avoid injury to the temporal branch of the facial nerve.

After dissection to expose the SOOF has occurred, suspension can be performed. This is accomplished with a horizontal mattress 2–0 suture placed from the lateral edge of the SOOF to the deep temporal fascia. The number and vector of suspension sutures placed in the SOOF will depend on the patient's anatomy and the goals of the surgeon for midface elevation.

After adequate midface lifting has been performed, the incision is closed with 4–0 suture in the deep dermis and 5–0 or 6–0 nylon in the skin. For incisions behind the hairline, skin staples can also be used. A compressive dressing is placed for 72 hours using gauze sponges and wraps to help prevent hematoma formation.

Fillers and Injectables

Commercially Available Products

There are multiple "off the shelf" fillers available for facial volume restoration. The main chemical components of fillers used in facial augmentation include hyaluronic acid gels (Restylane and Perlane, Medicis Pharmaceutical, Scottsdale, AZ; Juvederm, Allergan, Irvine, CA), poly-L-lactic acid (Sculptra, Sanofi-Aventis U.S., Bridgewater, NJ), calcium hydroxylapatite (Radiesse, Merz Aesthetics, San Mateo, CA), polymethyl methacrylate (Artefill, Suneva Medical, San Diego, CA), and silicone. The hyaluronic acid (HA) gel fillers are a good choice for patients who have never had any previous facial filler. Hyaluronidase can be injected to "reverse" or dissolve the HA filler if necessary. HA fillers can be injected into the tear trough to correct a deformity or into the dermis or deeper tissue of the melolabial fold to improve the aesthetic appearance of the midface. For patients with temporal wasting or a gaunt appearance of the midface, injectable poly-L-lactic acid may be used. Sculptra is injected deep, along the periosteum of the maxilla, and usually requires multiple injections to promote neocollagen formation and give patients increased facial volume. Calcium hydroxylapatite is a viscous, white filler that can be used for deep plane facial injection. It is not reversible and can cause firm nodules in the skin if injected too superficially. Lastly, the use of silicone for facial augmentation has been stigmatized by the severe complications associated with its misuse. If it is injected too superficially, or becomes infected, it is often difficult to reverse or correct.

Autologous Fat

The midface and periorbital areas can be treated with autologous fat injections to restore volume and promote a more youthful facial appearance (**Fig. 25.11a,b**). Autologous fat can also be used in other regions of the face, such as the lips and temporal hollows, to create volume and improve contour.[8]

Fat can be harvested from the lateral thigh and abdomen and injected into regions of the face that are volume deficient. The advantages of fat are that it is autologous tissue and there is the potential for long-lasting results. The disadvantages include the need for a donor site and the potential donor-site morbidity. The patient should be counseled that the duration of fat injection into the face can be variable, and for a large-volume restoration, more than one session of fat augmentation may be necessary.

The midface responds well to fat augmentation, and the surgeon can place fat in multiple layers to create a natural, rejuvenated appearance. The periorbital area should be injected very carefully because fat grafts survive well in this area, and the thin skin of the lower eyelid can produce visible and palpable irregularities. If fat is injected unevenly, or if lumps form, they can be very difficult to treat and sometimes require surgical excision. During treatment of the face, the fat injection cannula should be directed away from the globe. When obtaining fat from the donor site, care should be taken to avoid deep-tissue injury to thigh muscle, or into the peritoneum from abdominal harvest.

Botulinum Toxin

The use of botulinum toxin can help improve dynamic wrinkles in the face by providing a temporary denervation of muscles. Botulinum toxin acts to inhibit the release of acetylcholine from presynaptic motor terminals and has an effect in ~ 2 to 7 days following injection. The duration of chemical denervation is generally 3 to 4 months. Common sites of botulinum toxin injection include the glabella, forehead, and periorbital areas (**Fig. 25.12**).

Several different preparations of botulinum type A are commercially available and approved by the U.S. Food and Drug Administration (FDA). Botox Cosmetic (Allergan, Irvine, CA) is a form of onabotulinum toxin A and comes in 100 unit vials that can be diluted with normal saline. Dysport (Medicis Aesthetics, Scottsdale, AZ) is a form of abobotulinum toxin A and comes in 300 unit vials. It is important to realize that different brands of commercially available botulinum toxin are not equal in strength, duration, and effect per unit. The term "unit" is a proprietary measurement that differs between preparations of neurotoxin. For example, one unit of Botox Cosmetic

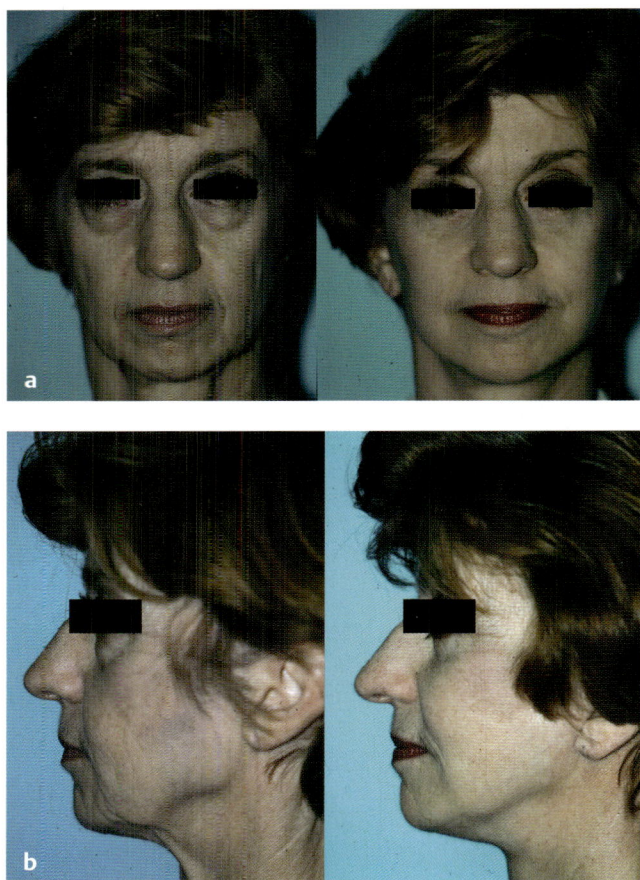

Fig. 25.11 Double contour. **(a)** Frontal preoperative and postoperative photographs are shown of a woman with a "double contour." (*Left*) The inferior eyelid fat has prolapsed anteriorly, and the cheek has descended. (*Right*) The patient has undergone a lower eyelid blepharoplasty with canthal tightening, a transblepharoplasty midface lift, a neck lift, and facial fat augmentation. **(b)** Lateral preoperative and postoperative photographs of the woman with a "double contour." (*Left*) The inferior eyelid fat has prolapsed anteriorly, and the cheek has descended. (*Right*) The patient has undergone a lower eyelid blepharoplasty with canthal tightening, a transblepharoplasty midface lift, a neck lift, and facial fat augmentation.

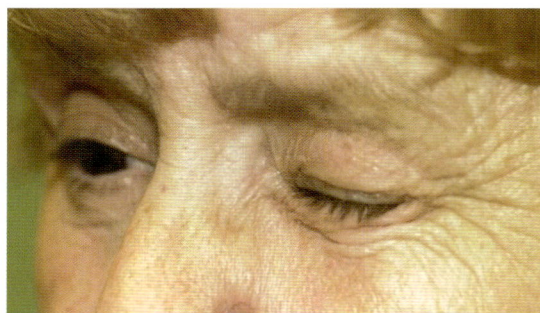

Fig. 25.12 Left hemifacial spasm. Blepharospasm can be treated with injections of botulinum toxin.

is roughly equivalent to 2.5 to 3 units of Dysport.[9] Xeomin is a form of incobotulinum toxin (Merz, Greensboro, NC) that comes in 50 unit and 100 unit vials. Xeomin has a similar dosing to Botox Cosmetic and is FDA-approved for cervical dystonia, blepharospasm, and the treatment of glabellar lines. The amount of toxin injected ultimately depends on how much normal saline is added to the crystalline product that is prepackaged in the vial. A more concentrated injection will have less diffusion potential but a higher risk of untoward side effects if imprecisely injected.

Postoperative Care

For surgical patients, postoperative care of wounds is important. Individuals who have undergone lower eyelid blepharoplasty should be advised to avoid strenuous activity for 3 weeks after the surgery to lessen the risk of postoperative bleeding, breaking of tension-bearing sutures, or wound dehiscence. Patients are instructed to avoid rubbing the eyelids and can apply ice to minimize bruising or edema. In cases of midface lifting, the patient may require a dressing for 72 hours to provide pressure to the temple or preauricular areas, which are most at risk for a hematoma.

Patients who have received filler or injectables should be counseled about the duration of effects and may also be instructed to perform postprocedural massage in the areas injected with filler. For those patients who receive botulinum toxin, it is generally recommended to have the head elevated for 4 hours after the injection.

Expected Results

Managing a patient's expectations is essential. Good communication can help foster satisfaction for both the patient and the surgeon. Open and honest discussion about the expected effects and limitations of a given procedure is always advisable. The surgeon should not "oversell" a procedure or product.

For many patients who desire a change to the lower eyelid and midface complex, the overlying skin is also bothersome. It is important to point out that wrinkles and the quality of the skin will persist even with stretching the skin from surgery.

Complications and Their Management

Even the most experienced and technically proficient surgeon will encounter complications. In surgery of the eyelid, malposition of the eyelid margin may occur (**Figs. 25.13** and **25.14**). Early eyelid malposition may respond to massage and time. Steroid injection may be necessary to treat granulomas or unfavorable scars.

In surgical approaches to the midface, nerve damage may result from injury to the temporal branch of the facial nerve or the infraorbital branch of the trigeminal. Nerve injuries may be short term or long lasting, and a patient should be followed closely to monitor for recovery. Patients who have undergone midfacial lifting may experience contour irregularities, suture granulomas, infection, or inadequate or unsatisfactory results. The overall goal in managing a patient with complications is to be involved in the process of recovery, available for frequent postoperative visits, and willing to refer or consult with colleagues if necessary.

Conclusion

Given the variety of possibilities for treating the lower eyelid and midface complex, the ultimate choice will depend on the wishes of the patient and the comfort level of the surgeon. Knowing the underlying anatomy and pathology leading to aesthetic changes guides interventions in the lower eyelid and midface complex.

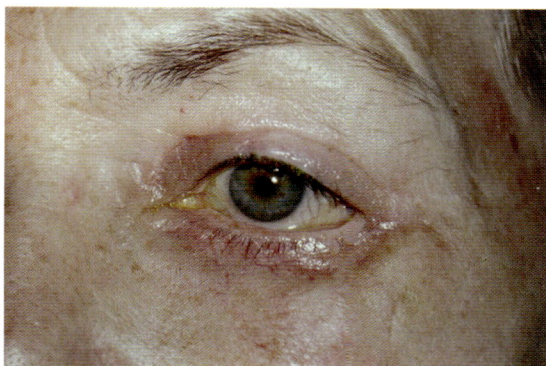

Fig. 25.13 Postoperative photograph taken 1 month after upper and lower eyelid blepharoplasty. Excess skin removal has resulted in lower eyelid malposition and ectropion.

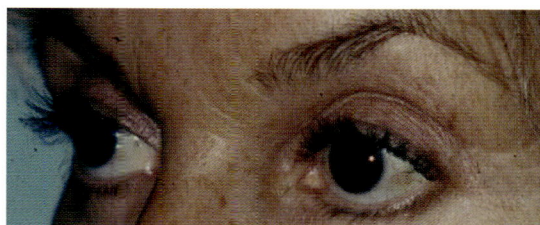

Fig. 25.14 Postoperative photograph of a patient who had overaggressive upper and lower eyelid blepharoplasty. The surgery has resulted in lower eyelid malposition and scleral show.

References

1. Paul MD, Calvert JW, Evans GRD. The evolution of the mid-face lift in aesthetic plastic surgery. Plast Reconstr Surg 2006;117(6):1809–1827

2. Coleman SR. The technique of periorbital lipoinfiltration. Oper Tech Plast Reconstr Surg 1994;1:120–134

3. Little JW. Three-dimensional rejuvenation of the midface: volumetric resculpture by malar imbrication. Plast Reconstr Surg 2000;105(1):267–285, discussion 286–289

4. Hester TR Jr, Codner MA, McCord CD, Nahai F, Giannopoulos A. Evolution of technique of the direct trans-blepharoplasty approach for the correction of lower lid and midfacial aging: maximizing results and minimizing complications in a 5-year experience. Plast Reconstr Surg 2000;105(1):393–406, discussion 407–408

5. Pitanguy I, Pamplona D, Weber HI, Leta F, Salgado F, Radwanski HN. Numerical modeling of facial aging. Plast Reconstr Surg 1998;102(1):200–204

6. Codner MA, Ford DT. Blepharoplasty. In: Thorne C, ed. Grabb and Smith's Plastic Surgery. 6th ed. Philadelphia, PA: Lippincott Williams & Wilkins; 2007:486–498

7. Pacella SJ, Codner MA. Anatomy of the upper and lower eyelids. In: Codner M, ed. Techniques in Aesthetic Plastic Surgery Series: Midface Surgery. Philadelphia, PA: Saunders; 2009

8. Coleman SR. Structural fat grafting: more than a permanent filler. Plast Reconstr Surg 2006;118(3, Suppl):108S–120S

9. Karsai S, Raulin C. Botox and Dysport: is there a dose conversion ratio in dermatology and aesthetic medicine? J Am Acad Dermatol 2010;62(2):346–347

26 Avoidance and Management of Complications Following Lower Eyelid Surgery

Farzad R. Nahai

Key Concepts

- An understanding of the anatomy and function of the eyelids is necessary for safety and avoidance of complications.

- It is important to appreciate the potential aesthetic and functional effects of lower lid surgery.

- The surgeon should be able to perform a thorough preoperative evaluation of the patient considering lid surgery.

- The canthal anchor is a critical aspect of lid surgery and plays a functional and aesthetic role.

- The common complications of lower eyelid surgery are addressed and methods to avoid them are presented.

Introduction

Aesthetic eyelid surgery is consistently one of the top five plastic surgery procedures performed yearly.[1] Lower eyelid aesthetic procedures are particularly effective at generating a more youthful appearance. The procedures are unique in that they have both *aesthetic* and *functional* consequences. If the procedures are performed well in the proper setting and on the right patient, beautiful and pleasing results can be obtained that maintain, and in some cases improve, proper lid function. Understanding the regional anatomy, performing a proper patient evaluation, and constructing a sound operative plan all play a significant role in avoiding complications in lower lid surgery. Nevertheless, complications do occur, and understanding how to recognize and treat them is crucial for positive outcomes.

Background: Basic Science of Procedure

The goal of lower lid aesthetic procedures is to restore a youthful appearance to the eyelid and maintain proper lid function. The youthful eye typically has smooth curves; an open, bright, and rested appearance; some degree of pretarsal lid show; a neutral or upward canthal tilt; and a lid–cheek junction that is smooth and without demarcation. There are many procedures for lower lid rejuvenation, and the most effective ones address each anatomical feature that contributes to an aged appearance (**Table 26.1**). It is up to the surgeon to ascertain the patient's desires and to conduct the physical exam and overall evaluation and to develop a surgical plan that will meet the patient's expectations while minimizing the risk of complications.

Pertinent Anatomy

The lower eyelid is divided into three layers, commonly referred to as the outer, middle, and posterior lamellae. The outer lamellae is made up of skin and the underlying orbicularis muscle, the middle lamella is the orbital septum, and the posterior lamellae is made up of the lower lid retractors and conjunctiva. The aperture of the eye is based on how the lids frame the globe. Normal lid position covers 1 to 2 mm of the upper and lower corneoscleral limbus, creating the medial and lateral scleral triangles, the lateral being slightly larger in general. Furthermore, the youthful eyelid generally has an upward canthal tilt, but not always (**Fig. 26.1**).

The orbicularis muscle serves two principal functional roles, for passive and purposeful eyelid closure and as a lacrimal pump that facilitates the progress of tears from the lacrimal gland, across the globe, out

Table 26.1 Surgical options in lower lid blepharoplasty

Spectrum of choices	Increasing complexity of procedure
Skin/muscle/orbicularis flap with fat redistribution, full cheek lift with primary spacer graft and canthal anchor	
Skin/muscle/orbicularis flap with fat redistribution and full cheek lift and canthal anchor	
Skin/muscle/orbicularis flap with fat redistribution and canthal anchor	
Skin/muscle/orbicularis flap with canthal anchor	
Skin/muscle take out	
Transconjunctival	
Skin pinch	

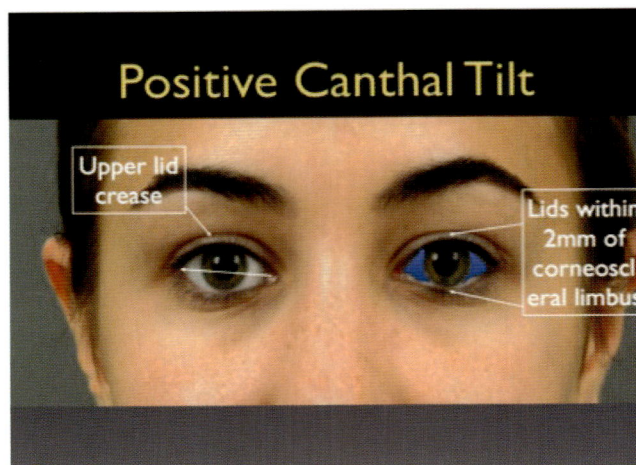

Fig. 26.1 Normal eye shape and lid position. The upper and lower lids should be within 1 to 2 mm of the corneoscleral limbus. Canthal tilt, the slope between the medial canthus and lateral canthus, is typically upward or neutral, but not always. The lateral scleral triangle is typically larger than the medial scleral triangle.

the lid punctum, and through the tear ducts into the lacrimal sac and nasal cavity. To further understand the orbicularis function, it can be divided based on anatomical location in two ways: (1) a concentric model, labeling the pretarsal, preseptal, and orbital orbicularis based on the underlying anatomy; and (2) an innervation-based model, based on the zygomatic branches of the facial nerve that innervate the extracanthal orbicularis and the buccal branches that innervate the inner-canthal orbicularis. This division in innervation (and, to a lesser degree, the division based on the concentric model of labeling) is reflected in a division of labor within the orbicularis. The extracanthal orbicularis (innervated diffusely by the zygomatic branches of the facial nerve) is responsible for purposeful and forceful eyelid closure (i.e., hard squinting in direct sunlight), whereas the inner-canthal orbicularis is responsible for minute-to-minute reflexive blinking that maintains the tear film and activates the lacrimal pump (**Fig. 26.2a–d**). Injury (surgical or otherwise) to the former mechanism has minimal functional impact; injury to the latter mechanism can have severely detrimental functional consequences.

For the lid to function properly in closure, three aspects must work together: a stimulus (the nerve), a motor (the muscle), and an anchoring mechanism (the canthal apparatus). The canthal apparatus is made up of the medial and lateral canthus (with direct bony attachments based on the canthal tendons) and the tarsoligamentous sling that spans

between them. When stimulated, the orbicularis muscle contracts in a horizontal fashion. However, the lid must traverse vertically across the convexity of the globe. The translation of a horizontal force into vertical movement of the eyelids is dependent on a stable and fixed medial and lateral canthus (**Fig. 26.3**), without which complete eyelid closure cannot be achieved, resulting in fish-mouth lid closure and beady-eye syndrome (**Fig. 26.4**).

■ Patient Selection

One of the most critical means by which to avoid complications from lower eyelid surgery is proper preoperative patient evaluation. This starts with taking a history that documents previous lid surgery, use of corrective lenses, previous refractive corneal surgery, and a history of dry eye. A history of dry eye requiring use of eye lubricants is an indication for preoperative punctal plugs to avoid severe dry eye postoperatively. Corneal refractive surgery temporarily renders the cornea insensate, inhibiting its protective mechanism. Thus, cosmetic eyelid surgery should be delayed for at least 6 months to minimize the risk of the corneal injury.

The physical exam includes an assessment of the Bell phenomenon, lid laxity, globe prominence, visual acuity, and midface vector. The Bell phenomenon, which is the upward tilt of the globe during lid clo-

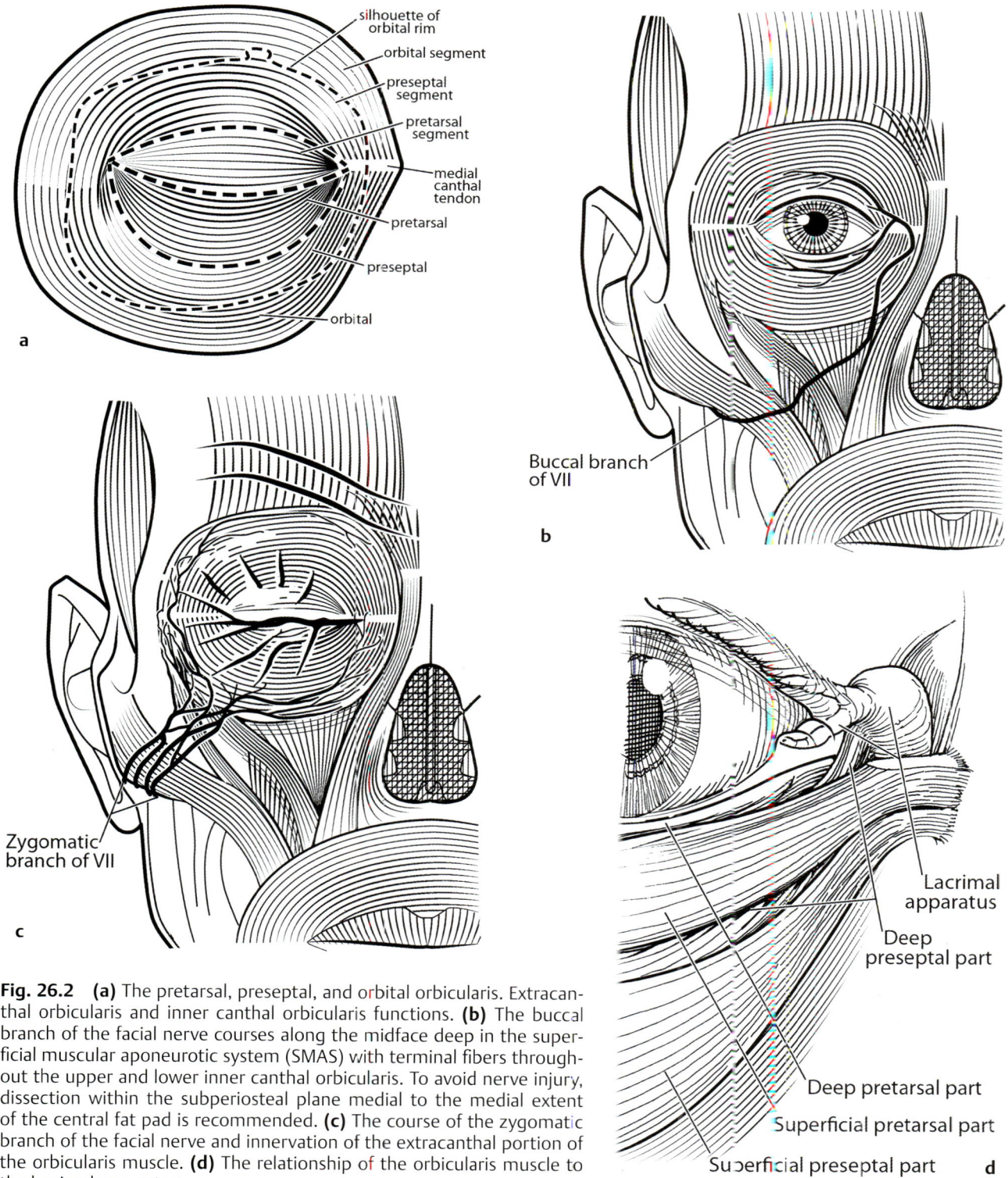

Fig. 26.2 **(a)** The pretarsal, preseptal, and orbital orbicularis. Extracanthal orbicularis and inner canthal orbicularis functions. **(b)** The buccal branch of the facial nerve courses along the midface deep in the superficial muscular aponeurotic system (SMAS) with terminal fibers throughout the upper and lower inner canthal orbicularis. To avoid nerve injury, dissection within the subperiosteal plane medial to the medial extent of the central fat pad is recommended. **(c)** The course of the zygomatic branch of the facial nerve and innervation of the extracanthal portion of the orbicularis muscle. **(d)** The relationship of the orbicularis muscle to the lacrimal apparatus.

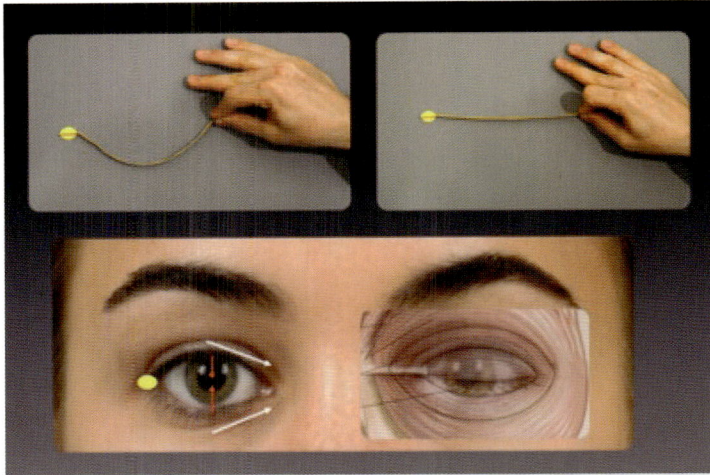

Fig. 26.3 A demonstration of eyelid mechanics and the importance of the canthal anchor. For the lid to close properly, three aspects of the lid must be working; the stimulus (nerve input), the motor (muscle contraction), and a fixed counter pull (the canthal anchor). Given the concentric orientation of the orbicularis muscle, it generates a horizontal force across the lid (*white lines*). In order for the horizontal force to translate into vertical motion of the lid (*red lines*), the muscle must have a fixed point that acts as a counter (*yellow dot*). That mechanical effect is demonstrated in the analogy of the rubber band (the lid) being pulled horizontally by the hand (the muscle) resulting in upward movement of the rubber band. Lack of an adequate canthal anchor can result in incomplete eyelid closure (fish-mouthing) and a rounded or small lateral scleral triangle (beady-eye syndrome).

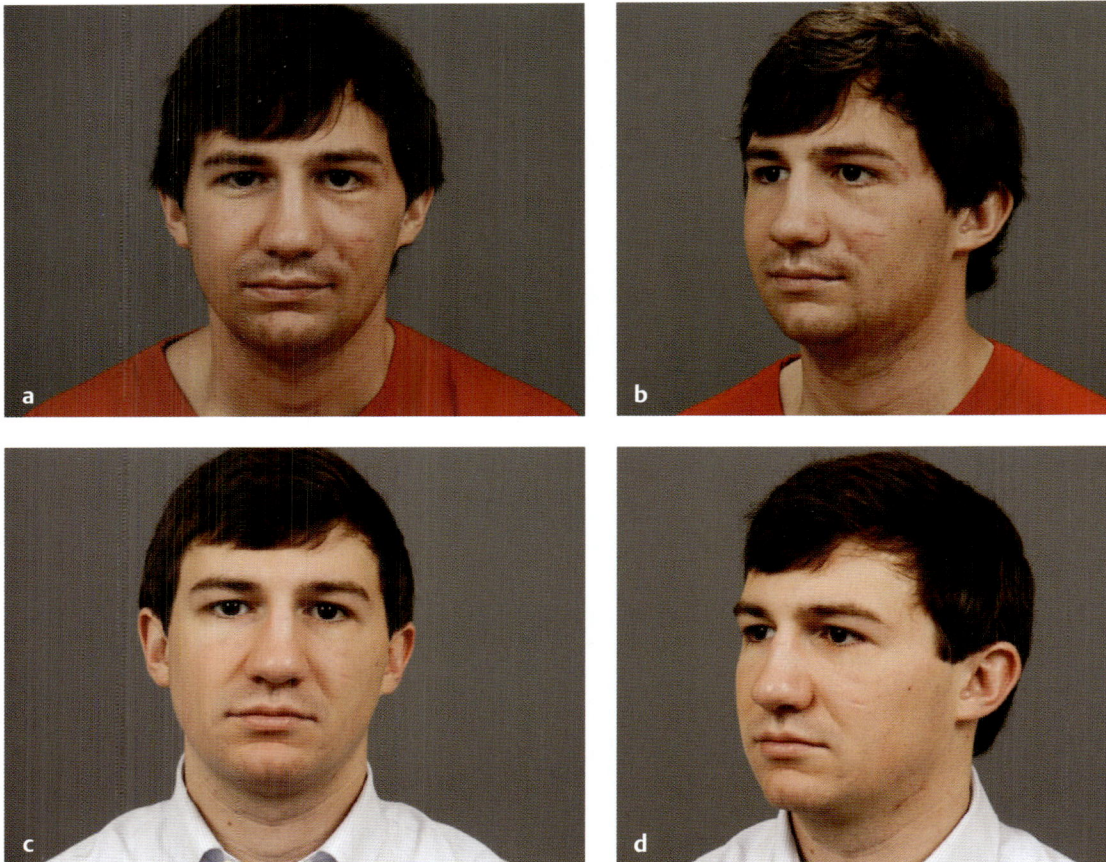

Fig. 26.4 **(a)** Lateral oblique and **(b)** anteroposterior views of a 29-year-old man who experienced trauma to his left orbit from a snowboarding accident. He had an initial procedure elsewhere to repair his orbital floor and zygoma fractures through an open lower lid approach. As a result he had left lower lid malposition. After several months of massage and conservative management, he had left lower lid reconstruction with an Enduragen spacer graft, canthopexy, and mid-face advancement through an open approach **(c)**. He is shown 6 months postoperatively **(d)**.

sure, is intact in ~ 80% of the population. This response is corneoprotective, and when it is not intact, the cornea is put at higher risk for exposure during the early postoperative recovery period when the eyelids can be stiff and prone to lagophthalmos and poor closure. Visual acuity can be easily assessed before surgery. When documented, it can be readily referenced in case any changes in visual acuity occur after surgery.

Most critical to avoiding lower lid complications are four clinical aspects: lower lid tone, globe position, midface vector, and prior lid surgery. Recognizing poor lower lid tone preoperatively and addressing it formally intraoperatively are key to avoiding lower lid malposition and ectropion. Scleral show (lid position below the level of the corneoscleral limbus) at baseline and distraction of the lower lid beyond 10 mm from the globe are de facto evidence of poor lower lid tone.

Another method to assess lower lid tone is the snap test. Normally, when the lower lid is distracted from the globe, it will snap back to baseline position on its own. In the patient with poor lower lid tone, the lid will not snap back on its own and will only take up a baseline position after an active blink (**Fig. 26.5**).

Globe position also affects lid position. A Hertel exophthalmometer can be used to measure the relative position of the globe to the bony orbit. Normal (euophthalmos) is 15 to 19 mm, enophthalmos is less than 15 mm, and exophthalmus is 20 mm or greater. The exophthalmic patient presents certain challenges to proper lid positioning and often requires special attention during lid surgery. Tightening the lower lid in a prominent-eye patient can easily lead to a clothesline effect of the lid position relative to the globe and result in lid malposition (**Fig. 26.6**).

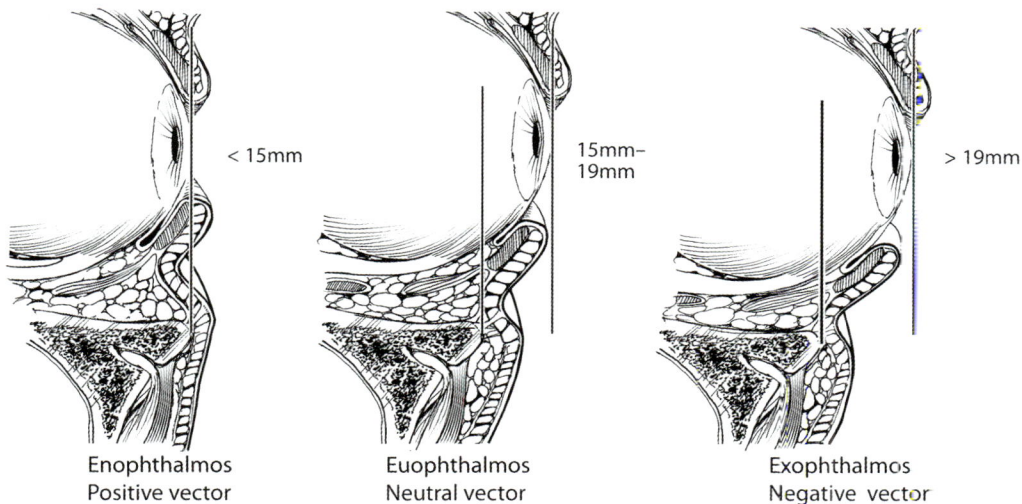

Poor lower lid tone

- Greater than 10mm of displacement with downward distraction
- Snap test: incomplete recovery of lower lid position

Fig. 26.5 An example of poor lower lid tone. The lid is displaceable > 10 mm away from the globe (*left*). A snap test that demonstrates incomplete recovery of the lid position (without blink) is indicative of poor lid tone (*right*).

The negative vector midface presents a similar challenge. Sometimes referred to as a polar bear midface, a heavy midface with a lack of midfacial skeletal prominence creates a negative vector slope and extra pull and downward drag on the lower lid.

Lastly, a history of previous eyelid procedures places the patient at significantly higher risk for postoperative complications. The presence of scar tissue, previous skin resection, skin resurfacing of the eyelid, prior canthal procedures, and even fat or filler injections, can all

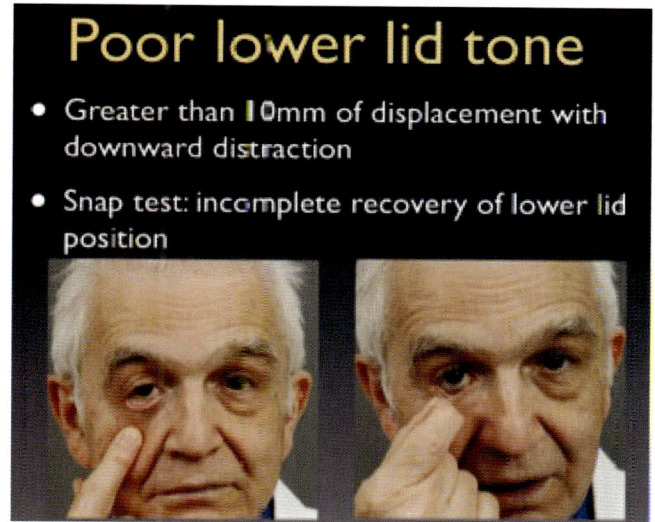

Enophthalmos
Positive vector

< 15mm

Euophthalmos
Neutral vector

15mm–19mm

Exophthalmos
Negative vector

> 19mm

Fig. 26.6 Differences in projection of the orbital rim relative to the projection of the globe.

conspire to make lid surgery more technically challenging and increase the risks of lid position and functional complications. Typically, secondary lid procedures should be performed more conservatively and with specific planning to address preexisting or intraoperative lid findings. Identifying these four clinical aspects and designing an operative plan to address them goes a very long way to minimizing lower lid complications.

■ Technical Aspects of Procedure

Once a thorough patient evaluation has been performed and the patient's goals have been taken into account, an operative plan can be constructed. There are many surgical options for aesthetic lower eyelid surgery (**Table 26.1**). In addition to patient factors, the operative plan must also take into account the surgeon's comfort level with a given procedure. Aspects of technique to consider during surgical planning are access incisions, tissue plane of dissection, the extent of dissection, management of the periorbital fat, canthal support, and concomitant procedures ▶**Video 26.1**.

Two of the common incisions used in lower lid blepharoplasty are transconjunctival (**Fig. 26.7a**) and subciliary with or without a lateral extension (**Fig. 26.7b,c**). The choice between these two approaches is driven principally by the quality of the lid skin, need for canthal tightening, and surgeon preference. In general, the best patients for a transconjunctival approach are younger, with limited skin excess and protruding periorbital fat. Some surgeons choose the transconjunctival approach to manage the fat then address crepelike or excess skin with resurfacing via laser or peel.

The subciliary approach allows the surgeon to resect lid skin and acts as an open pathway to address anatomical features of the aging eyelid more directly (**Fig. 26.8**). If a subciliary approach is used, there are two common planes of dissection, the subcuticular (skin only) and submuscular (skin–muscle flap). Rosenfield[2] has been a proponent of the skin-only "pinch" lower lid blepharoplasty and has reported very low complications and good results. The submuscular plane is commonly used because it is relatively avascular, affords direct access to underlying fat pads, and eventuates to the orbital rim for direct access to the midface; when the flap is advanced, it directly lifts the midface and supports the lower lid. For these reasons, it is the author's preferred plane of dissection.

The extent of dissection depends on how much periorbital aging is present and to what extent you want to address it. A decision is made at the level of the orbitomalar ligament to progress through it or not. Beyond the ligament and the orbital rim, there are differing extents to which dissection over the zygoma can be performed. The more extensive the dissection, the more of the midface is mobilized (and therefore affected by the lift), and the more postoperative swelling is induced. The subperiosteal plane of dissection over the midface is generally straightforward and safe as long as the operator avoids the infraorbital nerve, which is in a generally consistent anatomical location ~ 7 mm below the orbital rim in the midpupillary line.[3-5] When the orbitomalar ligament is released, it is critical to resuspend the mid-

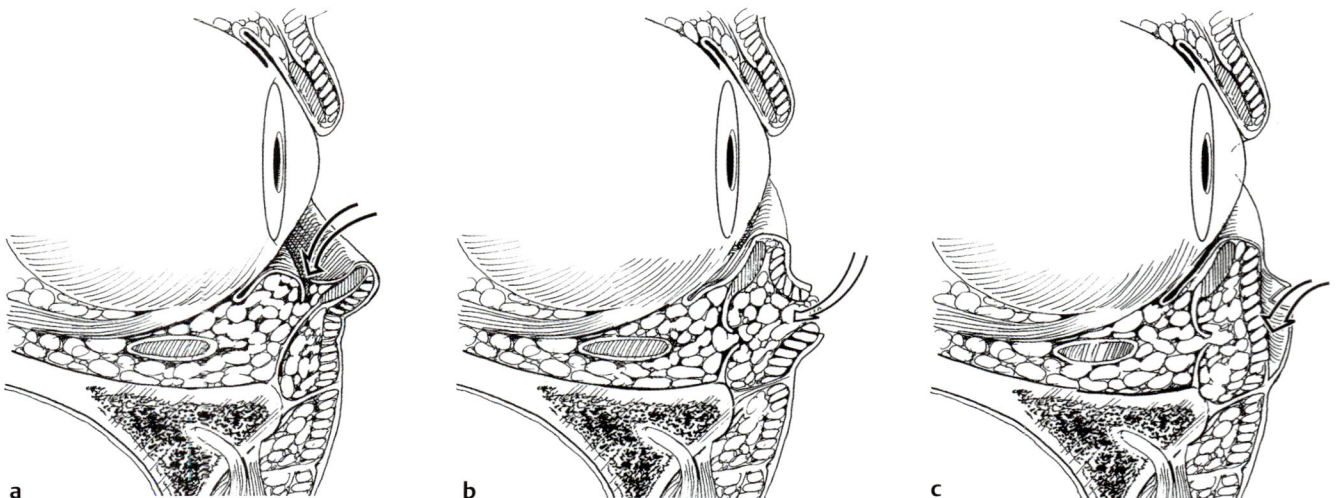

Fig. 26.7 **(a)** The transconjunctival approach. **(b)** The subciliary-submuscular approach. **(c)** The subciliary-subcuticular approach.

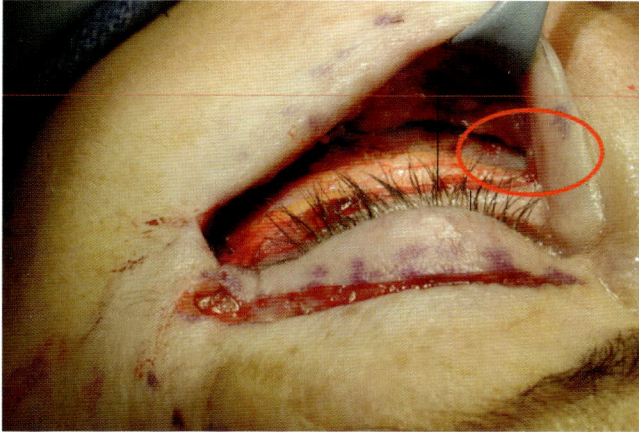

Fig. 26.8 An intraoperative view through a lower lid subciliary incision. The skin–muscle flap is raised, and the orbitomalar ligament has been incised. The orbital rim is demonstrated and a subperiosteal dissection has been performed. It is particularly important to avoid dissection within the soft tissue of the lower lid medial to the medial aspect of the central fat pad. The buccal branch of the facial nerve can be injured in the area outlined in red.

face. This can be done by suturing the orbicularis muscle to the fascia of the lateral orbital rim.

With exposure of the fat pads (via an open or transconjunctival approach), the fat can be left alone, partially resected, or released and redraped over the rim. The decision to resect or redrape is made based on the thickness of the overlying soft tissue layer, presence of a deep tear trough, and amount of fat present. In the case of secondary lid surgery, fat preservation is generally preferred because the fat has usually been manipulated previously.

Perhaps the most critical maneuver during lower lid blepharoplasty that minimizes the risks of complications is canthal anchoring. In the author's opinion, any lower lid procedure that includes a skin muscle flap or is being performed in the presence of one of the four clinical findings mentioned earlier (lid laxity, negative vector midface, prominent eyes,

or prior lower lid surgery) requires some form of canthal anchoring.

Canthal anchoring generally takes one of two forms, canthopexy or canthoplasty (**Fig. 26.9**). Canthopexy is tightening of the lateral canthal tendon in situ without canthal release or resection. Canthoplasty involves division of the lateral canthal apparatus, partial resection, then reanchoring. In either situation, the common goal of proper canthal anchoring is to preserve eye shape and the lateral scleral triangle, maintain adequate lower lid tone and position, and restore a youthful canthal tilt. Furthermore, the canthal anchor is the most effective means (although not the only factor) by which to avoid lid retraction and ectropion, problems with lid closure mechanics, and beady- or rounded-eye syndrome.

■ Complications and Their Management

By designing an operative plan to address the features of the eyelid that warrant rejuvenation or correction and by performing a thorough preoperative patient evaluation, most complications can be avoided. Nevertheless, despite adequate preparation, planning, and technical execution, complications can occur. Complications common to eyelid surgery are chemosis, lid malposition, lid-closure mechanical issues, eye-shape problems, dry eye, A-frame deformity and contour irregularities, injury to the inferior oblique muscle, injury to the buccal branch of the facial nerve, hematoma, and infection.

Basic Operating Room Safety

The use of corneal protectors is recommended for most, if not all, eyelid procedures. Corneal protectors are lined with ophthalmic lubricant or saline and are simply placed over the globe prior to injection of local anesthetic and surgical incision. This is a simple

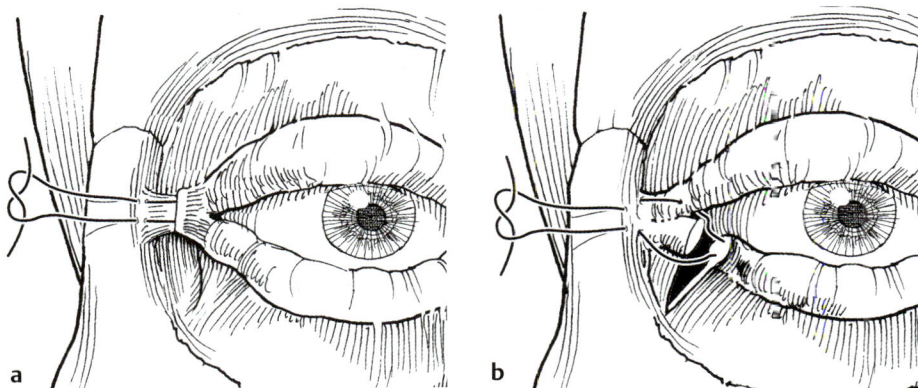

Fig. 26.9 Canthopexy **(a)** and canthoplasty **(b)**.

means for reducing the risk of corneal injury during eyelid surgery to almost nil. For procedures around the face being performed under local anesthetic and intravenous sedation, oxygen is often administered to the patient via a nasal cannula. Fires in the operating room have been reported based on the combination of oxygen (the oxidizer), electrocautery (the ignition source), and drapes (the fuel). The minimum amount of oxygen should be used to maintain proper blood oxygen saturation, and it should be allowed to escape and not collect under drapes. In addition, the electrocautery should be set to the lowest effective setting and used only when necessary to minimize the risk of operating room fires.

Chemosis

The pathophysiology of chemosis is not entirely understood, but it is believed to be related to eyelid trauma, local edema, exposure of the sclera, and alterations in lymphatic drainage from surgery. Classification and management strategies of chemosis have been previously described.[6] Chemosis identified in the operating room during the procedure should be managed one of two ways, depending on the severity. Severe chemosis that is herniating beyond the lid margin and interfering with lid closure should be treated by open drainage (conjunctivotomy) followed by topical steroids and temporary tarsorrhaphy suture. Less severe chemosis will generally resolve with tarsorrhaphy and topical steroids alone. Chemosis that is evident postoperatively and extends beyond 7 days after surgery despite topical steroids is treated by conjunctivotomy and 24 hours of patching. Some surgeons recommend their patients start steroid and antibiotic eye drops several days before lid surgery in an effort to minimize chemosis, though the effectiveness of this practice has not been proven.

Dry Eye

Dry eye is a serious condition that can be exacerbated by eyelid surgery, placing the cornea at risk for exposure keratitis. Identified before surgery, it can be ameliorated by placement of punctal plugs prior to surgery and liberal use of corneal lubricants. Temporary tarsorrhaphy sutures or soft contact lenses may be used for pathological exposure after surgery.

Contour Irregularities

Several types of contour irregularities can occur after eyelid surgery, usually due to overaggressive resection of the periorbital fat. In the upper eyelid, over-resection of the medial or central fat pad leads to a hollow appearance. Furthermore, minimal resection at the junction between the medial and central fat pad will result in an A-frame deformity, which is sometimes found at baseline in the aged patient. In the lower lid, if fat is resected, it should be done until flush with the orbital rim and no further. The lateral fat pad is more difficult to reach from the transconjunctival approach and sometimes can be seen as an irregular bulge in the lower lid following surgery. Areas of overresection can be treated with fillers or fat grafting, being sure to stay away from subdermal injections and injections in the pretarsal area. The safest place for filling is the subperiosteal space. Contour irregularities from underresection can be managed by reoperation. Although injection lipolysis has been investigated by some authors,[7,8] it is not approved by the U.S. Food and Drug Administration (FDA) and cannot be generally recommended unless within an investigational study protocol.

Injuries to Critical Structures

Injuries to critical structures can be avoided with keen knowledge of the eyelid and orbital anatomy and careful, meticulous technique. The use of a corneal protector was mentioned earlier. The buccal branch of the facial nerve is critical to baseline eyelid closure via activation of the inner-canthal orbicularis. The nerve courses along the midface deep to the superficial muscular aponeurotic system (SMAS), with terminal fibers throughout the upper and lower inner-canthal orbicularis (**Fig. 26.2b,c**). Within the medial orbit, the muscle and skin are very thin, and the buccal branch fibers can be easily injured if dissection veers into the soft tissue of the medial lid and orbit. To keep safe, it is highly recommended to dissect within the subperiosteal plane medial to the medial extent of the central fat pad.

An incidental injury to the inferior oblique muscle can occur.[9] The muscle is very small and has an oblique orientation between the central and nasal fat pads. Care must be taken during fat resection or redraping to identify and avoid the inferior oblique muscle. Temporary weakness can occur from the effect of the local anesthetic or transient/tangential trauma from the electrocautery and local edema. Permanent injury will lead to diplopia and inability to look upward during adduction. A typical complaint is double vision with an upward lateral gaze away from the affected side. Long-term diplopia or permanent injuries should be referred to a strabismus surgeon for evaluation.

Lower Lid Retraction

One of the most dreaded and debilitating complications of lower lid surgery is ectropion (the lesser form being lid malposition). This can occur for numerous reasons, including poor eyelid tone, prominent eyes, prior lid surgery, negative vector midface, excess skin resection, and lack of canthal support. Adequate canthal support is by far the most effective and robust means by which to avoid and prevent ectropion and malposition. Treatment of malposition is initially expectant. Taping, massage, and squinting exercises are very helpful means to improve lid position early and to buy time until a definitive procedure can be performed. This author recommends a minimum of 3 months and preferably closer to 6 months until reoperation is considered in these difficult cases. Scar tissue and edema can be dense in the lid, and to best set oneself up for success with revision surgery, the lid tissues should be soft, mobile, and stable. Furthermore, there is often an enormous amount of emotionality with these cases, feelings of guilt, betrayal, anger, and desperation that need to be managed and quelled before revision surgery.

Once the decision is made to repair the lid, a thorough assessment is performed for surgical planning, much like in the primary procedures. Patipa[10] has written an excellent article on the evaluation and management of lid malposition in the aesthetic patient. Several factors to consider are the approach (open subciliary vs transconjunctival), means of canthal anchoring (canthopexy versus canthoplasty ± drill hole orbitotomy), extent of midface dissection, and use of a spacer graft. Many of the features of the exam (in particular, lid mobility and ease of correction of lid position with digital manipulation, aka the Patipa test) are taken into account when one is constructing a plan (**Table 26.2**). Occasionally, in patients with multiple prior lower lid procedures, the periosteum on the inner aspect of the lateral orbital rim is damaged or absent and there is not adequate tissue to hold a suture reliably. In these cases, a drill hole orbitotomy is made through which the canthal anchoring suture is passed as a means of secure canthal fixation (**Fig. 26.10**). In practical terms, many of the cases seen are moderate or severe enough (i.e., a two-finger Patipa test or greater) to require using a spacer graft. The author's experience with cross-linked porcine acellular dermal spacer grafts in the lower eyelid has been previously reported.[11] A clinical example of lower lid repair is presented in **Fig. 26.4a–d**.

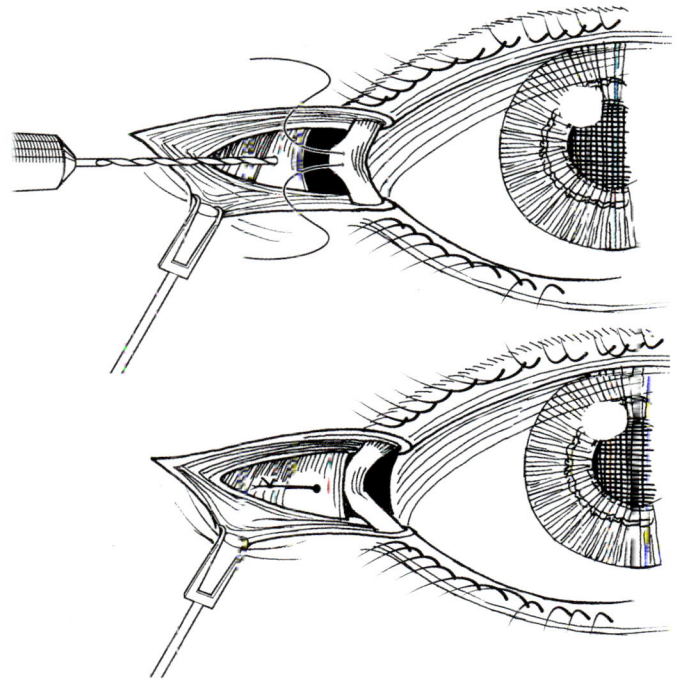

Fig. 26.10   Drill hole orbitotomy for canthal fixation.

Eye Shape and Closure

The integrity, or lack thereof, of the canthal anchor is also directly related to eyelid shape and closure mechanics. Adequate canthal support is necessary to maintain proper eye shape, specifically an open lateral scleral triangle. An example of a man with prior lower lid surgery and no canthal support demonstrates the beady-eye appearance of a small lateral scleral triangle (**Fig. 26.11**). Eyelid closure mechanics depend on three factors: a stimulus (the nerve), a motor (the muscle), and an anchoring mechanism (the canthal apparatus) (**Fig. 26.3**). Poor closure results in fish-mouthing. Correction of fish-mouthing is achieved with proper canthal anchoring, canthopexy, canthoplasty, or drill hole suspension, depending on the situation.[12]

Table 26.2 Decision table based on Patipa test

Procedure choice based on lid reposition test	One finger	Two finger	Three finger	Four finger
Proposed procedure	Canthopexy or canthoplasty	Prior + spacer graft	Prior + cheek lift, possible drill hole	All methods considered

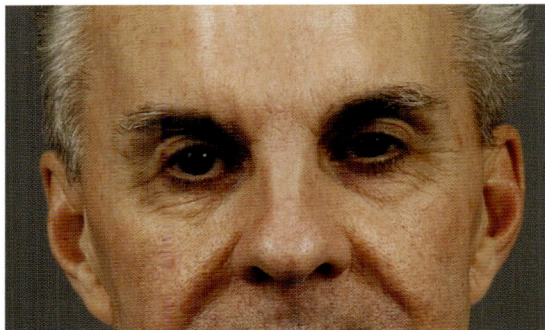

Fig. 26.11 The beady-eye appearance of a small lateral scleral triangle.

■ Conclusion

The avoidance and management of common complications in lower lid surgery have been reviewed. Recognition of key findings on the exam, proper patient evaluation, and good surgical planning and execution will keep surgeons and their patients safe and free of complications in most cases. A strategy and method for managing complications have been presented.

References

1. American Society for Aesthetic Plastic Surgery. Cosmetic Surgery National Data Bank data, 2008, 2009, 2010

2. Rosenfield LK. The pinch blepharoplasty revisited. Plast Reconstr Surg 2005;115(5):1405–1412, discussion 1413–1414

3. Singh R. Morphometric analysis of infraorbital foramen in Indian dry skulls. Anat Cell Biol 2011;44(1):79–83

4. Elias M, Sliva R, Pimentel M, Cardoso V, Rivello T, Babinski M. Morphometric analysis of the infraorbital foramen and accessory foramina in Brazilian skulls. Int J Morphol 2004;22(4):273–278

5. Boopathi S, Chakravarthy Marx S, Dhalapathy SL, Anupa S. Anthropometric analysis of the infraorbital foramen in a South Indian population. Singapore Med J 2010;51(9):730–735

6. Weinfeld AB, Burke R, Codner MA. The comprehensive management of chemosis following cosmetic lower blepharoplasty. Plast Reconstr Surg 2008;122(2):579–586

7. Rittes PG. The use of phosphatidylcholine for correction of localized fat deposits. Aesthetic Plast Surg 2003;27(4):315–318

8. Ablon G, Rotunda AM. Treatment of lower eyelid fat pads using phosphatidylcholine: clinical trial and review. Dermatol Surg 2004;30(3):422–427, discussion 428

9. Mowlavi A, Neumeister MW, Wilhelmi BJ. Lower blepharoplasty using bony anatomical landmarks to identify and avoid injury to the inferior oblique muscle. Plast Reconstr Surg 2002;110(5):1318–1322, discussion 1323–1324

10. Patipa M. The evaluation and management of lower eyelid retraction following cosmetic surgery. Plast Reconstr Surg 2000;106(2):438–453, discussion 454–459

11. McCord C, Nahai FR, Codner MA, Nahai F, Hester TR. Use of porcine acellular dermal matrix (Enduragen) grafts in eyelids: a review of 69 patients and 129 eyelids. Plast Reconstr Surg 2008;122(4):1206–1213

12. McCord CD, Ford DT, Hanna K, Hester TR, Codner MA, Nahai F. Lateral canthal anchoring: special situations. Plast Reconstr Surg 2005;116(4):1149–1157

27 Lip Rejuvenation

Brian P. Maloney

Key Concepts

- The upper and lower lips respond differently to cosmetic procedures.

- Many facial structures are involved with perioral aging.

- Skin resurfacing techniques, lip augmentation procedures, nasal base resection, and vermilion advancement are often combined to achieve perioral rejuvenation.

■ Introduction

Few other structures of the face carry such an important functional and aesthetic value as the lips. For thousands of years, the physical shape of the lips has had significant aesthetic connotations. Full lips are associated with beauty, fertility, health, and youth. Thin lips are associated with weakness, aging, and fragility. Even the fullest lips, however, will be subject to the many varied effects of the aging process in this anatomical region, resulting in loss of proportion and involution. Because of the special aesthetic and functional features of the lips, surgical rejuvenation of this area tests the skills of even the most experienced surgeons.

Many patients begin the consultation regarding lip rejuvenation with trepidation, for fear of receiving large unnatural features. Other patients may seek out cosmetic surgeons who prefer a more overdone or inflated look. It is important to discuss the patient's goals and determine if the goals are consistent with your aesthetic preferences. If the goals are not in agreement, the surgeon may elect not to operate on the patient. The patient's threshold for recovery, acceptance of possible complications, and realistic expectations are additional factors to evaluate.

■ Background: Basic Science of Procedure

The lip is not only an important aesthetic feature of the face, but also a very dynamic functional structure. Lip movements are an important element of speech, eating, digestion, and romance. Cosmetic alteration of the lips should therefore ideally seek to have minimal alteration of lip motion. When determining a treatment course, it is important to consider that the choice of procedures, combined with the patient's healing, may result in temporary, or rarely permanent alteration of lip function.

■ Pertinent Anatomy

The ideal lower third of the face extends from the nasal base to the inferior aspect of the chin. It can be further subdivided into an upper third, extending from the nasal base to the inferior aspect of the upper lip vermilion, and a lower two-thirds extending from the superior aspect of the lower lip vermilion down to the inferior aspect of the chin. The lateral view should reveal a gentle curve from the nasal base to the upper lip vermilion. The lips should have a slightly rounded contour when viewed from the side. This feature is commonly called the projection of the lips (**Fig. 27.1**).

Aesthetically, there is no ideal lip proportion relative to upper and lower lip projection. That is, some patients have a fuller lower lip than upper lip, others may be balanced, and some may have a fuller upper

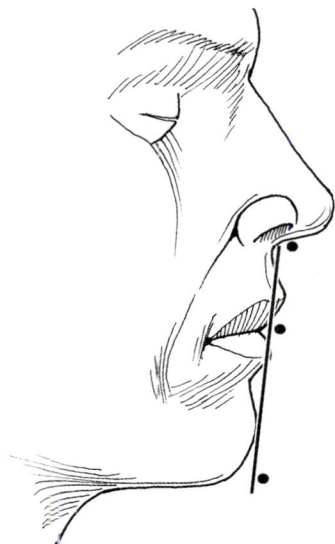

Fig. 27.1   Profile of the face. The lower third of the face is subdivided into the upper one-third and lower two-thirds. Also notice the aesthetic gentle curve of the upper lip to the white roll area.

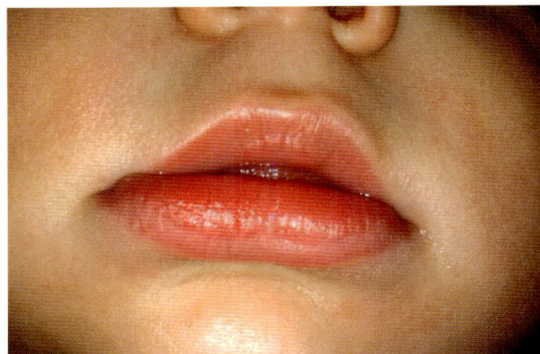

Fig. 27.2   Newborn lip showing the end result of the developmental differences between the upper and lower lips.

lip. Variations in the position of the underlying teeth, bone structure, and lip anatomy account for the multitude of lip variations.

The lip derives its unique shape from the fact that the upper lip forms from three subunits when viewed from the front. The condensation of these components results in a structure defined by two raised philtral ridges flowing from the nasal base to the vermilion-cutaneous junction. The ridges, combined with a central depression, the philtral sulcus, create the defining feature of the upper lip, known as the cupid's bow.[1–3]

The embryology of the lower lip is very different from the upper lip. The lower lip forms from two subunits that merge together, resulting in a smooth lip border (**Fig. 27.2**). The embryological differences result in two very different structures in regard to movement and response to surgical procedures. The upper lip flexes much more than the lower lip; therefore, it is less tolerant of lip procedures that restrict movement. Surrounding the lip vermilion-cutaneous junction is a raised non-hair-bearing white roll. This structure, originally described by Gilles and Kilner,[4] is believed to act as a reservoir of elastic elements that allow the lips the flexibility to perform their many actions.

The bulk of the lip is composed of a sphincteric muscle, the orbicularis oris, covered by a thin mucosal layer. The orbicularis muscle condenses at the corner of the mouth into a modiolus. A few superficial fibers of the orbicularis muscle insert directly into the undersurface of the dermis. The depressor

anguli oris is a small muscle that runs from the modiolus to the mandible; its path becomes more apparent with age due to frequent frowning. Both upper and lower lips act like curtains draped over the underlying teeth. Therefore, evaluation of the patient's occlusion and tooth size is an important part of the pretreatment examination.

The pink, or vermilion, portion of the lip is divided into a dry and wet surface separated by the "wet line" (**Fig. 27.3**). The dry vermilion is exposed to the air, and the wet vermilion is bathed by oral secretions. After lip rejuvenation, commonly a small portion of the wet vermilion may be exposed to the air and remain dry and flaky until it has an opportunity to adapt to its new position.

As the lips age, the cutaneous portion of the lips may develop actinic changes, such as thickening of the epidermis and lentigines. With repeated pursing of the lips, vertical and horizontal rhytids begin to appear. Philtral ridges and white rolls begin to flatten as the collagen breaks down, resulting in a longer upper and

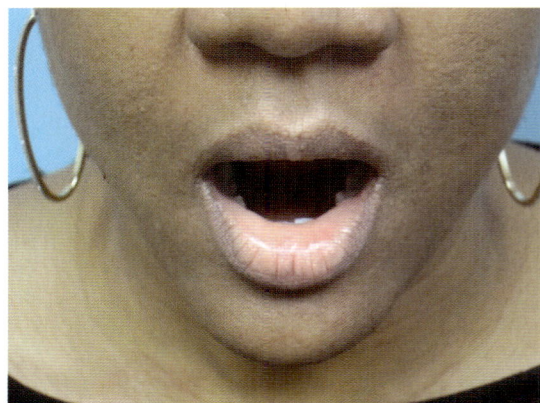

Fig. 27.3   A well demarcated "wet line" of the lower lip in an African American patient.

lower lip. As the upper lip lengthens, the ability to see the inferior aspect of the upper incisors disappears.

Lip volume, which peaked at puberty, begins to deflate. Therefore, the once full vermilion of the lips extending from commissure to commissure begins to shorten, losing the outer corners first, followed by loss of central volume. The amount of lip vermilion show begins to decrease as the lips lose volume and the white roll flattens. Rhytids begin to develop in the vermilion portion of the lip. As the vermilion portion of the lip loses volume, the cutaneous portion is generally losing volume from a decrease in subcutaneous fat and orbicularis muscle mass. This will commonly deepen the horizontal lines across the central upper lip and vertical lines surrounding the lips. Often the teeth, which have helped support and add projection to the lips, begin to decrease in vertical height, move, and turn inward. The supporting maxillary and mandibular bone also loses volume, contributing to the involution of the lower third of the face with age.

Repeated action of the depressor anguli oris, a small muscle at the corner of the mouth, combined with loss of soft tissue volume, results in a downturning of the lip corners. As this process occurs, the smooth jaw line of youth is erased and replaced with a wide, irregular jaw line (**Fig. 27.4**).

■ Patient Selection

Patients undergoing lip procedures should have realistic expectations. Physical examination involves an assessment of the overall proportions of the face, length of the upper and lower lip, definition of the lip structures, lip projection, amount of vermilion show on frontal and lateral views, quality of cutaneous and vermilion skin, amount of dental show, occlusion, and tooth appearance.

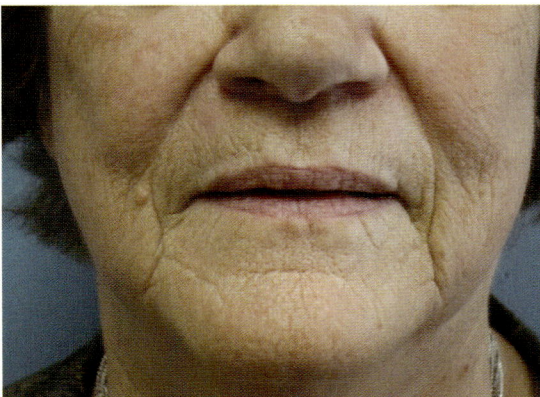

Fig. 27.4   The aging changes of the perioral region.

■ Technical Aspects of Procedure

Lip rejuvenation procedures are divided into four categories based on the patient's anatomy.

1. Rejuvenation of the perioral and vermilion skin
2. Lip augmentation
   a. Autogenous, hyaluronic acid (HA)
   b. Autologous fat transfer
   c. Acellular human dermal matrix
3. Long upper lip with adequate cupid's bow definition—nasal base resection
4. Long upper lip with poor cupid's bow definition—vermilion advancement

The first section touches on the importance of the quality of the overlying skin when rejuvenating the lip area. The next sections transition into structural changes that occur with the aging process. To achieve the desired lip rejuvenation, the cosmetic surgeon will often perform several lip procedures simultaneously.

■ Lip Anesthesia/ Patient Preparation

There are a variety of topical anesthetics currently available to apply to the cutaneous or vermilion lip. Care should be taken to check the patient's history of medication allergies. Choose topical anesthetic agents that will not interact with the patient's medications and have a low incidence of adverse reactions. Patients with a history of herpes simplex should receive systemic antiviral agents in the peri-procedure period.

Topical anesthesia can be further supplemented with topical ice, held directly on the lip until the lip is adequately chilled. With the advent of fillers containing lidocaine, the use of regional blocks has ceased in the author's practice, though the blocks do continue to be utilized in other practices. The very nervous patient could be placed on an anxiolytic agent and/or oral pain medication, to help make the procedure a more comfortable experience.

Excision techniques require the injection of a local anesthetic with epinephrine, mixed with hyaluronidase, to help minimize tissue distortion. If a HA filler is present or placed simultaneously, or if an acellular dermal matrix graft is used, hyaluronidase should not be used.

If a patient has a history of herpes simplex, then systemic antiviral treatment is initiated prior to the procedure.

■ Rejuvenation of the Perioral and Vermilion Skin

Patient Selection

The perioral skin aesthetic unit tends to be prone to rhytid formation due to the frequent muscle action of the area. Patients display a reactive thickening of the epidermis in response to years of sun and wind damage. Smoking also affects the appearance of the lips and leads to increased risks in any lip rejuvenation procedure. Nightly application of topical retinoids, coupled with daily use of sun protection, is often the first step in softening these actinic changes. As the aging process continues and exposure to environmental factors and lip pursing activities occur, perioral lines develop. In-office treatments for the perioral lines involve the use of botulinum toxin, fillers, and chemical peels.

Technical Aspects of Procedure— Botulinum Toxin Type A

Botulinum toxin type A is commonly used for the treatment of mild perioral rhytids, though it should be noted that this is a U.S. Food and Drug Administration (FDA) off-label use. It is important to understand the different types of botulinum toxins and use their appropriate doses. Generally, if onabotulinum toxin is used, 1 to 2 units are placed in the center of each lip rhytid. The technique involves placing the toxin immediately underneath the dermis in the middle of the wrinkle with a 30-gauge needle (**Fig. 27.5**). If treating a downturning corner of the mouth, 2 units of botulinum toxin can be placed 1 cm lateral and 1 cm inferior to the oral commissure. Injecting medial to this point or along the mandibular edge should

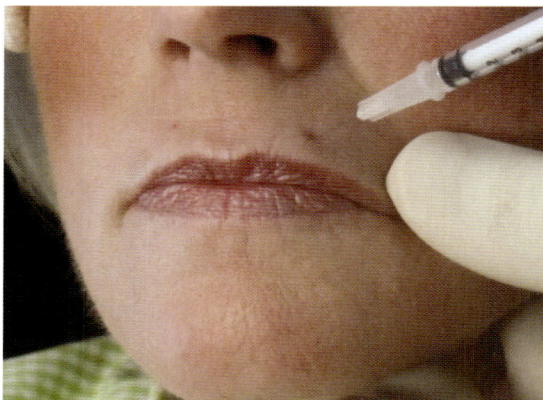

Fig. 27.5 Subdermal injection of botulinum toxin to the middle of an upper lip rhytid.

be avoided to minimize affecting the depressor labii inferioris. Inadvertent action of botulinum toxin on this muscle will cause the lower lip to rise up on that side. Patients should be advised that lip sphincter function may be affected, and the procedure should be avoided if this cannot be tolerated.

Postoperative Care—Botulinum Toxin Type A

Frequent pursing of the lips intermittently over the first 30 minutes will help the uptake of the botulinum toxin into the muscle. Patients generally notice softening of the rhytid within a few days, with continued improvement over the duration of the effect. Potential adverse effects include decreased lip movement with pursing, such as using a straw or performing similar activities. Patients with thin, cutaneous lips will be at higher risk for this complication. Some physicians will use only neuromodulators in this region when the patient is also having placement of an appropriate filler in the lips.

Patient Selection—Hyaluronic Acid

HA fillers are very versatile around the lip area. The filler can be placed in the mid to deep dermis to soften deep rhytids of the lips, redefine philtral ridges, and enhance the white roll. HA fillers should not be used in patients who have a history of allergic reactions to gram-positive bacteria or lidocaine. They are also contraindicated in patients with multiple severe allergic reactions or a history of anaphylaxis.

Technical Aspects of Procedure— Hyaluronic Acid

HA fillers can be used in combination with botulinum toxin for softening the deeper cutaneous lip lines. Placement of the filler into the rhytid first will avoid any distortion from initial placement of the toxin into the rhytid, allowing for accurate placement. The HA can also be used to add volume to cutaneous vertical and horizontal lines, the white roll, the philtral ridge, or the lip vermilion. When one is treating an ill-defined white roll or philtral ridge, the filler can be placed by threading the needle through the desired structure. Gentle pressure applied to the syringe will deposit filler upon withdrawal of the needle. Care is taken to make sure the plane of injection in the white roll is in a deep dermal location. Philtral ridge augmentation may require only deep dermal placement of filler, or subcutaneous placement as well, to achieve the desired effect. Cutaneous lines can be injected in a deep dermal plane in a threading or point technique or both (**Fig. 27.6**). Care is taken not to overfill the rhytids and create a ridge.

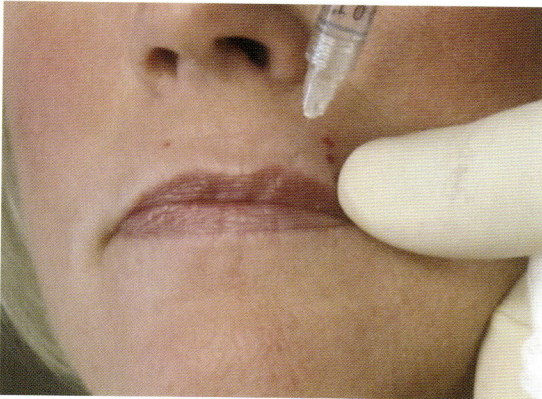

Fig. 27.6 Intradermal threading of a cutaneous lip rhytid.

Patient Selection and Technical Considerations—Resurfacing

Resurfacing of the perioral skin utilizing chemical peels or carbon dioxide (CO_2) laser can help improve actinic damage to the cutaneous and vermilion portions of the lip. To soften rhytids, the resurfacing technique needs to extend to the dermis. Microdermabrasion and Jessner peels are superficial peels that only penetrate the epidermis and can improve the complexion. The combination of a Jessner peel and 25 or 35% trichloracetic acid (TCA) produces a medium-depth chemical peel that penetrates through the papillary dermis. Patients who are the best candidates for the medium and deep chemical peels are those with the lighter skin types. The phenol peel and CO_2 resurfacing laser produce a deeper treatment with the most dramatic improvement. These techniques are described in depth in other portions of the book. To maximize the effect of the resurfacing procedure, the lip rhytids are pretreated 2 to 4 weeks prior to the procedure with botulinum toxin. One to two units of onabotulinum toxin, or an equivalent dose of another neuromodulator, are placed in the muscle ridge contributing to the cutaneous rhytid. Because laxity of the lip may occur, this should be limited to the portions of the upper lip that are inferior to the nose, avoiding those that are lateral to this.

■ Lip Augmentation Technique

Hyaluronic Acid Filler

Patient Selection

The goal of lip augmentation for most cosmetic patients is to add volume to the lip in a fashion to create a fuller consistent lip vermilion. Patients who had full lips when younger and who have lost volume are the ideal candidates. A patient with very thin lips generally cannot have adequate filler injected to create full lips with a natural look, though a noticeable improvement with a natural look is attainable. Patients with lips with a multitude of vermilion rhytids, indicating volume loss, are generally excellent lip augmentation candidates.

Technical Aspects of Procedure

Many outcomes are possible with lip augmentation. The final effect of the lip augmentation is determined by the three-dimensional placement of the filler. That is, if the goal is to increase lip projection, the filler is placed in an anterior plane (**Fig. 27.7**). Injections are laid down, end to end, creating a continuous chain of filler in a consistent plane. If the goal is to lengthen the lip, the tunnel of filler is placed inferiorly. If augmentation is desired in both areas, it can be placed in-between ▶ **Video 27.1**.

When performing a lip augmentation with a filler, this author stabilizes the lip by applying pressure to both commissures (**Fig. 27.8**). The needle is inserted beginning at the commissure in the desired plane. Injection is performed as the needle is withdrawn, allowing for greater control. The needle is reinserted with a slight overlap in the same plane, and filler is deposited upon withdrawal. Pressure on the syringe ceases when the needle is halfway exposed to

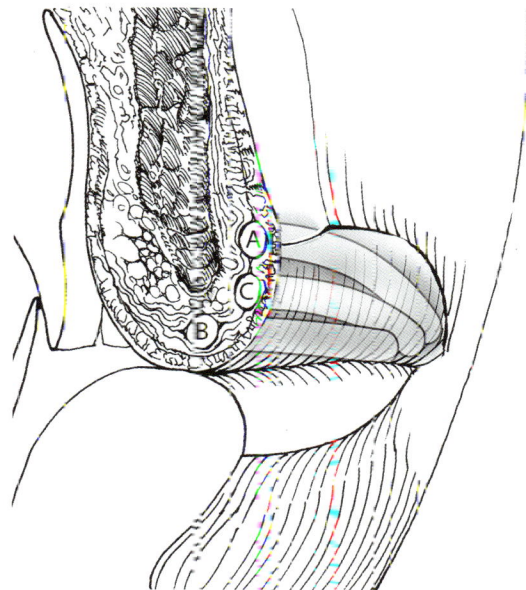

Fig. 27.7 Cross-section of the upper lip with various planes of augmentation. (A) Serial placement of a filler across the length of the lip to increase lip projection. (B) Placement of filler to lengthen the upper lip. (C) To increase volume and length, the tunnel can be placed between the two points.

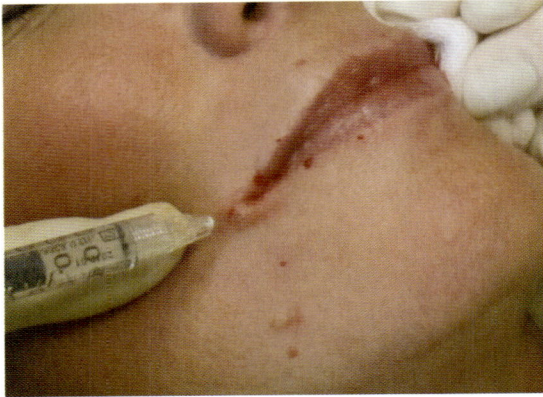

Fig. 27.8 Stabilizing the lip for injections by applying pressure over the commissures.

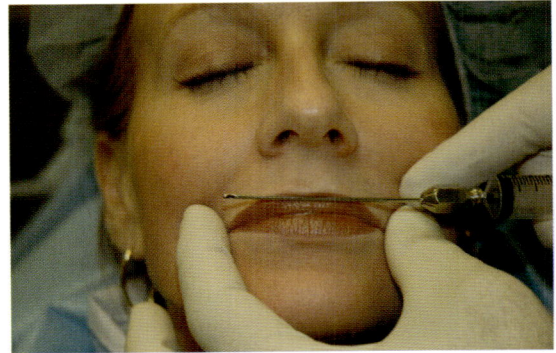

Fig. 27.9 Just prior to the insertion of a blunt-tip cannula into the lateral commissure. Both the upper and the lower lip and the corner of the mouth can be augmented through this single puncture site.

minimize any extravasations of filler superiorly. This process is repeated until the opposite commissure is reached. The end result is a series of "connected sausage links" in a continuous plane. This can be confirmed by palpation of the lip with thumb and index finger, or by visual inspection of the lip. Gentle massage should be performed to spread the filler through the tissues and connect the "links." The injection technique can also help diminish any preexisting, natural asymmetry of the lips.

Autologous Fat

Patient Selection

Autologous fat transfer is a popular technique for lip augmentation. This procedure is often used when other areas of the face need volume restoration.

Technical Aspects of Procedure

After preparing the fat, it is deposited in the lip with a round tip, side-port cannula inserted at the commissure, in a multiple back-and-forth fashion (**Fig. 27.9**). Additional fat can be placed in the triangular cutaneous subunit of the upper lip, making up the superior aspect of the nasolabial fold. Fat can also be placed into the downturning of the mouth. Given the variability in fat-grafting results, more than one session may be necessary to achieve the desired results.

Dermal Matrix

Patient Selection

Acellular dermal matrix augmentation of the lips can easily be performed in the office. Human dermal ma-

trix can be a long-lasting lip augmentation material, in which the host's tissue grows into the matrix.

Technical Aspects of Procedure

Local infiltration of lidocaine with epinephrine without hyaluronidase is necessary to prepare the lip. An incision is made in each commissure with a no. 15 blade. Tenotomy scissors are inserted and used to create a surgical pocket across the desired plane of the lip. The actual placement of the pocket depends on the goals of the procedure, similar to the placement of filler in the lips. The acellular dermal matrix graft is hydrated according to the manufacturer's directions. The matrix is prepared in a fashion that avoids any contact with surgical gloves and towels in order to minimize powder and fiber contamination. The matrix is trimmed to the desired size. Care should be taken to avoid making any slits in the matrix because this seems to damage the framework and cause more resorption. A curved tendon passer is inserted through the surgical pocket. The matrix is then grasped with the forceps and pulled into the pocket (**Fig. 27.10**). The free end of the matrix should be grasped with a forceps, and, once both ends are visible, pulled back and forth in the pocket to ensure central placement. The commissure incisions are closed with dissolvable sutures.

◾ Long Upper Lip with Adequate Cupid's Bow Definition— Nasal Base Resection

Patient Selection

Some people are born with a long upper lip; others acquire it over time as a result of the aging process as

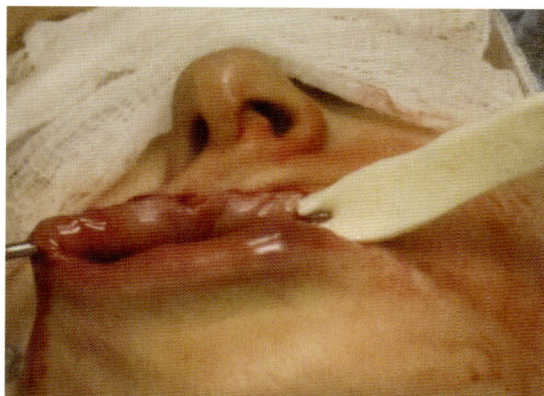

Fig. 27.10 Tendon passer inserted through commissure incisions and passing through an anterior plane of the upper lip. The white acellular dermal matrix is grasped by the passer at one end and a forceps on the other. Care is taken to avoid any contact with the surrounding tissues while pulling it into the tunnel.

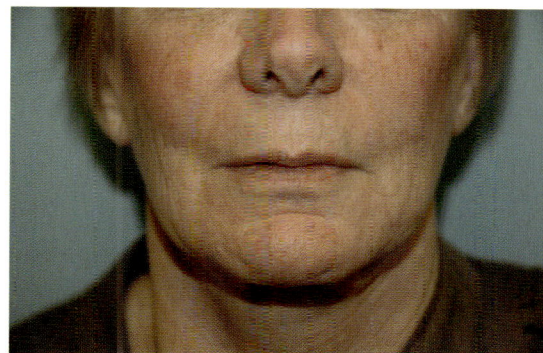

Fig. 27.11 The aging changes to the lip. Notice the actinic changes, lip rhytids, loss of vermilion volume, and lengthening of the upper lip resulting in no inc sor show.

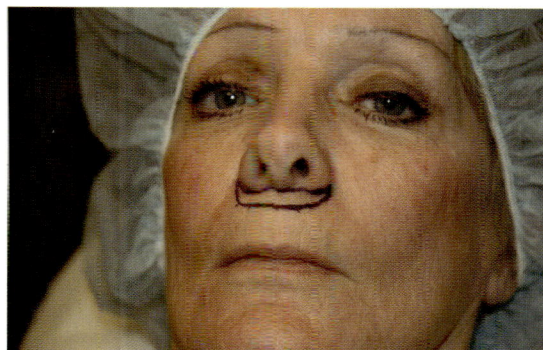

Fig. 27.12 A long upper lip with the gull wing excision marked along the nasal base.

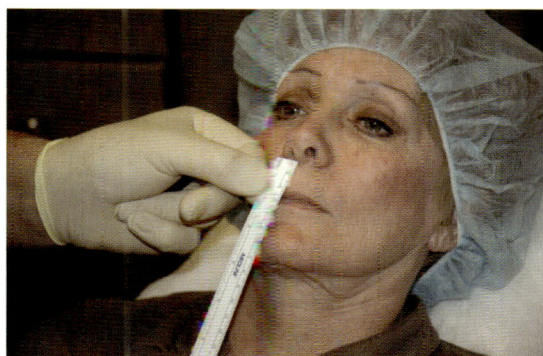

Fig. 27.13 The amount of skin to be excised from the upper lip can generally be calculated by measuring the thirds of the lower face.

previously described. Patients with a long upper lip generally have poor dental show; that is, no teeth are visible at rest (**Fig. 27.11**). Attempting to perform lip augmentation alone in a patient with a long upper lip can make the upper lip appear even longer. If a patient has a long upper lip and a gummy smile due to an elongated maxillary segment, nasal base resection is not recommended. If the distance from the lower lip to the chin makes up more than two thirds of the lower third of the face, nasal base resection may not be appropriate because it would further exaggerate this disproportion. The procedure shortens the cutaneous upper lip and can be combined with lip augmentation procedures if necessary. Realistic patients with no history of excessive scarring who are willing to accept a scar along the nasal base are candidates.

Technical Aspects of Procedure

The procedure is performed in an office setting under local anesthesia supplemented with oral anxiolytic or pain medication as needed for patient comfort ▶ Video 27.3. The gull wing incision is marked along the nasal base (**Fig. 27.12**). This will be the location of the final scar. The nasal base anatomy will generally dictate the location of the scar. The lower portion of the ellipse represents the amount of skin to be excised. The amount to be excised can be determined mathematically. In the midline, the length from the nasal base to the inferior aspect of the upper lip is measured (**Fig. 27.13**). The distance from the superior aspect of the lower lip vermilion to the inferior aspect of the chin is measured. A simple proportion with X (the ideal length of the upper lip segment) over the length of the lower lip segment equals 1

over 2 (the ratio of upper lip to lower lip segments ideally). The equation simplifies to the lower lip segment length divided by 2 to give us the ideal length of the upper lip. This number is subtracted from the actual length to give us the amount of excision necessary. Overcorrection by a millimeter is generally recommended. The patients are generally given a mirror and an opportunity to comment on the planned procedure after the lip is marked.

Lidocaine with epinephrine can be used for the procedure. If hyaluronidase is utilized, 9 mL of lidocaine 1% with epinephrine 1/100,000 is combined with 1 mL of hyaluronidase. The mixture is injected in the surgical area with a 30-gauge needle. Tension is applied to the upper lip, stabilizing it against the maxilla and teeth. A no. 15 blade is used to incise the ellipse of tissue. The deep dissection is in the subcutaneous plane (**Fig. 27.14**). Care is taken not to penetrate the intraoral mucosa. Homeostasis is obtained with limited electrocautery. Reconstruction of the defect involves placement of several 5–0 absorbable sutures in the deep dermal layer. Final wound edge approximation is accomplished with an absorbable 6–0 suture.

Postoperative Care

Ice or other cold compresses can be applied to the area for several hours following the procedure. Patients follow a moist wound-healing protocol, cleaning the incision six times a day with hydrogen peroxide and applying a topical antibiotic ointment for the first week. Patients are advised to avoid any stretching of the lip and to avoid chewy food for the first 2 weeks. Makeup can be applied at the end of the week if there is no crusting along the incision and the sutures are no longer present.

■ Long Upper Lip with Poor Cupid's Bow Definition— Vermilion Advancement

Patient Selection

Vermilion advancement[5] is a surgical procedure that helps to shorten the upper lip, increase definition of the cupid's bow area, and increase the amount of vermilion show of the upper or lower lips. The focus of the procedure is on creating an appropriate amount of vermilion show for the patient, not on shortening the upper lip to ideal proportions. This procedure can leave a visible scar, so only realistic patients willing to accept scarring along the vermilion-cutaneous junction are candidates for this procedure.

Technical Aspects of Procedure

The existing vermilion of the upper or lower lip is traced with a fine marking pen. Based upon the patient's goals for the procedure, points marking the

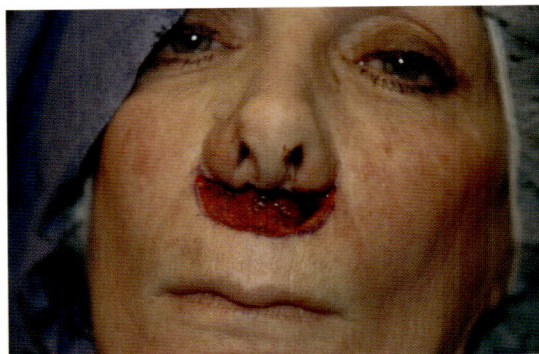

Fig. 27.14 The subcutaneous depth of the excision of the nasal base resection.

limits of excision are placed (**Fig. 27.15**). The highest points of the upper lip are the two peaks along the philtral ridges. The lowest points on the lower lip lie along parallel vertical lines with the high points of the upper lip. Based upon patient preferences and anatomy, the peaks along the cupid's bow can be angular or curved ▶ Video 27.2.

The lip(s) are injected with 1.0 to 1.5 mL of lidocaine with epinephrine in a subcutaneous plane. The lip is gently placed under tension against the underlying teeth. A no. 15 blade is used to incise the marked boundaries with a slight bevel outward (**Fig. 27.16**). Reconstruction is initiated by placing 6–0 fast-absorbing gut vertical mattress sutures along the philtral ridges and sulcus. Interrupted sutures may be placed in-between to complete the wound-edge approximation. The lateral incisions can be closed with a running locking 6–0 fast-absorbing suture (**Fig. 27.17**).

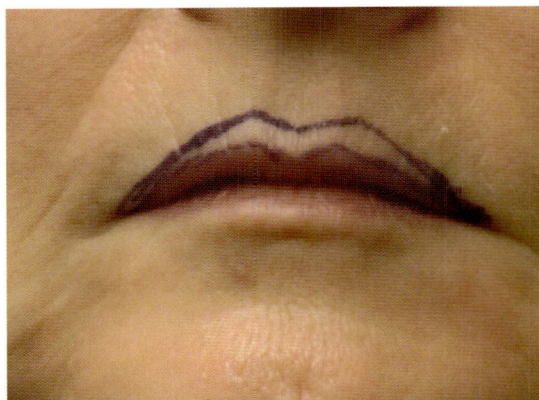

Fig. 27.15 The vermilion advancement is marked along the upper lip, with the high points along the philtral ridges. The incision flows laterally to the commissure and medially to a point above the philtral sulcus.

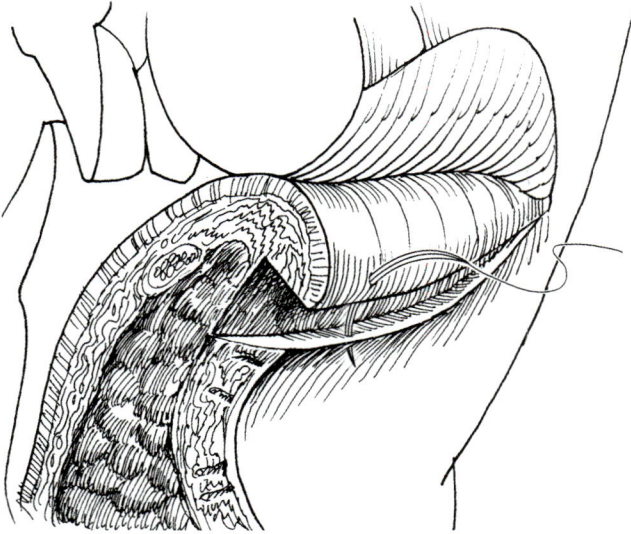

Fig. 27.16 Cross-section of the upper lip. The beveled edges and immediate subcutaneous plane of dissection are visible.

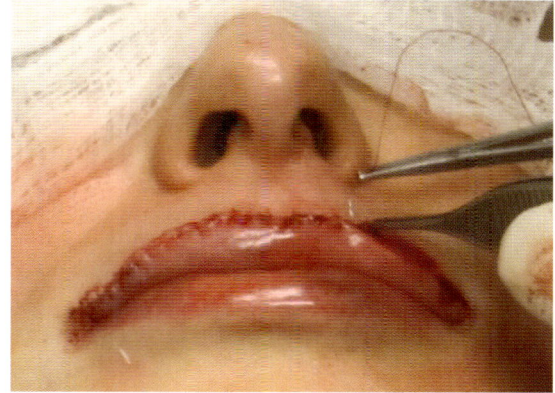

Fig. 27.17 Lip advancement closure showing interrupted sutures at key points in the cupid's bow area and running locking sutures laterally.

■ Postoperative Care

Due to the vascular and muscular nature of the lips, swelling is common. This can be reduced by applying ice or other cold compresses to the lips for several hours after the procedure. Patients may benefit from restricting their sodium intake for 3 days prior to the procedure and 2 days after the procedure. On rare occasions, a patient with a history of significant swelling may benefit from systemic steroids posttreatment.

If any healing wounds, such as incisions or laser resurfacing, are present, antiviral medication is continued until epithelialization is complete. A moist wound-care protocol, consisting of application of a topical antibiotic ointment six times a day, is followed for the first week.

One to two units of botulinum toxin type A can be placed at several points along the vermilion border to decrease movement of the lip following vermilion advancement or fat transfer. This helps to rest the area, relieving some of the tensions that could result in widening of the scars or failure of the fat to survive.

■ Expected Results

The expected results of lip rejuvenation vary, in any combination of obtaining a fuller, smoother, defined, or proportioned lip. The patient's goals, the basic anatomy, and the age-related changes that affect the lips, teeth, and facial bones all play a role and affect the surgeon recommendations for achieving these goals.

■ Complications and Their Management

Dry lips are not a complication, but they are a common patient complaint after lip augmentation as the wet vermilion rolls out and is exposed to the dry air. It may take several weeks for the mucosa to adapt to its new environment. Drinking lots of water and using lip balms may help to ameliorate this. Tartar-control and whitening toothpaste as well as certain mouth rinses may exacerbate the dryness.

Because fillers are the most common lip treatment, asymmetries are probably the most common complication of lip rejuvenation. Some asymmetries may be due to swelling or bruising, which can be corrected with massage or additional filler in the relatively smaller portion of the lip. Only on rare occasions is it necessary to use local placement of hyaluronidase, making an HA filler preferable for in-office lip augmentation. The degree of cross-linking and concentration of the HA will affect how much hyaluronidase to inject. Results are generally visible within 24 hours, and the procedure may be repeated every few days if necessary.

Asymmetries from autologous fat transfer are not unusual in the early stages. There is generally more swelling associated with this procedure, which can localize. Focal massage using the thumb and index finger will usually be sufficient to treat these irregularities. Any irregularities persisting beyond 6 weeks are treated with a low-dose triamcinolone injection, followed by massage.

Herpes simplex is best managed with peritreatment prophylaxis using antiviral agents. If a patient experiences an active breakout, doses may be increased, and a topical antiviral applied to the areas.

Angular cheilitis, dryness, flaking, and redness in the corner of the lips can also develop. This condition can represent a fungal overgrowth and is often treated with a topical antifungal cream. The use of periprocedure antibiotics, tartar-control toothpaste, and certain mouthwashes seems to predispose patients to this condition.

Widening of vermilion scars or loss of lip color following vermilion advancement can be treated with permanent cosmetics. If there is a localized widening, scar revision can be considered.

Persistence of perioral rhytids can be seen, due to thinning of the cutaneous and vermilion lip, coupled with significant actinic changes.

■ Conclusion

Rejuvenation of the lip area tests all the skills of the surgeon. The region, with its unique anatomy, is constantly in movement throughout daily life. As the aging process progresses, changes are often magnified by the frequent movement in the mouth area, as the vertical height of the teeth decreases, facial bones lose volume, and the skin and lip structures thin. If age-related changes are left unchecked, for most, the lower face appears to fall in toward the mouth. A multidisciplinary approach addressing each of the aging components generally offers the best outcomes in lip rejuvenation.

References

1. Moore K. The Developing Human. Philadelphia, PA: WB Saunders; 1977:156–174
2. O'Conner GB. Surgical formation of the philtrum and the cutaneous upsweep. Am J Cosmet Surg 1958;95:227–230
3. Mulliken JB, Pensler JM, Kozakewich HP. The anatomy of cupid's bow in normal and cleft lip. Plast Reconstr Surg 1993;92(3):395–403, discussion 404
4. Gilles HD, Kilner TP. Hare-lip: operation for correction of secondary deformities. Lancet 1932;223:1369–1375
5. McCollough EG, Maloney BP. Aesthetic lip advancement. Am J Cosmet Surg 1996;13:207–212

28 Otoplasty and Earlobe Rejuvenation

Edward H. Farrior

Key Concepts

- Otoplasty, the reshaping of the ear, must be performed by recreating absent normal architecture or reducing excesses to recreate a normal size, shape, and position of the ear.

- Fossa and eminence of the anterior and posterior surface of the ear need to be understood and recreated to yield a normal-appearing anatomically correct ear.

- Auricular hillocks of the first and second branchial arch form the external ear, primarily the third through fifth hillocks.

- Overdeveloped conchal bowl must be addressed in otoplasty through conchal reduction and setback with suturing.

- Earlobe reduction in conjunction with aging face surgery creates greater harmony and can help avoid a postsurgical incongruity.

- Stellate resection may be required for an earlobe reduction that addresses issues of height and width.

Introduction

Otoplasty is the reshaping of the ears. This routinely refers to correcting the protruding ears or lop ear deformity. Reshaping also occurs in the form of microtia repair on a grander scale and earlobe reduction or repair of iatrogenic deformities to a more minor degree.

Otoplasty most commonly involves the reduction of protruding ears. This usually includes the re-creation of normal cartilaginous contours on the anterior surface of the ear and reduction in the depth of the conchal bowl. Contour re-creation and depth re-duction of the bowl may occur in an isolated setting. However, they are most often found in association with one another and to varying degrees affect the protrusion of the ear away from the side of the head and the ideal postauricular angle or cephaloauricular angle of less than 45 degrees.[1] This chapter summarizes the abnormalities producing the protruding ear and their correction and addresses relatively simple solutions for the aging lobule and postsurgical lobular deformities.

Background: Basic Science of Procedure

Embryologically, the ear arises from the first and second brachial arch in the six auricular hillocks that form within the first and second branchial arches. The first three hillocks (1 through 3) are attributed to the first brachial arch, and the second three hillocks (4 through 6) are attributed to the second brachial arch. It is the general consensus that the bulk of the ear is formed from the third through fifth hillocks, that the sixth hillock contributes to the lobule and antitragus, and that the tragus and helical crus originate from the first and second hillocks.[2] Development of the pinna usually occurs during the first trimester of pregnancy, and as a consequence, deformities will have developed during this phase of embryological maturation.

Pertinent Anatomy

The lack of development of the external ear takes varying degrees and may result in microtia, the absence of most external anatomy including the external auditory canal, and, frequently, underdevelopment of the middle and inner ear. This is considered a third-degree deformity of the ear. The cupped ear deformity is a second-degree deformity and is most often represented by an undersized ear with reduced components. The superior helical margin, superior crus of the antihelix, and scaphoid fossa are most commonly affected. First-degree deformities of the ear are deformities of excess rather than of absence and are manifested by the protruding and overly large ear.

Lop ear deformity, or protruding ears, is inherited as an autosomal dominant gene with variable penetrance, with 59% of patients having a positive family history. Protruding ears affect 5% of the Caucasian race.

Abnormalities of the ear can also arise from iatrogenic and traumatic sources. One of the most frequently occurring iatrogenic abnormalities is the pixie ear deformity, which can be the result of a facelift (**Fig. 28.1**). There is a similar congenital variation in the degree of attachment of the lobule to the neck that can be released, if so desired, in the same fashion as the repair of the postsurgical pixie ear.

Abnormalities that are the consequence of aging may also affect the lobule, resulting in elongation and thinning. If these are not addressed at the time of a facelift, there will be a severe lack of harmony after completion of the facial rejuvenation, which may distract from an otherwise satisfactory result.

In performing otoplasty, it is imperative to realize that for each eminence there is a fossa, and that through re-creating the normal convexities and concavities of the auricular cartilage, the surgeon can create an ear that looks normal and will persist (**Fig. 28.2a,b**).

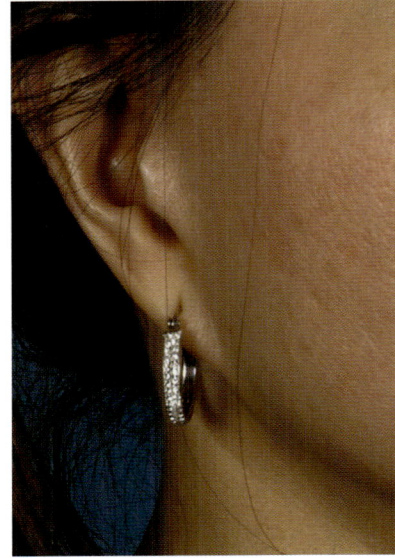

Fig. 28.1 Pixie ear deformity with effacement of the infralobular crease after facelift.

■ Patient Selection

Ears that protrude and may become the source of ridicule can be corrected as early as 5 to 6 years of age. There is evidence to suggest that teasing and harassment will begin when the patient enters elementary school. This, of course, may depend upon the degree of protrusion, the gender of the patient, and the hairstyle. The parents of males are more likely to seek correction at a younger age than those of females. There is an upper limit on the age at which an otoplasty can be performed. In the older patient, the cartilage will become more rigid and may require more aggressive surgical techniques.

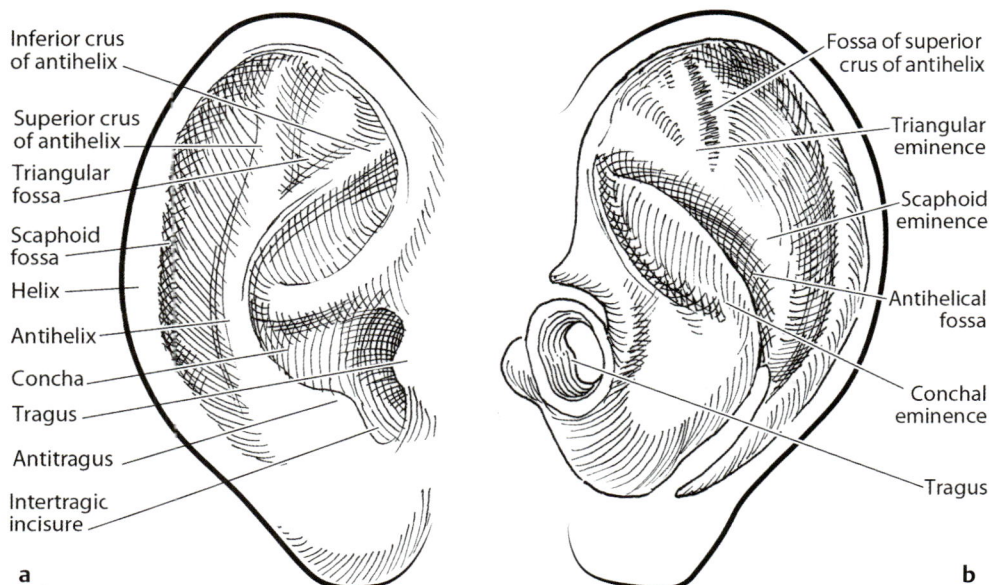

Inferior crus of antihelix

Superior crus of antihelix

Triangular fossa

Scaphoid fossa

Helix

Antihelix

Concha

Tragus

Antitragus

Intertragic incisure

a

Fossa of superior crus of antihelix

Triangular eminence

Scaphoid eminence

Antihelical fossa

Conchal eminence

Tragus

b

Fig. 28.2 Common external landmarks of pinna. **(a)** Lateral aspect. **(b)** Medial aspect.

Technical Aspects of Procedure

Lop Ear Deformity

Correction of the lop ear deformity takes many forms and has been covered extensively in the past.[3–6] This section summarizes the author's preferred techniques and offers an explanation for these choices ▶Video 28.1. Any technique must be customized to address the deformities that exist and neither over- nor undertreat.

In the author's practice, there is a 93% occurrence of absence or underdevelopment of the superior crus of the antihelix in patients with protruding ears. This may present in isolation, resulting in the protrusion of the superior pinna, or in conjunction with the absence or underdevelopment of the antihelix along its entire length; this occurs in 75% of the patients and will result in the protrusion of the entire helical margin. Protrusion of the entire helical margin in the absence or underdevelopment of the antihelix is almost universally associated with a prominent cauda helices, contributing to protrusion of the lobule. A deep conchal bowl that further exacerbates the protrusion occurs in ~ 45% of the author's patients.

Absence of the superior crus is the most straightforward deformity and the most consistently encountered. It is addressed through the excision of an ellipse of skin on the posterior surface of the ear over the desired fossa of the superior crus of the antihelix. This is determined by folding the ear to re-create the superior crus and identifying the corresponding position on the posterior surface. This can be accomplished by the placement of Keith needles through the ear from the anterior surface. Needles are placed at the junction of the superior and inferior crus of the antihelix in the fossa triangularis, the lateral conchal bowl at the junction of the superior and inferior crus, and the anterior margin of the scaphoid fossa (**Fig. 28.3a,b**). These are used as guideposts for the scoring of the posterior surface of the ear in the antihelical fossa, while avoiding incisions that would cross the inferior crus, a devastating error. After scoring, horizontal mattress sutures are placed from the scaphoid eminence to the eminence triangularis and the lateral conchal bowl, sequentially. These sutures are performed with a 4–0 Mersilene suture and are tightened to the desired projection, which is having the helical margin 1.5 to 2 cm off the mastoid at the junction of the superior and inferior crus.[7,8]

When absence of the antihelix in the entirety is present, the posterior skin excision is extended as an elliptical dumbbell inferiorly until the beginning of the lobule (**Fig. 28.4**). After skin excision is complete, the skin is dissected off the posterior surface of the cauda helices. Then 5 to 7 mm of the distal lateral margin of the skin is resected obliquely (**Fig. 28.5**). The scoring is then performed, extending down the

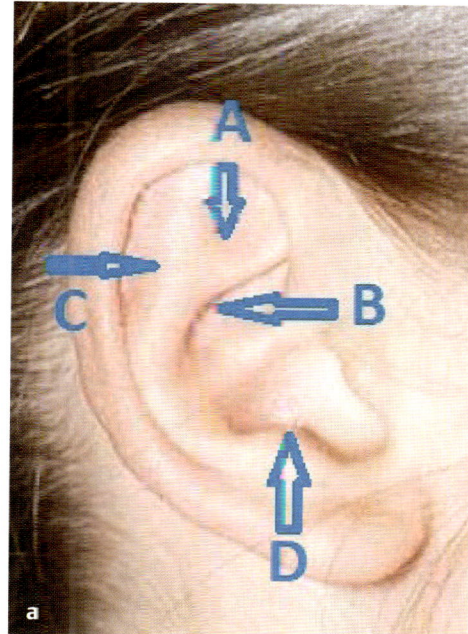

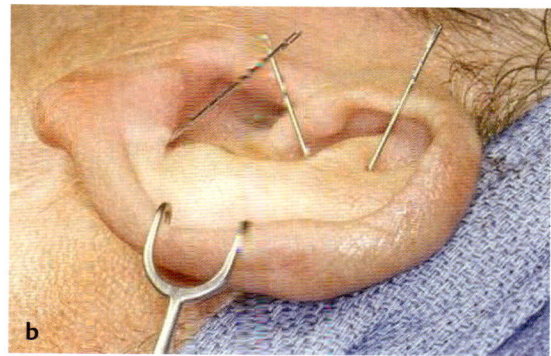

Fig. 28.3 Keith needle placement for the postauricular identification of anterior anatomical landmarks. Needles B and D are placed medial to the desired antihelix.

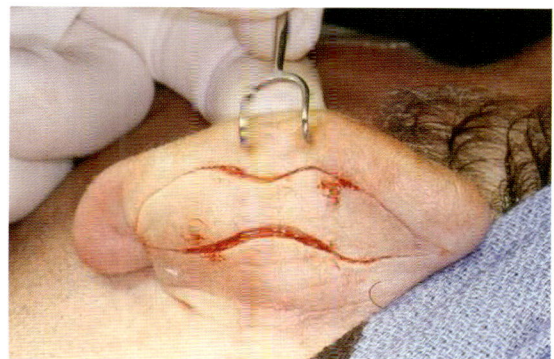

Fig. 28.4 Elliptical dumbbell excision on the posterior surface of the ear. This is narrower in the midportion to help avoid a telephone ear deformity.

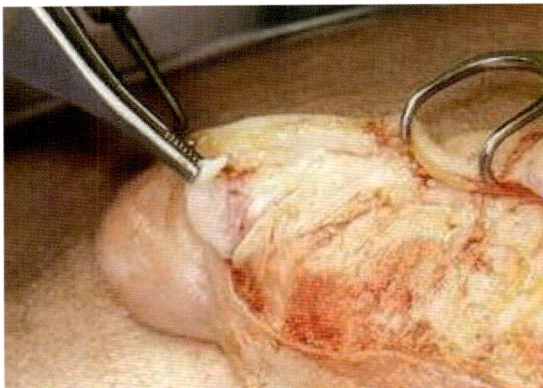

Fig. 28.5   Trimming of the cauda helicis.

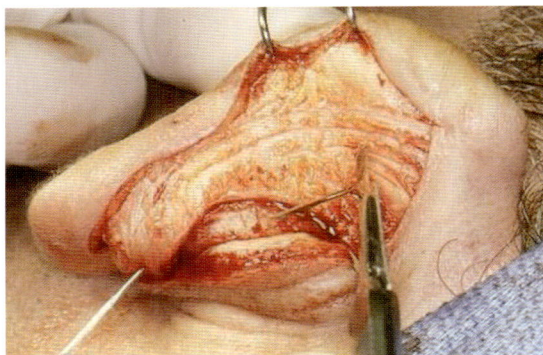

Fig. 28.6   Partial-thickness scoring of the posterior surface of the antihelix, the antihelical fossa.

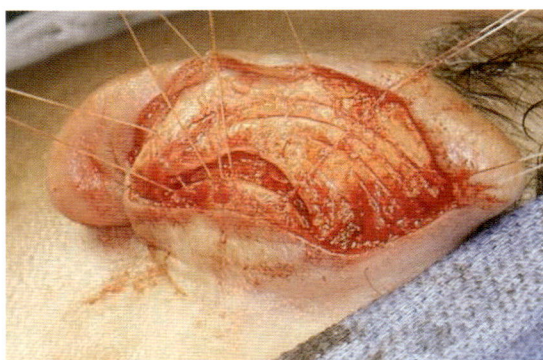

Fig. 28.7   Placement of mattress sutures radiating from the conchal bowl to the scaphoid eminence, including a suture from the fossa triangularis to the superior portion of the scaphoid eminence.

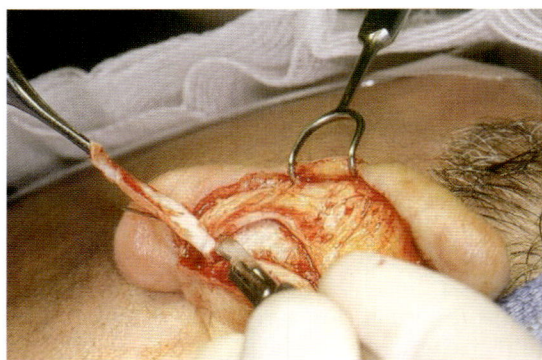

Fig. 28.8   Resection of an ellipse of the lateral conchal bowl and conchal reduction.

entire length of the antihelix (**Fig. 28.6**). Horizontal mattress sutures of 4–0 Mersilene are placed from the scaphoid eminence to the lateral conchal bowl (**Fig. 28.7**). The sutures all radiate from the external auditory canal. When one is placing the sutures, care is taken to avoid the skin on the anterior surface.

In the presence of a deep conchal bowl, conchal reduction or conchal setback needs to be executed. The author has found that conchal reduction is more reliable and results in much less postoperative pain and discomfort. With conchal setback alone, there is no re-creation of the antihelix in its absence.

To perform conchal reduction, the posterior surface of the cartilage is marked with transauricular Keith needles corresponding to the previously described locations, in addition to the placement of a needle at the lateral conchal bowl even with the antitragus (**Fig. 28.3a,b**). The index or middle finger is placed in the conchal bowl to palpate the deep surface of the conchal incision, and an ellipse of lateral bowl cartilage is resected, with the width dependent on need (**Fig. 28.8**). This defect is then incorporated into the posterior suturing. The additional sutures are placed from the scaphoid eminence in a horizontal fashion to the lateral, and subsequently, medial margin of the conchal bowl as a vertical suture (**Fig. 28.7**).

The postauricular incision is closed with a running locked 5–0 plain gut suture. Antibiotic ointment is applied to the incision, and mineral oil–impregnated cotton is placed in the postauricular sulcus, fossa triangularis, scaphoid fossa, concha cavum, and concha cymba (**Fig. 28.9**). Fluffed cotton 4 × 4 gauze is secured over the ears with a circumferential dressing encompassing both ears.

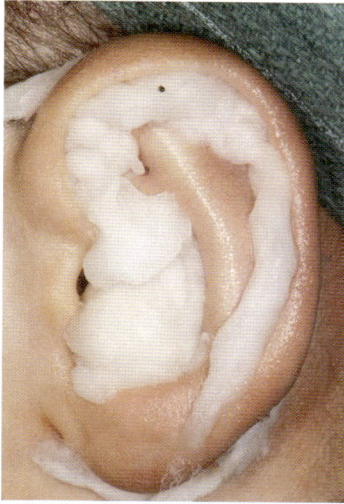

Fig. 28.9 Mineral oil–impregnated cotton placed in the post-auricular crease, fossa triangularis, scaphoid fossa, concha cavum, and concha cymba.

Appropriate applications of elliptical dumbbell excision of posterior auricular skin, cauda helicis trimming, conchal reduction, posterior scoring, and mattress suturing will lead to excellent, anatomically correct–appearing ears with little to no evidence of surgical correction. The margins of the cartilage are realigned when cartilage excision is performed. The incision is on the medial surface of the protruding portion of the pinna and is invisible to observers (**Fig. 28.10**; **Fig. 28.11a,b**).

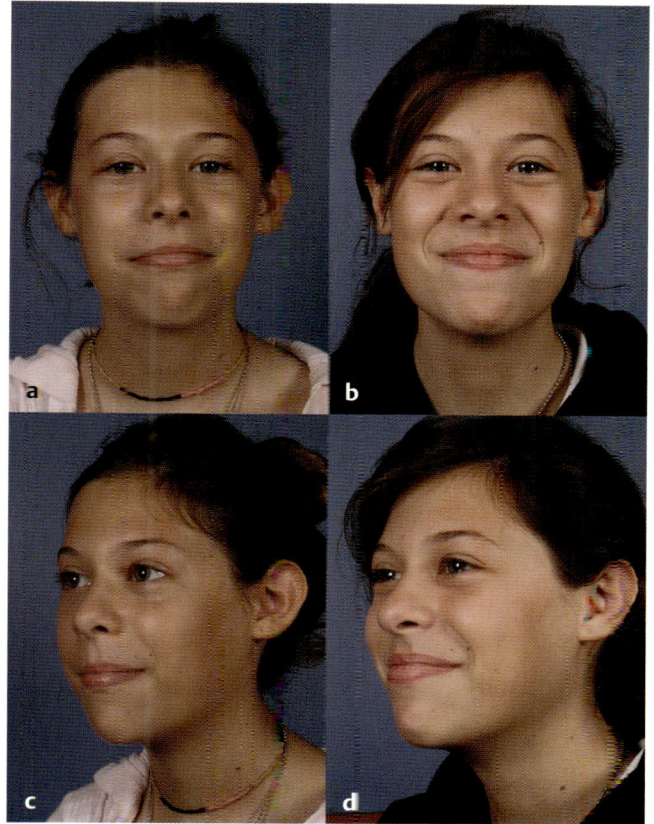

Fig. 28.10 Preoperative views (**a,c**) and postoperative views (**b,d**) at 12 months after conchal reduction, cartilage scoring, and suturing.

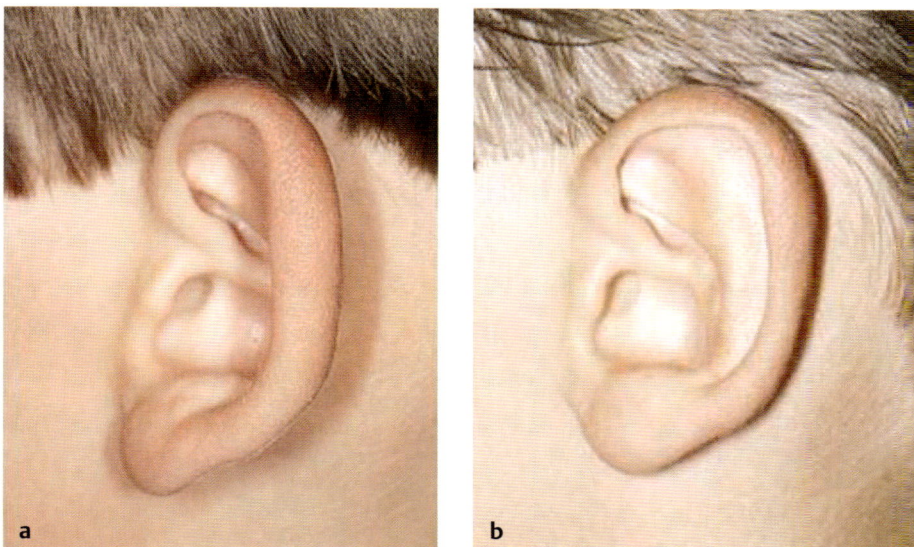

Fig. 28.11 Conchal setback with cartilage scoring and suturing. (**a**) Preoperative. (**b**) Twelve months postoperative.

Earlobe Abnormalities

Earlobe abnormalities may take many forms. They may be postsurgical in nature or the result of a congenital variation or the aging process. The most common variation is congenital attached lobules, and management is similar to the technique for correcting the postsurgical pixie ear deformity. The technique for correction of the senile and large lobule will depend upon the vertical and horizontal dimensions of the earlobe and the nature of the attachment of the lobule to the posterior face. The patient's desire, or lack thereof, to change the attachment is also relevant. With the large lobule, simple marginal excision, as described by Adamson and Litner, can be performed.[8]

With the normal-sized attached lobule, whether congenital or iatrogenic, the goal is achieving a more acute angle of attachment without a scar extending vertically into the neck. This is best achieved with a simple transposition flap created from the skin of the inferior margin of the lobule (**Fig. 28.12a,b**). This flap is repositioned into a postauricular recipient incision, maintaining all visible incisions in the postauricular sulcus and mastoid.

When the attached lobule is enlarged, and overall size reduction as well as release is desired, creativity is the key to a successful release and camouflaged scar. If this is being performed in conjunction with a facelift, avoiding a vertical, cervical incision is easy when lobular reduction is performed first, and the facelift flap trimming is executed to accommodate the repositioning of the earlobe (i.e., eliminating infralobular tension with minimal flap resection).

In both cases, reduction is achieved through a hemicrescentic resection of the lobule with the wider portion anterior at the lobular facial junction (**Fig. 28.13**). Superiorly and posteriorly on the lateral surface of the ear, the incision can be blended into the soft tissue furrow of the inferior extent of the scaphoid fossa. If the desired result is to reduce the overall size and release the lobule from its attachments to the posterior face and neck, it is then necessary to butterfly the inferior segment, creating a transposition flap (as in the release of the attached lobule in **Fig. 28.12a,b**) prior to creating the hemicrescentic excision.

For the lobule that is detached and of increased horizontal and vertical dimension, stellate excision is performed. This is planned to include any preexisting rhytids and will more than likely necessitate the repiercing of the ear after completion. With both the stellate and pie-shaped excision, the pattern is offset at the inferior margin of the lobule to prevent a circumferential scar and contracture between the anterior and posterior surface (**Figs. 28.14** and **28.15**).

■ Postoperative Care

The otoplasty dressing remains in place for 5 days but is removed for any complaints of discomfort, pain, or bleeding. After the dressing is removed, the patient is instructed to secure the ears while asleep for 6 weeks postoperatively. This can be accomplished with an athletic headband. The postauricular incision is cleaned with hydrogen peroxide and dressed with antibiotic ointment until the fast-absorbing sutures have resorbed. Swimming is allowed immediately after the head dressing is removed, but diving is prohibited for 6 weeks postoperatively. Patients are also forbidden from wearing athletic or recreational headgear (e.g., helmets) for 6 weeks.

With earlobe reduction, it is virtually impossible to dress the lobule. Patients are instructed to clean the surgical incisions with hydrogen peroxide and apply antibiotic ointment twice a day. If the ear is pierced at the time of the procedure, the 14-karat gold post remains in place for 6 weeks to allow epithelialization; it is then changed under the supervision of a nurse in the office.

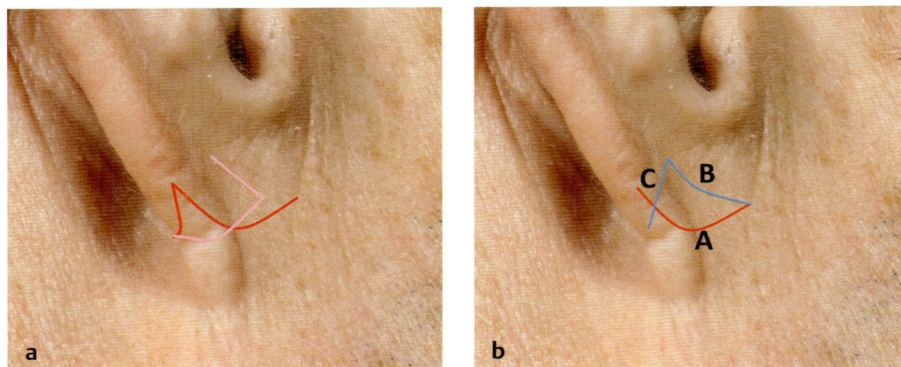

Fig. 28.12 Incision placement for release of the congenital attached lobule or postoperative pixie ear deformity (a). Postoperative (b) flap repositioning with line A representing the closure on the inferior lobule and lines B and C representing the postauricular closures.

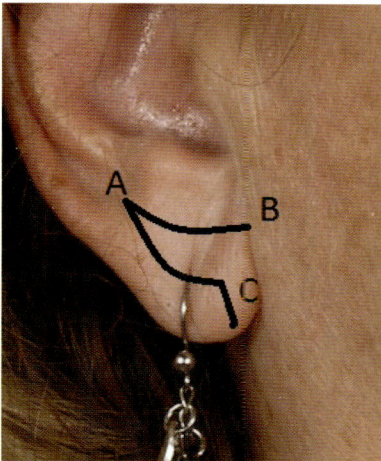

Fig. 28.13 Anterior incisions for simple crescentic earlobe reduction.

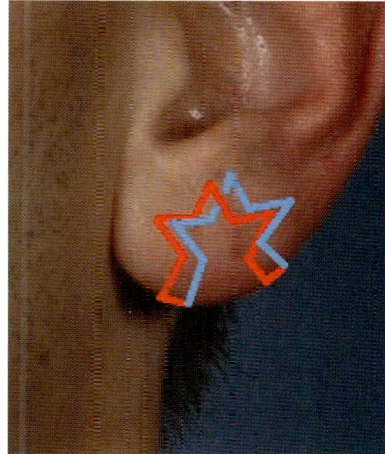

Fig. 28.14 Stellate excision of the oversized lobule with offset of the incisions on the anterior and posterior surface.

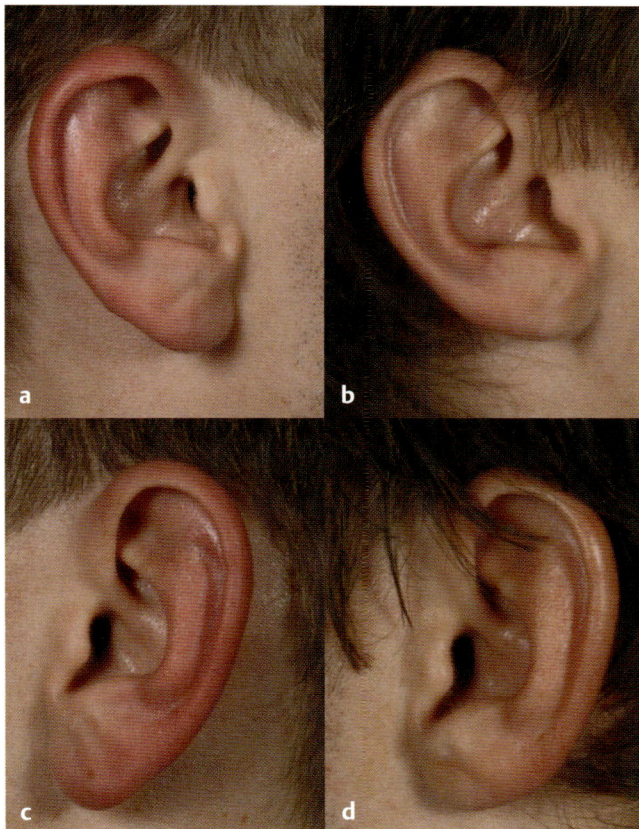

Fig. 28.15 Preoperative **(a,c)** and 12 months postoperative **(b,d)** after stellate lobular excision

■ Complications and Their Management

The rate of complications or adverse incidents is minimal with these procedures. The most common complication in an otoplasty may be the postoperative reflection of a preoperative asymmetry that is persistent. Therefore, it is imperative to point out any preoperative differences prior to surgery. They may or may not have been identified by the parents or patient before surgery, but they will indeed be noticed postoperatively. If an asymmetry exists, it can be addressed with local anesthesia on an outpatient basis. Most patients are initially counseled to avoid intervention for at least 12 months after surgery. Cartilaginous irregularities and granulations usually occur on the anterior surface of the ear overlying sutures and incisions. When performing a conchal setback, careful posterior suture placement must be performed to avoid anterior displacement of the posterior border of the external auditory canal.

The second-most-common complication is the extrusion of one of the contouring sutures. This may happen years after the original procedure. In most cases, the cartilage will have recontoured, and the protruding suture can be removed without consequence. Hypertrophic and keloid scar formation in the postauricular incision can occur and will more than likely require excision and scar repair but should initially be treated with intralesional steroid injections.

Postoperative hematoma can develop and necessitate evacuation. If it is left untreated, the likelihood of developing a wound infection is increased. This may lead to perichondritis and the possible loss of the affected ear's cartilaginous framework.

■ Conclusion

The graduated technique for otoplasty that incorporates a means of reducing conchal depth and re-creating the antihelix has served the author's patients well. The most consistent combination of surgical techniques involves reducing conchal depth through conchal reduction and re-creating the antihelix with scoring in the antihelical fossa on the posterior surface of the ear. This also includes the placement of vertical mattress sutures from the scaphoid fossa, approximating the lateral conchal bowl and medial antihelix.

Modifications of lobular size, position, and attachment may be performed as stand-alone procedures or as an adjunct to facial rejuvenation or otoplasty for the protruding ear (**Fig. 28.16**). Their use in facial rejuvenation patients can sometimes be synonymous with overall facial harmony. Ignoring an enlarged earlobe at the time of a facelift will create an inconsistent appearance postoperatively. These procedures are a safe and simple approach to enhancing outcomes from otoplasty and rhytidectomy, as well as simply reducing an enlarged lobule.

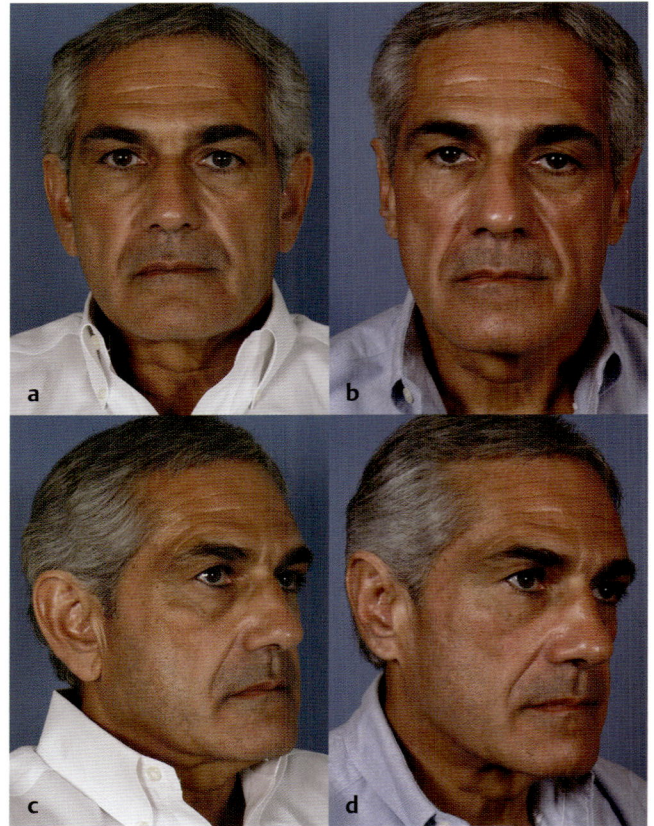

Fig. 28.16 Preoperative **(a,c)** and 12 months postoperative **(b,d)** after otoplasty with conchal reduction, cartilage scoring, and suturing accompanied by stellate earlobe reduction.

References

1. Richards SD, Jebreel A, Capper R. Otoplasty: a review of the surgical techniques. Clin Otolaryngol 2005;30(1):2–8
2. Rogers BO. Microtic, lop, cup and protruding ears: four directly inheritable deformities? Plast Reconstr Surg 1968;41(3):208–231
3. Farrior RT. Modified cartilage incisions in otoplasty. Facial Plast Surg 1985;2:109–118
4. Farrior RT. A method of otoplasty; normal contour of the antihelix and scaphoid fossa. AMA Arch Otolaryngol 1959;69(4):400–408
5. Mustarde JC. The correction of prominent ears using simple mattress sutures. Br J Plast Surg 1963;16:170–178
6. Furnas DW. Correction of prominent ears by conchamastoid sutures. Plast Reconstr Surg 1968;42(3):189–193
7. Larrabee WF, Kibblewhite D, Adams JB. Otoplasty. In: Smith JD, Bumsted R, eds. Pediatric Facial Plastic and Reconstructive Surgery. New York, NY: Raven; 1993:79–98
8. Adamson PA, Litner JA. Otoplasty technique. Facial Plast Surg Clin North Am 2006;14(2):79–87, v

29 Short-Incision Facelift and Necklift

Gregory J. Vipond and Harry Mittelman

Key Concepts

- A short-incision face-/necklift may result in a more rapid recovery than classic approaches. However, the extent of undermining must extend to the posterior edge of the ptotic superficial muscular aponeurotic system (SMAS) and platysma for adequate suspension.

- The multivector SMAS and platysmal suspension technique employs a customized, anatomical method of suspension that restores the ptotic tissue to a more youthful position.

- The use of a permanent, monofilament suture permits a means of permanent resuspension. However, to avoid sutures pulling through, the suspension must be reinforced with multiple interrupted or continuous sutures.

- The short-incision face-/necklift may be combined with a traditional submentoplasty for patients with significant anterior platysmal banding or liposis.

- A horizontal limb extension may be used if there is dimpling of the postauricular skin flap. This extension will not compromise the healing and will allow patients to wear their hair pulled back much more quickly than if there is a visible skin crease.

◼ Introduction

There has been a great deal of evolution with regard to surgical techniques to address the aging face and neck. The first facelift techniques involved subcutaneous elevation and removal of excess skin in the pretragal area. Unfortunately, there was limited long-term improvement in the cervicomental angle, and laxity due to ptosis of the deeper tissues was not addressed. In 1976, Mitz and Peyronie[1] introduced the superficial musculoaponeurotic system (SMAS). SMAS re-suspension, either through imbrications or plication, led to improvement in subcutaneous and cutaneous aging and also increased the longevity of that improvement. The next development was by Hamra, who pioneered both the deep plane lift and then the composite lift.[2,3] These innovations were designed to add additional rejuvenation to the melolabial fold and periocular areas. Following the trend of more invasive procedures came the subperiosteal lift.[4] Although the more aggressive procedures may have theoretical advantages, in terms of efficacy, over more conservative procedures, this has been an often debated subject, with proponents of the deeper-level lifts arguing better postoperative rejuvenation despite a longer recovery and greater risk of complications. Unfortunately, there have been very few meaningful studies to offer objective evidence to support either argument.[5] As with many areas of medicine, market forces and patient demand have led to a reversing trend back to more conservative procedures.

The lateral SMASectomy[6] and S-lift[7] both use a short incision with a predominantly vertical vector of SMAS suspension. The S-lift utilizes a preauricular incision to gain access to the SMAS and involves making a double purse-string suture to suspend the SMAS to the periosteum of the zygomatic arch. The principal limitation of this technique is the inability to adequately address platysma laxity and cervicomental angle.

The minimal access cranial suspension (MACS) lift was developed in 2001 by Tonnard and Verpaele and was an advance on the purse-string lifts.[3] It incorporates additional undermining of the lateral face and jowl and uses larger purse-string sutures to grasp the cranial border of the platysma. Submental liposuction is also used, where indicated, leading to improved results, especially in the heavier-volume face and neck. A further modification has been made through the addition of a third purse-string suture to attempt effacement of the malar fat pad and melolabial fold.[9]

In 2004, Brandy added another modification to the S-lift by incorporating postauricular and lateral neck undermining to achieve greater correction of the platysma–SMAS complex.[10,11] This lift became branded as the Quicklift. The Quicklift and the LifestyleLift, a limited-dissection SMAS/platysma plication, are among two of the more widely advertised face and neck lifts. Their brands imply a minimal degree of invasiveness, risk, and recovery, and through clever marketing, they are influencing the way the American population views facial rejuvenation.

Consequently, there is a greater awareness of facial rejuvenation surgical procedures, although the prospective patient is not necessarily better educated. Patients like the concept of a shorter recovery, natural look, and lower risk, and may be willing to sacrifice some degree of efficacy for this. In order for facial plastic surgeons to remain relevant, they must be able to speak to this demand and offer a similar procedure as part of their facial rejuvenation repertoire.

The multivector lift is a technique whereby the SMAS and platysma are re-suspended in a reverse pathophysiological manner. It appreciates that soft tissue descent with age is not a uniform process, and to achieve an effective, yet natural, result, the surgeon should attempt to restore the ptotic soft tissue to its youthful position (see ▶ **Video 29.1**). This chapter describes a technique employed by both authors for well over a thousand patients with a very high level of satisfaction and low level of morbidity, complications, and need for revision.

Background: Basic Science of Procedure

With age, there is increased laxity and loss of tone both in the superficial layers of the face, such as the epidermis and dermis, and in the deeper layers of the face, including the SMAS and platysma. There is also a change in underlying bone structure that affects the skeletal support of the overlying tissues. The principal layers involved in rhytidoplasty are the SMAS and platysma, with a smaller emphasis on the skin and adipose tissue. Without proper elevation of the SMAS and platysma, there will be insignificant postoperative improvement. The procedure would be a skin lift, which may look good during the early postoperative period in the presence of skin edema, but once the induration has resolved, there may be a quick return of the preoperative laxity.

In addressing the aging SMAS and platysma, the authors employ a multivector lift approach that appreciates that the descent of the subcutaneous soft tissue

does not occur in a uniform direction or amount throughout its distribution. Consequently, to reverse the aging process, it is appropriate to return each aspect of the SMAS and platysma to its former, youthful position throughout its entire distribution, rather than by an arbitrary amount or direction. While this approach may be more labor intensive than other methods of SMAS/platysma re-suspension, we believe it is more anatomically correct and beneficial in the long term. As the patient continues to age postoperatively, there is a natural recurrence of SMAS/platysmal descent without an operated or artificial appearance.

The concept behind minimal incision face-/necklifting is that, with appropriate patient selection, sufficient re-suspension of the SMAS/platysma complex can be achieved without extensive skin undermining. With a shorter skin flap, there is a hypothetical decreased recovery period with less edema and ecchymosis, less risk of hematoma and infection, shorter operative time, and smaller incisions. Many facial plastic surgery patients have jobs and do not have the luxury of a long postoperative recovery. Consequently, the option of having a procedure with a relatively short downtime is very appealing. Additionally, due to a shorter operative time with less undermining, the option of a decreased level of anesthesia, such as intravenous or oral conscious sedation with local anesthetic, can be attractive to the patient.

Pertinent Anatomy

The minimal-incision face-/necklift is a modification of the standard rhytidoplasty. The preauricular incision is made in a similar fashion, but the horizontal sideburn limb is often shorter. The postauricular incision may include a horizontal limb, but the decision is often made during skin redraping, depending on the degree of elastosis. The degree of skin undermining is determined by the location of the posterior edge of the platysma and ptotic SMAS (**Fig. 29.1a–c**). To properly elevate the SMAS and platysma, skin undermining must be performed, at a minimum, to the edge of these structures. Failure to adequately undermine and expose the SMAS and platysma will lead to insignificant soft tissue re-suspension and will essentially be a skin lift with poor efficacy and longevity.

Patient Selection

The ideal candidate for a minimal-incision face- and necklift is one with early signs of elasticity. In general, there is mild jowl formation with little anterior platysmal banding, submental elastosis, or liposis. Other concerns that should be taken into account

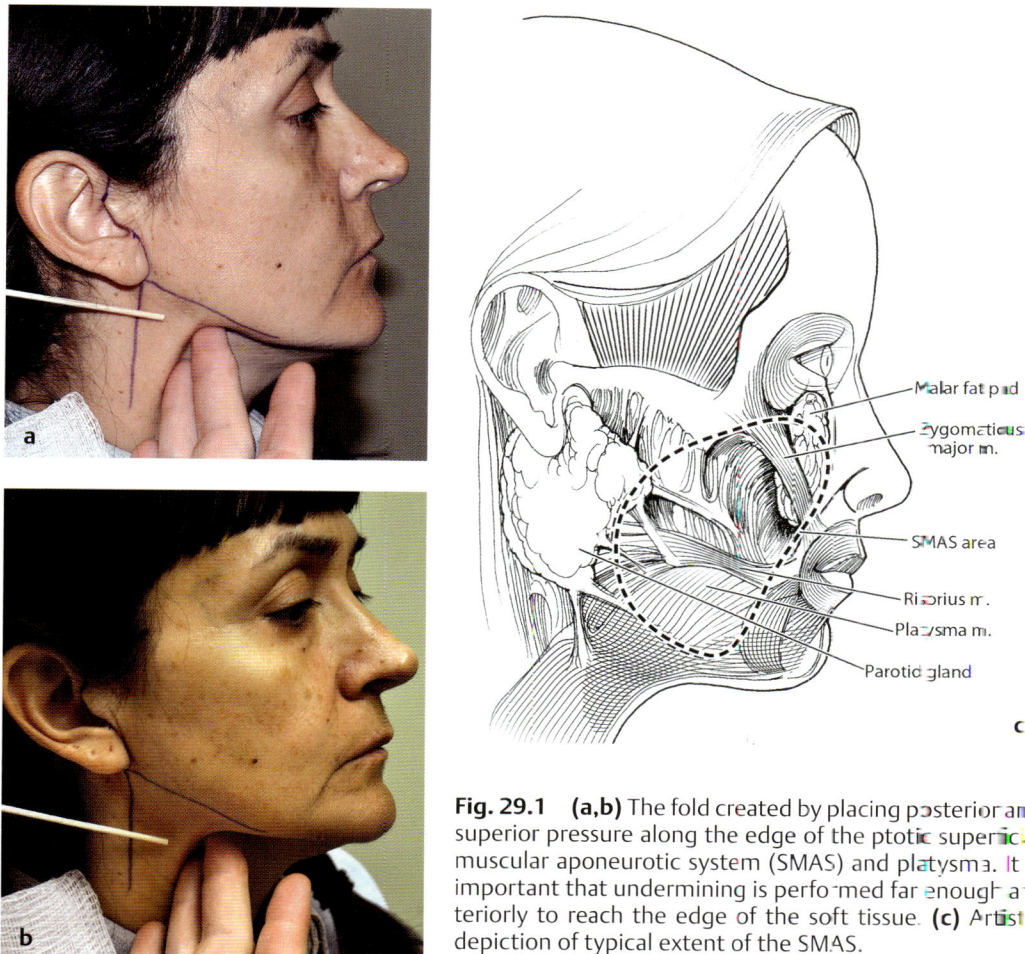

Fig. 29.1 **(a,b)** The fold created by placing posterior and superior pressure along the edge of the ptotic superficial muscular aponeurotic system (SMAS) and platysma. It is important that undermining is performed far enough anteriorly to reach the edge of the soft tissue. **(c)** Artist's depiction of typical extent of the SMAS.

include patients who desire a very conservative result and natural look, patients who do not want a horizontal segment of their postauricular incision, patients seeking a very short recovery time, patients seeking very modest, socially unnoticeable results, and patients with compromised blood supply, such as tobacco users and diabetics.

The typical age range for these patients is the late thirties to mid to late forties. However, patients who have undergone a prior rhytidoplasty with recurrence of facial and cervical elastosis are also potential candidates. An important aspect of a successful surgical outcome is preoperative counseling and setting of expectations. Minimal incision procedures often carry the benefit of a faster recovery and lower risk of complications but may not offer as dramatic a postoperative improvement as a more extensive procedure. Unsatisfied patients are often those who expect the improvement of a traditional procedure, but with the cost, recovery, and risk of a less extensive one.

If a patient does exhibit significant anterior submental elastosis and platysmal laxity, the procedure should be combined with a submentoplasty and an-

terior platysmal plication and liposculpting, as indicated. If there is significant skin flap dimpling with the anterior plication, connecting the undermined regions of the submental and preauricular skin flaps may help avoid contour irregularities.

■ Technical Aspects of Procedure

The patient is marked in an upright position, prior to the administration of any sedation or anesthetic. The authors feel that the upright position allows better visualization of the true position of facial and cervicomental laxity. Additionally, areas of potential liposculpting may be identified. If a submentoplasty is going to be performed, an incision is made in or just posterior to the submental crease in a curvilinear fashion to parallel the crease. This will help to avoid elevation of the lateral aspect of the incision with the rhytidoplasty to where it may become visible. The area of skin undermining is outlined along with any visible platysmal banding. Generally, dissection is performed to the thyroid notch inferiorly, and as far laterally as necessary to expose any platysmal banding.

The face- and necklift incision is then marked (**Fig. 29.2a–c**). It extends along the sideburn superiorly, inferiorly along the helical root, along the apex of the tragus, inferiorly along the perilobular crease, ascending postauricularly lateral to the postauricular crease, and making a lateral limb of variable length at the height of the helical root. The mandibular border and the anterior border of the sternocleidomastoid (SCM) muscle are marked along with any potential areas for facial liposculpting. The extent of soft tissue undermining, corresponding to the leading edge of the ptotic SMAS and posterior edge of the platysma, is marked. Depending on surgeon preference, a small area of hair along the sideburn and horizontal limb of the postauricular incision may be trimmed to facilitate the procedure and reduce the incidence of ingrown hair within the suture line. The remainder of the patient's hair is gathered within a bouffant cap and secured with paper tape (**Fig. 29.3**).

At this time, anesthesia is given. This may be oral sedation, intravenous sedation, or induction of general anesthesia. Once the patient is comfortably sedated or intubated, the local anesthetic is infiltrated. The authors prefer a mixture of 1% lidocaine and 0.5% bupivacaine in a 1:1 ratio. Epinephrine may be added to make a dilution of 1:150,000. Preservative-free anesthetic may cause less discomfort than the premixed lidocaine/bupivacaine with epinephrine. The anesthetic is infiltrated in a subcutaneous plane so that ballooning of the tissue is achieved. The order of infiltration is the same as the procedure: submen-

toplasty, right face and neck, left face and neck. The bouffant cap is resecured and hair retracted with paper tape. The patient is then prepped with a noniodine solution and draped sterilely.

Although the focus of this chapter is on the minimal-incision face- and necklift, for completeness the submentoplasty portion will be briefly described here. The submental incision is made and undermining is performed in a shallow subcutaneous plane. It is important to leave a modest amount of subcutaneous tissue on the superficial flap to improve the flap viability, decrease the incidence of postoperative skin flap discoloration and telangiectasias, and avoid skeletonization of the platysma and possible cobra-neck deformity. Laterally, along the margin of the mandible, it is important to divide the skin from its attachment to the anterior mandibular ligament. This helps reduce the incidence of banding along the prejowl sulcus with skin redraping following the rhytidoplasty. Once the skin flap has been elevated, the decision is made to perform liposculpting. In a thin neck, extremely conservative liposuction is performed only to assist in identifying the platysma. In heavier necks, more aggressive liposuction may be performed, and subplatysmal liposuction may also be required. This should be done conservatively to reduce postoperative cobra-neck deformity. It is important to feather the peripheral areas, especially lateral to the submental pocket, to ensure a smooth contour.

Anterior platysmal plication may be performed in all patients, except those with extremely wide lateral banding of more than 2.5 cm. The plication extends inferiorly at the hyoid bone and continues superior

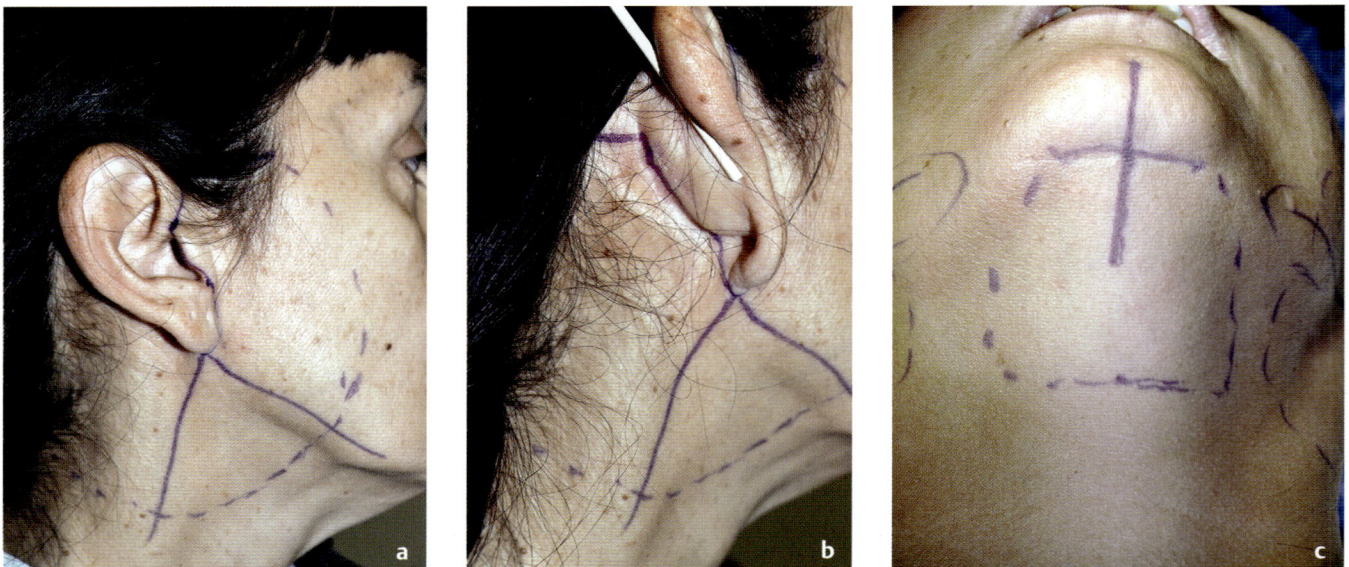

Fig. 29.2 Preoperative markings. **(a)** The preauricular incision and extent of proposed skin flap undermining. **(b)** The postauricular incision and extent of proposed skin flap undermining. **(c)** The submental incision and extent of proposed undermining.

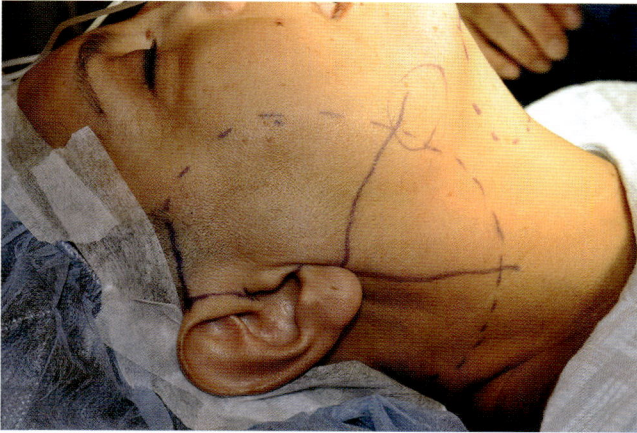

Fig. 29.3 The patient prior to injection of the local anesthetic.

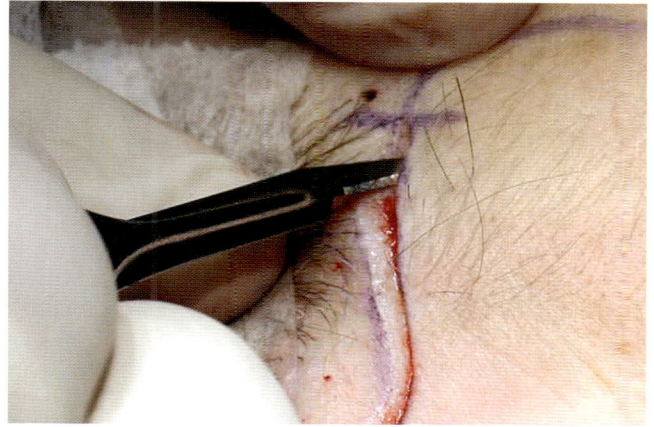

Fig. 29.4 The skin incision is made in a beveled fashion, perpendicular to the hair follicles, so that hair growth may occur through the incision.

to the junction of the platysma with the mentalis muscle. A 3–0 polypropylene suture is used in a simple continuous fashion and is tied so that the knot is buried beneath the platysma. If there is excess tissue bunching along the suture line, it may be trimmed or cauterized for contour. A bilateral horizontal back cut is made in the platysma just below the hyoid to disrupt the vertical platysmal band and to help create a hinge for posterior platysmal re-suspension. Meticulous hemostasis should be obtained, especially along the platysmal edges. Prior to skin redraping, a small horizontal skin ellipse (< 1 cm) may be excised along the inferior edge of the flap to improve the postoperative submental skin contour. The incision is carefully closed with 5–0 polypropylene in a continuous simple and vertical mattress fashion.

Rhytidoplasty usually starts on the right side of the face. The incision is made in a beveled fashion toward the flap side to promote hair growth through the incision (**Fig. 29.4**). Postauricular undermining is performed in a subcutaneous plane directly on the mastoid fascia and fascia of the SCM so that adipose tissue is left on the skin flap. In thin necks, it is extremely important to avoid injury to the great auricular nerve, which may have a superficial location in the inferior neck (**Fig. 29.5**). Preauricular undermining is performed directly on top of the SMAS (**Fig. 29.6**) so that there is adequate adipose tissue on the skin flap to help reduce any postoperative contour irregularity, ensure adequate skin flap blood supply, and help reduce the postoperative incidence of skin flap discoloration and telangiectasia development.

Once the skin flap has been elevated circumferentially, hemostasis is obtained. If a submentoplasty has been performed, a decision is made regarding the necessity of connecting the submental dissection and rhytidoplasty pockets. If there is submental skin

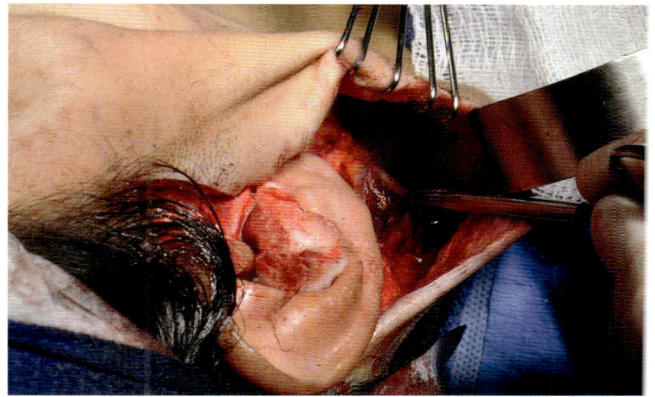

Fig. 29.5 In thin necks, the great auricular nerve may be seen with skin flap elevation.

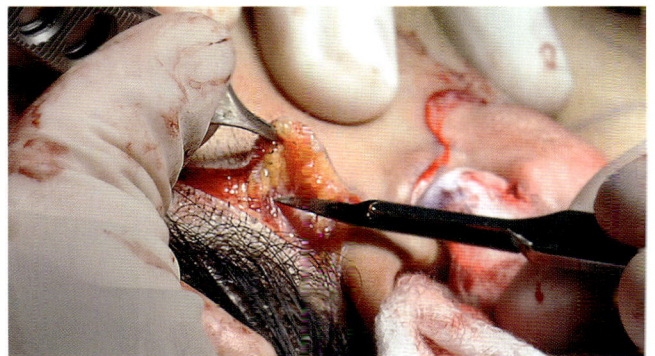

Fig. 29.6 The level of undermining for the preauricular flap is underneath the hair follicles and directly on top of the superficial muscular aponeurotic system.

dimpling from the anterior platysmal plication, the dissection pockets may be connected to assist with smooth skin redraping. Connecting the skin flaps is also beneficial in patients with heavier necks because a better-defined mandibular border is possible through improved liposculpting access.

Plication of the SMAS begins along the mandibular border. The edge of the ptotic SMAS is identified and then elevated in a posterior-superior vector to the anterior edge of the ear lobule. It is secured in a buried fashion with 3–0 polypropylene suture (**Fig. 29.7a,b**). This process is repeated approximately midway between the zygomatic arch and the mandible (**Fig. 29.8a,b**). The optimal vector of suspension should be determined by grasping the edge of the ptotic SMAS

and elevating it toward the auricle. The edge of the SMAS should elevate smoothly without dimpling. In general, the vector is slightly more posterior than superior at this point, and the SMAS is sutured in the same fashion. The next point of elevation is just inferior to the zygomatic arch and may achieve some effacement of the melolabial groove (**Fig. 29.9a,b**). This vector is mostly posterior and should complete the smooth SMAS elevation as a unit. A fourth plication suture is placed in the region of the malar fat pad and may be considered a "high SMAS" suture for melolabial fold effacement (**Fig. 29.10**).

Once the SMAS has been re-suspended, the repair is further reinforced, either with several buried, interrupted sutures (HM) or with a continuous 3–0 poly-

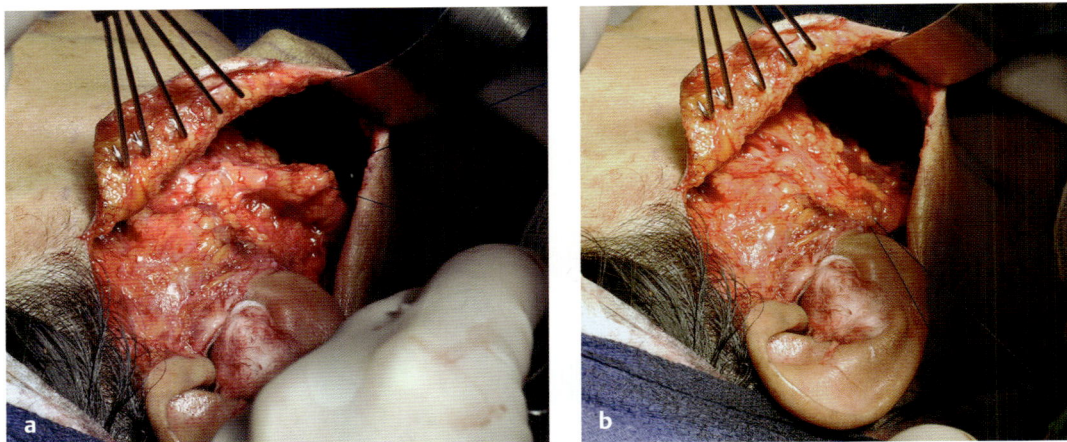

Fig. 29.7 The first suspension suture of the multivector superficial muscular aponeurotic system (SMAS) suspension. **(a)** The ptotic edge of the SMAS is grasped along the mandibular border and secured with 3–0 polypropylene suture. **(b)** The optimal vector of re-suspension is determined prior to tying the knot.

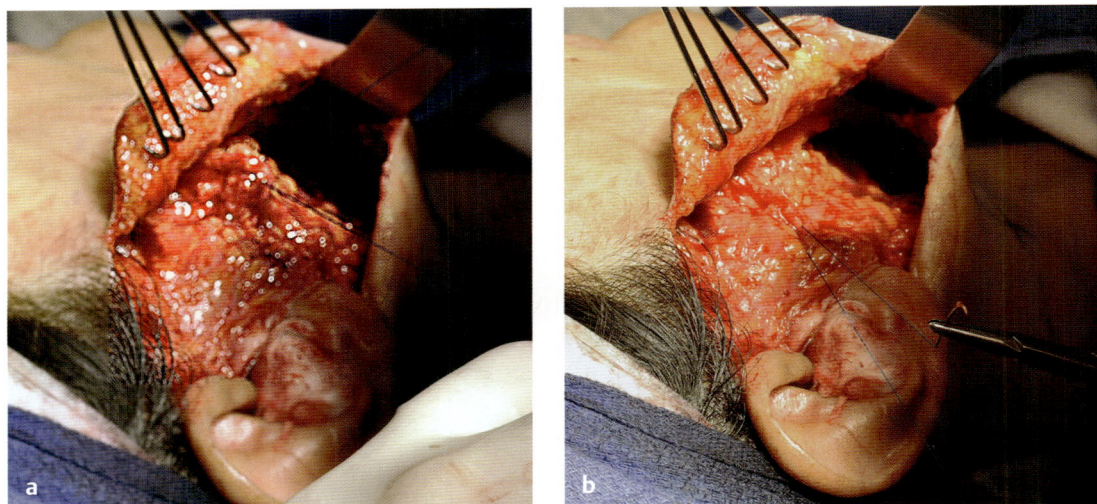

Fig. 29.8 The second superficial muscular aponeurotic system (SMAS) suspension suture. **(a)** The ptotic edge of the SMAS midway between the angle of the mandible and the zygomatic arch is grasped and secured with a 3–0 polypropylene suture. **(b)** The optimal vector of re-suspension is determined prior to tying the knot.

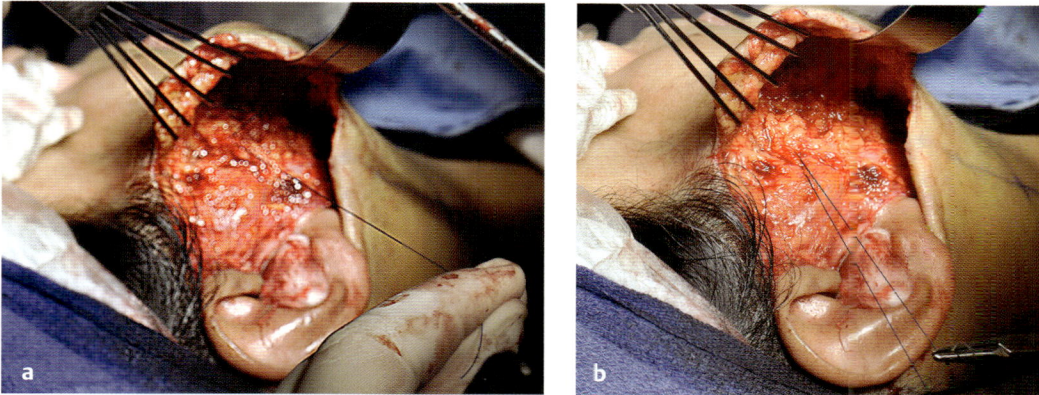

Fig. 29.9 The third superficial muscular aponeurotic system (SMAS) suspension suture. **(a)** The ptotic edge of the SMAS just below the zygomatic arch is grasped and secured with a 3–0 polypropylene suture. **(b)** The optimal vector of re-suspension is determined prior to tying the knot.

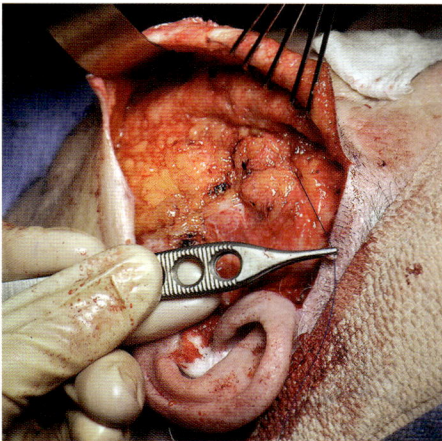

Fig. 29.10 The high superficial muscular aponeurotic system (high SMAS) suture. The edge of the malar fat pad has been grasped and secured to the zygomatic arch (note: this is the left side of the patient's face).

propylene suture with occasional locking sutures (GV) (see ▶Video 29.1). The use of polypropylene allows for permanent support with minimal tissue reaction. There may be a concern about monofilament sutures pulling through the soft tissue, though with the use of multiple sutures, this is less likely than if only several SMAS plication sutures are used.

After the SMAS plication, the platysma is elevated in a similar manner, proceeding in an inferior direction. The initial suspension is just below the angle of the mandible, and the posterior edge of the platysma is elevated in a posterior-superior vector to the edge of the SCM fascia and sutured in a buried fashion (**Fig. 29.11a,b**). Another plication suture is performed ~ 1.5 cm inferiorly with a slightly more posterior than superior vector (**Fig. 29.12a,b**). At the inferior edge of the dissection pocket, another suture is placed with a mostly posterior vector (**Fig. 29.13a,b**). As with the SMAS, the suspension is further reinforced with either additional interrupted sutures (HM) or a continuous suture with interval locking (GV).

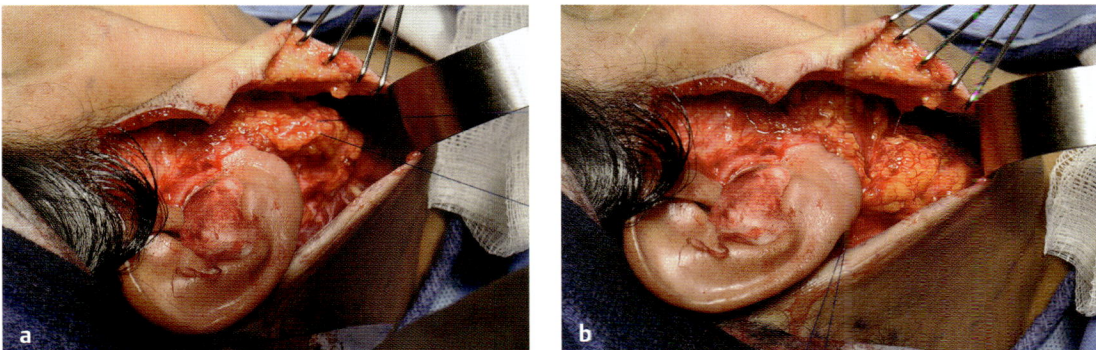

Fig. 29.11 The first platysmal plication suture. **(a)** The posterior edge of the platysma just inferior to the mandible is grasped and secured with a 3–0 polypropylene suture. **(b)** The optimal vector of re-suspension is determined prior to tying the knot.

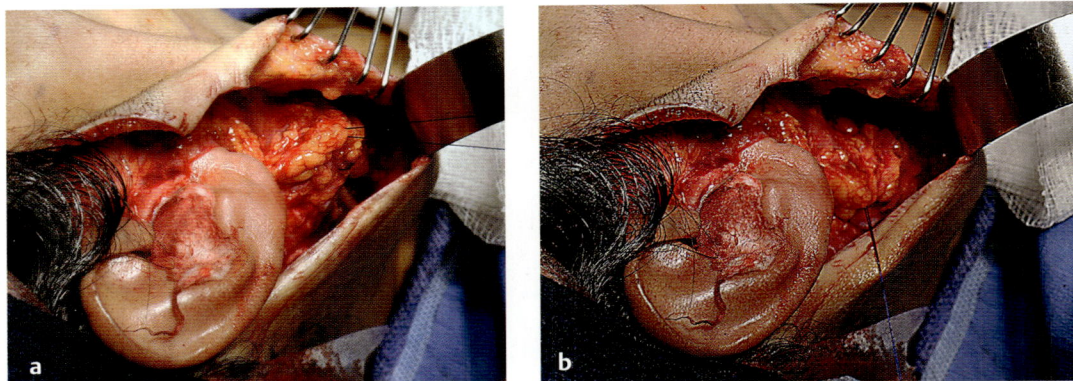

Fig. 29.12 The second platysmal plication suture. **(a)** The posterior edge of the platysma just inferior to the mandible is grasped and secured with a 3–0 polypropylene suture. **(b)** The optimal vector of re-suspension is determined prior to tying the knot.

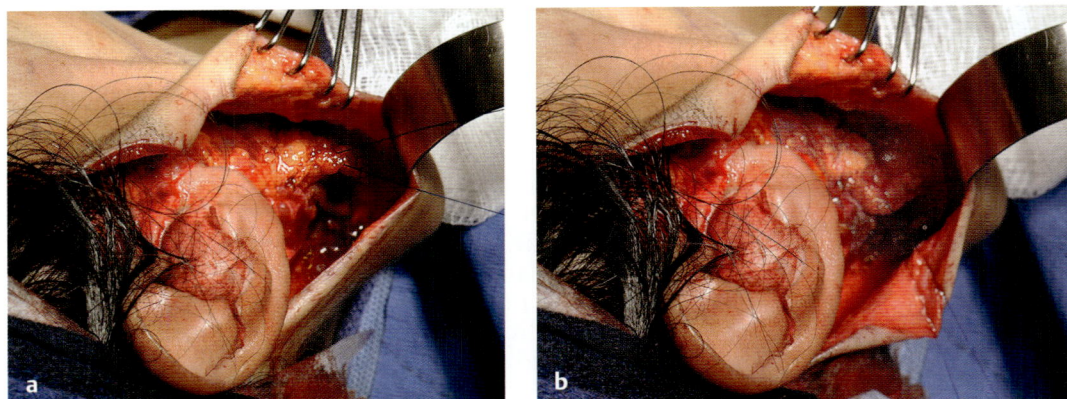

Fig. 29.13 The third platysmal plication suture. **(a)** The posterior edge of the platysma at the inferior edge of the dissection pocket is grasped and secured with a 3–0 polypropylene suture. **(b)** The optimal vector of re-suspension is determined prior to tying the knot.

After the plication is completed, any bunching along the suture line is trimmed. The skin flap is examined for any evidence of dimpling, which may be corrected by additional undermining. The need for liposculpting in the face and neck is also evaluated (**Fig. 29.14**). In general, it is performed in a conservative fashion with an emphasis on volume preservation. In a heavy neck, face and lateral neck liposculpting is performed prior to the SMAS and platysmal plication. Hemostasis is obtained prior to skin flap redraping.

Skin flap redraping begins preauricularly at the helical root. The skin is elevated in a posterior-superior vector, ensuring a smooth contour. With the assistant supporting the skin flap, a curved iris scissor is used to make a cut along the helix down to the apex of the helical root incision. The skin flap is reapproximated with a 5–0 polypropylene simple interrupted suture or staple (**Fig. 29.15**). The temporal tuft is now trimmed, and the subcutaneous tissue is reapproximated with two 5–0 polydioxanone (PDS, Ethicon, San Angelo, TX). The skin is then redraped over the auricle in a posterior-superior vector. The assistant supports the skin flap beneath the lobule, and the superior and inferior tragal borders are marked, along with the helical and perilobular margin. The skin is trimmed with curved iris scissors, carefully following along the edge of the preauricular incision. It is important to thin the supratragal skin so that there is a minimal amount of superficial adipose tissue on the flap (**Fig. 29.16**). This helps to avoid the appearance of a "fatty" tragus.

It is also important to avoid excess thinning of the flap because this can lead to tragal skeletonization and flap contraction. A buried 5–0 PDS suture is placed above and below the tragus. An anchor su-

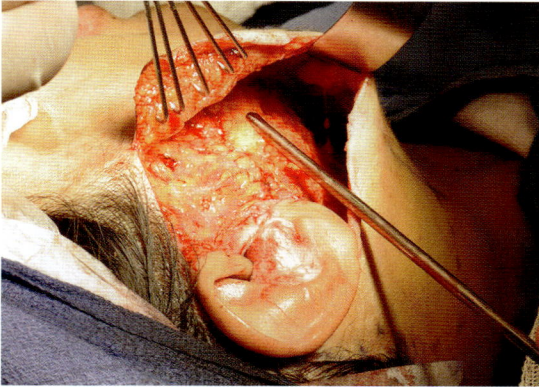

Fig. 29.14   The need for facial liposculpting is evaluated. It is extremely important to be conservative to avoid excessive hollowing.

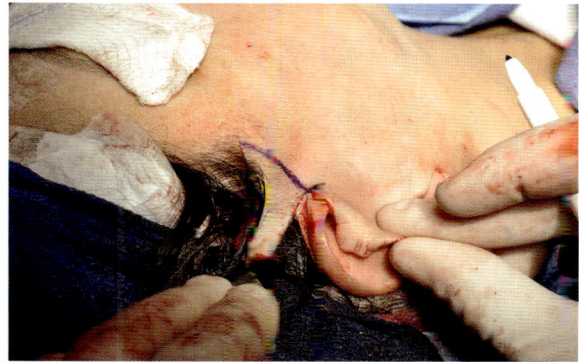

Fig. 29.15   Preauricular skin flap redraping begins at the helical root. The skin is smoothly laid back on the ear and a cut is made to the apex of the temporal tuft and helical root. This may be secured with a staple or interrupted suture.

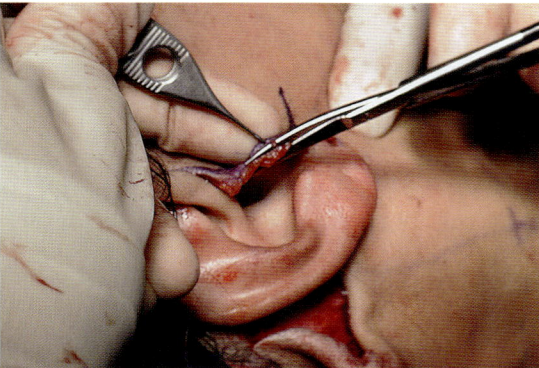

Fig. 29.16   Thinning of the tragal skin flap. The subcutaneous tissue overlying the tragus should be trimmed of all adipose tissue to avoid the postoperative appearance of a "fatty" tragus. It is essential to avoid excessive thinning of the dermis to avoid skin flap necrosis.

ture is placed at the apex of the lobule connecting the deep lobular tissue to the dermis of the skin flap using a 5–0 PDS or polypropylene suture. The skin is reapproximated using 5–0 polypropylene in a continuous simple with interval vertical mattress sutures for optimal reapproximation. Vertical mattress sutures are especially important along the anterior aspect of the lobule.

Postauricular skin flap redraping is done in a similar manner with the skin being elevated in an anterior-superior vector. The surgical assistant should retract the ear with one hand and then support the skin flap with another. The outline of the new skin edge is drawn and trimmed, ensuring that there is minimal skin tension (**Fig. 29.17**). A curved iris scissor is used to trim the flap, which is anchored

at the apex of the postauricular sulcus with one simple, interrupted 5–0 polypropylene suture. A buried 5–0 PDS suture is placed at the midportion of the horizontal limb of the postauricular suture, suspending the subcutaneous tissue of the skin flap to the mastoid fascia. An additional 5–0 PDS suture is placed at the posterior aspect of the lobule to offer further support. At this point, it is necessary to evaluate the lateral aspect of the incision for any standing cutaneous deformity. If present, a vertical limb, along or just inside the hairline, may be necessary to avoid skin dimpling. The epidermis is reapproximated with a continuous polypropylene suture in a simple and interval vertical mattress fashion (**Fig. 29.18**). By placing several vertical mattress sutures along the postauricular sulcus, the incidence of poor tissue union upon suture removal is much reduced. Although rarely used postoperatively, a quarter-inch Penrose drain may be placed between the sutures along the postauricular sulcus. This stays in place until the conclusion of the case, when it is removed before applying the pressure dressing.

The procedure is then repeated in an identical fashion for the contralateral side. After the skin incisions have been sutured, the undermined pre- and postauricular skin flaps are aggressively milked to remove any excess serosanguinous fluid. The Penrose drains are removed, and a compressive dressing is placed. Occasionally, a Penrose drain may be needed until the pressure dressing is removed the following day, especially in patients with above-average intraoperative blood loss, hypertension, or significant collections underneath the skin flaps at the conclusion of the case. It is important to explain that these patients may see more drainage on the dressing so that they are not alarmed.

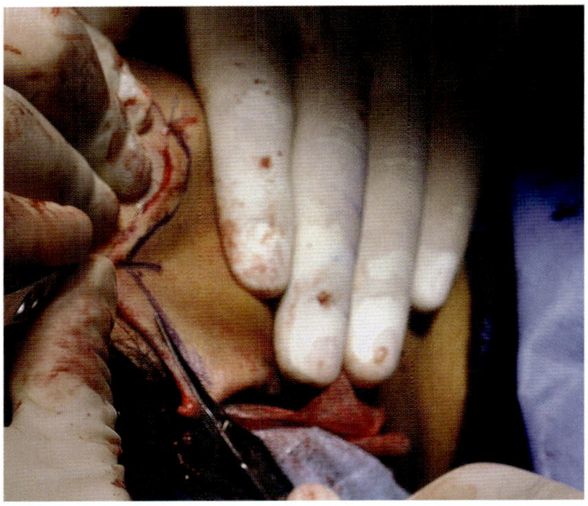

Fig. 29.17 Redraping the postauricular skin flap. The skin is laid back over the ear in an anterior-posterior direction and the new skin edge is marked.

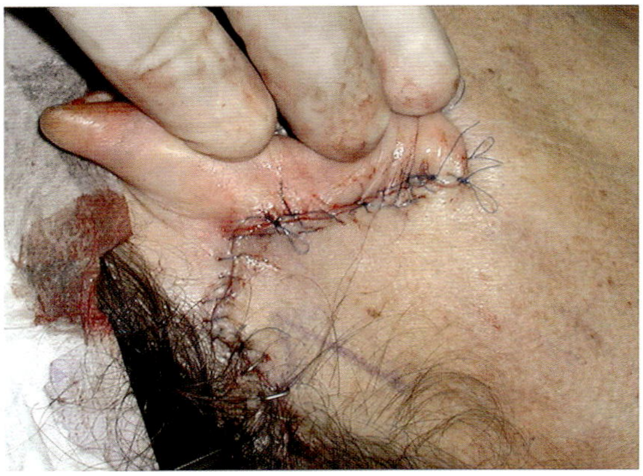

Fig. 29.18 The reapproximated postauricular incision.

■ Postoperative Care

At the conclusion of the procedure, a compressive gauze dressing is placed. The patient is discharged with a family member after reviewing overnight care instructions, ensuring that the patient sleeps on his or her back, upright at a 45 degree angle; that the patient has filled all postoperative prescriptions for analgesia, antibiosis, and insomnia; and that the patient has a return appointment for the next day to remove the dressing. An on-call number for any overnight questions should also be given to the family member.

On postoperative day 1 (POD 1), the compressive dressing is removed. The skin flaps are examined for any evidence of hematomas or seromas, venous congestions, or epidermolysis. Basic wound care is performed and demonstrated/explained to the patient. Incisions are to be cleaned three times a day with warm water and a very thin layer of petroleum jelly placed to avoid desiccation. Patients are also instructed to ice the pre- and postauricular skin flaps for 20 minutes every waking hour for the next 48 hours. Thereafter, a warm compress may be placed on any ecchymosis to help hasten resolution. The patients are also instructed to wear a supportive nylon/spandex strap as much as possible over the first week to support the readhering skin flaps. It is also helpful to review with the patient signs of a possible hematoma/seroma and contrast them with normal postoperative induration and edema. The patient is discharged after answering any questions, confirming a follow-up appointment in 1 week for suture removal, and emphasizing that patients are free to return at any time if there are any concerns.

On postoperative day 7 (POD 7), the patient returns for suture removal. All permanent sutures are removed. If there is any sign of actual or potential incisional separation, tissue adhesive or Steri-Strips (3M, St. Paul, MN) may be placed. The patient is also instructed to be careful with manipulation of the earlobes, especially when changing clothes. Any ecchymosis may be treated with warm compresses and, in some circumstances, may be quickly improved with intense pulsed light (IPL) treatment. At this point, the support strap need only be worn at night for 1 additional week.

On postoperative day 14 (POD 14), the patient returns for a brief evaluation. The incisions are inspected for early signs of hypertrophy or milia, and patients may begin to use topical scar therapies. Patients are also instructed to begin gentle massage over the skin flaps several times a day in the following manner: for the preauricular skin flap, the patient is instructed to use the flat portion of the first few fingers along from the corner of the mouth back toward the ear; for the postauricular skin flap, the patient uses the flat portion of the fingers and sweeps in an anterior-superior direction toward the back of the ear. In this manner, tension is never placed on the incision or on the SMAS/platysmal plication sutures. If there is any residual ecchymosis, IPL may be used a second time.

From this point onward, the follow-up is similar to that for other facial plastic surgical procedures. The patient is typically seen at 4 weeks, 2 months, 3 months, 6 months, and 1 year postoperatively. However, the patient may be seen more frequently if needed.

■ Expected Results

When the patient is seen on POD 1, there is often mild to moderate anterior facial edema due to the compressive bandage. It is also common to see mild supraclavicular ecchymosis, and less frequently, ecchymosis along the commissure–mandibular groove. Hematomas are seen in less than 10% of patients, and if present, usually are less than 5 mL. If present, they are aspirated with a needle and syringe, and a modified pressure dressing may be placed. The patient is seen each day for repeat aspiration until the fluid collections have resolved.

The incisions heal quickly and often demonstrate minimal erythema after suture removal. With the use of topical agents and camouflage makeup application, they are virtually undetectable.

The majority of edema and dark ecchymosis resolves by the end of the first week, coinciding with suture removal. There is often palpable induration and tenderness over the areas of the plication sutures preauricularly and inferiorly over the SCM muscle. By the end of the second week, there should be very little visible ecchymosis or edema. There is often palpable edema over the plication sites, but the patient should be reassured that it is invisible to all but the closest friends and family (**Fig. 29.19a–c**). By the end of the first month, there is usually only minimal palpable edema around the plication sutures, and the majority of tissue edema has resolved (**Fig. 29.20a–c**).

Over the first postoperative year, the edema within the skin flaps and the SMAS/platysma will resolve. This can manifest as a return of skin laxity, although with reassurance and proper early patient education, this change will not be alarming or unexpected. Ad-

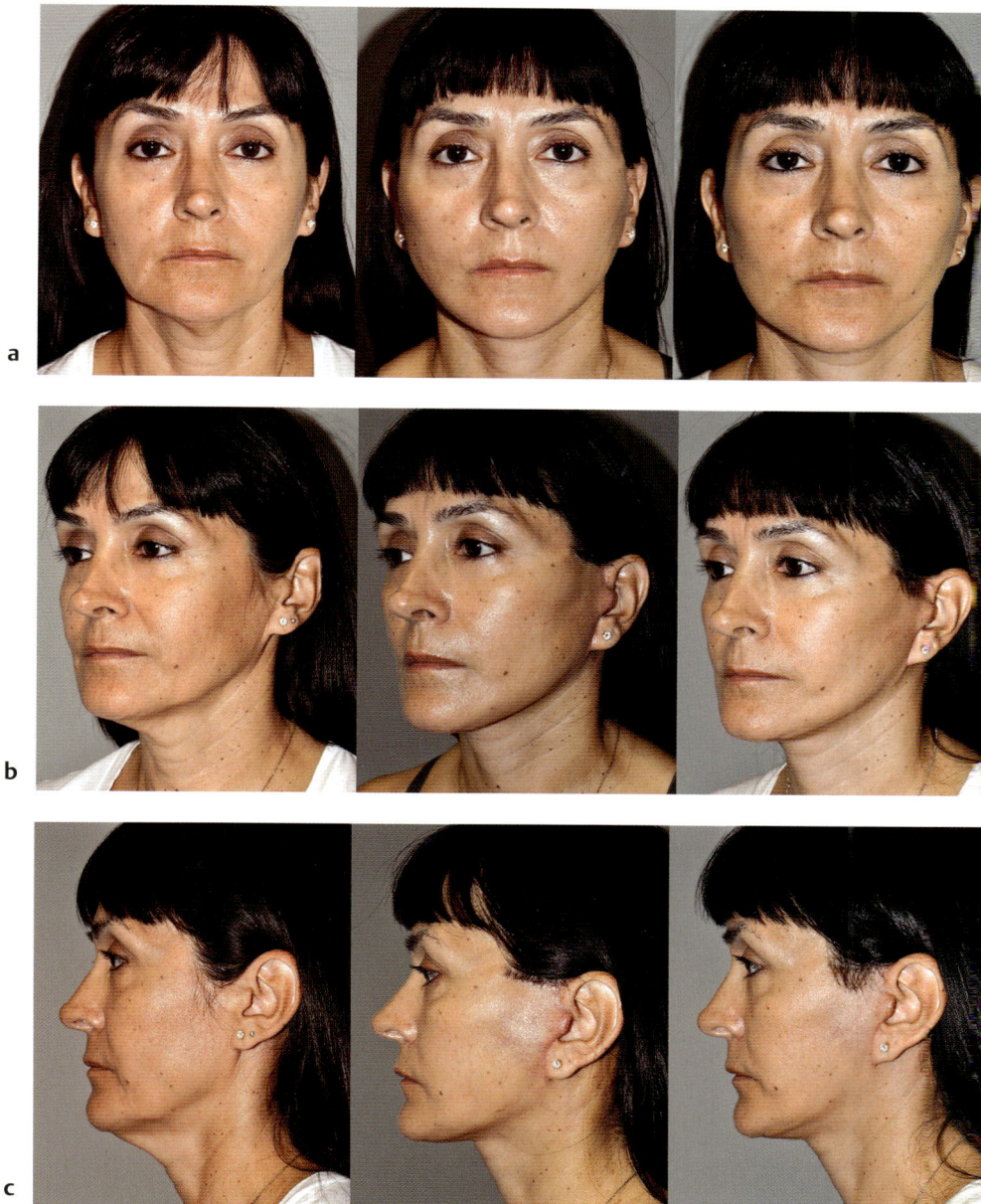

Fig. 29.19 (a) Preoperative (*left*) anteroposterior (AP) view, 2 week postoperative (*center*) AP view, 4 week postoperative (*right*) AP view. (b) Preoperative (*left*) left oblique view, 2 week postoperative (*center*) left oblique view, 4 week postoperative (*right*) left oblique view. (c) Preoperative (*left*) left lateral view, 2 week postoperative (*center*) left lateral view, 4 week postoperative (*right*) left lateral view.

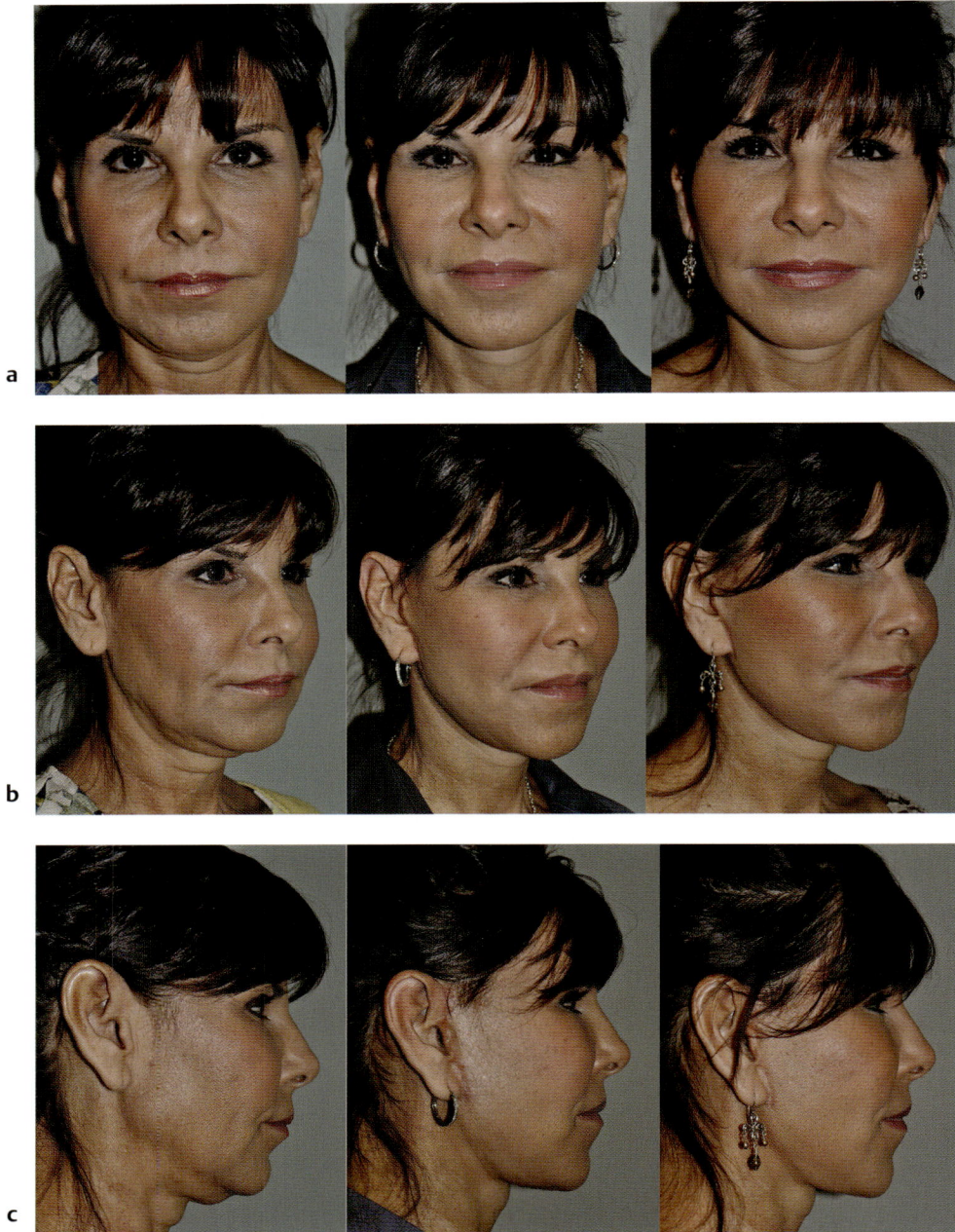

Fig. 29.20 (a) Preoperative (*left*) anteroposterior (AP) view, 2 week postoperative (*center*) AP view, 4 week postoperative (*right*) AP view. (b) Preoperative (*left*) right oblique view, 2 week postoperative (*center*) right oblique view, 4 week postoperative (*right*) right oblique view. (c) Preoperative (*left*) right lateral view, 2 week postoperative (*center*) right lateral view, 4 week postoperative (*right*) right lateral view.

ditionally, any changes in skin flap color due to intraoperative disruption in blood supply should resolve. Occasionally, especially in patients with thin, fair skin, some darkening or bronzing of the skin may be seen. This is more likely due to a small amount of venous congestion and resolves as the venous supply strengthens and returns to its preoperative state.

With regard to aesthetic improvement, one can expect significant early improvement in jowl formation and skin laxity. Additionally, there may be a noticeable reduction in the depth of the commissure–mandibular groove and melolabial groove. However, this is often a consequence of tissue edema, and with its

resolution, there is some return of the groove depth. It is important to adequately counsel patients preoperatively and early in the postoperative period so that this change is expected and not seen as a surgical failure.

Significant anterior platysmal banding may be ameliorated with a posterior SMAS and platysmal plication, but often the anterior bands will remain visible, though less apparent and in a more posterior position. If there is significant preoperative submental liposis, elastosis, and platysmal banding, then a minimal incision face-/necklift should be combined with an anterior submentoplasty and platysmaplasty.

Patients will frequently ask about the lifespan or longevity of the procedure. One useful strategy is to ask them to review old photographs and compare them to their new postoperative appearance. If one assumes that aging is more or less linear, then the age difference between the two matching appearances is roughly the length of time until patients return to their preoperative appearance. It is very important to avoid giving patients a guaranteed amount of rejuvenation. Even though patients will continue to age after the procedure, they will always look relatively more rejuvenated than if they had not had the procedure.

Complications and Their Management

Complications can be classified into intraoperative, early postoperative, and late postoperative. Intraoperative complications are similar to those seen in more extensive facelift and necklift surgery and include poor skin flap design, hemorrhage, and neurovascular and SMAS damage. Early postoperative complications include hematoma/seroma, wound infection, skin flap vascular compromise and necrosis, and wound dehiscence. Late postoperative complications include hypertrophic scars/keloids, contour irregularities, lobule malposition, and alopecia. Management is similar to that taken for more extensive procedures.

For poor skin flap design, if there is a standing cone deformity ("dog ear") at the anterior edge of the temporal tuft incision, a vertical extension along the sideburn may correct this. If there is difficulty in reapproximating the postauricular skin flap, extending the horizontal limb of the incision or making a vertical limb that extends inferiorly just inside the hair line will help. Judicious use of buried long-term absorbable sutures will help reduce suture line tension. Fortunately, if there is any skin flap breakdown, it is most frequently seen in the postauricular flap, and healing, even if suboptimal, will be hidden by the ear or hair.

Intraoperative hemorrhage may be the result of hypertension, preoperative use of antihemostatic medications and herbal supplements, inadequate vasoconstriction, or vessel injury. The treatment of hypertension can be addressed by the anesthesiologist and should be properly screened during the preoperative appointment. Additionally, the use of medications or herbal supplements that interfere with platelet aggregation or coagulation should be addressed preoperatively and discontinued, when possible, at least 1 week pre- and postoperatively. In the case of widespread bleeding, field infusion of local anesthetic containing a vasoconstrictor will help.

Firm pressure applied with gauze for several minutes also helps stop most small blood vessel bleeding. More persistent bleeding should be carefully cauterized with bipolar or monopolar cautery to avoid thermal injury to facial nerve branches and to the SMAS/platysma or skin flaps.

Large-vessel injury, although very rare, may be seen more commonly in secondary procedures because normal tissue planes are often obscured by scar tissue, and vessels may be found within sheets of scar tissue. If there is large-vessel injury and repair is not possible, the vessel should be suture ligated with a permanent suture to reduce the risk of delayed hemorrhage. With such ligation, there may be increased edema and induration on that side during the early postoperative period. In the event of significant intraoperative blood loss, it may be helpful to place a drain to help reduce the accumulation of fluid underneath the skin flap. The primary author (GV) prefers to use a quarter-inch Penrose drain inbetween the sutures along the vertical aspect of the postauricular incision. If a drain is placed, an extra gauze roll may be used to absorb any excess drainage. The patient is also educated regarding the possibility of visible serosanguinous drainage to decrease any anxiety. The drain is typically removed the next day, and no additional wound treatment is necessary However, if there appears to be some mild incisional delayed healing/dehiscence at the time of suture removal, a Steri-Strip (3M), tissue adhesive, or suture may be placed.

Damage to neural structures, such as the great auricular nerve (GAN) or branches of the facial nerve should be repaired with a fine monofilament suture Fortunately, anesthesia from GAN damage often decreases with time. Weakness to the branches of the facial nerve due to neuropraxia will resolve with time, although the patient requires a great deal of reassurance.

Interruption of the SMAS layer may occur during elevation of the skin flaps or during placement of the SMAS plication sutures If possible, such disruptions should be sutured together to help avoid any inherent weakness in the re-suspension of the SMAS. The primary author (GV) prefers to use a small, monofilament, nonabsorbable suture such as 5–0 polypropylene. Once the disruption is repaired, multivector suspension may continue in the same manner as for an uninjured SMAS.

Seromas and hematomas are generally seen in the immediate postoperative period. If minor, they may be treated with needle aspiration in the office and placement of a focal pressure dressing. Patients should be seen each day after discovery for repeat evaluation and drainage until the fluid collection has resolved. If the hematoma is significant, the patient should have the skin flap explored, the hematoma evacuated, and the flap bed irrigated before reapproximating the incision. Occasionally, a limited opening can be performed and a small liposuction cannula (2 or 4 mm) can be used to evacuate the clot. With this less invasive approach, it is still essential to irrigate the wound bed. A complete pressure dressing should be placed, and the patient should return the following day for wound inspection. It is important to reassure the patient that the presence of a hematoma should not change the final result; it merely delays the resolution of edema and ecchymosis. Preoperative counseling should include discussion of the risk of hematoma as well as preventive measures and treatment.

Wound infection is a rare complication, occurring in less than 2% of the primary author's (GV) practice. Risk factors include patients with immune deficiencies, diabetes mellitus, vascular insufficiency, poor hygiene, and poor oxygen delivery to the skin (e.g., use of nicotine, living at high altitude). To reduce the risk of postoperative infection, patients are given preoperative antibiotics, either oral or intravenous, depending on the procedural anesthesia. The antibiotics are continued postoperatively until suture removal. It is important to monitor the patients for potential side effects of antibiotic use, such as allergy or gastrointestinal complaints. If there is any concern about potential infection, the skin flaps must be evaluated for evidence of seroma or abscess. If present, they must be drained and the fluid sent for culture to aid in antibiotic selection. The patient should be placed on a second-line antibiotic for at least 1 week and should be frequently reevaluated.

Skin flap vascular compromise may be suspected on POD 1 after pressure dressing removal. It is usually seen at the apex of the pre- or postauricular incisions and peritragally. It presents as a duskiness or violaceous hue at the superficial level of the skin flap and is due to venous congestion of the skin flap. If present, any associated seromas or hematomas must be drained. Sometimes, it is helpful to make several perforations in the overlying skin with an 18-gauge needle. The skin flap may be milked, and some of the excess venous blood may be released. In the absence of major hematoma, starting the patient on low-dose aspirin may help by improving microthrombi within the venous circulation. Frequent patient follow-up and counseling are essential. If the venous congestion progresses to skin flap epidermolysis or eschar, then conservative wound care should be initiated. In general, an acceptable cosmetic outcome may be achieved through healing by secondary intention. It is imperative to stress sun protection to help reduce the risk for postinflammatory hyperpigmentation. After the eschar has resolved, fractional carbon dioxide (CO_2) laser resurfacing over the area may help to improve skin texture and discoloration.

The incisions should be closely monitored in the postoperative period for signs of scar hypertrophy or keloid formation. Fortunately, with proper incision design and closure and good postoperative wound care, the incidence of unsatisfactory incisions is low. If suspected, early injection with triamcinolone may abort the abnormal wound healing response. Alternatively, the use of topical silicone-containing ointments or the use of silicone sheeting may help. Reexcision may be performed, but the primary author prefers to wait a minimum of 3 months postoperatively.

Contour irregularities are common in the early postoperative period and are due to uneven swelling within the SMAS or skin flap level. Reassurance, massage, and patience are important. If there is focal induration after the first 4 weeks, a conservative dose of triamcinolone (10 or 20 mg/mL) may be injected into the offending area. Steroid injection should be conservative to avoid potential complications of fat or dermal atrophy and telangiectasias. Mild persistent contour irregularities in the form of skin tethering may be treated with subdermal release with the use of a 16- or 18-gauge needle. If significant contour irregularity persists beyond the sixth postoperative month, skin flap exploration with reevaluation of the SMAS or platysmal plication and skin flap redraping may be required.

Lobule malposition is best treated by intraoperative prevention through proper perilobular incision design, minimizing perilobular tension in skin flap redraping, and ensuring excellent lobule support in incisional closure. Occasionally, lobule attachment may be temporary due to induration around the lobule, and watchful waiting or conservative triamcinolone injection may help. If the lobule attachment persists beyond the third postoperative month, a lobule revision with a V-Y advancement may be performed.

Incisional alopecia may be the result of poor incision design, excessive use of cautery and follicular injury, or wound edge tension. Often, the hair loss may be telogen effluvium and will resolve after the first 3 months. However, if it is permanent and cosmetically disfiguring, then follicular unit grafting may help camouflage the alopecia.

■ Conclusion

With the increase in demand by patients for less invasive procedures, shorter recovery, and more natural results, the short-incision face- and necklift is an attractive option. Although patients are more educated about treatment options for rejuvenation, it is important for them to understand the limitations of nonsurgical treatments and how only a surgical procedure can address fat, skin, and soft tissue laxity. Although there are many techniques that propose excellent rejuvenation with minimal incisions, risk, recovery, and complication, their methods to address soft tissue ptosis may be suboptimal. Using the multivector technique of SMAS and platysmal plication, an individualized, anatomical rejuvenation is possible. Although the recovery and expense of a short-incision face- and necklift may be greater than many nonsurgical options, the benefit of a lasting resuspension of the SMAS and platysma certainly compensates for any perceived disadvantages. Thus, the short-incision face- and necklift is an essential component of the facial plastic surgeon's repertoire.

References

1. Mitz V, Peyronie M. The superficial musculo-aponeurotic system (SMAS) in the parotid and cheek area. Plast Reconstr Surg 1976;58(1):80–88
2. Hamra ST. The deep-plane rhytidectomy. Plast Reconstr Surg 1990;86(1):53–61, discussion 62–63
3. Hamra ST. Composite rhytidectomy. Plast Reconstr Surg 1992;90(1):1–13
4. Ramirez OM. The subperiosteal rhytidectomy: the third-generation face-lift. Ann Plast Surg 1992;28(3) 218–232, discussion 233–234
5. Chang S, Pusic A, Rohrich RJ. A systematic review of comparison of efficacy and complication rates among face-lift techniques. Plast Reconstr Surg 2011;127(1):423–433
6. Baker DC. Lateral SMASectomy. Plast Reconstr Surg 1997;100(2):509–513
7. Saylan Z. The S-lift for facial rejuvenation. Int J Cosmet Surg 1999;7(1):18–23
8. Tonnard P, Verpaele A. The MACS-lift short scar rhytidectomy. Aesthet Surg J 2007;27(2):188–198
9. Verpaele A, Tonnard P, Gaia S, Guerao FP, Pirayesh A. The third suture in MACS-lifting: making midface-lifting simple and safe. J Plast Reconstr Aesthet Surg 2007;60(12):1287–1295
10. Brandy DA. The QuickLift: a modification of the s-lift. Cosmet Dermatol 2004;17:351–360
11. Brandy DA. The revised QuickLift: featuring an encircling double purse-string plication technique with blunt neck/jowl undermining and small submental tuck for tightening of the sagging SMAS platysma and skin. Am J Cosmet Surg 2004;22(4):223–232

30 Liposuction and Minimally Invasive Fat Reduction

T. Gerald O'Daniel and Ron Hazani

Key Concepts

- A thorough understanding of the fat compartments is essential in determining which facial procedure will provide the optimal outcome.

- Liposuction of the neck alone in patients with fat deep to the platysma will result in less than optimal outcomes.

- Treating the neck in isolation when the lower third has advanced aging will result in suboptimal outcomes.

- Conventional liposuction and selective laser lipolysis provide comparable results in the isolated treatment of the preplatysmal fat compartments of the neck.

- Laser lipolysis is a powerful tool for sculpting the fat compartments above the jawline and for secondary liposuction of the neck and in the fibrous fat compartments overlying the parotid gland and lateral neck.

■ Introduction

The beauty of the face and neck is defined by the contours and balance of adjacent structures. Patients presenting with concerns related to their facial shape are affected by the intrinsic nature of their facial anatomy. As patients age, the intrinsic factors are further influenced by weight gain or loss, loss of the facial bony skeleton, and loss of skin elasticity-due to environmental factors, such as sun and smoking. Aesthetic contouring of the face can be achieved by the addition and subtraction of volume and the rearrangement of displaced volume, as well as by tightening the supporting structures and excision of redundant tissues. Fillers or volumizers can replace and augment areas of deficiency.[1-4] Repositioning of displaced volume can be readily achieved with formal surgical lifts.[5] The removal of volume as an isolated procedure can improve the contours of the face and neck, particularly in the younger patient and in highly selected older patients. Typically, a combination of procedures is required to restore the aesthetic shape and balance in the aging patient.

This chapter focuses on liposuction and laser-assisted lipolysis to reduce fat and improve the face and neck contour. As emphasized here, appropriate patient selection is the key factor to a successful outcome.

■ Background: Basic Science of Procedure

Liposuction of the face has historically been confined to the neck and the portion of the jowl that extends below the face–neck interface.[6-8] In 1989 McKinney and Cook[6] suggested that liposuction of the jowls and nasolabial folds be done concomitantly with facelift procedures, but the suggestion was met with limited acceptance. Traditional liposuction techniques above the jawline can lead to contour irregularity because of cannula size, difficulty in selectively removing fat from individual compartments, and variable overlying skin response. Some surgeons have difficulty achieving predictably smooth contours, even with microsyringe liposuction. In the neck, the fat below the jawline can sometimes consist of a greater amount of fibrous tissue that makes liposuction cannula passage difficult. Over all, though, the authors have found conventional liposuction utilizing cannulas 3 mm and smaller to be equally as effective as laser lipolysis in managing the preplatysmal fat.

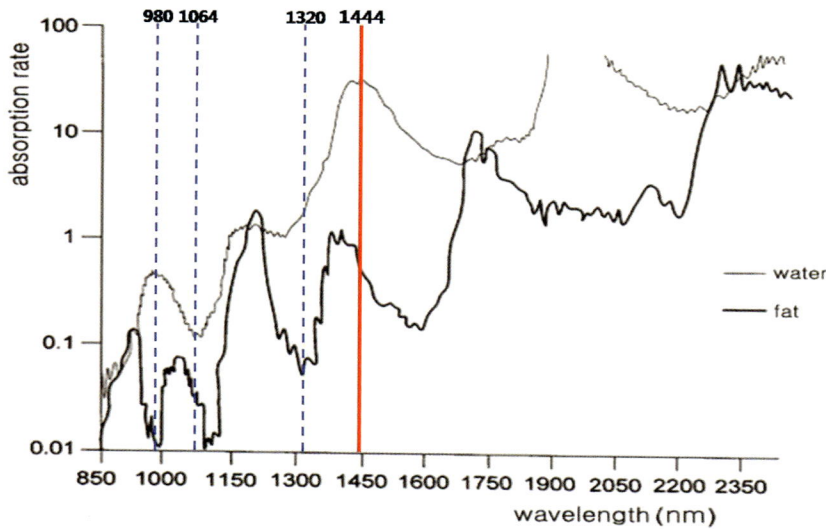

Fig. 30.1 Fat and water optical absorption curves for various laser wavelengths currently used for laser lipolysis, shown as vertical lines. (From Holcomb JD. Facelift adjunctive techniques: skin resurfacing and volumetric contouring. Facial Plast Surg Clin North Am 2009;17:505–551. Used with permission.)

Several new laser applications on the market target the fat of the body and the face.[9-14] Depending on the laser wavelength, there is variable specificity for fat and water (**Fig. 30.1**).[15] Selective lipolysis of the targeted fat compartment for regional contouring can lead to less risk of nonspecific collateral tissue damage, such as in the overlying skin.

A selective laser expands options for a multimodality and individualized approach to the treatment of the aging face by shaping the jowl and neck fat, tightening the overlying skin, and targeting other areas of fatty irregularities in the perioral area. As our understanding of the aging face is evolving in relation to volume shifts, volume loss, and volume accumulation, one can more specifically target treatment to the variable regional changes within the same face. In other words, the approach to the aging face can include volume removal with direct excision, traditional liposuction, and laser-assisted lipolysis, as well as volume addition with autologous fat, filler, and alloplastic implants, in addition to repositioning facial fat and muscles with various midface and necklift procedures.

■ Pertinent Anatomy

Fat Compartments of the Face

The subcutaneous fat of the face has long been considered to be a unified confluent mass. Historically, great attention has been paid to the process of skin aging, laxity, loss of elasticity, and sun damage. Recent studies of the face and its underlying adipose layer reveal a mosaic of subcutaneous fat compartments with distinct boundaries and associated findings relating to the process of aging.[16-18] In their landmark study, Rohrich and Pessa[16] describe the partitioning of subcutaneous fat of the face in multiple independent anatomical compartments (**Fig. 30.2a,b**). Facial fat is therefore divided into discrete facial subunits corresponding to several fat compartments found in each facial region. Examples of such regions are the forehead, the periorbital area, the cheeks, and the jowls.

The forehead is a collection of three anatomical units, including central, middle, and lateral-temporal cheek fat. Periorbital fat is also divided into three distinct regions: superior, inferior, and lateral. In the cheek, what has been referred to as malar fat is composed of the following three separate compartments: medial, middle, and lateral-temporal cheek fat. The nasolabial fold nonetheless, is a discrete unit with distinct anatomical boundaries.

Retaining Ligaments

Histology of the septal boundaries between the several adjacent fat compartments demonstrates a fibrous condensation of connective tissue that forms diffusion barriers. The septa originate from underlying fascia and insert into the dermis of the skin. These septa form an interconnecting framework that limits shearing forces on the face and provides a retaining system for the face. Perforating vessels arising from the deep arteries of the face travel through these septa to supply the skin and define the overlying vascular territories, or angiosomes, of the face.[19]

This chapter expounds on the anatomy of the lower face and neck because volume reduction and liposuction of the nasolabial, jowl, and submental fat has demonstrated significant improvement in the contouring of the face.

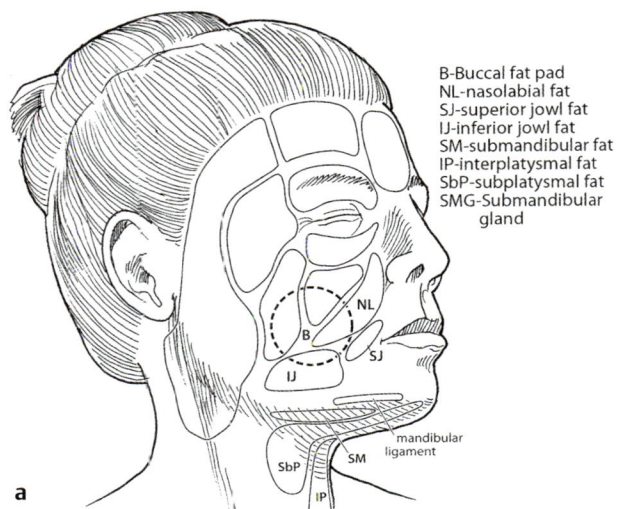

Fig. 30.2 Fat compartments in the face and neck. **(a)** Facial subcutaneous fat compartments. NL, nasolabial fat; B, buccal fat pad; SJ, superior jowl fat; IJ, inferior jowl fat; SM, submandibular fat; SpP, supraplatysmal fat; IP, interplatysmal fat; SbP, subplatysmal fat; SMG, submandibular gland. **(b)** Drawing depicting neck supraplatysmal and subplatysmal fat compartments.

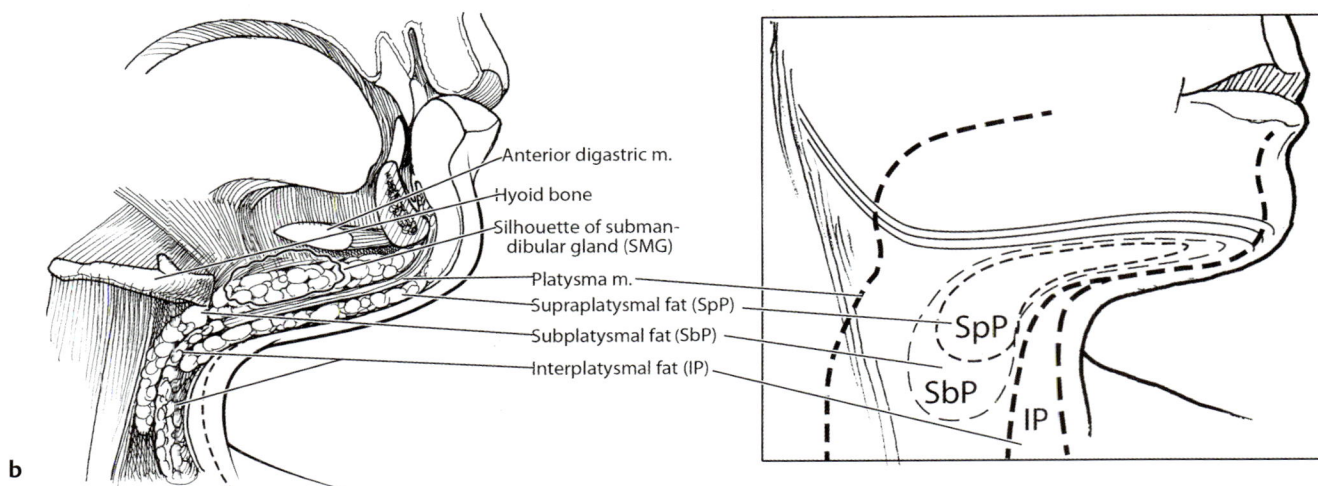

Nasolabial Fat Compartment

The nasolabial fat lies anterior to medial cheek fat and overlaps the jowl fat. The orbicularis-retaining ligament represents the superior border of this compartment. Nasolabial fat can be noted medial to the deeper fat of the suborbicularis fat compartment. The lower border of the zygomaticus major muscle is adherent to this compartment.[16]

With aging, the fullness in the nasolabial fold represents a form of pseudoptosis. The volume of the nasolabial fat compartment is preserved while the superficial cheek fat compartment deflates and accentuates the appearance of a prominent fold.[19]

The Jowl

In the lower face, the jowl fat has been defined as a collection of overlapping subcutaneous fat compartments above and below the mandibular border. Two subcutaneous compartments above the mandibular border make up the substance of the jowl fat, a superior compartment and an inferior compartment.[17]

The superior jowl compartment clinically appears as the most inferior extension of the nasolabial fold. Anteriorly, it consistently approximates the oral commissure. Posteriorly, it relates to at least two regions: superiorly to the fat overlying the malar hollow and inferiorly to the inferior jowl fat pad. Despite the proximity of buccal fat to the jowl, it represents an anatomically separate compartment deep to the jowl fat. Buccal fat does not contribute to the location or degree of jowling.[17]

The inferior jowl fat compartment rests inferior and posterior to the superior jowl fat compartment. Superiorly, it abuts the superior jowl fat pad and fat from the malar region. Anteriorly, the superior jowl fat descends to meet it. The posterior border is the fat overlying the parotid-masseteric fascia. Inferiorly, the subcutaneous fat reaches the mandibular border. The inferior jowl fat overlaps the submandibular fat pad caudally.

The mandibular septum is the superior border to the submandibular fat compartment located immediately below the border of the mandible. It borders the inferior jowl fat compartment superiorly. Anteriorly, it relates to fat in the submental area, and posteriorly it relates to fat that descends across the border of the mandible from the parotid-masseteric region. The inferior border of this compartment relates to the fat over the sternocleidomastoid muscle.[17]

Submental Fat Compartments

Adipose tissue in the anterior neck is located in three different layers. It is described in relation to the superficial cervical fascia that splits and encases the platysma in the submental region. The supraplatysmal fat is found within the subcutaneous tissue and contains greater amount of fat in the submental region as compared with the surrounding fat.[19]

Between the medial edges of the platysma muscles and inferior to the level of their decussation exists a more fibrous fatty tissue. The consistency of this interplatysmal fat compartment is related to the hyoid ligament and its attachment to the hyoid bone, the perihyoid fascia, and the anterior digastric muscles. Therefore, interplatysmal fat removal is likely to require direct excision, whereas liposuction techniques are usually reserved for the supraplatysmal fat compartment.

Deep to the platysma muscles and extending over to the medial wall of the submandibular gland capsule is a compartment of fat that is superficial to the anterior digastric muscles. This subplatysmal fat can be abundant, in some patients extending down to the suprasternal notch.[20]

The Facial Nerve

Facial nerve paralysis is a rare but dreaded complication following aesthetic facial procedures. In the lower face and neck, the marginal mandibular nerve and the cervical branch of the facial nerve are both subplatysmal, where injury can be avoided if the plane of dissection remains superficial to the platysma muscles.

Laterally, the marginal mandibular nerve is well protected by the substance of the parotid gland. Anterior to the anterior edge of the parotid, it courses deep to the superficial muscular aponeurotic system (SMAS) layer and, in most patients, below the border of the mandible. Beyond the facial vessels, the marginal mandibular nerve is located above the mandibular margin and can be damaged as the platysma thins anteriorly. Paresis of the mandibular nerve presents as weakness of the lower lip depressors.[19]

The cervical branch exits the parotid gland at its caudal tip and then splits to superior and inferior branches. Both branches enter the platysma laterally and course within the muscle. Injury to the cervical branch can present as pseudoparalysis of the marginal mandibular nerve, because the platysma cofunctions with the lower lip depressors as a depressor of the corner of the mouth.[21]

Superficial Veins

The superficial venous system in the neck is, for the most part, subplatysmal and therefore is rarely a concern during minimally invasive procedures such as suction lipolysis of the subcutaneous tissues. One exception is the path of the external jugular vein along the posterior border of the platysma. In the lateral neck, the external jugular vein is protected only by a thin veil of superficial cervical fascia[21] and requires great care not to bluntly injure the vein with a suction cannula.

The anterior jugular vein is found in the subplatysmal layer along the medial aspect of the platysma muscle. It courses within the subplatysmal fat and occasionally connects with the common facial vein with a communicating branch lying along the anterior border of the sternomastoid muscle.[20] Due to the anatomical relationship of these venous structures to the deep fat compartments, caution is recommended when one is attempting to remove fat from the subplatysmal layer.

■ Patient Selection

Laser-assisted volumetric contouring is most effective in the lower third of the face and neck. A thorough evaluation of the fat, skin, muscle, and subplatysmal structures will determine which operation is appropriate to address the patient's concerns. The fat layer is the most important layer affected by the laser energy, and its removal has the most dramatic effect on the neck and jowl fat compartment. Accurate localization of the fat in either the supraplatysmal or subplatysmal plane is paramount in the treatment of the neck. Pinching the submental fat compartment at rest and then having the patient grimace will help evaluate the position of fat. If the pinched fat volume does not diminish, it is suggestive that the majority of the fat is supraplatysmal; if it does reduce in volume, then there is a significant volume of fat in the subplatysmal plane. Fat that is predominantly positioned in the supraplatysmal plane suggests that laser-assisted liposuction alone will yield a satisfactory result. When there is substantial subplatysmal fat, laser liposuction alone will potentially produce a suboptimal outcome.

The platysma and deep platysmal structures are then evaluated. When an obtuse cervicomental angle is accompanied by platysmal bands at rest or on animation, an open neck approach is generally necessary to create a pleasing neck. Subplatysmal structures need to be evaluated to determine the presence of ptotic submandibular glands. Care must be taken, and the patient made aware, that the glands might become more visible after removal of the supraplatysmal fat alone.

Evaluation of the skin determines the presence or absence of excess skin, the quality of the skin, and the elasticity of the skin. Excess skin, in general, is considered when it extends below the hyoid cartilage. Poor quality skin and lack of elasticity suggest that a full-incision face- and necklift is required for an optimal outcome. Skin that does not extend below the hyoid cartilage and has reasonable quality and residual elasticity responds nicely after laser lipolysis alone.

The jowls are evaluated in relationship to the cervicofacial interface. If the jowl fat pad extends into the neck and there is minimal ptosis of the compartment superiorly at the submalar transition area, then isolated laser lipolysis can be very effective in improving the jawline. When there is significant ptosis of the jowl fat compartment below the jawline with loss of volume at the submalar transition, then an elevation of the jowl fat with or without laser-assisted lipolysis of the jowl fat compartment will give the most favorable outcome.

■ Technical Aspects of Procedure

Unless otherwise indicated, the following discussion of laser-assisted lipolysis employs the 1,444 nm neodymium:yttrium-aluminum-garnet (Nd:YAG) laser (AccuSculpt, Lutronic, Princeton Junction, NJ), which is reported to be highly specific for subcutaneous fat and water ▶ **Video 30.1**.[15,22]

Preoperative Preparation and Planning

All patients undergo a preoperative history and physical. Patients over the age of 50, and any patients with a significant medical condition, are cleared by their personal physician. Medicines that interfere with platelet function, as well as all nutraceutical supplements, are discontinued 2 weeks prior to surgery. A list of these agents is sent to the patient along with all the preoperative instructions, postoperative instructions, and informed consents 3 weeks prior to surgery to allow adequate time for review.

The most important aspect of an optimal outcome is determining which combination of techniques is most suitable for the patient from the criteria described in the patient selection section. With the patient in the

upright position and utilizing the preoperative five position photos of the patient in repose, the contour irregularities are marked as a topographical map for the fat to be removed and any volume deficits that are to be augmented (**Fig. 30.3**).

Anesthesia

Patients undergoing isolated laser lipolysis of the jowls and melolabial folds and limited neck area can be treated in the office setting with oral sedation. All other patients, with the exception of patients undergoing adjunctive rhinoplasty (who are anesthetized with a general endotracheal anesthesia), are anesthetized with a protocol utilizing dexmedetomidine (Precidex, Hospira, Lake Forest, IL) as the primary sedative.[23] Effort is made to limit the use of intraoperative narcotics because they commonly increase the postoperative nausea and vomiting rate. After proper sedation is achieved under monitored anesthesia care, utilizing 0.25% lidocaine and 1:400,000 epinephrine, a total of 6 to 10 mL of tumescent anesthetic solution is administered to each jowl region and melolabial fold. When the neck is treated, ~ 100 mL of solution is infiltrated into the neck from mandibular angle to angle. When using a 1,444 nm wavelength laser, a conservative amount of injection is used because of this laser's affinity to water. With its

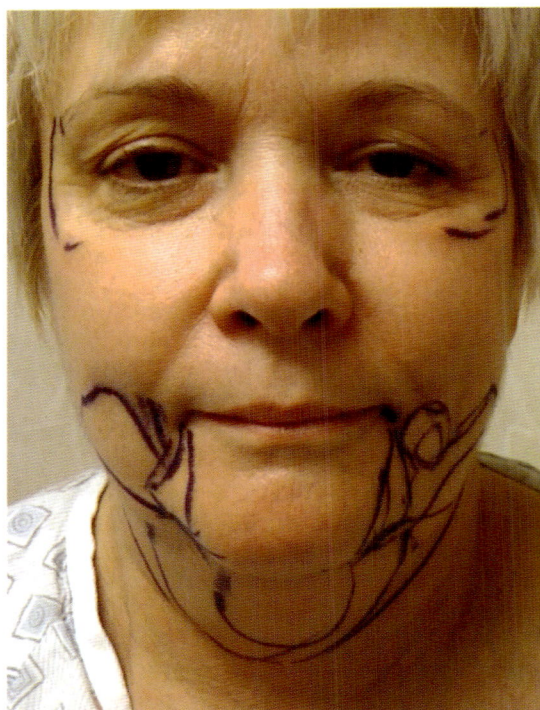

Fig. 30.3 Patient shown with preoperative topographical markings for selective laser-assisted lipolysis and micro–fat grafting.

high selectivity for water, use of adequate amounts of tumescent solution will enhance thermal confinement and further minimize the possibility of nonspecific tissue injury. Approximately 200 mL is used in the rest of the face when a lower facelift is also being performed.

Surgical Technique

Although the technique is similar to that utilized with other devices, this section is based on the usage of the 1,444 nm Nd:YAG laser. The entrance wound for the laser fiber is created with an 18-gauge needle, and the fiber is passed into the subcutaneous plane below the dermis. Using up to 200 J at 7.5 W, the 600 µm laser tip is passed over the jowl, delivering the laser energy in a gridlike fashion (**Fig. 30.4**). The tip is passed under the dermis to undermine the jowl skin as well as to subcise and release the marionette lines and other pre-jowl rhytids. This will facilitate skin tightening by delivering heat to the undersurface of the skin. It is important to maintain constant motion of the laser in the subcutaneous tissues at all times to avoid creation of irregularities from uneven energy delivery and injuring the skin from concentrated laser energy. The laser-aiming beam is easily visible through the skin to allow visualization of the laser tip position. The deeper layer of the jowl fat is sculpted with the 1,444 nm laser by pinching the area to be lasered and delivering the energy into the deeper fatty tissues.

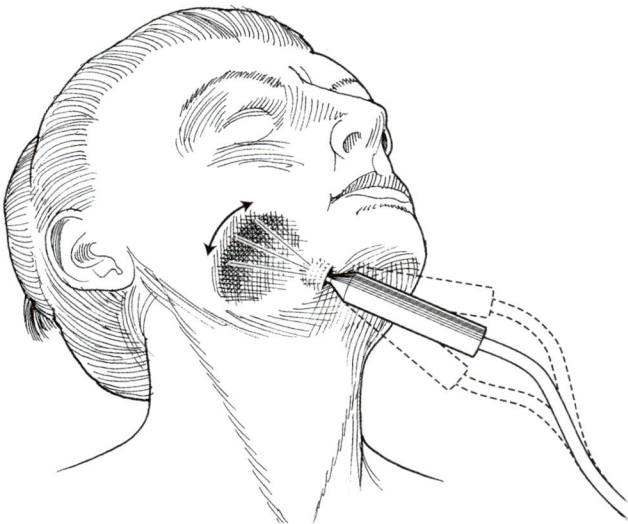

Fig. 30.4 Laser fiber is passed in a gridlike fashion, undermining the fat compartment skin initially then passed in a similar fashion into the deeper layer of fat. The surgeon should be careful to avoid important anatomical structures such as the marginal mandibular nerve.

The transition from the jowl fat pad to the submalar fat pad is achieved with feathering of the laser energy. A total of 200 to 400 J is delivered into the fat pad, with the end point determined by palpable reduction in the fat thickness. A triport syringe 18-gauge aspirator is used to remove only the emulsified fat. When indicated, the laser energy is then delivered in similar fashion to the melolabial folds through a different entrance wound in the nasolabial crease, delivering 150 to 300 J followed by triport aspiration of the emulsified fat only.

Attention is then turned to treatment of the neck. Approximately 3,000 J of energy is delivered through three different ports, one submental and one behind each earlobe. The energy is once again delivered in a gridlike fashion, with superficial undermining first performed, followed by the delivery of energy to the deeper supraplatysmal fat by pinching the fatty layer and passing the fiber continuously and uniformly through each port. After the desired palpable reduction in thickness of the fatty layer has been achieved, the emulsified fat is removed with syringe triport suctioning or with a 2.4 mm Mercedes tip liposuction cannula with wall or machine suction.

If the laser-assisted liposuction is an isolated procedure, the dressings are applied. Otherwise, attention is directed to the other procedures to be concomitantly performed. In the case of neck- and facelift, we begin next the open neck approach to the management of the submental supraplatysmal fat, subplatysmal fat, and jowl fat pad that extends below the cervical–facial interface. The remaining fat overlying the platysma and ptotic jowl fat pad are further refined with careful direct excision. The subplatysmal fat contouring is performed to allow proper correction or creation of the cervical mental angle. A corset platysmaplasty is then performed, with paramedian sutures placed when needed to further smooth the neck contour. When indicated, fat grafting to the midface and periorbital region is then performed prior to a high lamellar SMAS facelift. After successful midface suspension has been accomplished with the facelift, the final fat contouring in the neck is performed and the skin is further released to allow smooth redraping. After excision and closure of the skin, the final fat grafting is performed in the geniomandibular groove and pre-jowl sulcus to create a smooth transition from the chin to the posterior jawline.

All open procedures have a drain placed. Two-inch foam tape is placed under the chin and along the mandibular border to help eliminate the accumulation of serous fluid and prevent the formation of a seroma in the submental triangle. A bulky pressure dressing is applied for 24 hours, and the patient is discharged home with instructions.

■ Postoperative Care

If a concomitant facelift is performed, the drains are removed the next day. The sutures and foam tape are removed on postoperative day 6. Utilizing adhesive remover facilitates foam tape removal (Detatchol Adhesive Remover, Ferndale Laboratories, Ferndale, MI). Dermatolymphatic massage within the first 2 postoperative weeks assists with the resolution of soft tissue edema along the mandibular border and neck.

■ Expected Results

Laser lipolysis can be a powerful tool in refining the outcomes of facial contouring procedures. The key to success is the appropriate matching of the operative procedure with the patient's anatomical deformity. The following patient examples cover the range of applications for laser-assisted volumetric contouring we are currently using in facial aesthetic surgery.

Isolated Laser-Assisted Liposuction

This 42-year-old patient had concerns related to the fullness in the lower third of her face and early formation of jowls (**Fig. 30.5**). On examination, she has fat predominantly in the supraplatysmal layer, apparent skin excess confined to the suprahyoid neck, and excellent skin quality. The treatment of the supraplatysmal fat and jowl fat compartment that extends below the neck–face interface with laser-assisted lipolysis and suctioning creates a pleasing cervicomental angle and a refined jawline. A similar result can be expected utilizing conventional small cannula liposuction.

Isolated Suction with Pre-Jowl Implant

This 27-year-old patient presented with concerns related to the lack of refinement of her jawline and shape of her lower face (**Fig. 30.6**). She has predominantly supraplatysmal fat that is the main contributing factor to her obtuse cervicomental angle. In addition, there is a lack of volume in the pre-jowl sulcus that creates the illusion of a weak chin and excess jowl fat, particularly in the oblique and anterior views. A balanced lower facial profile is created with laser-assisted lipolysis and suctioning of the neck and lower jowl compartment, with volume added to the pre-jowl sulcus utilizing a pre-jowl silicone implant.

Isolated Suction with Buccal Fat Pad Removal

This 34-year-old patient complained of poor definition of the lower two thirds of her face despite a high lean body mass (**Fig. 30.7**). She is without skin redundancy and fat is confined to the supraplatysmal plane. Removal of fat was performed in the neck utilizing conventional small cannula liposuction, and bilateral buccal fat pads were removed to give a more angular appearance to her lower face.

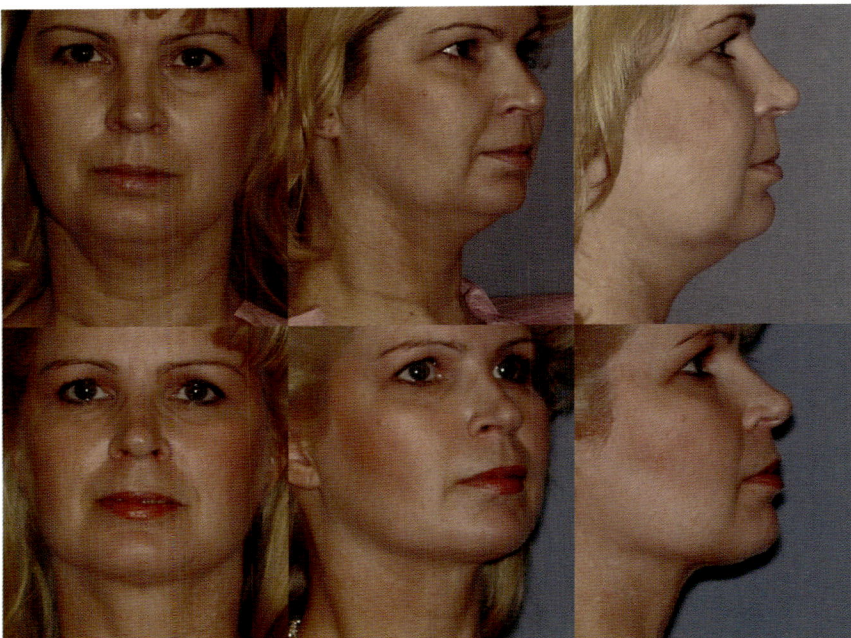

Fig. 30.5 Patient shown 1 year after isolated laser-assisted liposuction of the neck.

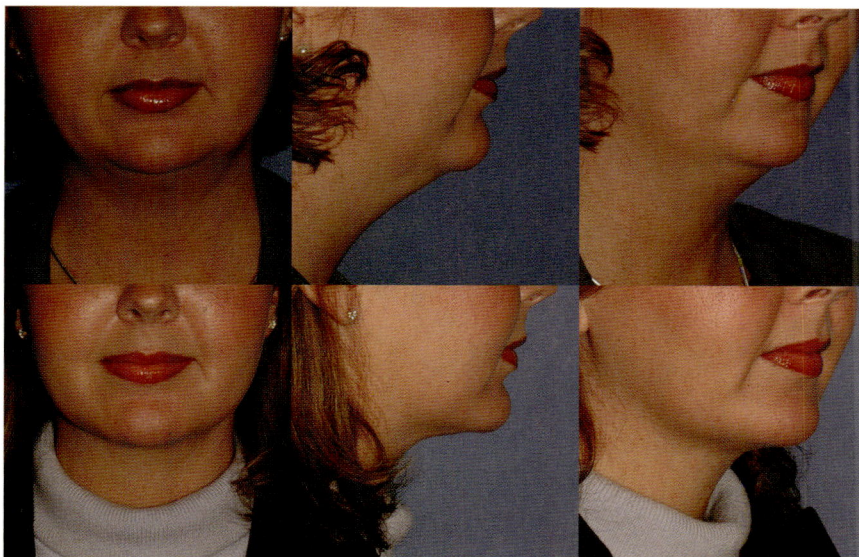

Fig. 30.6 Patient shown after placement of a pre-jowl sulcus silicone implant through a submental incision and laser-assisted liposuction of the neck.

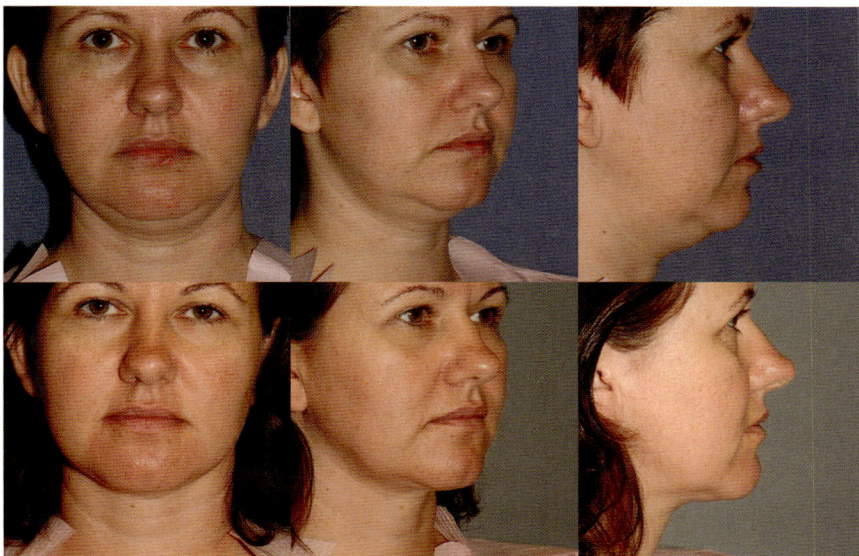

Fig. 30.7 Patient after isolated conventional liposuction with buccal fat pad removal.

Lipolysis and Necklift with Pre-Parotid Fat Reduction

This is a 50-year-old man 1 year postoperatively after presenting with concerns related to fullness in the lower third of his face (**Fig. 30.8**). The submental fat was predominantly in the subplatysmal plane, and the jawline was obscured by the jowl fat compartment and the dense fat layer in the pre-parotid area. The neck was treated with laser-assisted lipolysis of the supraplatysmal fat. Direct sculpting of the subplatysmal fat and a platysmal corset was performed through a submental incision. Laser lipolysis was used to reduce the fullness of the dense fat layer overlying the parotid and jawline. The use of the 1,444 nm laser for the reduction of the denser layer

of fat over the parotid gland has been a particular advancement over traditional liposuction because of the ease of melting the fat while passing the 600 μm laser fiber into the fibrofatty tissue.

Lipolysis and High Lamellar Facelift

This 52-year-old patient presented with the typical finding in lower facial aging (**Fig. 30.9**). All compartments of the face and neck are affected. There is ptosis of the midface, an accumulation of fat in the jowl fat compartments with ptosis of the inferior fat compartment over the jawline, loss of volume in the pre-jowl sulcus, and redundancy of skin in the neck with platysmal bands present at rest. She is shown 14 months after treatment consisting of laser lipoly-

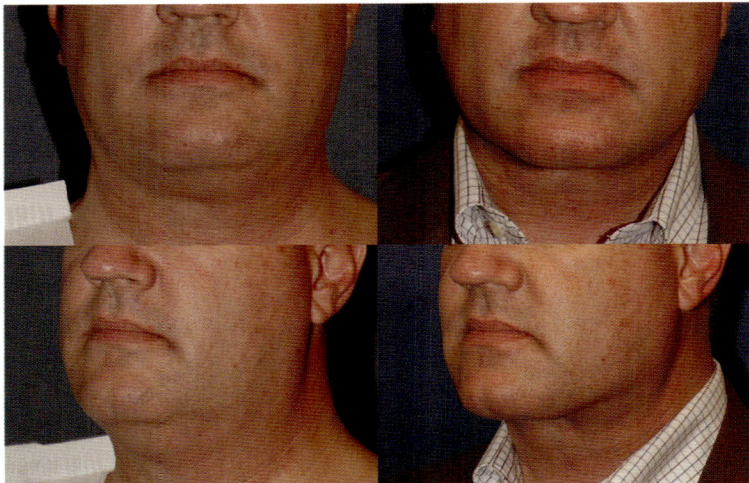

Fig. 30.8 A 50-year-old patient is shown 1 year after laser-assisted lipolysis of the jowl and pre-parotid fat with an open necklift.

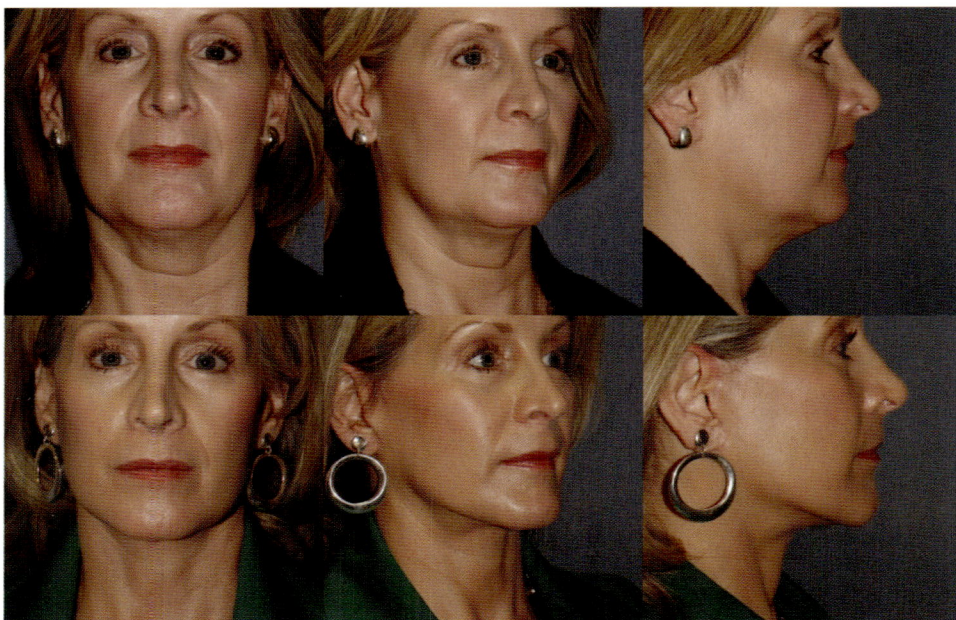

Fig. 30.9 A 52-year-old patient is shown 14 months after laser-assisted lipolysis of the jowl fat pad, high lamellar facelift, an open necklift, and pre-jowl sulcus fat grafting.

sis of the jowl fat compartment above the jawline, open neck treatment sculpting of the supraplatysmal and subplatysmal fat with a corset platysmaplasty, high lamellar facelift, and micro-fat injections to the pre-jowl sulcus and geniomandibular groove.

Lipolysis and Facelift with Perioral Contouring of the Irregularities

This patient in her sixties is shown 24 months after a high lamellar facelift, open neck treatment sculpting of the supraplatysmal and subplatysmal fat with a corset platysmaplasty, and micro-fat injections to the pre-jowl sulcus and geniomandibular groove

(**Fig. 30.10**). She also had laser-assisted lipolysis for reduction of the jowl fat pads above the jawline. The medial aspect of the superior jowl fat compartment just lateral to the corner of the mouth, which has been previously difficult to treat, has been effectively reduced to allow a smooth transition from the perioral fat compartments into the submalar and medial cheek fat compartment.

Sculpting of Face and Nasolabial Folds

This patient in her fifties wanted refinement in the lower two thirds of her face (**Fig. 30.11**). With age she had experienced a loss of shape to her lower face

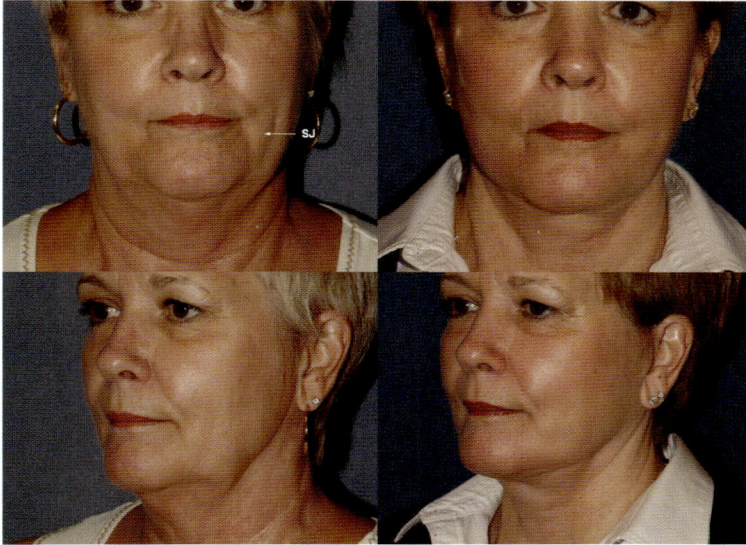

Fig. 30.10   Patient shown 24 months after laser-assisted lipolysis of perioral irregularities of the medial superior jowl fat pads (SJ) with high lamellar facelift and open necklift.

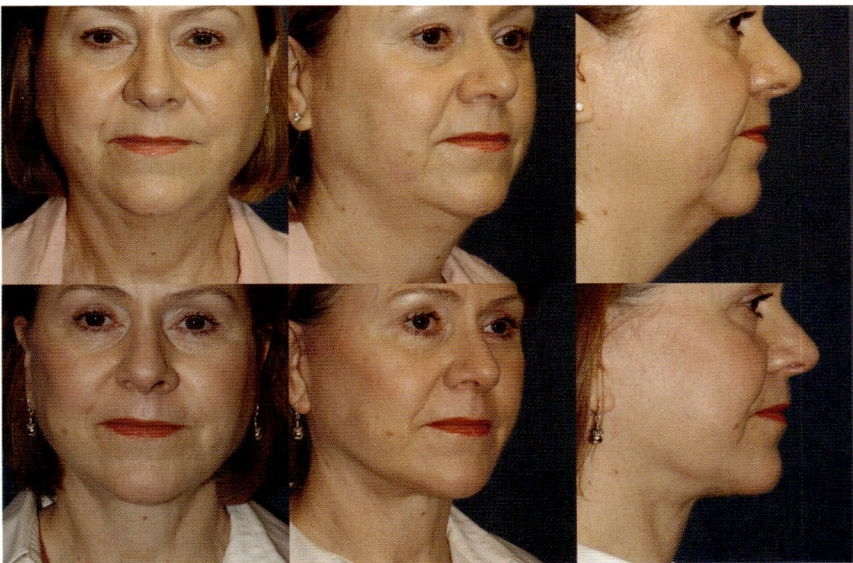

Fig. 30.11   This patient in her fifties presents with loss of shape to her lower face with ptosis and of the midface fat compartments and accumulation of volume in her jowl fat pads and neck. She is shown 9 months after laser lipolysis to the jowl fat pads with facelift and upper lid blepharoplasty achieving a smoother transition from the lower third into the malar region.

secondary to the ptosis of the midface fat that blends into the increased accumulation of fat in the jowl fat compartment. The inferior jowl fat compartment extended into the neck, and with the increased neck fat and laxity of the platysmal muscle, created a blunting of the mandibular margin and loss of the face–neck interface. She is shown 14 months after upper lid blepharoplasty, a high lamellar facelift, open-neck sculpting of the supraplatysmal and subplatysmal fat with a corset platysmaplasty, and micro-fat injections to the pre-jowl sulcus and geniomandibular groove. Laser-assisted lipolysis was performed in the jowl fat compartments with the laser energy extended into the submalar region to create a transition between the medial cheek fat compartments and the

superior jowl fat compartment, thus improving the submalar triangle aesthetics.

Laser-Assisted Lipolysis to Improve Lower Third Facial Asymmetry

This patient in her fifties presents with lower facial asymmetry with significant fullness in the left jowl fat compartment as compared with the right (**Fig. 30.12**). She also has bilateral upper eyelid ptosis. She is shown 9 months after a high lamellar facelift, open neck treatment sculpting of the supraplatysmal and subplatysmal fat with a corset platysmaplasty, and micro-fat injections to the pre-jowl sulcus and ge-

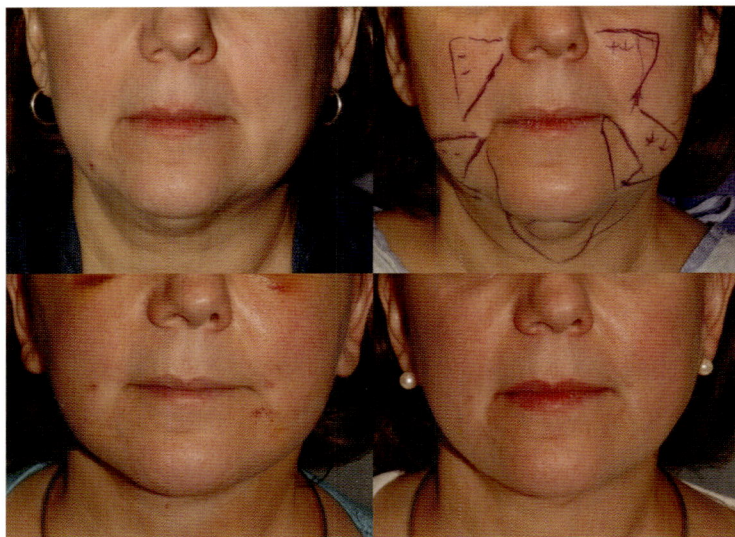

Fig. 30.12 This patient has preoperative facial asymmetry with significant fullness in the left jowl fat compartment. She is shown with preoperative markings, 1 week postoperative, and 9 months after a high lamellar facelift, open neck treatment, and micro-fat injections to the pre-jowl sulcus and geniomandibular groove.

niomandibular groove. Twice the amount of laser-assisted energy was delivered to the left jowl fat compartment as compared with the right to reduce the degree of soft tissue asymmetry.

■ Complications and Their Management

Bleeding is the most common complication encountered in facial aesthetic surgery. The result of bleeding during and after surgery ranges from ecchymosis to hematoma. The incidence of hematoma after isolated laser liposuction is rare, whereas the incidence of hematoma after concomitant neck or facelift ranges from 1 to 10%.

Minimization of the incidence of a hematoma after surgery begins with the preoperative management of hypertension and the avoidance of medications and supplements that affect bleeding. Intraoperative use of α_2 agonists, including clonidine, given orally as a preoperative medication, or dexmedetomidine (Precidex, Hospira) given as an intravenous drip during surgery, has been shown to assist in the modulation of intraoperative blood pressure as well as recovery room blood pressure. The authors have routinely used Precidex in facial aesthetic cases for 8 years, with a hematoma rate of less than 1% in over a thousand cases. Most hematomas after face- and necklift procedures occur in the recovery room and within the first 12 hours postoperatively.[24] Control of blood pressure, pain, postoperative nausea and vomiting, anxiety, and excessive movement will assist in the reduction of hematomas. Drains and pressure dressings have not proven effective in preventing hematomas and can increase the risk of skin loss from

excessive pressure from such a dressing in the face of an expanding hematoma.

Early detection and treatment of a postoperative hematoma are imperative to prevent adverse sequelae. Undetected and untreated expanding hematomas can lead to skin slough and even airway compromise. Most hematomas are treated with removal of sutures. Evacuation of all clots is followed by irrigation of all clot material, with reclosure over drains (**Fig. 30.13**). Small collections can be treated with needle evacuation, understanding that contour irregularities, prolonged bruising, and swelling can occur with retained blood.

Infections are unusual in facial aesthetic procedures. However, any early signs of infection such as cellulitis warrant treatment initially with antibiotics and drainage at the first sign of a fluid collection, with culture and sensitivity of the fluid. Recurrent collections are treated with early irrigation and drainage with placement of a drain (**Fig. 30.14**). Infections can delay wound healing and result in contour irregularities.

Seroma formation can occur, particularly in the neck after an open lipectomy. The dependent nature of the submental skin makes the submental triangle susceptible, particularly in men. Seromas are initially treated with needle aspiration with a culture and sensitivity performed on the aspirate. Because seromas are prone to recurrence, the authors see the patient frequently and are quick to place a 7 French drain via a small stab incision into the seroma (**Fig. 30.15**). Inadequately treated seromas can lead to prolonged thickening of the skin and subcutaneous tissue that may require steroid injections to soften the tissue.

The biggest risk of laser lipolysis of the face is overheating of the facial skin, with deformity and scar-

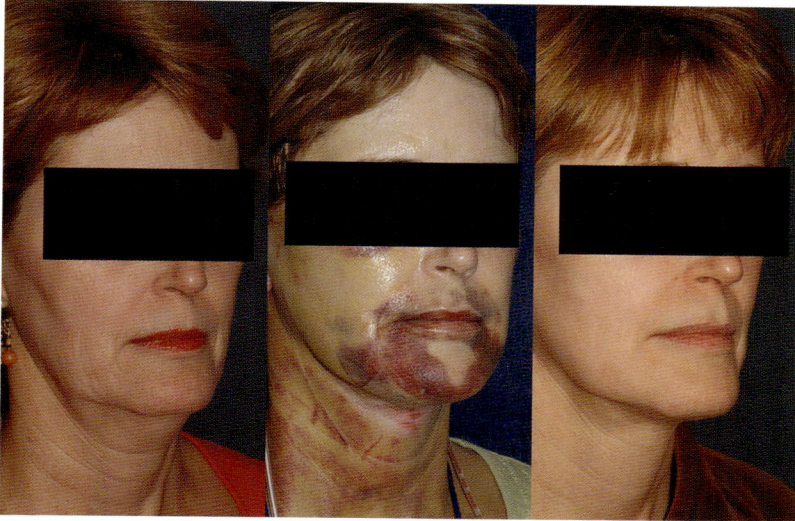

Fig. 30.13 Middle picture shows patient 1 day after evacuation of a large hematoma, and the right photo shows the final result, not affected by early intervention for the hematoma.

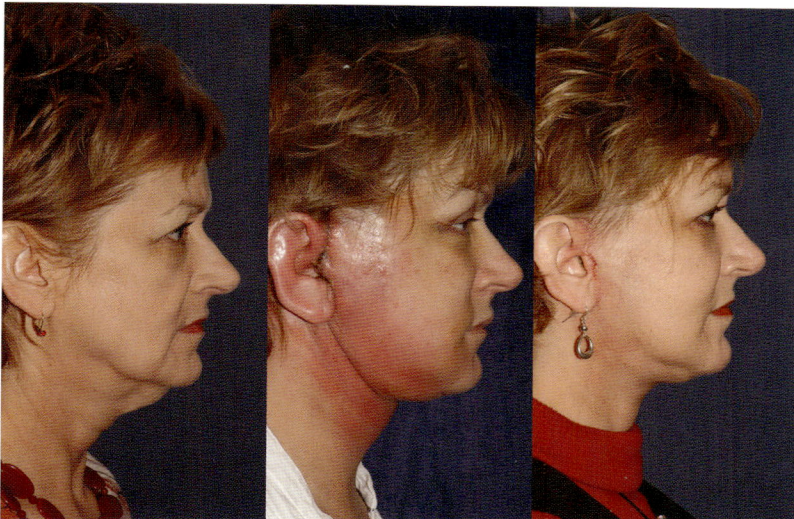

Fig. 30.14 Patient shown on postoperative day 5 with cellulitis and fluid collections over the entire right face and neck. The picture on the right is 5 weeks after resolution of infection and shows resolving contour irregularity in the submental triangle.

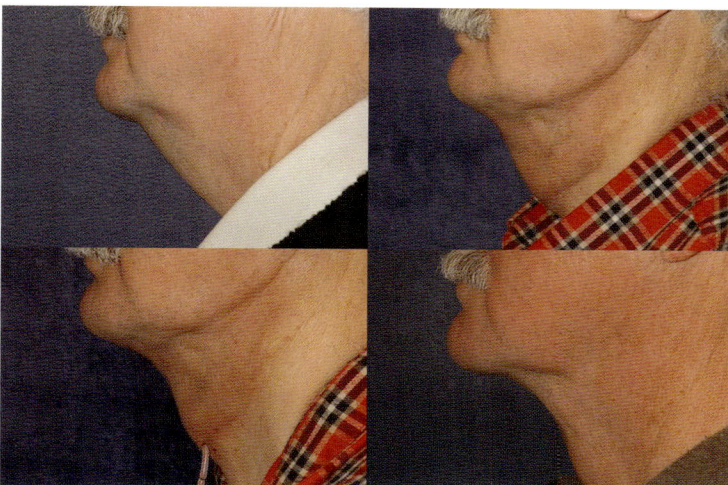

Fig. 30.15 A man presenting with a significant fluid collection after an open necklift with laser-assisted lipolysis of the jawline (*upper right photo*), immediately after drain placement and 8 months after resolution of the seroma.

ring from the burn. Thermal injury to overlying skin is always a risk when an energy-delivery device is used in the subdermal plane. The high specificity of fat and water to the 1,444 nm laser wavelength and short pulse duration may reduce the risk of thermal injury to the skin as compared with the other commercially available laser wavelengths at 1,064 nm and 1,320 nm. In our personal experience with over 200 patients on whom we utilized the 1,444 nm laser in facial procedures, we have not experienced a thermal injury. Early clinical reports from other early adopters of the 1,444 nm laser have reported the occurrence of minor second-degree burns at the laser fiber entry site that healed uneventfully.

Contour irregularities can result from excessive or uneven energy delivery to the targeted fat compartment. Irregularities can also occur with overly aggressive removal of the lipolysis fat with the triport aspirator. Contour deformities will become apparent as the postsurgical edema begins to resolve (**Fig. 30.16**). Temporary improvement can be achieved with injection of fillers, such as hyaluronic acid or calcium hydroxylapatite (CaHA) microspheres. Permanent correction can be achieved with autologous fat injection.

Undercorrection is not necessarily a complication but can lead to an unsatisfied patient. It is critical that preoperative evaluation determine the appropriate procedure or combination of procedures that address the concerns of the patient and the true deformity based on the patient selection criteria. For example, submental fullness treated with laser lipol-ysis as an isolated procedure when the majority of the fat is located in the subplatysmal plane will not completely correct an obtuse cervicomental angle.

Injury to the facial nerve is very rare in treatment of the lower third of the face. Nerve injury with isolated laser lipolysis of the jowls and neck has not been reported. The nerve is at risk when a concomitant facelift procedure is performed. The risk of permanent injury is less than 0.1%. Diminished movement in the lower lip on depression can be seen when fat is injected into the geniomandibular groove and prejowl depression. Full range of motion returns as the postoperative swelling diminishes.

■ Conclusion

As our understanding of the facial fat compartments and the variable impact each compartment has on the facial contours improves, a more individualized approach to treatment is evolving. Selective laser lipolysis has added another tool to assist in the refinement of outcomes of procedures to improve the contours of the lower third of the face and neck based on these variable findings within the fat compartments. It allows the safe volumetric contouring of the facial fat compartment and neck by delivering an energy that is selective to fat and water, thus reducing the risk of collateral tissue injury and adverse outcomes. Patient selection based on the anatomical findings is critical for optimal outcomes.

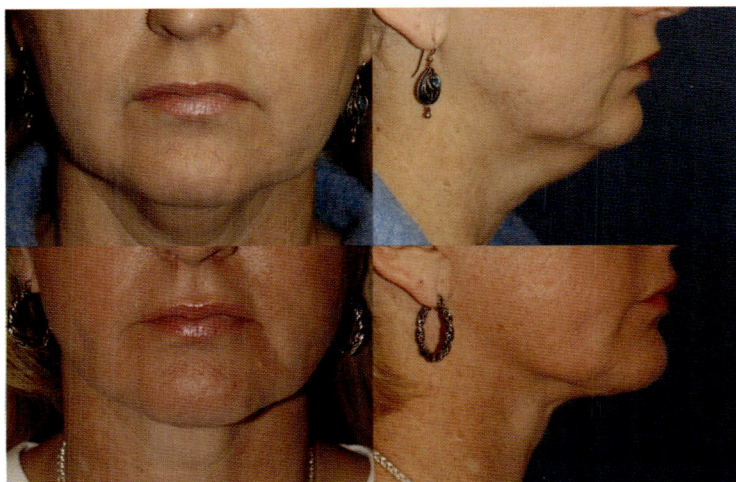

Fig. 30.16 This patient is shown 6 months after laser lipolysis with facelift and necklift. The right jowl fat compartment shows dimpling from overlasering.

References

1. Fitzgerald R, Vleggaar D. Facial volume restoration of the aging face with poly-L-lactic acid. Dermatol Ther 2011; 24(1):2–27

2. Fitzgerald R, Vleggaar D. Using poly-L-lactic acid (PLLA) to mimic volume in multiple tissue layers. J Drugs Dermatol 2009;8(10, Suppl):s5–s14

3. Vleggaar D, Fitzgerald R. Dermatological implications of skeletal aging: a focus on supraperiosteal volumization for perioral rejuvenation. J Drugs Dermatol 2008;7(3):209–220

4. Fitzgerald R, Graivier MH, Kane M, et al. Update on facial aging. Aesthet Surg J 2010;30(Suppl):11S–24S

5. Stuzin JM, Baker TJ, Gordon HL. The relationship of the superficial and deep facial fascias: relevance to rhytidectomy and aging. Plast Reconstr Surg 1992;89(3):441–449, discussion 450–451

6. McKinney P, Cook JQ. Liposuction and the treatment of nasolabial folds. Aesthetic Plast Surg 1989;13(3):167–171

7. Asken S. Microliposuction and autologous fat transplantation for aesthetic enhancement of the aging face. J Dermatol Surg Oncol 1990;16(10):965–972

8. Langdon RC. Liposuction of neck and jowls: five-incision method combining machine-assisted and syringe aspiration. Dermatol Surg 2000;26(4):388–391

9. Goldman A. Submental Nd:YAG laser-assisted liposuction. Lasers Surg Med 2006;38(3):181–184

10. Cook WR Jr. Laser neck and jowl liposculpture including platysma laser resurfacing, dermal laser resurfacing, and vaporization of subcutaneous fat. Dermatol Surg 1997;23(12):1143–1148

11. Sasaki GH, Tevez A. Laser-assisted liposuction for facial and body contouring and tissue tightening: a 2-year experience with 75 consecutive patients. Semin Cutan Med Surg 2009;28(4):226–235

12. McBean JC, Katz BE. A pilot study of the efficacy of a 1,064 and 1,320 nm sequentially firing Nd:YAG laser device for lipolysis and skin tightening. Lasers Surg Med 2009; 41(10):779–784

13. Badin AZ, Gondek LB, Garcia MJ, Valle LC, Flizikowski FE, de Noronha L. Analysis of laser lipolysis effects on human tissue samples obtained from liposuction. Aesthetic Plast Surg 2005;29(4):281–286

14. Khoury JG, Saluja R, Keel D, Detwiler S, Goldman MP. Histologic evaluation of interstitial lipolysis comparing a 1064, 1320 and 2100 nm laser in an ex vivo model. Lasers Surg Med 2008;40(6):402–406

15. Holcomb JD. Facelift adjunctive techniques: skin resurfacing and volumetric contouring. Facial Plast Surg Clin North Am 2009;17(4):505–514, v

16. Rohrich RJ, Pessa JE. The fat compartments of the face: anatomy and clinical implications for cosmetic surgery. Plast Reconstr Surg 2007;119(7):2219–2227, discussion 2228–2231

17. Reece EM, Pessa JE, Rohrich RJ. The mandibular septum: anatomical observations of the jowls in aging—implications for facial rejuvenation. Plast Reconstr Surg 2008; 121(4):1414–1420

18. Pilsl U, Anderhuber F. The chin and adjacent fat compartments. Dermatol Surg 2010;36(2):214–218

19. Nahai F. The Art of Aesthetic Surgery. 2nd ed. St. Louis, MO: Quality Medical Publishing; 2011

20. Feldman JJ. Neck Lift. St. Louis, MO: Quality Medical Publishing; 2006

21. Mathes S. Plastic Surgery. 2nd ed. Philadelphia, PA: Elsevier; 2006

22. Tark KC, Jung JE, Song SY. Superior lipolytic effect of the 1,444 nm Nd:YAG laser: comparison with the 1,064 nm Nd:YAG laser. Lasers Surg Med 2009;41(10):721–727

23. O'Daniel TG, Shanahan PT. Dexmedetomidine: a new alpha-agonist anesthetic agent for facial rejuvenation surgery. Aesthet Surg J 2006;26(1):35–40

24. Grover R, Jones BM, Waterhouse N. The prevention of haematoma following rhytidectomy: a review of 1078 consecutive facelifts. Br J Plast Surg 2001;54(6):481–486

31 Hair Transplantation

Agata K. Brys and Daniel E. Rousso

Key Concepts

- Male pattern androgenic alopecia is a hereditary problem due to the effects of dihydrotestosterone on the terminal hairs. The use of 5α-reductase inhibitors to stop testosterone conversion to dihydrotestosterone can reduce hair loss.

- Hair transplantation is a viable option for hair restoration. Best results are seen in men who are over 25 years of age, with stabilized hair loss, coarse, wavy hair, and minimal contrast of skin and hair color. Donor-site density and scalp laxity also influence results.

- Follicular unit transplantation is the gold standard in hair transplant surgery, producing natural, lasting results. Variations of the technique include donor strip harvesting and follicular unit extraction.

Introduction

Human concern with hair loss dates back to prehistoric times. Primitive remedies for baldness were quite imaginative, ranging from camel dung to stump water. Ancient Egyptians used castor oil to promote hair growth. Bhringaraj and amla oils were used in Asia. Since then, significant advancements in hair restoration have occurred.

In 1882, autologous hair transplantation was first shown to be feasible in animals by J. Dieffenbach, a German doctoral student. Fifty years later, Okuda described the first hair transplants in humans.[1] He used punch grafts to treat alopecia in burn victims. However it was not until the 1950s, when Dr. Norman Orentreich described the first hair transplant for male-pattern baldness using punch grafting, that attention was given to hair replacement surgery.[2]

This treatment was based on the principle of donor dominance, which states that hairs maintain their innate ability to grow as they would have in their donor site.

Early transplants involved large numbers of hairs in each graft, sometimes referred to as plugs. Unfortunately, this could lead to an apparent "doll's head" appearance. To obtain more natural-appearing results, smaller grafts were developed, called minigrafts, which included three or more hair follicles, and micrografts, which had one to two hair follicles. J.T. Headington is credited with describing the follicular unit as an anatomical entity, and his work gave credence to using smaller grafts. In 1988, Dr. Robert Limmer performed the first pure follicular unit transplantation.[3] Since that time, the procedure has become the gold standard in hair transplant surgery, producing natural, lasting results.

Background: Basic Science of Procedure

All hair follicles are formed by gestational week 22. At this time, there are 5 million follicles on the body, of which 1 million are on the head, and 100,000 are on the scalp. As the size of the body increases with age, no new hair follicles are added, and the density of the existing follicles decreases.

The hair follicle is derived from both the ectoderm and the mesoderm. The hair matrix cells and the melanocytes originate from ectoderm, whereas the arrector pili, dermal papilla, follicular sheath, and blood vessels are mesodermal derivatives. The primary hair germ begins as an epithelial bud that protrudes into the dermis and is driven by the dermal papilla. Together, the papilla and the epithelial cells make up the hair bulb. The components of the hair follicle include the sebaceous gland and duct, the apocrine gland and duct, and the attachment point of the arrector pili muscle (**Fig. 31.1**).[4]

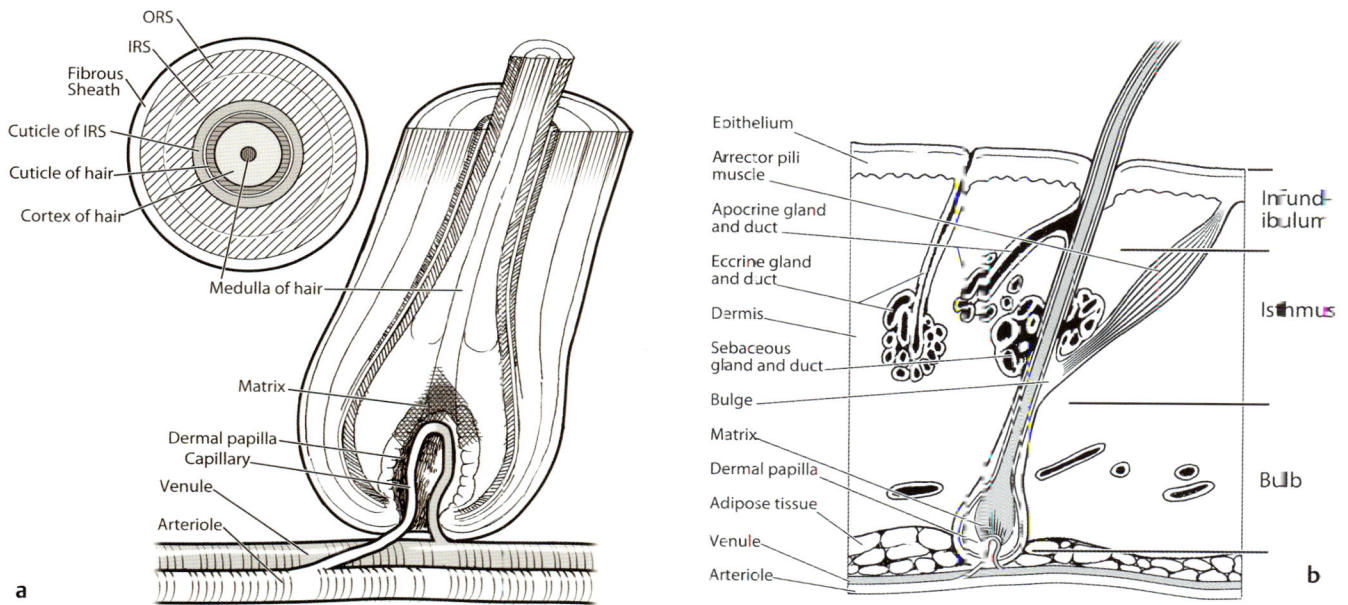

Fig. 31.1 Hair follicle anatomy. Labeled structures include epithelium, dermal papilla, sebaceous gland and duct, apocrine gland and duct, arrector pili muscle, outer root sheath (ORS), inner root sheath (IRS), medulla, matrix, cortex, and dermal papilla. **(a)** Cross-section through hair bulb and hair follicle. **(b)** The hair follicle is divided into three parts: infundibulum—from the entrance of the sebaceous duct to the follicular ostium; isthmus—from the insertion of the arrector pili muscle to the sebaceous duct; bulb—from the base of the follicle to the insertion of the arrector pili muscle.

The hair follicle can be divided into three parts. The superior portion is the infundibulum, which runs from the entrance of the sebaceous duct to the follicular ostium. Apocrine cells may empty into the infundibulum. The middle portion extends from the insertion of the arrector pili muscle to the sebaceous duct and is called the isthmus. The inferior portion is the bulb, which extends from the base of the follicle to the insertion of the arrector pili muscle. It contains melanocytes and the hair matrix with cells responsible for hair growth. The hair bulb surrounds the papilla, which influences the activity within the hair matrix. Keratinization of cells within the hair matrix forms the hair shaft. Vellous hair lacks the innermost portion of the shaft, the medulla. A follicular unit is composed of one to four terminal hairs, with or without several villous follicles, associated sebaceous glands, the arrector pili muscles, and a common vascular and neural plexus, and is surrounded by a connective tissue sheath (**Fig. 31.2**).

The follicular life cycle has three phases: anagen, catagen, and telogen (**Fig. 31.3**). The anagen phase is the phase of active growth, which lasts ~ 3 to 4 years. Most hairs in the scalp are in the anagen phase. The catagen phase is a 2 to 3 week involutional stage in which the inferior portion of the follicle ascends to the level of the attachment of the arrector pili muscle. The telogen phase represents a resting period and lasts ~ 3 months. With aging, the number, rate of growth, and diameter of hair shafts decline. In predisposed individuals, the terminal hairs of the adult scalp can undergo involutional miniaturization (become vellus), and the percentage of telogen hairs increases.

Alopecia

There are multiple causes of hair loss, including trauma, burns, neoplasms, autoimmune disorders, chemotherapy, and dermatologic conditions. However, the most common form in both men and women is androgenic alopecia. Androgenic alopecia can present as male-pattern androgenic alopecia (MPAA), female-pattern androgenic alopecia (FPAA), or diffuse androgenic alopecia. Other causes of hair loss that can mimic pattern hair loss include acute and chronic telogen effluvium, diffuse or reverse ophiasis alopecia areata, and early cicatricial alopecia.

Telogen effluvium is characterized by massive hair loss as a result of early entry of hairs into the telogen phase,[5] often secondary to emotional or physiological stresses. A variety of causes exist, including eating disorders, fever, childbirth, chronic illness, major surgery, anemia, severe emotional disorders, crash diets, hypothyroidism, and drugs.[6] Hair loss lags the

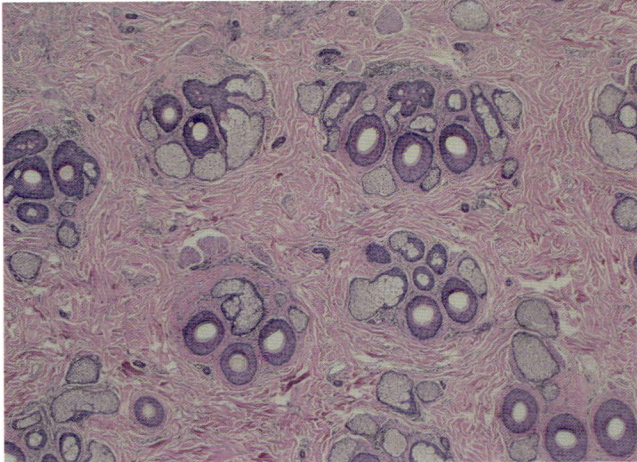

Fig. 31.2 Follicular units composed of one to four terminal hairs, with or without several villous follicles, associated sebaceous glands, the arrector pili muscles, a common vascular and neural plexus, surrounded by a connective tissue sheath. Hematoxylin-eosin, ×25. (From Rousso DE, Presti PM. Follicular unit transplantation. Facial Plast Surg 2008;24:381–388. Used with permission.)

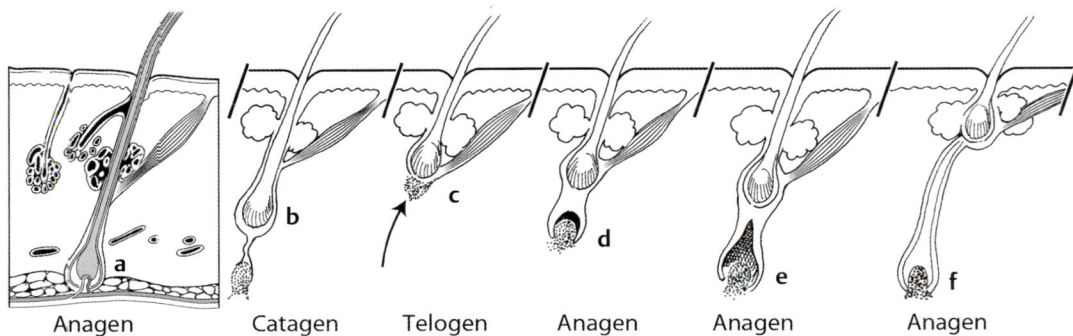

| Anagen | Catagen | Telogen | Anagen | Anagen | Anagen |

Fig. 31.3 The follicular life cycle is divided into three phases: anagen, catagen, and telogen. Anagen phase **(a,d–f)** consists of active hair growth. Catagen phase **(b)** is a stage of involution, in which the inferior portion of the follicle ascends to the level of the attachment of the arrector pili muscle. Telogen **(c)** represents a resting period.

inciting event by ~ 3 months. Anagen effluvium is the pathological loss of anagen hairs. Classically, it is caused by radiation therapy to the head and systemic chemotherapy, especially with alkylating agents.[7]

Alopecia areata is an immunologically driven condition, often triggered by stress, that causes patchy hair loss, which can range from diffuse thinning to extensive areas of baldness with "islands" of retained hair. On exam, the hair will have an exclamation point appearance, becoming narrower along the length of the strand closer to the base. The diffuse form mimics telogen effluvium and FPAA.

Cicatricial alopecias involve inflammation directed at the upper part of the hair follicle, which leads to destruction of the stem cell and the associated sebaceous gland. The hair follicle is then replaced with scar tissue, and permanent hair loss results. Causes include lichen planopilaris, frontal fibrosing alopecia, central centrifugal alopecia, lupus, pseudopelade (Brocq), folliculitis decalvans, tufted folliculitis, and dissecting cellulitis. There are also many infectious and inflammatory causes of alopecia. Some of the more common infectious causes include dermatophytes and syphilis. These present with a patchy "moth eaten" alopecia.[8] Hair loss in trichotillomania is typically patchy, as compulsive hair pullers tend to concentrate the pulling in selected areas. Often, short stubble hairs are present.

Pathophysiology

MPAA has been recognized as an androgen-dependent hereditary disorder since the 1940s.[9] MPAA was noted to be absent in men castrated before puberty, but developed in 12 castrated men who were treated with testosterone. Men who lack androgen receptor expression also do not develop MPAA.[10] However, it is dihydrotestosterone (DHT) that plays the dominant role in MPAA. DHT causes terminal hairs in the frontal and vertex/crown areas to become vellus, while at the same time causing vellus hairs to become terminal in the beard, mustache, chest, and upper pubic region. The enzyme responsible for converting free testosterone into DHT is 5α-reductase. Of the two isoforms of 5α-reductase, type II is expressed in androgen-dependent tissues, such as the prostate and hair follicle, and plays a role in MPAA. Men with deficiency of 5α-reductase do not develop MPAA.[11] Men with androgenic alopecia typically have higher levels of 5α-reductase, lower levels of total testosterone, higher levels of unbound/free testosterone, and higher levels of total free androgens, including DHT.[12] Current forms of medical treatment for MPAA aim to inhibit 5α-reductase activity. Men should be warned that anabolic steroids or supplemental androgens may increase hair loss.

MPAA is caused by the genetic sensitivity of hair follicles to DHT, causing the hairs to miniaturize and have a shorter lifespan, therefore preventing the individual from producing hair normally. Approximately 50% of all men are affected by MPAA, and there is a strong hereditary predisposition. The inheritance pattern is most likely polygenic.[13] Sons of men with MPAA have an increased frequency of MPAA, whereas sons of nonbalding men have a decreased risk of MPAA.[14,15] There is a maternal effect on MPAA, but it is less defined.

Clinical hair loss in classic male-pattern baldness follows a well-defined pattern, consisting of hair recession in the frontotemporal region and loss of hair at the vertex. These areas of loss gradually enlarge and coalesce until the entire front, top, and vertex of the scalp are bald. The stages of hair loss were originally described by Hamilton[16] and then modified by Norwood (**Fig. 31.4**).[17] The Norwood classification is as follows: Class I represents an adolescent or juvenile hairline resting on the upper brow crease. Class II hairline is 1.5 cm above the upper brow crease with some temporal recession. This is a mature hair line. Class III is the earliest stage of male hair loss and is characterized by a deepening temporal recession. Class III vertex represents early hair loss in the vertex. Class IV is continued hair loss in the frontal and vertex regions, but with a solid band of hair across the top separating the front and vertex. Class V is continued balding in the frontal and vertex regions with thinning of the bridge of hair separating the two areas. Class VI is the complete loss of the connecting bridge of hair, with a resulting single large bald area on the front and top of the scalp. The hair on the sides of the scalp remains relatively high. Class VII patients have extensive hair loss with only a rim of hair around the sides and rear. The Norwood Class A patterns are characterized by a front-to-back progression of hair loss, without the connecting bridge across the top of the scalp and a more limited hair loss on the vertex, even when advanced.

Usually, women do not suffer classic male-pattern baldness, but 30 to 40% of women are affected by hair loss. Women more commonly have diffuse central thinning[18] or frontal accentuation,[19] otherwise known as the "Christmas tree" pattern. Although the entire scalp is at risk of alopecia, recession at the temples is less likely than in men, and women tend to maintain the position of their hairlines. Female-pattern alopecia was classified by Ludwig in 1977 into three stages: mild, moderate, and extensive (**Fig. 31.5**).[18] Stage I is mild, with thinning in the crown but preservation of the frontal hairline. Stage II patients have significant widening of the midline part and noticeably decreased volume. Type III patients have diffuse thinning with a see-through look on the top of the scalp.

The role of androgens in FPAA is less straightforward. As already described, FPAA differs in distribution from MPAA. This is due to the fact that aromatase breaks down testosterone to estrogen and prevents the effects of DHT. The affected women typically do not have signs of hyperandrogenism and do not respond to treatment with 5α-reductase inhibitors.[20]

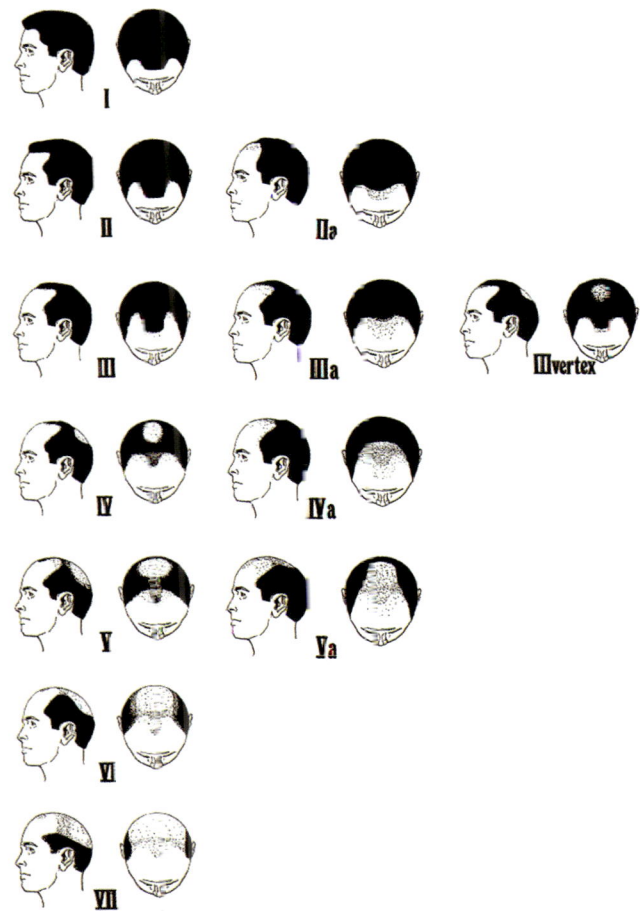

Fig. 31.4 Norwood classification of male-pattern baldness. (From Norwood OT. Male-pattern baldness: classification and incidence. South Med J 1975;68(11):1359–1365. Used with permission.)

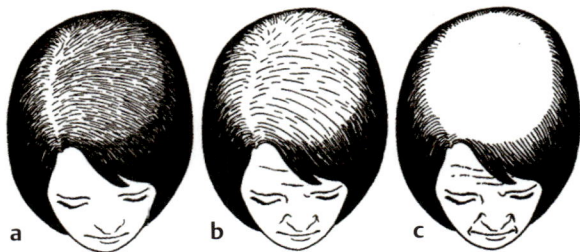

Fig. 31.5 Ludwig classification of female pattern baldness. **(a)** Stage I, perceptible hair loss with thinning in the crown, but preservation of the frontal hairline. **(b)** Stage II, significant widening of the midline part and noticeably decreased volume. **(c)** Stage III, diffuse thinning. (From Ludwig E. Classification of the types of androgenetic alopecia (common baldness) occurring in the female sex. Br J Dermatol 1977;97:247–254. Used with permission.)

There is a smaller subset of women who present with a more typical male pattern of hair loss. These women may be suffering from hyperandrogenism and need to be evaluated for other signs or symptoms of hyperandrogenism, including hirsutism, moderate to severe or treatment-refractory acne, irregular menses, infertility, and galactorrhea. Women with male-pattern hair loss in the presence of signs of hyperandrogenism may respond to treatment with finasteride or cyproterone acetate.[21,22] In addition, a family history should be obtained from the patient, although it may not be as clear as with males.

Medical Treatment

Before therapy is offered, a correct diagnosis must be made. Infections and autoimmune conditions must be identified and treated. Laboratory evaluation in men with androgenic alopecia is minimal. One may consider thyroid testing if the hair loss is diffuse and not following the typical MPAA pattern. Men on a strict vegetarian diet may be deficient in iron, and an iron evaluation may be warranted.

Women should have their thyroid-stimulating hormone (TSH) and serum ferritin levels tested. Deficiencies in either can cause telogen effluvium.[23,24] Iron deficiency can interfere with medical treatment of FPAA.[25] Women with clinical signs of hyperandrogenemia should undergo serological studies. These tests should include free and total testosterone and dehydroepiandrosterone sulfate. If galactorrhea is present, prolactin levels should be checked.

A scalp biopsy is indicated in men with female-pattern hair loss, diffuse hair loss, or scalp changes consistent with cicatricial alopecia. Women benefit from a scalp biopsy to exclude chronic telogen effluvium, diffuse alopecia areata, or cicatricial alopecia.

The topical and oral treatments for androgenic alopecia are numerous. Of these, topical minoxidil (Rogaine, McNeil-PPC, Lititz, PA) and oral androgen modifiers have been found to be effective. Minoxidil, a piperidinopyridine derivative initially used as a vasodilator to treat hypertension, was noted to increase hair growth in 70% of the patients taking the medication for hypertension. The action of minoxidil is not fully understood, but it might increase blood flow to the scalp or stimulate hair follicle growth through growth factor modification. Topical minoxidil applied every night in a 2 or 5% solution has been shown to be effective over 4 to 6 months.[26] Discontinuation of treatment leads to loss of gained hair over 3 to 4 months.[27] Initially, patients may observe an increase in hair loss because hairs are induced into anagen and telogen hairs are shed. Minoxidil is safe for use by both men and women, although the 5% solution may cause unwanted facial hypertrichosis in females. Therefore, it is recommended for women to use the 2% solution. Minoxidil used within days of hair transplantation can delay the typical shedding seen after hair transplantation and may shorten the period needed for hair grafts to regrow. There are minimal side effects associated with minoxidil use, and they are typically dermatologic in nature. The 5% solution is more likely than the 2% solution to cause scalp irritation, dryness, scaling, itching, or redness.

Drugs that interfere with type II 5α-reductase, such as finasteride, have been approved by the U.S. Food and Drug Administration (FDA) to treat hair loss in men. These medications, such as Proscar (Merck, Whitehouse Station, NJ), were originally used to treat prostate hypertrophy and were incidentally noted to improve hair loss. They work by reducing production of DHT, thus limiting the action of DHT on scalp hair follicles, but having no intrinsic steroid activity. Recommended dosage of finasteride (Propecia, Merck) is 1 mg daily.[28] Increases in hair counts are seen within the first year of use; following this, there is a plateau of hair growth, but there is also a continued decrease in hair loss. The decreased DHT levels also reduce prostate-specific antigen (PSA), and it is recommended that any PSA value should be doubled for men taking finasteride.[29] In men, side effects are limited to decreased libido, erectile dysfunction, and decreased ejaculate volume. These were noted in 1.8% of men ages 18 to 41 versus 1.1% in those on placebo and were reversible with cessation of medication.[30]

Because DHT is necessary for embryonic sexual differentiation and virilization of the male embryo, finasteride is contraindicated in women of childbearing age. No risk is seen to the fetus or the mother from semen of men taking finasteride.[31] A 1 year, double-blind, placebo-controlled, randomized, multicenter trial of finasteride in postmenopausal women did not show increase in hair growth or decrease in the progression of hair thinning.[20] Better results are seen in women with a male pattern of hair loss and evidence of hyperandrogenism.[32] All women of childbearing age using 5α-reductase inhibitors or antiandrogens need to use effective birth control. Oral contraceptives have the additional benefit of lowering serum androgens.

Spironolactone is an aldosterone antagonist employed in clinical practice as a potassium-sparing diuretic used to treat high blood pressure. Spironolactone is used off-label to treat alopecia and hirsutism in females. It decreases production and blocks the effect of androgens at the cellular level. Birth defects are possible with this medication, and a form of birth control is recommended when taking this medication. Small, uncontrolled studies with spironolactone show efficacy of spironolactone in women who have hyperandrogenism.[33] The minimum effective dose to treat hair loss is 100 mg daily. Doses above 100 mg a day are associated with uterine bleeding and a possible risk of developing breast cancer.[34]

In Europe, cyproterone acetate is approved for women with alopecia, high ferritin levels, or clinical evidence of hyperandrogenism. It is an androgen receptor–binding molecule that competes with DHT. Combining 100 mg cyproterone acetate with 50 μg ethinyl estradiol on days 5 to 25 of the menstrual cycle helps decrease side effects. Combination products of oral contraceptives and a small amount of cyproterone acetate exist but are not available in the United States.

Grooming

No patient undergoing hair restoration surgery should ignore the benefits of hair styling. A consultation with a hair stylist can maximize the effect of the transplantations, and most patients benefit from the use of a hairstyling blow dryer. Those with thin, straight hair can benefit from a permanent body treatment. The use of topical scalp concealers such as COUVRé or Toppik hair-building fibers (Spencer Forrest, Los Angeles, CA) can give additional benefit by deflecting light away from thin areas.

Surgical Treatment

The basic principle in hair restoration surgery is to redistribute the existing hairs to give the scalp the appearance of increased hair density. This can be achieved through transplantation, flaps, or scalp reductions. Hair transplantation has become the gold standard of hair restoration surgery. Initial methods involved the use of punches to remove large areas of donor hair and to place them in the areas of alopecia. Currently, smaller transplants are used to provide a more natural result.

■ Patient Selection

Although almost every patient is a candidate for some form of hair replacement procedure, there are certain factors that make some patients better surgical candidates.[35] These factors include age, pattern of alopecia, heredity, hair density in donor area/fringe, hair and skin color, hair texture, and scalp laxity. Very few absolute contraindications to surgery exist, especially if one does not count lidocaine allergy, active autoimmune, inflammatory or infectious disease, and inadequate health status to undergo this type of surgical procedure.

Age

No minimum age limit exists for hair replacement, but experience has demonstrated that patients younger than their early twenties may be less content with the results gained. Waiting for the patient to mature tends to dissipate unrealistic expectations of hair density and allows the patient to accept a more mature hairline. It also allows the surgeon to better evaluate the progressive nature of the patient's alopecia and to determine the final pattern of hair loss. Younger patients with premature alopecia also tend to have progressive hair loss and less impressive gains from restoration surgery.

Pattern of Alopecia

Androgenic alopecia is progressive; therefore the pattern of alopecia at the time of presentation is only a snapshot in time. The rate of alopecia progression is unknown. The Hamilton–Norwood and Ludwig classifications are helpful for communication purposes but do not predict the pattern of hair loss for the patient. It is important to determine the rate of progressive hair loss and to evaluate the patient's family history to better predict the patient's possible future hair loss.

Heredity

Because androgenic alopecia has both maternal and paternal hereditary influences, information about the pattern of hair loss on both the maternal and the paternal sides of the family tree can help in estimating the patient's future hair loss. For example, a patient with hair loss presenting in the early twenties and a family history of extensive alopecia on both the maternal and paternal sides will likely continue to lose hair and may be limited in reconstructive options.

Hair Density in Donor Area/Fringe

Occipital hair density will determine the number of grafts that can be harvested per each session. Patients with advanced alopecia but with excellent density in the donor area can be candidates for hair transplantation with good results. Patients with poor density may only be candidates for restoration of an isolated frontal forelock. One cannot expect to obtain or even attempt to achieve full coverage in patients with type VII alopecia.

Hair and Skin Characteristics

The apparent density of hair following hair transplantation is affected by the characteristics of the hair and scalp. Coarse, wavy hair appears denser than limp, fine hair (**Fig. 31.6**). A strong contrast between the hair and skin color decreases the apparent density of hair. Light hair against a background of light skin appears denser than does dark hair against light skin. A light-skinned individual with dark hair will have a harder time camouflaging the hair transplants and achieving a natural result unless a greater number of grafts is used. On the other hand, a light-skinned patient with curly gray or blond hair will have an apparently better result.

Scalp Laxity

Evaluation of occipital scalp laxity will determine whether graft harvest is reasonable, especially in patients who have undergone prior transplantation.

Patients with significant laxity may be candidates for alopecia reduction. Those with very limited laxity could benefit from scalp expansion or extension prior to undergoing any surgery. In our observation, intraoperative use of hyaluronidase can decrease closure tension in patients with poor scalp laxity (pers. comm., Carlos Puig).

Patient Counseling

It is imperative that hair restoration physicians develop open communication with their patients and counsel them about the appropriateness of hair restoration surgery. Based on the patient's expectations and the evaluation of the patient's age, pattern of alopecia, hereditary history, hair density in donor area/fringe, hair and skin color, hair texture, and scalp laxity, realistic goals can be developed. Each patient needs to be advised that significant changes in density will often require more than one or two transplant sessions. A thorough discussion of the risks and benefits of surgery should also occur at the preoperative visit.

Hairline design should be decided preoperatively with the patient's input. Low hairlines and blunted frontotemporal gulfs are to be avoided because these will result in an unnatural appearance. The anterior hairline should be set 7.5 to 9 cm above the glabella (**Fig. 31.7**). The contour of the hairline can be flared, rounded hemioval, flat, or slightly rounded. In addition, the hairline can be drawn with an irregular in-and-out microcontour. Feathering of smaller, single-hair follicular unit grafts anterior to the hairline allows for further blending of the hairline.

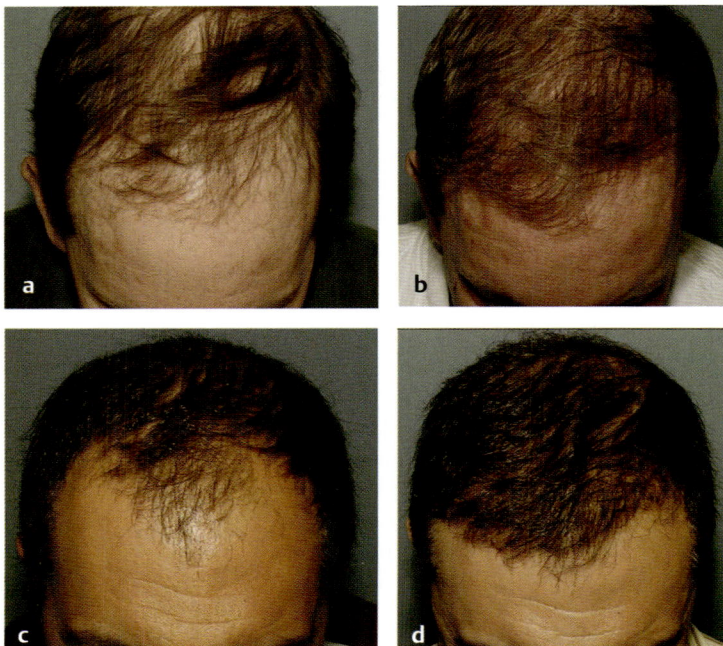

Fig. 31.6 Preoperative **(a,c)** and postoperative **(b,d)** views of hair transplantations. Each patient had one transplant session with 1,500 follicular unit transplants. The patient in **(a)** and **(b)** has finer hair. The patient in **(c)** and **(d)** has coarser hair, giving the appearance of a denser transplant result.

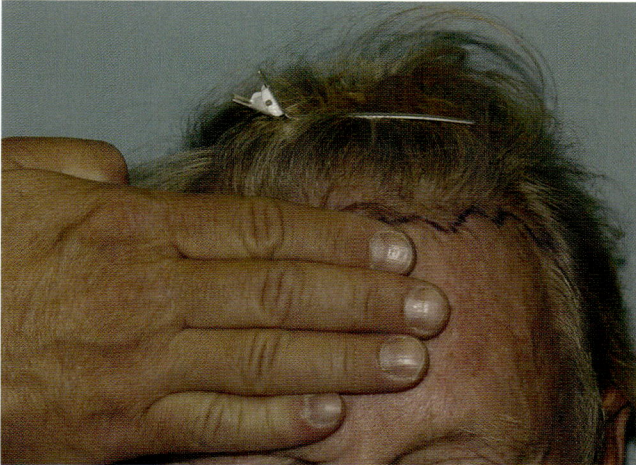

Fig. 31.7 The anterior hairline should be set 7.5 to 9 cm above the glabella. This may be more easily examined if the surgeon knows the width of his/her own palm. The contour of the hairline is rounded, but can also be flared, rounded hemioval, or flat, and drawn with an irregular in-and-out microcontour.

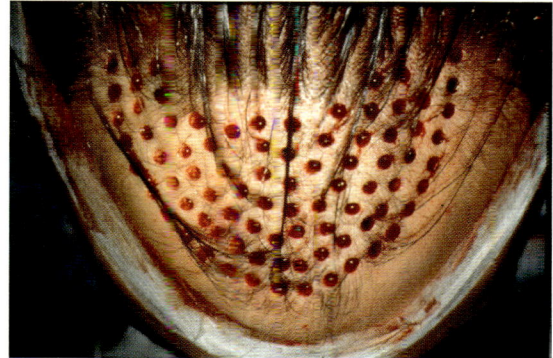

Fig. 31.8 Intraoperative view of recipient sites created for punch grafts. These are staggered and require repeat procedures to fill in the ungrafted area.

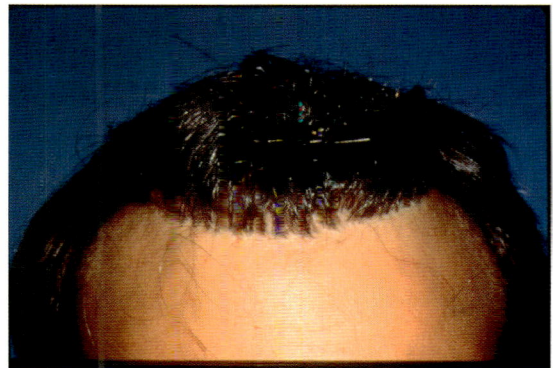

Fig. 31.9 Postoperative result following four punch grafting sessions. This patient achieved excellent density, and with proper hairstyling can achieve a very natural result. However, certain situations, such as wet hair, give a "doll's head" appearance.

■ Technical Aspects of Procedure

Punch Grafts

In the 1950s, the work of Norman Orentreich popularized the use of punch grafts for hair restoration. The use of a 4 mm round punch graft, with 12 hairs per graft, was the standard treatment through the 1980s. Excellent density could be achieved with repeat sessions, but the effect often resulted in a tufted, unnatural appearance. The procedure involved punching out donor hair from the fringe area using hand- or power-driven punches. The use of power tools greatly hastened the process. The grafts were taken ~ 1 mm apart, and the donor sites were allowed to heal by secondary intention. Care had to be taken to align the punch with the angle of the hair shaft to minimize follicle transection. Next, punches were performed in the recipient area to make room for the harvested hair-bearing donor plugs (**Fig. 31.8**). These were typically made slightly smaller than the hair-bearing donor plugs and were spaced apart to allow adequate blood flow to the hair graft. Complete hair restoration using punch grafts required a minimum of three sessions to evenly fill out the recipient area. With these repeat sessions, excellent density could be achieved, though the result was often an unnatural "doll's head" appearance, with significant scarring in the donor area (**Fig. 31.9**).

The current treatment for patients presenting with the unsightly appearance of plugs is to partially punch out the plugs and redistribute the removed hair anterior and posterior to the plug reduction sites.[36] Scar revision can be performed to the donor site if adequate scalp laxity is present. In addition, the patients may be candidates for follicular unit grafting to help camouflage the plugs.

Follicular Unit Transplantation

The alternative to the 4 mm punch graft was to use higher numbers of much smaller grafts. Initially, minigrafts containing 3 to 12 hairs and micrografts containing 1 to 2 hairs were used (**Fig. 31.10**). Currently, individual follicular units containing 1 to 4 hairs are being transplanted ▶ **Video 31.1** (**Fig. 31.11**). The transplant of individual follicular units minimizes the transfer of non-hair-bearing tissue and therefore allows for maximal density of hair distribution. There is also a decrease in trauma to the recipient area because the need to create large recipient sites is obviated.

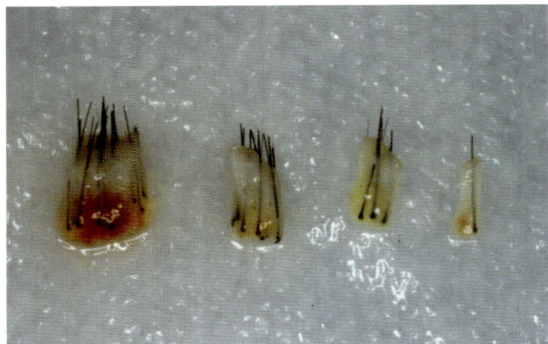

Fig. 31.10 View of various-sized grafts prior to placement. 4 mm square graft (*far left*), minigrafts (*center left and right*) containing between 3 and 12 hairs, and a micrograft (*far right*) containing fewer than 3 hairs.

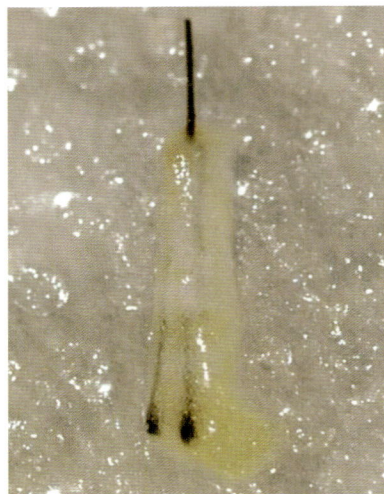

Fig. 31.11 Close-up of a follicular unit transplant. (From Rousso DE, Presti PM. Follicular unit transplantation. Facial Plast Surg 2008;24:381–388. Used with permission.)

Anesthesia

Follicular unit transplantation can be performed under strictly local anesthesia or local with mild sedation. Thirty minutes prior to injection of local anesthesia, the patient is typically given 10 to 20 mg of oral diazepam, depending on the patient's habitus and experience with benzodiazepines. Supraorbital, occipital, and postauricular nerve blocks are performed with 2% lidocaine with 1:100,000 epinephrine. This is followed by a ring block using 1% lidocaine with 1:100,000 epinephrine. The scalp is then infused subdermally with 1% lidocaine with 1:100,000 epinephrine.

Strip versus Follicular Unit Extraction

The traditional method of harvesting donor hair is by harvesting a strip of tissue from the occipital scalp. The density of the occipital scalp will determine the number of grafts that can be obtained. The average density in Caucasians is 1 FU/mm^2 (~ 175 to 275 hairs/cm^2).[37] The densest area of the occipital scalp and possibly the parietal scalp is chosen, and the proposed donor site is trimmed with scissors, leaving a 2 mm stub of hair to allow easier determination of the angle that the hair exits the scalp (**Fig. 31.12**). This aids in preventing transection of the follicles during harvesting. Harvesting of the strip in a block fashion can be performed with a no.10 blade (**Fig. 31.13**). The superior incision is beveled parallel to the direction of hair growth. The inferior incision is overbeveled, leaving deepithelialized follicles in the inferior portion of the scalp. This creates a trichophytic incision and allows for hair growth through the resulting scar (**Fig. 31.14**). Alternatively, a multibladed knife can be used for strip harvesting (**Fig. 31.15**). This method places multiple incisions paral-

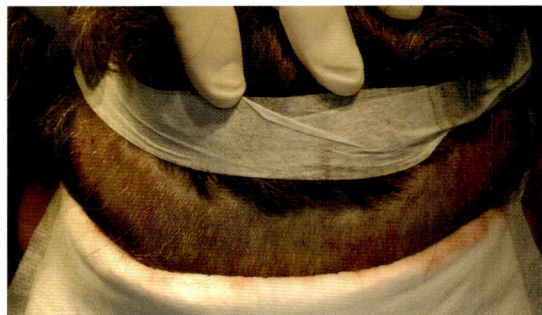

Fig. 31.12 The donor area consists of the densest hair-bearing areas of the occipital scalp and possibly the parietal scalp. The hair is trimmed with scissors, leaving a 2 mm stub of hair to allow easier determination of the angle at which the hair exits the scalp. (From Rousso DE, Presti PM. Follicular unit transplantation. Facial Plast Surg 2008;24:381–388. Used with permission.)

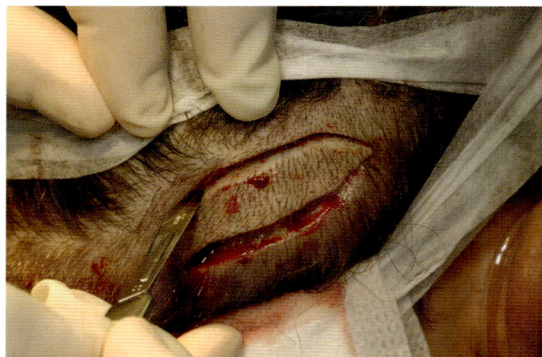

Fig. 31.13 Harvesting of the strip in a block fashion can be performed with a no. 10 blade. (From Rousso DE, Presti PM. Follicular unit transplantation. Facial Plast Surg 2008;24:381–388. Used with permission.)

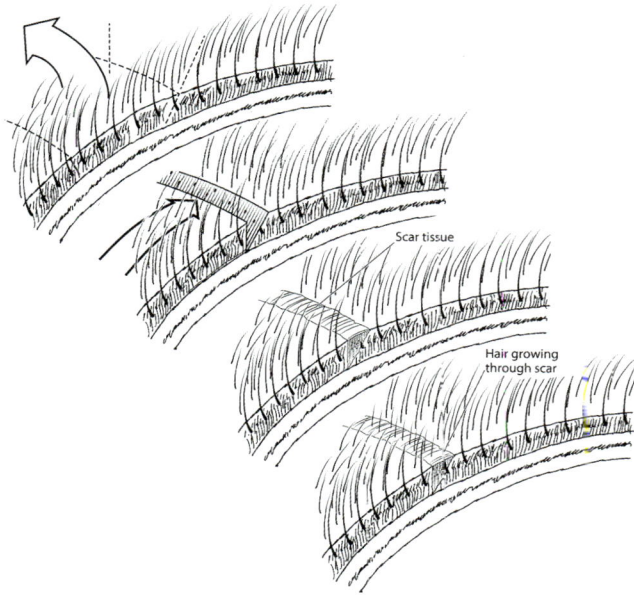

Fig. 31.14 Trichophytic incision. The superior incision is beveled parallel to the direction of hair growth. The inferior incision is overbeveled, leaving deepithelialized follicles in the inferior portion of the scalp. This allows for hair growth through the resulting scar.

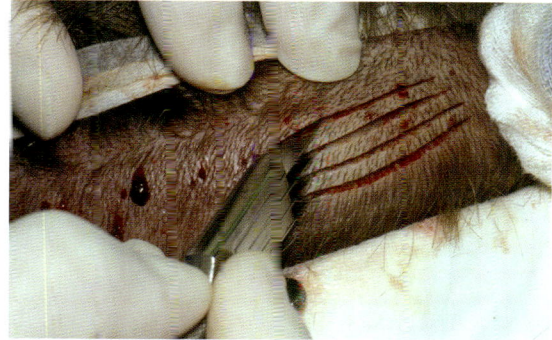

Fig. 31.15 The strip can be harvested either as a block excision or with a multibladed knife, as shown.

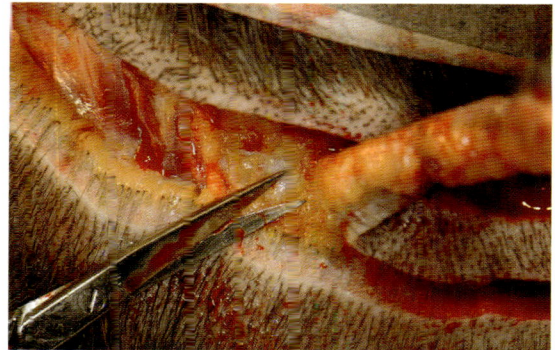

Fig. 31.16 Strip elevation is made in the deep subcutaneous plane, above the plane of the occipital arteries and nerves. (From Rousso DE, Presti PM. Follicular unit Transplantation. Facial Plast Surg 2008;24:381–388. Used with permission.)

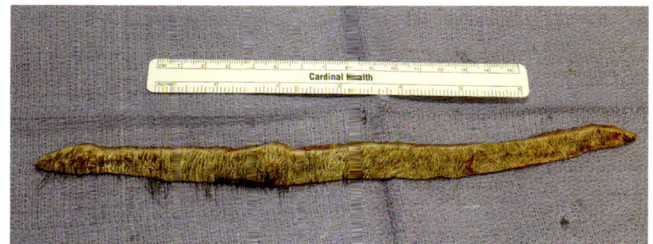

Fig. 31.17 The harvested strip of hair.

lel to the direction of hair growth. However, its use increases the incidence of transection of the follicles and graft loss. To obtain a trichophytic closure with this method, one needs to return to the area and remove a strip of superficial skin from one side, leaving the hair bulbs in place.

Once the incisions are made, the strip is sharply dissected in the deep subcutaneous plane, above the plane of the occipital arteries and nerves (**Fig. 31.16**). The typical dimensions of the strip are 18 to 22 cm in length by 1 to 1.5 cm in width (**Fig. 31.17**).[38] The harvested strip is passed to the hair technician team, who dissect it into slivers that are one follicular unit thick, which can be more easily dissected into individual follicular unit grafts. The donor site defect is closed with a running locking 2–0 Prolene suture (Ethicon, Somerville, NJ). The suture is placed intradermally to avoid the hair follicle bulbs (**Figs. 31.18** and **31.19**). Stainless steel autostaples can also be used; however, in the authors' opinion, this is more uncomfortable for patients. The beveling performed allows a trichophytic closure that is easily concealed if hair length is maintained at ≥ 1 cm.

Alternatively, an individual follicular unit graft can be extracted from the scalp using a 1 mm punchlike instrument without the need for microscopic dissection. This method is called follicular unit extraction (FUE). The donor area is the entire possible donor zone in the occipital and parietal region, as well

as the low supraauricular region and neck, where smaller-caliber hairs can be obtained.[39] The entire donor area needs to be shaved prior to harvesting to allow better visualization and access. If the patient is concerned about shaving the area, then intervening strips of hair-bearing scalp can be left between the shaved areas, or the hair can be cut short on only the follicular units to be extracted. Both modifications

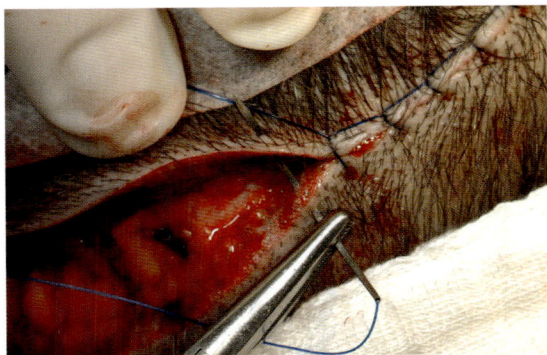

Fig. 31.18 A running locking 2–0 Prolene suture (Ethicon) is placed intradermally to close the donor site defect. (From Rousso DE, Presti PM. Follicular unit Transplantation. Facial Plast Surg 2008;24:381–388. Used with permission.)

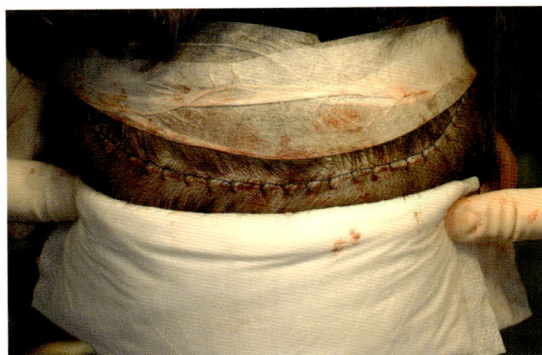

Fig. 31.19 Closed donor site scalp incision.

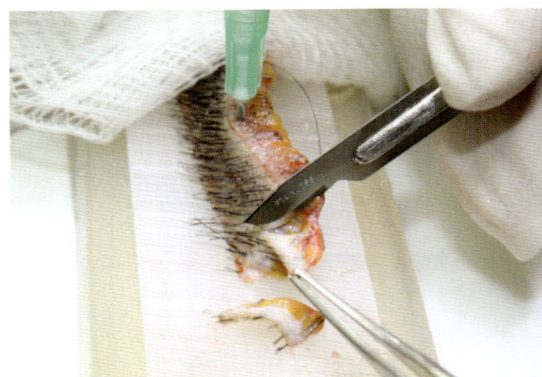

Fig. 31.20 The harvested strip is initially dissected into slivers that are the thickness of a single follicular unit, which can be more easily dissected into individual follicular unit grafts.

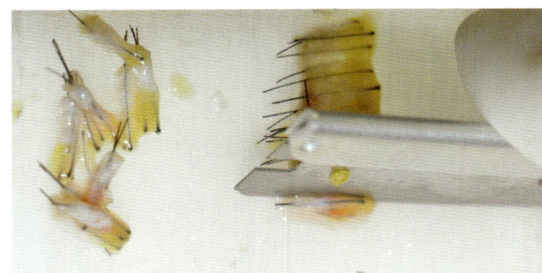

Fig. 31.21 The slivers are dissected into follicular unit grafts.

are more time consuming, and care must be taken to ensure a random distribution of extraction sites.

The follicular extractions are performed with either a sharp or a dull dissecting punch of variable sizes, and the graft is removed with a forceps. The key is to align the punch with the angle of the hair shaft and presumably the follicles. Because the alignment of the hair follicle may not mimic the angle of the hair shaft, there is a risk of follicle transection with this method. Depending on the type of punch used, transection rates vary from 1.3% to more than 10%.[39]

The key benefit to follicular unit extractions is the absence of a linear scar in the donor site. No sutures are necessary, and there may be less postoperative discomfort. The disadvantages include an increased risk of follicular damage during the extraction, which can lead to suboptimal growth of the hair transplant.[40] The removed graft also has a decreased amount of surrounding fat and is at risk for desiccation while awaiting placement.

Follicular Unit Preparation

Once the strip is harvested, it is passed to the hair technicians for preparation. Throughout the process until placement, the grafts are kept moist in saline-soaked nonadherent gauze (Telfa, Kendall, Mansfield, MA). The harvested strip is initially dissected into single-follicular-unit-thick slivers under the microscope (**Fig. 31.20**). The slivers are then dissected into follicular unit transplants (**Fig. 31.21**).

Recipient Site Creation

The recipient sites can all be created prior to initiating implantation. Alternatively, they can be made along with placement of grafts, the so-called stick and place technique. The authors prefer to make all

of the recipient sites initially, prior to placing the grafts. This method gives the surgeon complete control over hairline placement, and the positioning and direction of each graft, and it gives time for the hair technicians to start dissecting the grafts.

A lightening knife handle with an SP-90 or SP-91 blade (Swann-Morton, Sheffield, England) or a 1.3 or 1.5 mm Minde knife with a 40 degree angle knife

(Surgical Specialties, San Juan, PR) is used to create precise stab incisions (**Figs. 31.22** and **31.23**). Attention is given to the surrounding hair growth to angle the incisions along the natural pattern of hair growth. The incisions are feathered along the anterior hairline.

Placement

The grafts are meticulously placed into the individual slits with fine jeweler's forceps (**Fig. 31.24**). One set of forceps can be used to open the slit and another to place a graft, but this is not necessary. Attention must be given to prevent already-placed grafts from extruding by avoiding undue tension and preventing bleeding. Hemostasis can be achieved with reinjection of 1% lidocaine with 1:50,000 epinephrine. Graft extrusion can also occur from large graft sizes, shallow recipient sites, and scar tissue at the recipient site (**Fig. 31.25**).

Megasessions

A traditional hair transplant session usually uses 2,000 or fewer grafts. During a megasession, 3,000 to 4,500 grafts may be placed, and a super megasession consists of over 4,500 grafts. Dramatic results can be obtained in one session but require significant operating time and a sufficient number of well-trained staff. One of the disadvantages of megasessions includes decreased graft survival because grafts are not inserted in a reasonable amount of time. Some patients are not candidates for a megasession due to inadequate donor hair density or scalp laxity.

Complications

Infection is a rare entity with follicular unit transplantation but can occur in less than 1% of cases. Perioperative use of antibiotics is routine. Bleeding is most commonly seen in the occipital region. By keeping the strip dissection in the deep subcutaneous plane, the occipital arteries can be avoided. Punch harvesting, such as follicular unit extraction,

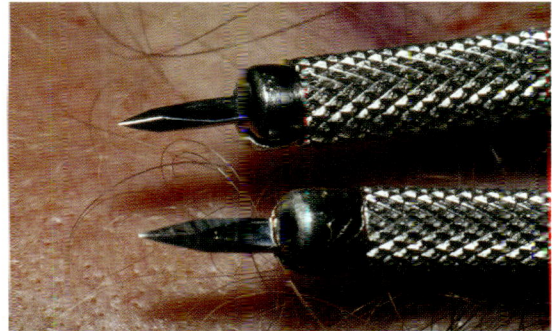
Fig. 31.22 A lightering knife handle with an SP-90 (*upper*) or SP-91 (*lower*) blade.

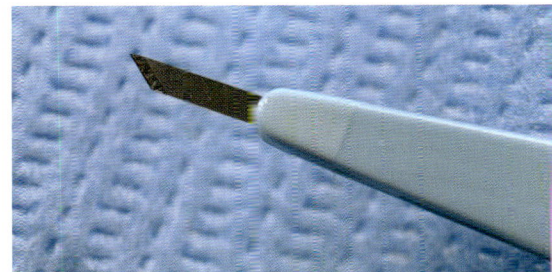
Fig. 31.23 A 1.3 Minde knife with a 40-degree-angle knife.

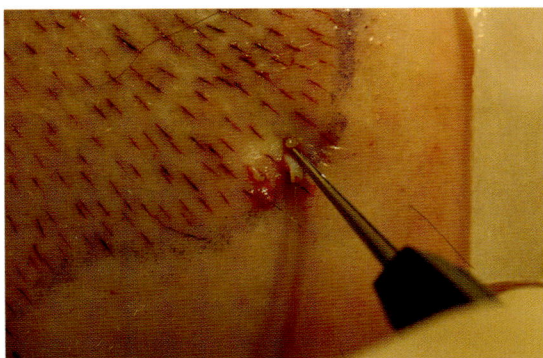
Fig. 31.24 Placement of a follicular unit transplant using a fine jeweler's forceps. (From Rousso DE, Presti PM. Follicular unit transplantation. Facial Plast Surg 2008;24:381–388. Used with permission.)

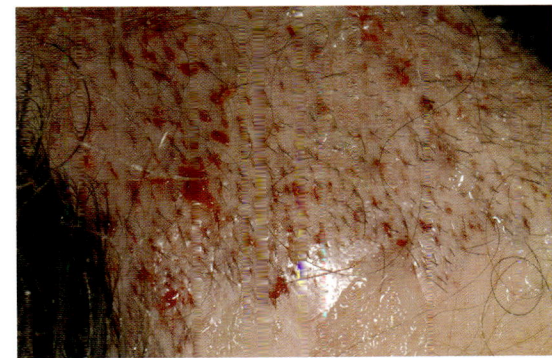
Fig. 31.25 View of scalp after placement of all transplants.

can rarely result in an arteriovenous fistulas. These can be encountered in repeat surgery and should be treated with suture ligation. If bleeding occurs after the patient has left the operating room, the patient is advised to apply manual pressure. Bleeding in the recipient spaces can be controlled with pressure or injection of 1% lidocaine with 1:50,000 epinephrine. Patients need to be forewarned about the possibility of postoperative edema, especially with extensive grafting. Edema can be decreased by maintaining 30-degree head elevation at night and with the use of oral prednisone during the first postoperative week.

Graft survival can diminish with prolonged exposure to dry, dehumidified air. All precautions should be taken to keep the grafts constantly bathed with saline prior to implantation. Prolonged time outside of the body also affects graft survival. Grafts kept out of the body for 6 hours have a 92% survival rate, and this rate decreases ~ 1% for each additional hour.[41] Any additional trauma, such as during placement, can also decrease graft survival. Placement of graft below the level of the epithelium can cause epithelial inclusion cysts and ingrown hairs to form.

Scarring is rarely a concern with small follicular unit grafting. In African Americans predisposed to keloids, a waiting period of 3 months after the initial session is adequate time to assess for any possible keloid formation prior to continuing with further transplant sessions.

Two to three months postoperatively, patients may experience a significant number of ingrown hairs as the transplanted hairs are growing. These can simply be uncapped in the office. If folliculitis develops, it may be treated with oral antibiotics, such as tetracycline.

Flaps

With the success and natural results obtained with hair transplants, flaps have become a less popular method of treating alopecia. However, there is a subset of patients who are excellent candidates for flap surgery. Patients with alopecia restricted to the frontal area are most ideal candidates. In addition, there are advantages to flaps over transplants. The results achieved are seen immediately. The blood supply is maintained to the hair follicles, therefore there is no associated hair loss secondary to follicles going into telogen phase. The hairs continue to grow throughout the process. Also, a higher density of hair can be achieved than with transplants.

Axial and Random

Flaps were initially described for scalp reconstruction in 1897 by Tillmanns.[42] They can be divided into axial and random flaps. Axial flaps are based on specific arteries and include the Juri flap, the temporoparietal

occipital (TPO) flap, and the temporoparietal (TP) flap. These are based on the superficial temporal artery.[43] The Juri and TPO flaps are twice delayed to ensure flap viability and, with a length of 25 cm, are designed to span the entire frontal hairline. The Juri flap is 4 cm wide, whereas the TPO flap is 3 cm wide. This modification allows easier turning of the base of the flap with less tendency for a lateral standing cone deformity. It also facilitates closure of the donor area. The Mayer and Fleming modification of the Juri flap makes the anterior hairline irregular, and gives a softer appearance.[44]

The TP flap is also based on the superficial temporal artery but is shorter, at 15 cm. For complete creation of a frontal hairline, it needs to be combined with a flap from the contralateral side.[44] Because the blood supply is primarily axial in nature, no delay procedure is required. Although the TPO flap is preferred, there are certain situations where the TP flap is the procedure of choice.[45] Patients with scarring that could interfere with blood flow to the distal tip of the TPO flap can undergo the shorter flap with less risk of flap compromise. Also, the TP flap can be used as salvage surgery for those with distal necrosis of longer flaps. Patients with poor results from punch grafts can also be salvaged with the TP but not the TPO flap due to the significant scarring in the occipital donor area.

The disadvantage to both the TPO and the TP flap is the posterior superior direction of hair growth, which can complicate styling. To overcome this issue, random blood supply flaps have been proposed. These are based more superiorly and result in hair growth directed anteriorly and inferiorly. Random flap procedures include those by Dardour,[46] Nataf et al,[47] and Frechet.[48] Because the blood supply of random flaps is not as predictable as that of axial flaps, problems with tip necrosis and early telogen are more likely to occur. These flaps are also shorter; therefore bilateral flaps need to be used to span the entire frontal hairline. It is possible to use tissue expanders prior to flap creation to improve results.[49] However, patients seeking cosmetic surgery may not be as tolerant of the deformity that is associated with tissue expanders, especially toward the end of the expansion process.

Alopecia Reduction

Alopecia reduction techniques allow the surgeon to excise the balding scalp and close the defect by advancing the temporal and parietal scalp. Alopecia reduction procedures are limited by the degree of scalp laxity. Excessive wound closure tension is associated with widening of the scar and possible necrosis, as well as the stretch-back phenomenon, which is the tendency of the remaining bald scalp to expand after a reduction. Often, complete excision of the bald area requires a series of reduction procedures, with 3 months between procedures to allow for scalp relaxation. The time between procedures can be shortened with the use of tissue expanders or extenders. These devices apply forces that stimulate mechanical creep, an increase in connective tissue between the cells, as well as biological creep, an increase in cell division.

A tissue expander is a Silastic balloon implanted under the skin adjacent to the area of alopecia that is inflated with a series of percutaneous injections of saline into a self-sealing port over a course of 8 to 10 weeks (Model SRE-RD-640s, Specialty Surgical Products, Inc., Victor, MT).[50] Although tissue expanders can allow for complete excision of the bald area with one reduction procedure, the deformity that the patient has to endure limits its use in cosmetic procedures (**Fig. 31.26**). As an alternative, Frechet[51] introduced the scalp extender in 1993. This device is a Silastic band with two series of hooks that are engaged into the undersurface of the scalp at the time of the initial reduction procedure (Frechet extender, France). It is left in place for 4 weeks, allowing for continuous horizontal traction force and tissue stretch with minimal cosmetic deformity. At 4 weeks, the device is removed and a more complete reduction procedure can be performed.

Various patterns of alopecia excisions have been proposed, with the midline sagittal ellipse pattern being the most simple. Placing the elliptical incision in a paramedian position or in a reverse J fashion provides for easier scar camouflage. Other patterns include a Mercedes or a horseshoe (**Fig. 31.27**). These patterns differ in the resulting direction of hair growth and the position of the scar and are individualized to each patient's pattern of hair loss. The incision is made through the galea, and the scalp is undermined to the superior attachments of the auricles and the nuchal line in the subgaleal plane. The flaps are advanced, and excess alopecic scalp is excised, followed by tension-free wound closure in two layers.

The extensive scalp lift continues the undermining beyond the nuchal line into the nape of the hairline, with ligation of the occipital arteries to maximize mobility.[52] The extensive scalp lift permits much

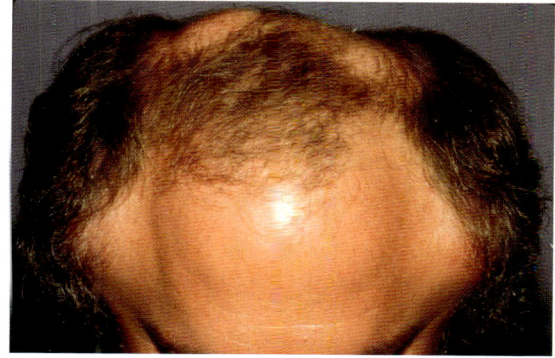

Fig. 31.26 The deformity with use of tissue expanders can prevent its use in cosmetic procedures.

greater mobility of the hair-bearing scalp but is associated with an incidence of occipital hair-bearing scalp necrosis. Mangubat[5] has modified this procedure to preserve the occipital artery and eliminate the incidence of necrosis.

Patients with crown balding are excellent candidates for scalp reduction and obtain results superior to transplantation alone. In general, scalp reduction is usually followed by hair transplantation to complete the restoration and to camouflage the scar area.

■ Postoperative Care

Following hair transplantation, hairline advancement, or scalp reduction, the patient is sent home with a nonadhesive dressing covering the scalp. This is removed the morning after surgery during the first postoperative appointment. The patient is to shower daily with lukewarm water and use baby shampoo starting the second night after surgery. Patients are told to gently pat the scalp with the balls of their

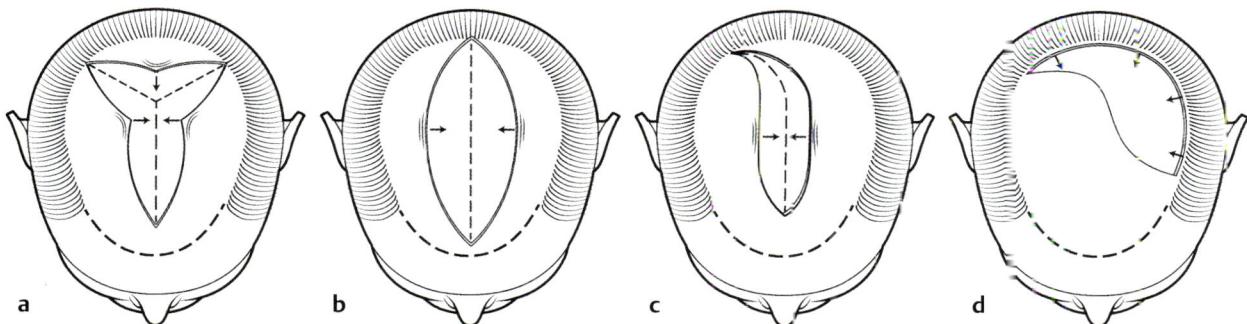

Fig. 31.27 Various patterns of alopecia excisions. (**a**) Mercedes. (**b**) Midline sagittal ellipse. (**c**) Reverse J. (**d**) Parasagittal.

fingertips during shampooing. Additionally, the patients are to apply witch hazel four to six times a day to the graft and donor sites, or the reduction incision, until all scabs and crusts are gone. Patients can expect some hair to fall out along with the scabs. To help decrease edema, patients are encouraged to sleep with their head elevated 30 to 40 degrees using pillows, a wedge cushion, or a recliner for 2 weeks. Patients are also restricted from heavy exercise for 2 weeks and should not bend over at the waist to pick up objects. Patients may use a hair dryer on a cool setting only and may comb hair with a clean wide-tooth comb, not a brush. Sutures and staples are removed on postoperative day 10.

Patients are told to contact the clinic and report any temperature elevations, sudden swelling or discoloration, excessive bleeding, discoloration from the wound edges or other evidence of infection, and development of any drug reaction.

Patients may expect the transplanted grafts to fall out ~ 4 weeks postoperatively. The graft hair will remain in telogen, the resting phase, for ~ 3 months and enter anagen to begin regrowth thereafter. Initially, the hair will be very fine, but as the hair grows longer, it will become similar to the hair texture and color in the donor area. Within 5 to 6 months postoperatively, patients can expect to have hair that is long enough to style and comb.

■ Conclusion

No other area in cosmetic surgery has undergone as much transformation in the past 20 years as hair restoration surgery. Today's methods of follicular unit transplantation can provide most patients with excellent, natural-appearing results that are indistinguishable from naturally occurring hair (**Figs. 31.28** and **31.29**). Proper patient selection and counseling are crucial for a successful outcome. Women can also achieve excellent results with follicular unit grafting but need to be evaluated preoperatively for underlying endocrine abnormalities.

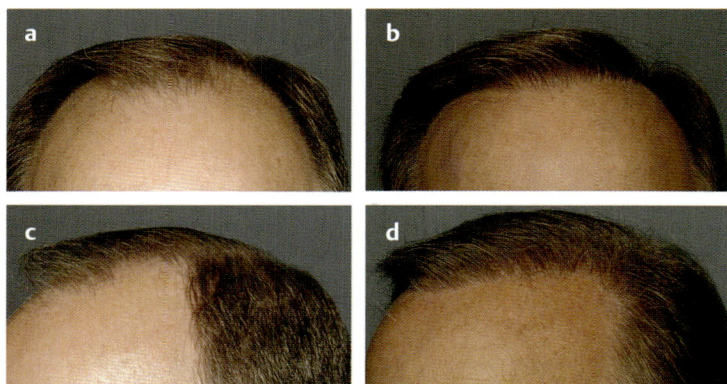

Fig. 31.28 Preoperative **(a,c)** and postoperative **(b,d)** views of a 45-year-old man who underwent three hair transplantation sessions, showing the pleasingly natural results that can be achieved.

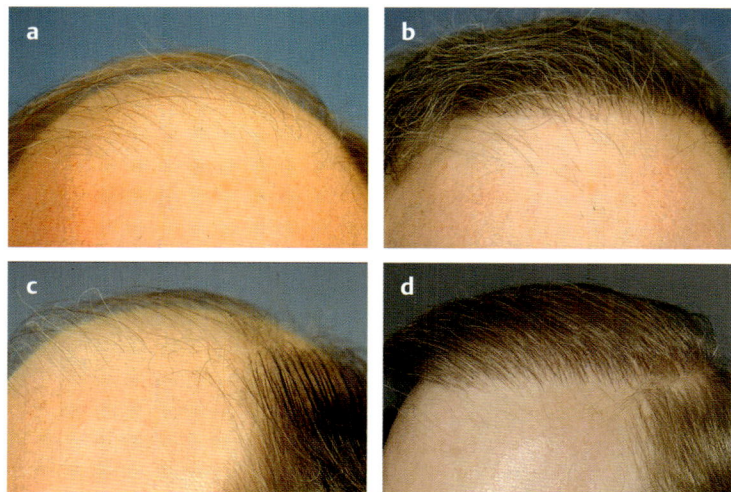

Fig. 31.29 Preoperative **(a,c)** and postoperative **(b,d)** views of a 52-year-old man who underwent three hair transplantation sessions, showing the natural results that can be achieved.

References

1. Okuda S. Clinical and experimental studies of transplantation of living hairs. Jpn J Dermatol Urol 1939;46:135–138
2. Orentreich N. Autografts in alopecias and other selected dermatological conditions. Ann NY Acad Sci 1959;83:463–479
3. Limmer BL. Elliptical donor stereoscopically assisted micrografting as an approach to further refinement in hair transplantation. J Dermatol Surg Oncol 1994;20(12):789–793
4. Hashimoto K. The structure of human hair. Clin Dermatol 1988;6(4):7–21
5. Marks JG, Miller J. Lookingbill and Marks' Principles of Dermatology. 4th ed. Philadelphia, PA: Elsevier; 2006:263
6. Fitzpatrick TB, Freedberg IM. Fitzpatrick's Dermatology in General Medicine. 6th ed. New York, NY: McGraw-Hill; 2003
7. James WD, Berger TG, Elston D. Andrews' Diseases of the Skin: Clinical Dermatology. 10th ed. Philadelphia, PA: Saunders; 2005
8. Olsen EA. Infectious, physical, and inflammatory causes of hair and scalp abnormalities. In: Disorders of Hair Growth: Diagnosis and Treatment. New York, NY: McGraw-Hill; 2003:87–123
9. Hamilton JB. Male hormone stimulation is prerequisite and an incitant in common baldness. Am J Anat 1942;72:451–480
10. Griffin JE, Wilson JD. The androgen resistance syndromes: 5-α-reductase deficiency, testicular feminization and related syndromes. In: Scriver CR, Beaudet AL, Sly WS, Valle D, eds. The Metabolic Basis of Inherited Disease. 6th ed. New York, NY: McGraw-Hill; 1989:1919–1944
11. Imperato-McGinley J, Guerrero L, Gautier T, Peterson RE. Steroid 5α-reductase deficiency in man: an inherited form of male pseudohermaphroditism. Science 1974;186(4170):1213–1215
12. Stárka L, Cermáková I, Dusková M, Hill M, Dolezal M, Polácek V. Hormonal profile of men with premature balding. Exp Clin Endocrinol Diabetes 2004;112(1):24–28
13. Küster W, Happle R. The inheritance of common baldness: two B or not two B? J Am Acad Dermatol 1984;11(5 Pt 1):921–926
14. Birch MP, Messenger AG. Genetic factors predispose to balding and non-balding in men. Eur J Dermatol 2001;11(4):309–314
15. Ellis JA, Stebbing M, Harrap SB. Genetic analysis of male pattern baldness and the 5α-reductase genes. J Invest Dermatol 1998;110(6):849–853
16. Hamilton JB. Patterned loss of hair in man; types and incidence. Ann N Y Acad Sci 1951;53(3):708–728
17. Norwood OT. Male pattern baldness: classification and incidence. South Med J 1975;68(11):1359–1365
18. Ludwig E. Classification of the types of androgenetic alopecia (common baldness) occurring in the female sex. Br J Dermatol 1977;97(3):247–254
19. Olsen EA. The midline part: an important physical clue to the clinical diagnosis of androgenetic alopecia in women. J Am Acad Dermatol 1999;40(1):106–109
20. Price VH, Roberts JL, Hordinsky MJ, et al. Lack of efficacy of finasteride in postmenopausal women with androgenetic alopecia. J Am Acad Dermatol 2000;43(5 Pt 1):768–776
21. Shum KW, Cullen DR, Messenger AG. Hair loss in women with hyperandrogenism: four cases responding to finasteride. J Am Acad Dermatol 2002;47(5):733–739
22. Vexiau P, Chaspoux C, Boudou P, et al. Effects of minoxidil 2% vs. cyproterone acetate treatment on female androgenetic alopecia: a controlled, 12-month randomized trial. Br J Dermatol 2002;146(6):992–999
23. Freinkel RK, Freinkel N. Hair growth and alopecia in hypothyroidism. Arch Dermatol 1972;106(3):349–352
24. Hard S. Non-anemic iron deficiency as an etiologic factor in diffuse loss of hair of the scalp in women. Acta Derm Venereol 1963;43:562–569
25. Rushton DH, Ramsay ID. The importance of adequate serum ferritin levels during oral cyproterone acetate and ethinyl oestradiol treatment of diffuse androgen-dependent alopecia in women. Clin Endocrinol (Oxf) 1992;36(4):421–427
26. Olsen EA, Dunlap FE, Funicella T, et al. A randomized clinical trial of 5% topical minoxidil versus 2% topical minoxidil and placebo in the treatment of androgenetic alopecia in men. J Am Acad Dermatol 2002;47(3):377–385
27. Olsen EA, Weiner MS. Topical minoxidil in male pattern baldness: effects of discontinuation of treatment. J Am Acad Dermatol 1987;17(1):97–101
28. Price VH, Menefee E, Sanchez M, Ruane P, Kaufman KD. Changes in hair weight and hair count in men with androgenetic alopecia after treatment with finasteride, 1 mg, daily. J Am Acad Dermatol 2002;46(4):517–523
29. Guess HA, Gormley GJ, Stoner E, Oesterling JE. The effect of finasteride on prostate specific antigen: review of available data. J Urol 1996;155(1):3–9
30. Kaufman KD, Olsen EA, Whiting D, et al; Finasteride Male Pattern Hair Loss Study Group. Finasteride in the treatment of men with androgenetic alopecia. J Am Acad Dermatol 1998;39(4 Pt 1):578–589
31. Physicians' Desk Reference. 5th ed. Montvale, NJ: Thomson PDR; 2003:56
32. Shum KW, Cullen DR, Messenger AG. Hair loss in women with hyperandrogenism: four cases responding to finasteride. J Am Acad Dermatol 2002;47(5):733–739
33. Burke BM, Cunliffe WJ. Oral spironolactone therapy for female patients with acne, hirsutism or androgenic alopecia [letter]. Br J Dermatol 1985;112(1):124–125
34. Leavitt M. Understanding and management of female pattern alopecia. Facial Plast Surg 2008;24(4):414–427
35. Rousso DE. Hair replacement surgery and transplantation. Curr Opin Otolaryngol Head Neck Surg 1997;5:209–213
36. Vogel JE. Hair restoration complications: an approach to the unnatural-appearing hair transplant. Facial Plast Surg 2008;24(4):453–461
37. Bernstein RM, Rassman WR. Follicular unit transplantation: 2005. Dermatol Clin 2005;23(3):393–414, v
38. Rousso DE, Presti PM. Follicular unit transplantation. Facial Plast Surg 2008;24(4):381–388
39. Harris JA. Follicular unit extraction. Facial Plast Surg 2008;24(4):404–413
40. Rassman WR, Bernstein RM, McClellan R, Jones R, Worton E, Uyttendaele H. Follicular unit extraction: minimally invasive surgery for hair transplantation. Dermatol Surg 2002;28(8):720–728
41. Limmer BL. Recipient site grafts and incision. In: Unger WP, Shapiro R, eds. Hair Transplantation. New York, NY: Marcel Dekker; 2004:383–533

42. Tillmanns H. Textbook of Surgery 1897, Tilton. Cited in Hunt HL. Plastic Surgery of the Face and Neck. Philadelphia, PA: Lea and Febiger; 1926

43. Juri J. Use of parieto-occipital flaps in the surgical treatment of baldness. Plast Reconstr Surg 1975;55(4):456–460

44. Mayer TG, Fleming RW. Aesthetic and Reconstructive Surgery of the Scalp. St. Louis, MO: Mosby; 1992:93–181

45. Rousso DE. The use of scalp flaps for frontal alopecia. Facial Plast Surg Clin North Am 1994;2(2):183–202

46. Dardour JC. Treatment of male pattern baldness with one-stage flap. Aesthetic Plast Surg 1985;9(2):109–112

47. Nataf J, Elbaz JS, Pollet J. Étude critique des transplantations du cuir chevelu et proposition d'une optique. Ann Chir Plast 1976;21:199–206

48. Frechet PJ. A new method for correction of the vertical scar observed following scalp reduction for extensive alopecia. J Dermatol Surg Oncol 1990;16(7):640–644

49. Anderson RD. The expanded "BAT" flap for treatment of male pattern baldness. Ann Plast Surg 1993;31(5):385–391

50. Kabaker SS, Kridel RW, Krugman ME, Swenson RW. Tissue expansion in the treatment of alopecia. Arch Otolaryngol Head Neck Surg 1986;112(7):720–725

51. Frechet P. Scalp extension. J Dermatol Surg Oncol 1993;19(7):616–622

52. Brandy DA. The bilateral occipito-parietal flap. J Dermatol Surg Oncol 1986;12(10):1062–1066

53. Mangubat EA. Preservation of the occipital artery during extensive scalp lifting. Am J Cosmetic Surg 1997;14:161–166

Index

Note: Page numbers followed by *f* and *t* indicate figures and tables, respectively.

A

AbobotulinumtoxinA, 189, 254. *See also* Botulinum
      neuromodulator(s)
  storage of, 190
Accutane. *See* Isotretinoin
Acetone, degreasing with
  for Hetter chemical peel, 61
  for medium-depth chemical peel, 52, 52*f*
  for superficial chemical peel, 44
Acne
  after laser skin resurfacing, 104, 133
  chemical peel for, 47, 48*t*
  in Fitzpatrick types IV–VI, skin care regimen for, 85, 85*t*
  superficial chemical peel for, 43–44
  treatment of, 11, 13
Actinic keratoses
  chemical peel for, 47, 48*t*
  photodynamic therapy for, 96
Acyclovir, prophylactic, 51, 104
Adato Sil-ol 5000, 158–159
Adhesive, allergic reaction to, 214, 215*f*
Aesthetic units, of face, 99, 100*f*, 139, 139*f*, 178, 178*f*, 179*t*
Aging
  extrinsic factors affecting, 1
  facial, 1–5
    ethnic differences in, 1
    and perception of age, 1–2
    progression of, 1, 2*f*
  intrinsic factors affecting, 1
  of skin
    extrinsic factors affecting, 9
    intrinsic factors affecting, 9
AHAs. *See* Alpha hydroxy acid(s)
Airway, assessment of, 20, 21*f*
ALA. *See* Aminolevulinic acid
Alar-facial crease, 178*f*
Alfenta. *See* Alfentanil
Alfentanil, 25
  intravenous, dosing guidelines for, 24, 24*t*, 25
  pharmacology of, 25
Aloesin, 12
Aloe vera, 11–12
Alopecia, 315–319
  androgenic. *See* Androgenic alopecia
  cicatricial, 316

  evaluation of patient with, 318
  incisional, with short-incision facelift and necklift, 298
  infectious causes, 316
  moth eaten appearance, 316
  reduction techniques, 326–327, 327*f*
Alopecia areata, 316
α_2-agonists, 24–25
Alpha hydroxy acid(s), 14. *See also specific acid*
  for acne, in Fitzpatrick types IV–VI, 85*t*, 86
  as humectants, 10
  peel, 43, 47, 81
    mechanism of action of, 81
    patient selection for, 82
American Society of Anesthesiologists, classification of anesthesia risk, 20, 21*t*
Aminolevulinic acid, 91
  in photodynamic therapy, 96–97
Amnesia, with benzodiazepines, 24
Amphadase, for hyaluronic acid filler removal, 230
Anagen effluvium, 316
Analgesia. *See* Anesthesia; Sedation
Androgenic alopecia, 315
  diagnosis of, 318
  diffuse, 315
  female pattern, 315, 317–318
  genetics of, 319
  male pattern, 314–315
    genetics of, 317
    Norwood classification of, 317, 317*f*
    pathophysiology of, 315–317
  medical treatment of, 318–319
Anesthesia. *See also* General anesthesia; Local anesthesia
  complications of, 26–27
  for endonasal rhinoplasty, 199
  fasting before (NPO guidelines), 21, 22*t*
  for hair transplantation, 322
  for Hetter chemical peel, 61–62
  for laser-assisted lipolysis, 304–305
  for laser skin resurfacing, 100–101
  levels of, 30, 30*t*
  for lip rejuvenation, 269
  for medium-depth chemical peel, 51
  nasal, 199
  patient assessment for, 20, 21*f*, 21*t*

Anesthesia *(continued)*
  recovery after, 21
    Phase I, 21
    Phase II, 21
  risk of, ASA classification of, 20, 21*t*
  for soft tissue filler injection, 168
  for surgical scar revision, 139–140
  twilight, 20
  for upper eyelid blepharoplasty, 239
Angular cheilitis, postoperative, 276
Anterior cutaneous nerve(s), of thorax
  anatomy, 38, 38*f*–39*f*
  block
    area of anesthesia with, 39
    technical aspects of, 38–39, 39*f*
Anterior ethmoidal nerve
  anatomy, 33
  block
    area of anesthesia with, 33
    technical aspects of, 33
Antibiotic(s)
  with medium-depth chemical peel, 51, 53
  prophylactic, for laser skin resurfacing, 100
Antiemetics, 25–26, 26*t*
Antioxidant(s)
  antiwrinkling effects of, 13
  for Fitzpatrick types IV–VI, 85*t*, 86
  photoprotective effects of, 14
Antiviral(s)
  prophylactic, 44, 46, 51, 61, 100, 104, 135, 174, 269, 275
    ophthalmic, 78
  therapy with, 66, 78, 275
  topical, 275
Anxiolysis, 23, 23*t*
Anzemet. *See* Dolasetron
Aprepitant, 26*t*
Aquaphor, postprocedure application
  with ablative resurfacing, 15
  with medium-depth chemical peel, 53
  with superficial chemical peel, 45
Arbutin, 12
Arrhythmia(s)
  from cardiotoxicity of local anesthetics, 39–40
  with phenol peel, 66, 75–78
Artefill, 147, 167, 253
  for facial augmentation, 171
Articaine, with epinephrine, maximal dosage, 39, 39*t*
Ativan. *See* Lorazepam
Atropine, for cardiotoxicity of local anesthetics, 39
Auriculotemporal nerve
  anatomy, 31*f*, 36, 36*f*
  block
    area of anesthesia with, 36
    technical aspects of, 36
Avage, 13
Avobenzone, 14
Azelaic acid, for Fitzpatrick types IV–VI, 86

B

Bacitracin, postprocedure application, for Hetter chemical
  peel, 62

Baker formulation, original ("classic"), 58–59, 58*t*
Baker-Gordon solution, 58, 58*t*, 68, 68*t*, 71
Baldness. *See also* Alopecia; Hair loss
  female-pattern, Ludwig classification of, 317, 318*f*
  male-pattern, Norwood classification of, 317, 317*f*
Basal cell(s), 43, 43*f*
Baumann Skin Type Indicator, 8
Baumann Skin Typing System, 8
  parameters used for, 8, 9*t*
Beady-eye syndrome, 258, 260*f*, 263, 266*f*
Bell phenomenon, 258–261
Belotero, 148
Benzodiazepine(s), 24
  administration, for Hetter chemical peel, 61
  reversal of, 24, 27
Benzoin, allergic reaction to, 214
Beta-blocker therapy, for hemangiomas, 112
Beta hydroxy acid, 15
  peel, 81
Birthmark, 107
Bleeding. *See also* Hematoma
  after endonasal rhinoplasty, 205
  intraoperative, with short-incision facelift and necklift, 297
Blepharoplasty
  definition of, 233
  historical perspective on, 233
  lower eyelid, 247–256
    canthal anchoring in, 263, 263*f*, 265, 265*f*
    complications of, 255, 255*f*
    options for, 257, 258*t*
    patient selection for, 250–251
    postoperative care, 255
    results, 255
    subciliary approach, 262–263, 262*f*–263*f*
    subciliary-subcuticular approach, 262, 262*f*
    subciliary-submuscular approach, 262, 262*f*
    technical aspects of, 251–252
    transconjunctival approach, 251, 251*f*, 262–263, 262*f*
    transcutaneous approach, 252
  upper eyelid, 233–246
    anatomical considerations in, 233–235, 234*f*–235*f*
    anesthesia for, 239
    complications of, 241
    hemostasis for, 241
    incision for, 239
    indications for, 233
    patient selection for, 235–236, 236*f*
    postoperative care, 241
    preoperative evaluation for, 237–238
    removal of strip of orbicularis in, 240
    results, 241, 242*f*–246*f*
    skin marking for, 238–239, 239*f*
    skin removal in, 239–240, 240*f*
    technical aspects of, 238–241
    wound closure, 241, 241*f*
Blindness
  after autologous fat transfer, 187
  dermal filler embolization in ophthalmic artery and, 156
Blistering, with laser hair removal, 122

BLU-U device, 96–97
Bone(s), facial, age-related changes in, 3
Botox, 189
Botox Cosmetic, 189, 254. *See also* Botulinum
  neuromodulator(s)
    for brow rejuvenation, 227–228, 227*f*–228*f*
    reconstitution of, 192–193
Botulinum neuromodulator(s)
    for blepharospasm, 254*f*, 255
    for brow rejuvenation, 227–228, 227*f*–228*f*
    contraindications to, 192
    for cosmetic use, 189
    for glabellar lines, 255
    injection
      complications of, 195–196
      postoperative care, 195
      technique for, 193–195
    for periocular rhytids, 247, 254
    for perioral rhytids, 269, 269*f*
    properties of, 189–190
    reconstitution of, 192–193
    therapy with
      patient selection for, 192
      technical aspects of, 192–195
    units of, 254–255
Botulinum toxin
    for cosmetic use, 189
    FDA indications for, 189
    in perioral rejuvenation, 151–153
Bowman-Birk inhibitor, 13
Brow(s)
    aesthetics of, 216, 217*f*
    age-related changes in, 3, 218–220, 219*f*–220*f*
    asymmetry, 234, 236, 236*f*–237*f*
    attractiveness, characteristics of, 217–218, 218*f*
    augmentation, dermal fillers for, 149–150, 150*f*
    autologous fat transfer to, 179, 180*f*–181*f*
    botulinum neuromodulator injection for, 193, 193*f*
    cable suture suspension of, 230
    descent of, 218–219, 219*f*–220*f*
    elevation of, 219–220
    female, 217, 217*f*, 218, 234, 234*f*
    Golden Proportion for, 218, 218*f*
    ideal, 217, 217*f*, 234, 234*f*
    male, 217, 217*f*, 218, 234, 234*f*
    muscular anatomy, 190–191, 190*f*
    position, 234, 234*f*
      emotions conveyed by, 218, 219*f*
    ptosis, 234
      after botulinum neuromodulator injection, 195, 230
    rejuvenation
      complications of, 230–231
      patient selection for, 220–221
      postoperative care, 230
      technical aspects of, 221–230
    shape of, 217
    surgical results and, 220
    unattractive, characteristics of, 218, 219*f*
Brow lift
    direct, 223, 223*f*
    lateral, 226, 226*f*

options for, 238, 238*f*
    transblepharoplasty approach, 225–226, 225*f*
BSTI. *See* Baumann Skin Type Indicator
BSTS. *See* Baumann Skin Typing System
Buccal fat pad, 302, 302*f*
Buccal nerve
    anatomy, 31*f*, 36, 37*f*
    block
      area of anesthesia with, 37
      technical aspects of, 37
Buccal space, autologous fat transfer to, 180
Buccinator muscle, 190*f*
Bunny lines, 191, 194
Bupivacaine, 22, 22*t*, 29, 30*t*
    + lidocaine, 22–23
    maximal dosage, 39, 39*t*

C
CaHA. *See* Calcium hydroxylapatite
Calcium hydroxylapatite
    as filler, 147–148, 167, 167*t*, 228–229, 253
      for acne scars, 153–154
      for buccal atrophy, 151
      complications of, 156
      for facial augmentation, 169, 170*f*
      for mandibular arc restoration, 151
      nodules caused by, 230
    midface injection, technique for, 169
Canthopexy, 263, 263*f*
Canthoplasty, 263, 263*f*
Captique, 228
Carbocaine. *See* Mepivacaine
Cardiac arrhythmias. *See* Arrhythmia(s)
Catapres. *See* Clonidine
Cellulitis, postoperative, 310, 311*f*
Cephalexin, administration, with medium-depth chemical
    peel, 51, 53
Cervical plexus (C$_2$, C$_3$)
    anatomy, 38, 38*f*
    block
      area of anesthesia with, 38
      technical aspects of, 38
Cervicomental angle, age-related changes in, 4, 4*f*
Chamomile, 11
Cheek
    as aesthetic subunit, 178*f*, 179*t*
    autologous fat transfer to, 180–181, 181*f*
    soft tissue of, age-related changes in, 4
Chemexfoliation. *See* Chemical peel(s)
Chemical peel(s), 5
    agents for. *See specific agent*
    classification of, 48–49, 48*f*–49*f*
    combination, technical aspects of, 84–85
    contraindications to, 50, 51*t*, 60
    deep. *See* Deep chemical peel(s)
    depth of penetration of, 43, 43*f*, 48–49, 48*f*–49*f*, 68–69,
      81, 81*f*
    for Fitzpatrick types IV–VI
      postoperative care, 85
      results, 85–88, 87*f*–89*f*
    Hetter, 57–67. *See also* Hetter chemical peel(s)

Chemical peel(s) *(continued)*
 historical perspective on, 57–58
 indications for, 47, 48*t*, 82
 medium-depth. *See* Medium-depth chemical peel(s)
 patient selection for, 60, 82
 in perioral region, 270
 scientific principles of, 47, 57–58, 69, 81
 skin preparation for, 82
 superficial. *See* Superficial chemical peel(s)
Chemodenervation, for brow rejuvenation, 227–228,
  227*f*–228*f*
Chemosis, 264
Chin
 autologous fat transfer to, 185, 186*f*
 botulinum neuromodulator injection for, 195
 muscular anatomy, 190*f*, 192
Chromophore(s), 125
 definition of, 109
 targeted in laser hair removal, 117–118
Citric acid, 14
Cleansing agents, for skin care, 9
Clonidine, 25
Cocaine
 adverse effects and side effects of, 31
 as anesthetic, 22–23, 22*t*, 29, 30*t*, 31
  historical perspective on, 29
 dosage, 30*t*
 maximal dosage, 39, 39*t*
 toxicity of, 31
Coenzyme Q10, photoprotective effects of, 14
Coffeeberry, photoprotective effects of, 14
Collagen
 age-related changes in, 2–3, 50
 retinoids and, 13
 synthesis of, 13
 ultraviolet radiation exposure and, 2
 in wound repair, 125
Collagen stimulant(s), for Fitzpatrick types IV–VI, 85*t*,
  86
Compazine. *See* Prochlorperazine
Connell's sign, 220
Conscious sedation. *See* Sedation, moderate (conscious)
Corneal protection, in eyelid surgery, 263–264
Corrugator supercilii muscle, 190, 190*f*, 191, 191*f*
Corticosteroid(s)
 with laser treatment of scars, 128
 mechanism of action of, 10–11
 topical
  chronic use, adverse effects of, 11
  for sensitive skin, 10–11
Croton oil, 58
Crow's feet, 3–4, 191
 botulinum neuromodulator injection for, 194, 195*f*
Cupid's bow, 268
 adequate definition, with long upper lip, nasal base
   resection for, 272–274, 273*f*–274*f*
 poor definition, with long upper lip, vermilion
   advancement for, 274, 274*f*–275*f*
Cupped ear deformity, 277
Cyclooxygenase (COX) inhibitors, therapeutic uses of, 11
Cyproterone acetate, 319

D
Dantrium. *See* Dantrolene
Dantrolene, for malignant hyperthermia, 26
Decadron. *See* Dexamethasone
Deep chemical peel(s), 48, 49*f*, 68–79, 81, 81*f*
 complications of, 75–79
 contraindications to, 69
 depth of penetration of, factors affecting, 68
 healing time for, 69
 patient selection for, 69
 postoperative care, 72
 results, 72–75, 74*f*–77*f*
 technical aspects of, 71–72, 72*f*–73*f*
Degreasing
 for Hetter chemical peel, 61
 for medium-depth chemical peel, 52, 52*f*
 for superficial chemical peel, 44
Deoxyarbutin, 12
Depressor anguli oris muscle, 190*f*, 192, 268
Depressor labii inferioris muscle, 190*f*
Depressor septi muscle, 191–192
Dermabrasion, 5. *See also* Microdermabrasion
 depth of penetration, 69
 for scars, 144–145
  after rhinoplasty, 212, 215
 for transcolumellar scar, 212
DermalAID, 72
Dermal-epidermal junction, 43, 43*f*, 82
 age-related changes in, 43
Dermal filler(s), 147–157. *See also specific filler*
 embolization of, 155–156
 inflammatory reactions with, 156
 lidocaine plus epinephrine mixed with, 148, 148*f*, 149
 nodules caused by, 156, 156*f*, 230
 for treatment of facial imperfections
  complications of, 155–156, 155*f*–156*f*
  needles for, 148
  technical aspects of, 149–154
 and Tyndall effect, 150, 155, 155*f*, 173
Dermal matrix, for lip augmentation, 271, 272*f*
Dermatitis, after laser skin resurfacing, 133
Dermis
 age-related changes in, 2–3, 43, 50
 anatomy, 43, 43*f*, 50, 50*f*, 82, 125
 elastotic degeneration of, 2
 papillary, 43, 50, 81, 81*f*
 reticular, 43, 50, 81, 81*f*
 ultraviolet radiation exposure and, 2
Dexamethasone, 26*t*
Dexmedetomidine
 intravenous
  adverse effects and side effects of, 25
  dosing guidelines for, 24, 24*t*
 pharmacology of, 25
Diazepam, 24
 sedation with, for Hetter chemical peel, 61
Dihydrotestosterone, and male-pattern androgenic
  alopecia, 316–317
Diplopia
 after botulinum neuromodulator injection, 196
 after eyelid surgery, 264

Diprivan. *See* Propofol
Documentation
 of acne scars, 160
 of nasal defects, 160
 for superficial chemical peel, 44
Dolasetron, 26*t*
Doll's head appearance, 314, 321, 321*f*
Double contour, 254*f*
Dramamine administration, for Hetter chemical peel, 61
Drill hole orbitotomy, 260*f*, 265
Dry eyes, 258, 264
 after botulinum neuromodulator injection, 196
DUSA Pharmaceuticals, website, 96
Dyschromia(s), 2. *See also* Hyperpigmentation;
  Hypopigmentation
 in Fitzpatrick types IV–VI, skin care regimen for, 85, 85*t*,
  86, 86*f*
 superficial chemical peel and, 44
Dysport, 189, 254. *See also* Botulinum neuromodulator(s)
 for brow rejuvenation, 227
 reconstitution of, 193
Dysrhythmia(s). *See* Arrhythmia(s)

E
Ear(s)
 abnormalities
  age-related, 278
  iatrogenic, 278, 278*f*
  traumatic, 278
 age-related changes in, 278
 embryology of, 277
 external anatomy, 278*f*
 protruding, 277–278. *See also* Lop ear deformity
  correction, patient selection for, 278
 reshaping of, 277. *See also* Otoplasty
 undersized, 277–278
Ear deformity(ies)
 first-degree, 278
 second-degree, 277–278
 third-degree, 277
Earlobe(s)
 abnormalities, 282
 with attached lobule, release, 282, 282*f*
 lobular malposition, with short-incision facelift and
  necklift, 298
 reduction, 282–284, 283*f*–284*f*
Ecchymosis, with fillers for facial augmentation, 172
Ectropion, 264–265
Edema, after autologous fat transfer, 187
Eflornithine hydrochloride cream, in hair removal, 122
Elevess, 228
Elta, postprocedure application, for Hetter chemical peel, 62
Elure, 13
Emblicanin, 12
Emend. *See* Aprepitant
EMLA, 31
Emollients, 9–10
 postprocedure application, for Hetter chemical peel, 62
Emulsion(s)
 oil-in-water, 9
 water-in-oil, 9

Enophthalmos, 261, 261*f*
Ephedrine, for cardiotoxicity of local anesthetics, 39
Epidermis
 age-related changes in, 43
 anatomy, 43, 43*f*, 50, 50*f*, 82, 123
 dyskaryotic changes, 2
 ultraviolet radiation exposure and, 2
Epinephrine
 added to local anesthetic, 23, 29
 adverse effects and side effects of, 30
 contraindications to, 30
 dosage, 30*t*
 maximal dosage, 39, 39*t*
 pharmacology of, 30
Erythema
 after deep chemical peel, 78, 78*f*
 after Hetter chemical peel, 66
 after laser hair removal, 122
 after laser skin resurfacing, 104
 after laser treatment of scar, 133
 after medium-depth chemical peel, 56
 after superficial chemical peel, 43–46
 post-laser, 15
Ethanol, in Jessner's solution, 49, 49*t*
Eucerin, postprocedure application
 for Hetter chemical peel, 62
 with medium-depth chemical peel, 53
Exfoliant(s), for Fitzpatrick types IV–VI, 85*t*, 86
Exophthalmos, 261, 261*f*
External jugular vein, anatomy, 303
External nasal nerve
 anatomy, 31*f*, 33, 34*f*
 block
  area of anesthesia with, 33
  technical aspects of, 33
Eye(s)
 age-related changes in, 3–4
 corneal protection for, in eyelid surgery, 263–264
 globe position, 261, 261*f*
 normal shape, 257, 258*f*
 protection, in laser treatment, 115
Eyebrow(s). *See* Brow(s)
Eyelid(s)
 abbreviations used in, 69, 70*t*
 age-related changes in, 3–4
 biomechanics of, 258, 260*f*, 265
 canthal anchor of, 258, 260*f*, 263, 263*f*, 265, 265*f*
 closure mechanics, 258, 260*f*, 265
 contour irregularities, 264
 fish-mouthing, 258, 260*f*, 265
 lower
  age-related changes in, 248–249
  anatomy, 248
  autologous fat transfer to, 180, 180*f*–181*f*
  blepharoplasty, 247–256
  botulinum neuromodulator injection for, 194
  common problems of, 250*t*
  excessive skin of, 249, 249*f*
  horizontal laxity, 249, 250*t*
  lamellar structure of, 248, 249*f*, 257
  malfunction, 258, 260*f*

Eyelid(s), lower *(continued)*
    malposition, 260*f*, 261, 264–265
    retraction, 264–265
    revision surgery, 260*f*, 265
        planning, 265, 265*t*
    rounding (lateral inferior rotation) of, 237
    surgery
        aesthetic considerations in, 257
        anatomical considerations in, 257–258, 258*f*–259*f*
        complications of, avoidance and management of,
            257–266
        functional considerations in, 257
        patient selection for, 258–262
        technical aspects of, 262–263
    tone, 261, 261*f*
  normal position, 257, 258*f*
  photoaging of, 191
  positive canthal tilt of, 257, 258*f*
  prior surgery, and risk of postoperative complications,
    261–262
  ptosis, after botulinum neuromodulator injection, 195–196
  shape, 265, 266*f*
  surgery on
    corneal protection during, 263–264
    injury to critical structures in, 264
    operating room safety in, 263–264
  upper
    anatomy, 233–235, 234*f*–235*f*
    autologous fat transfer to, 180
    blepharoplasty, 233–246
    external landmarks of, 234–235, 235*f*
    lamellar structure of, 234, 234*f*
    pinch test, 238–239
    preoperative evaluation, 237
    skin of, 235

F
Face
  aesthetic units of, 99, 100*f*, 139, 139*f*, 178, 178*f*, 179*t*
  lower, dermal fillers for, 151, 151*f*
Facelift(s). *See also* Midface lift; Short-incision facelift and
    necklift
  abbreviations used in, 69, 70*t*
  historical perspective on, 285–286
  McCollough classification of, 69, 70*t*
Facial muscle(s), anatomy, 190, 190*f*
Facial nerve
  anatomy, 303
  buccal branch, 259*f*, 264
  cervical branch, 303
  injury, 312
  zygomatic branch, 259*f*
Facial rejuvenation, 5–6
Facial thirds, 233–234, 234*f*
Fasting, pre-anesthesia, 21, 22*t*
Fat
  autologous transfer, 147, 149, 175
    aspiration cannula for, 176–177
    cell survival theory of, 176
    complications of, 186–187
    donor site for, 176

embolization, 187
facial subunits for, 178, 178*f*, 179*t*
fat processing for, 177, 177*f*
grafting technique for, 178
historical perspective on, 175
host cell replacement theory of, 175–176
injection, 179–184
  for lip augmentation, 271, 271*f*
  to mandible, 151, 151*f*
  for midface rejuvenation, 248, 254, 254*f*
negative pressure and, 177
overcorrection with, 186–187
patient preparation for, 178
in periorbital region, 229
postoperative care, 186
results, 186
scientific principles of, 175–176
technical aspects of, 176–185
tumescent fluid for, 176
undercorrection with, 186–187
facial
  age-related changes in, 3
  compartmentalization of, 175. *See also* Fat
    compartment(s)
  orbital. *See* Orbital fat
  transfer, in facial rejuvenation, 6
Fat compartment(s)
  of face and neck, 175, 301, 302*f*
    anatomy, 301
    septal boundaries, 301
  interplatysmal, 302*f*, 303
  nasolabial, 302, 302*f*
  orbital. *See* Orbital fat, compartments
  submandibular, 302*f*, 303
  submental, 302*f*, 303
  subplatysmal, 302*f*, 303
  supraplatysmal, 302*f*, 303
Fatty acid(s), essential, 10
Fentanyl, 25, 30
  intravenous
    dosing guidelines for, 24, 24*t*, 25
    precautions with, 25
  pharmacology of, 25
Feverfew, 11
  photoprotective effects of, 14
Filler(s), 253. *See also* Dermal filler(s); *specific filler*
  autogenous. *See* Fat
  for brow rejuvenation, 228–230, 228*f*–229*f*
    embolization, 230
  for facial augmentation, 166–174
    anesthesia for, 168
    complications of, 172–174, 174*f*
    duration of effects, 167
    historical perspective on, 166
    hypersensitivity reaction with, 172, 174, 174*f*
    injection-site reactions with, 172
    patient selection for, 167
    preparation for, 168
    scientific principles of, 166
    selection of, by facial region, 167, 167*t*
    technical aspects of, 167–172

ideal, characteristics of, 158, 167
for midface rejuvenation, 248, 253
in midface rejuvenation, 247
nonautogenous, 6
requirements for, 158
in rhinoplasty, 212–214, 213f–214f
for soft tissue volume restoration, 166–174
Finasteride, 318–319
Fish-mouthing, of eyelid, 258, 260f, 265
Fitzpatrick skin types, 50, 51t, 60, 80
age-related changes in, 80
and resurfacing, 99
sun exposure and, 80
type IV
characteristics of, 80
skin rejuvenation for, 80–90
type V
characteristics of, 80
skin rejuvenation for, 80–90
type VI
characteristics of, 80
skin rejuvenation for, 80–90
Flowers sign, 220
Fluid collection(s), postoperative, 310, 311f. See also
Hematoma; Seroma
Flumazenil, 24, 27
5-Fluorouracil, with laser treatment of scars, 128
Follicular unit(s), 314–315, 316f
sizes of, 321, 322f
Foramen ovale, 31
Foramen rotundum, 31
Forehead
as aesthetic subunit, 178f, 179t
autologous fat transfer to, 179
botulinum neuromodulator injection for, 193–194, 194f
creases (lines) on, muscle activity causing, 220
height of, 216
muscular anatomy, 190f, 191
wrinkling of, 3
Forehead lift, subcutaneous, 224, 224f
Foreheadplasty
endoscopically assisted, 222–223, 222f–223f
open, 221–222
coronal incision for, 221, 221f
trichophytic incision for, 222, 222f
FPAA. See Androgenic alopecia, female pattern
Fractional photothermolysis, scientific principles of, 98–99
Frontalis muscle, 3, 190, 190f, 191

G
General anesthesia, 23, 23t
patient selection for, 20
for surgical scar revision, 140
Geometric broken line closure, for scar revision, 141, 143f
GHK-Cu, 10
Ginseng, 11
Glabella, 178f
autologous fat transfer to, 179, 180f–181f
vertical lines in, 4
Glabridin, 12
Glogau photoaging classification, 50, 51t, 60, 60t

Glycerin, as humectant, 10
Glycolic acid, 14, 43
for Fitzpatrick types IV–VI, 86
peel, 81, 81f
mechanism of action of, 81
patient selection for, 82
technical aspects of, 83
for postinflammatory hyperpigmentation, 66
pretreatment, for superficial chemical peel, 44
Glycyl-L-histidyl-L-lysine-Cu²⁺, 10
Granisetron, 26t
Grapeseed extract, photoprotective effects of, 14
Grapeseed oil, 10
Great auricular nerve, 31f
Green tea, photoprotective effects of, 14

H
HA. See Hyaluronic acid
Hair, vellous, 315
Hair cycle, 118, 315, 316f
anagen phase, 315, 315f
catagen phase, 315, 316f
telogen phase, 315, 316f
Hair follicle(s). See also Follicular unit(s)
anatomy, 118, 314, 315f
bulb of, 315, 315f
depth of, 118
and hair growth, 118
infundibulum of, 315, 315f
isthmus of, 315, 315f
life cycle of, 118, 315, 316f
number of, on body, 314
Hairline design, in hair restoration, 320, 321f
Hair loss, 314. See also Alopecia; Baldness
in cancer treatment, 316
causes of, 315
evaluation of patient with, 318
progression of, 319
reduction of, 314
surgical treatment of, 319
in women, 317
Hair removal
intense pulsed light therapy for, 94–96, 117, 120
laser treatment for, 117–123
anatomical basis of, 117–118
blistering caused by, 122
combined with eflornithine hydrochloride, 122
complications of, 122
patient education for, 113, 120, 121t
patient selection for, 118
postoperative care, 120–122, 121t
results, 122
technical aspects of, 118–120
Hair restoration. See also Hair transplantation
flaps for, 326
historical perspective on, 314
Hair transplantation, 314–330
donor area for, hair density in, 320
follicular unit
anesthesia for, 322
complications of, 325–326

Hair transplantation, follicular unit *(continued)*
  donor area for, 322, 322*f*
  follicular unit extraction for, 323–324
  follicular unit preparation in, 324, 324*f*
  and folliculitis, 326
  graft placement for, 325, 325*f*
  graft survival after, 326
  historical perspective on, 314
  and ingrown hairs, 326
  megasessions for, 325
  recipient site creation for, 324–325, 325*f*
  and scarring, 326
  strip extraction for, 322–323, 322*f*–323*f*
  technical aspects of, 321–326
hair characteristics and, 320, 320*f*
hairline design for, 320, 321*f*
hair styling and, 319
historical perspective on, 314
patient age and, 319
patient counseling about, 320
patient selection for, 319–320
pattern of alopecia and, 319
postoperative care, 327–328
punch grafts for, 321, 321*f*
results, 328, 328*f*
scalp laxity and, 320
skin characteristics and, 320
technical aspects of, 321–326
Helioplex, 14
Hemangioma(s), 108
  biology of, 108
  classification of, 112
  epidemiology of, 111–112
  involution of, 112
  laser treatment of, 110, 110*f*, 111–112, 111*f*–112*f*
  pathophysiology of, 112
Hematoma, postoperative, 310, 311*f*
  with short-incision facelift and necklift, 297–298
Hemoglobin, as cutaneous chromophore, 125
Herpes simplex virus (HSV), outbreaks
  with fillers for facial augmentation, 174
  with laser skin resurfacing, 104, 133–135
  postoperative, 56, 66, 275
  prophylaxis, 44, 46, 56, 61, 275
  treatment of, 66, 78, 275
Hetter chemical peel(s), 57–67
  anesthesia for, 61–62
  complications of, 66
  degree of frosting with, classification of, 61, 62*t*
  depth of penetration, 59
  eye care during, 62
  formula for, 59, 59*t*
  healing after, 63, 66
  historical perspective on, 57–59
  patient selection for, 60
  postoperative care for, 62
  pretreatment for, 60–61
  results, 63, 63*f*–65*f*
  scientific principles of, 57–59
  subunits of face and, 61–62
  technical aspects of, 60–62
  technique for, 61–62, 62*f*, 62*t*

HQ. *See* Hydroquinone
Humectants, 9–10
Hyaluronic acid
  as filler, 147–148, 167, 167*t*, 253
    for acne scars, 153–154, 153*f*
    advantages of, 147
    for facial augmentation, 168–169, 169*f*
    for lip augmentation, 153, 153*f*, 270–271, 270*f*–271*f*
    for lip rejuvenation, 269, 270*f*
    in lower eyelid, 150
    for orbital hollowing, 228, 229*f*
    for perioral region, 151–153, 152*f*
    in periorbital region, 149
    properties of, 147
    removal, 230, 253
    for traumatic scar, 154
    and Tyndall effect, 150, 155, 155*f*, 173
  as humectant, 10
Hyaluronidase
  added to local anesthetic, 32
  for hyaluronic acid filler removal, 230, 253
  intraoperative use, in hair transplantation, 320
Hydrelle, 168, 172
Hydrocortisone, for postinflammatory
    hyperpigmentation, 66
Hydroquinone, 12
  for Fitzpatrick types IV–VI, 86
  for postinflammatory hyperpigmentation, 66
  pretreatment, 15
    for Hetter chemical peel, 61
    for laser skin resurfacing, 100
    for medium-depth chemical peel, 51
    for superficial chemical peel, 44
Hydroxy acid(s), 14–15. *See also* Alpha hydroxy acid(s);
    Beta hydroxy acid
Hylaform, 148, 228
Hyperandrogenism, in women, 317–319
Hyperpigmentation
  after deep chemical peel, 78
  after Hetter chemical peel, 63, 66
  after medium-depth chemical peel, 56
  after superficial chemical peel, 45–46
  in Fitzpatrick types IV–VI, 86, 87*f*
  with laser hair removal, 122
  with laser treatment of vascular lesions, 110–111
  postinflammatory, 15, 66, 81–82, 88–89
    after laser skin resurfacing, 104
    after laser treatment of scar, 133
    in Fitzpatrick types IV–VI, 88, 89*f*
  spotty, 2
  treatment of, 11–13
Hypersensitivity, with fillers for facial augmentation, 172,
    174, 174*f*
Hypopigmentation
  after deep chemical peel, 78
  after Hetter chemical peel, 66
  after laser skin resurfacing, 104
  after laser treatment of scar, 133
  after laser treatment of vascular lesions, 110–111
  after superficial chemical peel, 46
  postpeel, 46, 66, 78, 89

I

Ibuprofen, 11
Ichthyosis, treatment of, 14
Idebenone, photoprotective effects of, 14
IncobotulinumtoxinA, 189, 255. *See also* Botulinum
       neuromodulator(s)
  storage of, 190
Infection(s)
  after autologous fat transfer, 187
  after chemical peel, 46
  after endonasal rhinoplasty, 205
  after Hetter chemical peel, 66
  after laser skin resurfacing, 104, 133–135
  after short-incision facelift and necklift, 298, 310, 311*f*
  with fillers for facial augmentation, 172
  and inflammatory skin nodules with dermal fillers, 156
  postoperative, 310, 311*f*
Inferior alveolar nerve, block, 37
Inflammation, topical treatment of, 11
Infrabrow, 216, 217*f*
  autologous fat transfer to, 181*f*, 228, 229*f*
  fillers for, 228–230, 228*f*–229*f*
Infraorbital foramen, 33–34, 34*f*–35*f*
Infraorbital nerve
  anatomy, 31*f*, 33, 34*f*–35*f*
  block
    area of anesthesia with, 34
    technical aspects of, 33–34
Infratrochlear nerve
  anatomy, 31*f*, 33
  block
    area of anesthesia with, 33
    technical aspects of, 33
Inner limbus line, 34*f*
Intense pulsed light, 91–97
  advantages of, 16
  characteristics of, 110
  complications of, 16, 97
  equipment for, 92–93
  historical perspective on, 91
  indications for, 16
  and lasers, comparison of, 91
  technique for, 16
  therapy with
    contraindications to, 91–92
    documentation of, 93, 95
    for erythema, 78, 114
    and hair, 92
    for hair removal, 94–96, 117, 120
    pain with, 92
    patient education and consent for, 92
    patient selection for, 91–92
    for pigmented lesions, 93–94, 94*f*
    and pigmented nevi, 92
    for port-wine stain, 113
    postprocedure care, 92
    safety considerations with, 93
    and tattoos, 92
    technical aspects of, 92–96
    for telangiectasia, 94, 114
    test spots, 92, 94–95
    for vascular lesions, 94, 95*f*, 110

Intercostal nerve(s), anatomy, 38, 38*f*
Intralipid rescue, for cardiotoxicity from local anesthetic
       overdose, 23, 27
Iopidine ophthalmic drops, for levator ptosis, 230
IPL. *See* Intense pulsed light
Isotretinoin, as contraindication to chemical peel, 60, 62

J

Jawline, autologous fat transfer to, 181*f*
Jessner's peel, 15, 82
  enhanced, 85
  modified, patient selection for, 82
  technical aspects of, 83–84
Jessner's solution, 43, 81, 81*f*
  components of, 49, 49*t*, 81, 81*t*
  modified, component of, 81, 81*t*
Jowl(s), fat compartments of, 302–303, 302*f*
Jowling, development of, 4
Juri flap, 326
Juvederm, 228, 253
Juvederm Ultra/Juvederm Ultra Plus, 147–148, 167*t*
  duration of effects, 143
  for lip augmentation, 153
  in lower eyelid, 150
  for traumatic scar augmentation, 154*f*
Juvederm Ultra XC/Juvederm Ultra Plus XC, for facial
      augmentation, 68

K

Keloid(s), 126
  laser treatment of, 128–129
  pathogenesis of, 125
  with short-incision facelift and necklift, 298
Kerastick Krusher, 96
Keratoses. *See also* Actinic keratoses
  pigmented, 2
Ketalar. *See* Ketamine
Ketamine
  intravenous
    adverse effects and side effects of, 25
    dosing guidelines for, 24, 24*t*
  pharmacology of, 25
Kojic acid, 12
  for Fitzpatrick types IV–VI, 86
Kytril. *See* Granisetron

L

Lacrimal nerve
  anatomy, 31*f*, 33
  block
    area of anesthesia with, 33
    technical aspects of, 33
Lactic acid, 14, 43. *See also* Jessner's solution
  mechanism of action of, 14
  peel, 81
Lanolin, 10
Laser(s)
  alexandrite, 110–111
    treatment, for hair removal, 120
  apparatus for, 108, 108*f*
  argon, characteristics of, 111
  biophysics of, 108

Laser(s) *(continued)*
  carbon dioxide (CO_2), 98
    characteristics of, 111
    helium-neon aiming beam for, 111
  characteristics of, 109–111
  chromophore absorption peak and, 109
  diode, 110–111
    treatment, for hair removal, 120, 120f
  duty cycle of, 109
  effects on tissue, 108–109, 109f, 125. *See also* Selective
      photothermolysis
  energy density (fluence) of, 109
  erbium, 99
  erbium-doped yttrium-aluminum-garnet (Er:YAG), 98
  eye injury caused by, 115
  fractional/fractionated, 98
    ablative, 98–99, 125, 129–131, 130f, 132
      devices, 127t
    devices for, 126, 127t
    equipment, 101
    nonablative, 98–99, 125, 129–131, 130f, 132
      devices, 127t
    in prevention of scar formation, 128
    treatment, for facial scars, 124, 129–131
  historical perspective on, 107
  infrared, 99, 110–111
  and intense pulsed light, comparison of, 91
  neodymium:yttrium-aluminum-garnet (Nd:YAG), 99
    characteristics of, 110–111
    for laser-assisted lipolysis, 304
    treatment
      for hair removal, 119, 119f
      for hemangioma, 112, 112f
      for venous malformations, 113, 114f
  potassium titanyl phosphate (KTP), characteristics of,
      110
  power density of, 109
  properties of, 109
  pulsed dye, 109–110
    chemical hazards associated with, 115
    treatment
      for facial scars, 124–125, 128–129
      for hemangioma, 112
      for port-wine stain, 113, 113f
      for telangiectasia, 114
  pulsed energy, 109
  Q-switched, 109, 126
  red, 110–111
  ruby, treatment, for hair removal, 120
  safety precautions with, 101, 115, 128
  therapy with
    for facial scars, 124–137, 144, 145f
      mechanism of action of, 125
    for hair removal, 117–123
    for vascular lesions, 107–116
      technical aspects of, 109–114
  wavelength of, 109
    ablative, 125, 126t
    and fat and water optical absorption, 301, 301f
    nonablative, 125, 126t
  yttrium-scandium-gallium-garnet (YSSG), 98

Laser-assisted lipolysis, 301
  anesthesia for, 304–305
  complications of, 310–312, 311f–312f
  contour irregularities after, 312, 312f
  and facelift, with perioral contouring, results, 308, 309f
  with high lamellar facelift, results, 307–308, 308f
  to improve lower third facial asymmetry, results, 309–310,
      310f
  isolated
    with pre-jowl implant, results, 306, 307f
    results, 306, 306f
  and necklift, with pre-parotid fat reduction, results,
      307, 308f
  patient selection for, 303–304
  planning for, 304, 304f
  postoperative care, 306
  preparation for, 304
  principles of, 301, 301f
  results, 306–310, 306f–310f
  and sculpting of face and nasolabial folds, results,
      308–309, 309f
  surgical technique for, 305, 305f
  technical aspects of, 304–305, 304f–305f
  thermal injury in, 310–312
  undercorrection with, 312
Laser skin resurfacing, 5
  ablative, 98, 129–132
    complications of, 132, 134t
  anesthesia for, 100–101
  for atrophic scars, 129–130, 129f–130f
    technical aspects of, 128–129
  complications of, 104–105
  contraindications to, 100
  depth of penetration, 69
  fractionated technologies, 98–106, 129–131, 130f–131f,
      132
  historical perspective on, 42, 98, 99f
  and infraorbital region, 102
  and mandibular region, 102
  in neck and décolleté area, 101–102
  nonablative, 98, 129–132
    complications of, 132, 134t
  patient education for, 100
  patient selection for, 99–100
  in perioral region, 270
  postoperative care, 102
  preconditioning for, 100
  preoperative preparation for, 100
  results of, 102, 103f
  technical aspects of, 100–102
  wavelengths for, 126, 126t
Lateral SMASectomy, 285
Lay peelers, 57–58
Lentigines
  chemical peel for, 47
  intense pulsed light therapy for, 93–94, 94f
  photodynamic therapy for, 96
LET, 31
Levator aponeurosis, of upper eyelid, 234, 234f
Levator labii superioris aleque nasi muscle, 190f
Levator labii superioris muscle, 190f

Levator palpebrae superioris muscle, 234, 234f
  dehiscence, 236f–237f
Levator ptosis, with brow chemodenervation, 230
Levulan Kerastick, 96–97
Licorice extract, 11–12
Lidocaine, 22, 22t, 29, 30t
  + bupivacaine, 22–23
  dosage, 30t
  and epinephrine, mixing, 148, 148f, 149
  with epinephrine, maximal dosage, 39, 39t
  maximal dosage, 39, 39t
  with medium-depth chemical peel, 51
  topical, 31
LifestyleLift, 286
Ligament(s), facial, 3, 3f
Lightening agent(s), for Fitzpatrick types IV–VI, 85t, 86
LightSheer laser, 120
Lignin peroxidase, 13
Linoleic acid, 10
Lip(s)
  aesthetic connotations of, 267
  age-related changes in, 4–5, 6f, 268–269, 273f
  anatomy, 267–269
  asymmetries, postoperative, 275
  augmentation, 270–271
    dermal fillers for, 152f, 153, 153f
  autologous fat transfer to, 184–185, 185f
  color loss in, postoperative, 276
  dryness, postoperative, 275
  embryology of, 268
  functions of, 267
  intramuscular block for, 34–36, 35f
    area of anesthesia with, 36
    technical aspects of, 36
  laser skin resurfacing for, 270
  lower, autologous fat transfer to, 181f
  projection of, 267–268
  rejuvenation, 267–276
    aesthetic considerations in, 267
    anatomical considerations in, 267–269
    anesthesia for, 269
    complications of, 275–276
    functional considerations in, 267
    patient preparation for, 269
    patient selection for, 269
    postoperative care, 275
    procedures for, 269
    results, 275
    technical aspects of, 269
  upper
    autologous fat transfer to, 181f
    long
      with adequate cupid's bow definition, nasal base
        resection for, 272–274, 273f–274f
      with poor cupid's bow definition, vermilion
        advancement for, 274, 274f–275f
    sensory innervation of, 34
  vermilion of
    dry, 268
    rejuvenation, 269–270
    scars, widening of, 276

  wet, 268, 268f
  volume, age-related changes in, 269
  wet line of, 268, 268f
  white roll of, 268
Lipectomy, suction-assisted, 5
Lipivage system, 176–177
Lipolysis, laser-assisted. See Laser-assisted lipolysis
Liposculpture, facial
  development of, 175–176
  technical aspects of, 176–185
Liposuction, 5
  facial, 300
    complications of, 310–312, 311f–312f
    patient selection for, 303–304
  isolated, with buccal fat pad removal, results, 306,
    307f
Lipothene, 31
Liquid injectable silicone, 160
  for acne scars, 153–160
    results, 162, 162f–163f
  advantages of, 159
  for herpes zoster scars, results, 163, 164f
  injections (for soft tissue augmentation), 158–165
    complications of, 164
    postoperative care, 160
    results, 160–164
    technical aspects of, 160
  for nasal defects, 158–159
    results, 160–161, 161f–162f
  properties of, 159
  for surgical scars, 160
    results, 163, 163f
LIS. See Liquid injectable silicone
LMX cream, with medium-depth chemical peel, 51–52
Local anesthesia. See also Regional block(s)
  advantages of, 28
  complications of, 39–40
  disadvantages of, 29
  historical perspective on, 29
  patient selection for, 20, 29–30
  for surgical scar revision, 140
  types of, 28
Local anesthetic(s), 22–23, 22t
  adverse effects and side-effects of, 23, 39–40
  allergic reactions to, 23, 30
  amide, 22t, 23, 29, 30t
  cardiotoxicity of, 23, 27, 39–40
  clearance of, 29
  ester, 22–23, 22t, 29, 30t
  injection
    intraneural, 40
    technique for, 32
    vasovagal response to, 40
  maximal dosage, 39, 39t
  mechanism of action of, 22, 29
  overdose, 27
  peripheral neurotoxicity caused by, 40
  pharmacokinetics of, 29
  pharmacology of, 22t, 29, 30t
  systemic absorption of, 29
  tachyphylaxis to, 40

Local anesthetic(s) (continued)
    topical, 31
        formulations, 31
    toxicity
        CNS symptoms of, 27, 39
        systemic, treatment of, 39–40
Lop ear deformity, 278
    correction, technical aspects of, 279–282, 279f–281f
Lorazepam, 24
Lower face, dermal fillers for, 151, 151f
Ludwig classification, of female-pattern baldness, 317,
        318f
Luer Lock, female-to-female adapter, 148, 148f, 149
Lunchtime peel. See Glycolic acid
Lycopene, photoprotective effects of, 14

M
MACS. See Minimal access cranial suspension (MACS) lift
Malar edema, with fillers for facial augmentation, 173–174
Malar eminence, 178f
    autologous fat transfer to, 180
Malic acid, 14
Malignant hyperthermia, 26–27
Mallampati classification, 20, 21f
Mandible
    angle of, autologous fat transfer to, 180–181, 182f
    autologous fat transfer to, 151, 151f
Mandibular ligament, 3, 3f
Mandibular nerve, 31, 31f
    blocks, 36
Mandibular ramus, autologous fat transfer to, 180–181
Marcaine. See Bupivacaine
Marginal mandibular nerve, anatomy, 303
Marionette groove(s), 178f
    autologous fat transfer to, 183f, 184, 184f–185f
Marionette line(s). See Marionette groove(s)
Masseteric-cutaneous ligament, 3, 3f
Masseter muscle, 190f, 192
    botulinum neuromodulator injection for, 195
Mastisol, allergic reaction to, 214, 215f
Matrix metalloproteinase (MMP), in photoaging, 13
Maxillary nerve, 31, 31f
    blocks, 33–36
McCollough Facial Rejuvenation Classification System, 69,
        70t, 71f
    abbreviations used in, 69, 70t
Medium-depth chemical peel(s), 43, 48, 49f, 69, 81, 81f
    agents for, 49
    complications of, 56
    contraindications to, 50, 51t
    historical perspective on, 47
    indications for, 47, 48t
    patient selection for, 50
    postoperative care for, 53, 54t
    pretreatment for, 51
    results of, 53, 54f–55f
    scientific principles of, 47
    technical aspects of, 51–53, 52f–53f
Melanin
    liposomal spray, 122
    production of, 82

as target in laser hair removal, 117–118
as target in laser treatment of scars, 125–126
Melanocyte(s), 43, 82
    ultraviolet radiation exposure and, 2
Melanosome(s), 11
Melanosome-transfer inhibitor(s), 12–13
Melanozyme, 13
Melasma, 82
    chemical peel for, 47, 48t
    superficial chemical peel and, 44
    treatment of, 12
Melolabial fold
    autologous fat transfer to, 182f
    dermal fillers for, 151
Melomental fold, dermal fillers for, 151, 153f
Mentalis muscle, 190f, 192
Mental nerve
    anatomy, 31f, 37, 37f
    block
        area of anesthesia with, 37
        technical aspects of, 37
Mentolabial crease, 5
Mentolabial sulcus, 178f
Mepivacaine, 29
    maximal dosage, 39, 39t
Metabisulfite, 30
Methylparaben, 30
Mexoryl, 14
MH. See Malignant hyperthermia
MH Hotline, 27
Miami Peel, 15
Microdermabrasion
    for Fitzpatrick types IV–VI, postoperative care, 85
    indications for, 16, 82
    patient selection for, 82
    in perioral region, 270
    principles of, 16
    results of, 16
    scientific principles of, 81
    skin preparation for, 82
    technical aspects of, 84
Microtia, 277
Midazolam, 24, 30
    for seizures from local anesthetic toxicity, 39
Midface
    age-related changes in, 248–249
    anatomy, 248
    biconvexity of, 4
    common problems of, 250t
    dermal fillers for, 151, 151f
    descent of, 3, 249, 250t
    polar bear, 261
    rejuvenation, 247–256
        complications of, 255
        historical perspective on, 247–248
        patient selection for, 250–251
        postoperative care, 255
        preauricular approach, 247
        principles of, 247–248
        results, 255
        transblepharoplasty approach, 247

transtemporal approach, 247
  volume restoration in, 248
Midface lift
  transblepharoplasty approach, 252, 252f–253f
  transtemporal approach, 252–253
Midface vector, 261, 261f. *See also* Negative vector
Midforehead lift, 224–225, 225f
Milia, 79
  after chemical peel, 46
  after laser skin resurfacing, 104, 133
Mineral oil, 9–10
Minimal access cranial suspension (MACS) lift, 285–286
Minoxidil, 318
MMPs. *See* Matrix metalloproteinase (MMP)
Moisturizer(s), 9. *See also* Natural moisturizing factor(s)
Monitored anesthesia care, 20
Monitoring, during office-based procedures, 21
MPAA. *See* Androgenic alopecia, male pattern
Müller's muscle, 234, 234f
Mushrooms, in topical preparations, 11
Mylohyoid nerve, anatomy, 37
Myobloc, 189

N
Naloxone, 25, 27
Narcan. *See* Naloxone
Naropin. *See* Ropivacaine
Nasal defect(s)
  external, anatomy, 159
  liquid injectable silicone for, 158–159
    results, 160–161, 161f–162f
Nasalis muscle, 190f, 191
  botulinum neuromodulator injection for, 194
Nasojugal groove, 178f
  autologous fat transfer to, 180
Nasolabial fold(s), 178f
  age-related changes in, 302
  autologous fat transfer to, 181–182, 181f, 183f
  deepening of, 4
Nasolabial region, age-related changes in, 4
Natural moisturizing factor(s), 8–9, 14
Nausea and vomiting, postoperative, 25–26
Navoban. *See* Tropisetron
Neck
  as aesthetic subunit, 178f, 179t
  autologous fat transfer to, 185
  botulinum neuromodulator injection for, 195
  muscular anatomy, 192
  superficial venous system of, 303
Necklace lines, 192
  botulinum neuromodulator injection for, 195
Negative vector, 249, 250f, 250t, 261, 261f
Nerve injury, in midface surgery, 255
Neuroma, postoperative, 231
Neuromodulator(s), 189–196. *See also* Botulinum
    neuromodulator(s)
  contraindications to, 192
  facial muscles targeted by, 190, 190f
  mechanism of action of, 189
Niacinamide, 12
NMDA receptor antagonist. *See* Ketamine

NMF. *See* Natural moisturizing factor(s)
Nonsteroidal anti-inflammatory drugs (NSAIDs), for
    UVB-induced inflammation, 11
Norwood classification, of male-pattern baldness, 317,
    317f
Nose. *See also* Nasal *entries*
  aesthetics of, 193
  age-related changes in, 4, 5f
  anatomy, 198
  cartilage irregularities, after rhinoplasty, 210–211,
    211f–212f
  muscular anatomy, 191–192
NPO guidelines, 21–22t

O
Oatmeal, 11
Occlusives
  for basic skin care, 9–10
  in postoperative care, 15
  postprocedure application, with medium-depth
    chemical peel, 53
  postprocedure use, after ablative resurfacing, 15
Olive oil, 10
Onabotulinum tox n, 6
Onabotulinumtoxin A, 189, 254. *See also* Botulinum
    neuromodulator(s)
  storage of, 190
Ondansetron, 26t
Ophthalmic artery, dermal filler embolization in, 156
Ophthalmic nerve, 31, 31f–32f
  blocks, 32–33
Opioid(s), 25
  adverse effects and side effects of, 25
  overdose, 27
  pharmacology of, 25
  reversal of, 25, 27
Oral commissure(s)
  botulinum neuromodulator injection for, 194–195
  dermal fillers for, 151
Orbicularis oculi muscle, 190, 190f, 191, 191f, 234, 234f,
    235, 235f, 257–258
  extracanthal, 258, 259f
  functions of, 257–258
  inner-canthal, 258, 259f
  innervation of, 258, 259f
  and lacrimal apparatus, 259f
  orbital, 258, 259f
  preseptal, 258, 259f
  pretarsal, 258, 259f
Orbicularis oris muscle, 190f, 192, 268
  age-related changes in, 4–5
Orbital fat
  bulging, 235
  compartments, 235, 235f, 248, 249f, 301
  inferior prolapse, 249, 250t, 251, 251f
  pseudoherniation, 237, 238f
  pseudoprolapse, 249, 250t
  removal, in upper eyelid blepharoplasty, 240–241, 240f
Orbital hollowing, filler for, 228, 229f
Orbital rim, lower, autologous fat transfer to, 181f
Orbitomalar ligament, 248, 249f

Otoplasty, 277
    clinical applications of, 277
    complications of, 283–284
    patient age and, 278
    patient selection for, 278
    postoperative care, 282
    principles of, 277
    results, 281f, 282, 284, 284f
    technical aspects of, 279–282

P
Para-aminobenzoic acid, 23, 30
Patipa test, 265, 265t
PCA Peel, 15
PDT. See Photodynamic therapy
Peanut oil, 10
Peau d'orange, 192, 195
Peel(s). See also Chemical peel(s)
    historical perspective on, 42, 47
Perfecta laser, 110
Periocular area, musculature of, 190f, 191, 191f, 248,
        248f
Perioral region
    as aesthetic subunit, 178f, 179t
    age-related changes in, 268–269, 269f
    autologous fat transfer to, 179–180, 180f, 181–185
    botulinum neuromodulator injection for, 194–195
    dermal fillers for, 151–153, 152f
    muscular anatomy, 190f, 192
    skin rejuvenation in, 269–270, 269f–270f
Periorbital region
    abbreviations used in, 69, 70t
    as aesthetic subunit, 178f, 179t
    age-related changes in, 3–4
    dermal fillers for, 149–150, 150f
Perlane, 147–148, 167t, 228, 253
    for facial augmentation, 168
Petrolatum, 9–10
Phenergan. See Promethazine
Phenol-croton oil formulation. See also Hetter chemical
        peel(s)
    Baker-Gordon, 58, 58t
    original ("classic") Baker, 58–59, 58t
Phenol peel, 47
    complications of, 66
    contraindications to, 69
Phenol peeling, Brown's three doctrines of, 58
Photoaging, 2, 47
    Glogau classification, 50, 50t, 60, 60t
    histopathology of, 47, 48f
    prevention of, 13
    superficial chemical peel and, 44
Photodamage
    in Fitzpatrick types IV–VI, skin care regimen for, 85, 85t,
        86, 86f–88f
    photodynamic therapy for, 96
Photodynamic therapy, 91
    complications of, 97
    contraindications to, 92
    indications for, 96
    patient selection for, 92

principles of, 96
    technique for, 96–97
Photoprotection, after medium-depth chemical peel, 56
Photothermolysis. See also Selective photothermolysis
    fractional
        for scars, 132
        scientific principles of, 98–99
    in laser treatment of facial scars, 125
Phytic acid, 14
Pigmentary aberration(s). See also Dyschromia(s);
        Hyperpigmentation; Hypopigmentation
    after deep chemical peel, 78
    after laser skin resurfacing, 104
    chemical peel for, 47, 48t
    with laser hair removal, 122
    superficial chemical peel and, 44
Pigmented lesions, intense pulsed light therapy for,
        93–94, 94f
Pigment Plus Peel, 15
Pixie ear deformity, 278, 278f
Platysma-auricular ligament, 3, 3f
Platysmal bands, 4, 4f, 192
    botulinum neuromodulator injection for, 195
Platysma muscle, 190f, 192
PLLA. See Poly-L-lactic acid
PMMA. See Polymethyl methacrylate
Poly-L-lactic acid, as filler, 147–149, 167, 167t, 228–229, 253
    for acne scars, 153–154
    for buccal atrophy, 151
    complications of, 156
    embolization in ophthalmic artery, 156
    for facial augmentation, 169–171, 171f
    inflammatory nodules caused by, 156, 156f, 230
    for mandibular arc restoration, 151
    for soft tissue atrophy, 154, 155f
    for temporal region, 150, 150f
Polymethyl methacrylate, as filler, 147, 149, 167, 167t, 253
    for acne scars, 153–154
    complications of, 156
    embolization in ophthalmic artery, 156
    for facial augmentation, 171
PONV. See Postoperative nausea and vomiting
Port wine stain, 108
    intense pulsed light therapy for, 94
    laser treatment of, 110–113, 113f
Postoperative care, for skin, 15
Postoperative nausea and vomiting
    prophylaxis, 25–26
    risk factors for, 25
Postpeel erythema syndrome, 78, 78f
Prejowl(s), 178f
    autologous fat transfer to, 180–181, 181f
Preparation H, postprocedure application, with medium-
        depth chemical peel, 53
Prescar
    definition of, 126
    laser therapy for, 128
Presyncope, with local anesthetic injection, 40
Prevelle, 228
Prevelle Silk, 148, 168–169
Prilocaine, 29

Procaine, 29, 30*t*
Procerus muscle, 3, 190, 190*f*, 191, 191*f*
Prochlorperazine, 26*t*
Promethazine, 26*t*
Propecia, 318
Propofol
  antiemetic effects of, 25–26
  intravenous, dosing guidelines for, 24–25, 24*t*
  pharmacology of, 24
  for seizures from local anesthetic toxicity, 39
Propranolol, for hemangiomas, 112
Propylene glycol, as humectant, 10
Proscar, 318
Puragen, 168–169
Pyruvic acid, 43

Q
Quicklift, 286

R
Radial lip lines, botulinum neuromodulator injection for, 194
Radiesse, 147–148, 167, 228–229, 253
  for facial augmentation, 169, 170*f*
5α-Reductase
  and androgenic alopecia, 317
  inhibitors of, 318–319
Regional block(s)
  of chest, 38–39
  of face, 31–37
  of neck, 38
Relaxed skin tension lines
  in face, 139, 139*f*
  scar alignment with, 139–140, 140*f*
Remifentanil, 25
  intravenous, dosing guidelines for, 24, 24*t*
  pharmacology of, 25
Renova, 13
Resorcinol. *See also* Jessner's solution
  peel, 43, 47
  toxicity, 90
Respiratory depression, management of, 27
Restylane, 147–148, 167*t*, 228, 253
  for acne scars, 153–154, 153*f*
  duration of effects, 148
  for facial augmentation, 168–169, 169*f*
  for lip augmentation, 153
  in periorbital region, 149
Resveratrol, photoprotective effects of, 14
Reticular vein(s), laser treatment of, 110–111
Retin-A. *See* Tretinoin
Retinoic acid
  peel, 43
  for postinflammatory hyperpigmentation, 66
  pretreatment, for laser skin resurfacing, 100
Retinoid(s)
  pretreatment, 15
  topical
    for acne, 13
    antiwrinkling effects of, 13–14
    mechanism of action of, 13

Retinol, 13–14
  pretreatment, for medium-depth chemical peel, 51
Retinyl palmitate, 13–14
Rhinophyma, chemical peel for, 47, 48*t*
Rhinoplasty
  and allergic reaction to adhesive or tape, 214, 215*f*
  columellar show after septal shortening for, 211–212, 213*f*
  complications of, 214–215
  endonasal, 197–208
    advantages of, 197
    alar cartilage delivery in, 202–203, 204*f*
    anatomical considerations in, 198
    anesthesia for, 199
    cartilage delivery technique for, 198, 202–203, 204*f*
    cartilage-splitting incision for, 199, 201*f*–202*f*
    complications of, 205
    directed techniques for office setting, 205
    dorsal approach in, 203, 204*f*
    dorsal reduction and augmentation in, 204
    dressings for, 205
    graft placement and fixation in, 204–205
    historical perspective on, 197
    indications for, 197
    instruments for, 198, 198*f*
    intercartilaginous incision for, 199, 201*f*
    marginal incision for, 199, 200*f*–201*f*
    osteotomies in, 203–204
    patient preparation for, 199
    patient selection for, 198
    planning for, 197
    postoperative care, 205
    preoperative photographs for, 198
    results, 205, 206*f*–207*f*
    retrograde approach to tip for, 202, 202*f*
    for revision, 205
    splints for, 205
    surgical approach for, 199–205
    technical aspects of, 198–205
  fillers in, 212–214, 213*f*–214*f*
  historical perspective on, 197
  malposition after, 210, 210*f*
  nasal bone alignment after digital pressure technique for, 210, 210*f*
  nonsurgical, 158, 160–161, 161*f*–162*f*
  office techniques for, 209–215
  revision
    early postoperative procedures, technical aspects of, 209–210
    late postoperative procedures, 210–212
    office techniques for, 209–215
  scar management after, 212
  scarring caused by, 214–215, 215*f*
  skin complications after, 214, 215*f*
  taping after, 209
Rhytids. *See also* Wrinkling
  chemical peel for, 47, 48*t*
  perioral
    botulinum toxin A for, 270, 270*f*
    dermal fillers for, 151, 152*f*, 270, 271*f*
    persistence of, 276
    skin resurfacing for, 271

Rhytids *(continued)*
  periorbital, 250*t*
  persistent
    after chemical peel, 79
    in perioral region, 276
Risorius muscle, 190*f*, 192
Rogaine, 318
Romazicon. *See* Flumazenil
Ropivacaine, 29, 30*t*
  maximal dosage, 39, 39*t*
Rosacea
  corticosteroids and, 11
  intense pulsed light therapy for, 94, 95*f*
  treatment of, 11
Rounded-eye syndrome, 263
RSTLs. *See* Relaxed skin tension lines

S
Safflower oil, 10
Salicylic acid. *See also* Jessner's solution
  for acne, in Fitzpatrick types IV–VI, 85*t*, 86
  mechanism of action of, 11
  peel, 15, 43, 47, 81, 81*f*
    for acne, 43
    mechanism of action of, 81
    patient selection for, 82
    technical aspects of, 83
Salicylism, 81, 83, 89
Scabies, treatment of, 11
Scalp
  expansion, 320, 327, 327*f*
  flaps
    axial, 326
    random, 326
  laxity, and hair transplantation, 320
  reduction, 326–327, 327*f*
Scar(s)
  acne, 126
    boxcar, 126
      dermal fillers for, 153–154, 153*f*
      laser resurfacing for, 128, 129*f*
    dermal fillers for, 153–154, 153*f*
    icepick, 126
      laser resurfacing for, 128, 129*f*
    laser resurfacing for, 129–130, 129*f*–130*f*
    laser treatment of, 126
    liquid injectable silicone for, 158–160
      results, 162, 162*f*–163*f*
    quartile grading system for, 130, 130*t*
    rolling, 126
      dermal fillers for, 153–154, 153*f*
    types of, 126, 159–160
    valley, dermal fillers for, 153–154, 153*f*
  anatomical location of, and laser treatment, 124
  atrophic, 126
    laser resurfacing for, 129–130, 129*f*–130*f*
    laser treatment of, 126
  burn, laser treatment of, 132, 132*f*
  chemical peel for, 47, 48*t*
  color of, and laser treatment, 124
  dermabrasion for, 144–145

  dermal fillers for, 153–154
  donor site, after autologous fat transfer, 187
  early, laser treatment of, 126–128
  formation of, 138
  herpes zoster, liquid injectable silicone for, results, 163, 164*f*
  hypertrophic, 126
    laser treatment of, 126, 128*f*
    with short-incision facelift and necklift, 298
  laser treatment of, 124–137, 144, 145*f*
    adjunctive corticosteroids with, 128
    adjunctive 5-fluorouracil with, 128
    complications of, 132–135, 134*t*
    historical perspective on, 124
    outcomes with, factors affecting, 124–125
    patient selection for, 126–128
    postoperative care, 129–130
    relation of scar type to preferred treatment modality, 132, 134*t*
    results, 130–131, 131*f*
    technical aspects of, 128–130
  maturation of, improvement with, 138
  nonsurgical treatment of, 144–145
  pathogenesis of, 125
  prevention of, 128
  psychological considerations with, 139
  revision of, characteristics improved by, 138
  surgical
    liquid injectable silicone for, 160, 163, 163*f*
    nonablative fractional photothermolysis for, 132
  surgical treatment of, 138–146
    by direct excision, 140, 140*f*
    geometric broken line closure for, 141, 143*f*
    patient selection for, 139
    postoperative care, 145
    results, 145–146
    technical aspects of, 139–143
    tissue expander in, 143, 144*f*
    tissue transfer for, 141–143, 143*f*
    by w-plasty, 141, 143*f*
    by z-plasty, 140–141, 141*f*
  tracheotomy, direct excision of, 140, 140*f*
  transcolumellar, after rhinoplasty, dermabrasion for, 212
  traumatic
    dermal filler for, 154, 154*f*
    laser treatment of, 132, 132*f*
    liquid injectable silicone for, 160
  types of, 124
Scarring
  after laser skin resurfacing, 105, 135
  with Hetter chemical peel, 66
  hypertrophic
    after chemical peel, 56
    after deep chemical peel, 79
  with laser hair removal, 122
  with laser treatment of vascular lesions, 110–111
  rhinoplasty-related, 214–215, 215*f*
Scleral show, 261
Scleral triangle(s)
  lateral, 257
  medial, 257

Scopolamine, 26*t*
Sculptra, 147, 167, 229–230, 253
  complications of, 156
  for facial augmentation, 169–171, 171*f*
Seborrheic dermatitis, treatment of, 11
Sedation, 20. *See also* Opioid(s)
  deep, 23–24, 23*t*
  for Hetter chemical peel, 61
  intravenous
    dosing guidelines for, 24, 24*t*
    equipment for, 21
  levels of, 23–24, 23*t*, 30, 30*t*
  with medium-depth chemical peel, 51–52
  minimal, 23, 23*t*
  moderate (conscious), 23, 23*t*, 30, 30*t*
  for surgical scar revision, 140
Sedative(s), 23–25, 24*t*
  intramuscular administration of, 24
  intravenous administration of. *See* Sedation,
    intravenous
  oral administration of, 24
  overdose, 27
Seizure(s), from local anesthetic toxicity, 39
Selective photothermolysis, 91, 109, 117, 125
Selenium, 11
Sensorcaine. *See* Bupivacaine
Sensory nerve, postoperative complications in, 231
Septisol, 58
  facial cleansing, with medium-depth chemical peel, 52
Septocaine. *See* Articaine
Seroma, postoperative, 310, 311*f*
  with short-incision facelift and necklift, 297
Short-incision facelift and necklift, 285–299
  historical perspective on, 285–286
  multivector SMAS and platysmal suspension technique
    for, 286
    anatomical considerations in, 286, 287*f*
    complications of, 297–298
    contour irregularities after, 298
    and intraoperative hemorrhage, 297
    large-vessel injury in, 297
    lobule malposition after, 298
    neurovascular injury in, 297
    and poor skin flap design, 297
    postoperative care, 294
    principles of, 286
    results, 294–297, 295*f*–296*f*
    seroma/hematoma after, 297–298
    skin flap vascular compromise and necrosis after, 298
    SMAS damage in, 297
    technical aspects of, 287–293, 288*f*–294*f*
    wound infection after, 298
  patient selection for, 286–287
Silastic sheet(s), topical application, for scar revision, 145
Silicone. *See also* Liquid injectable silicone
  cream, for scar revision, 145
  as filler, 167*t*, 253
    for acne scars, 153–154
  for lip augmentation, 172, 172*f*–173*f*
    overinjection, 172, 173*f*
  sheet, topical application, for scar revision, 145

Silikon 1000, 158–159, 167
  complications of, 172, 173*f*
  for facial augmentation, 171–172, 172*f*–173*f*
Skeleton, facial, age-related changes in, 3
Skin
  adnexal structures, 50, 50*f*
  aging
    extrinsic factors affecting, 9
    intrinsic factors affecting, 9
  anatomy, 50, 50*f*, 81*f*, 82, 125. *See also* Dermis, anatomy;
    Epidermis, anatomy
  dry, in Baumann Skin Typing System, 8
    skin care for, 9–10
  facial
    age-related changes in, 2–3, 9
    anatomy, 50, 50*f*
    resurfacing of, 5, 69
    surgical tightening of, 5
  hydration, 9–10
  necrosis, with fillers for facial augmentation, 172–173
  nonpigmented, in Baumann Skin Typing System, 9
  oily, in Baumann Skin Typing System, 8
  pigmented, in Baumann Skin Typing System, 8–9
    skin care for, 11–13
  rejuvenation, for Fitzpatrick types IV–VI, 80–90
    complications of, 88–90
    results, 85–88, 86*f*–89*f*
  resistant, in Baumann Skin Typing System, 8
  resurfacing of, abbreviations used in, 69, 70*t*
  sensitive, in Baumann Skin Typing System, 8
    topical treatments for, 10–11
    types of, 10, 10*t*
  thickness, age-related changes in, 2
  types
    Fitzpatrick classification, 50, 51*t*, 60, 80
    and resurfacing, 99
  unwrinkled, in Baumann Skin Typing System, 9
  wrinkled, in Baumann Skin Typing System, 9
    prevention of, 13
    skin care for, 13–15
Skin care
  for dry skin, 9–10
  for Fitzpatrick types IV–VI, 85, 85*t*
  for pigmented skin, 11–13
  postoperative, 15
  preprocedure, 15
  for sensitive skin, 10–11
  for wrinkled skin, 13–15
Skin flap(s), for scar revision, 141–143
Skin graft(s), for scar revision, 141–143, 143*f*
Skin polisher(s), 69
Skin typing, 8
S-lift, 285–286
SMAS. *See* Superficial musculoaponeurotic system (SMAS)
Smoking, and chemical peel, 60
Snap test, of lower lid tone, 261, 261*f*
Sodium bicarbonate, added to local anesthetic, 23, 32
Sodium hyaluronate, as humectant, 10
Soft tissue atrophy, dermal fillers for, 153–154, 155*f*
Solar lentigines, superficial chemical peel and, 44
SOOF. *See* Suborbicularis oculi fat pad

Sorbitol, as humectant, 10
Soy, as melanosome-transfer inhibitor, 13
Soybean trypsin inhibitor, 13
Soymilk, 13
SPF. *See* Sun Protection Factor
Spider telangiectasia(s), laser treatment of, 114
Spironolactone, 319
Steroid injections
    for scar management, 230–231
    for supratip problems after rhinoplasty, 209, 210*f*
Stratum basale, 43, 43*f*, 50, 50*f*
Stratum corneum, 43, 43*f*, 50, 50*f*, 82
Stratum granulosum, 43, 43*f*, 50, 50*f*
Stratum lucidum, 43, 43*f*, 50, 50*f*
Stratum spinosum, 43, 43*f*, 50, 50*f*
Sublimaze. *See* Fentanyl
Submalar space, autologous fat transfer to, 180, 182*f*
Suborbicularis oculi fat pad, 248, 249*f*
Succinylcholine, for seizures from local anesthetic toxicity,
    39
Sugar(s), as humectants, 10
Sulfa allergy, and Hydrelle, 172
Sulfacetamide, in topical preparations, 11
Sulfur, in topical preparations, 11
Sunburn, treatment of, 11
Sun exposure
    avoidance, after Hetter chemical peel, 63
    and chemical peel, 60
    and Fitzpatrick skin types, 80
Sunflower oil, 10
Sunlight. *See* Ultraviolet radiation
Sun Protection Factor, 14
Sunscreen, 13–14
    avoidance, after Hetter chemical peel, 63
    chemical blocker type, 14
    for Fitzpatrick types IV–VI, 85*t*, 86
    physical blocker type, 14
    preprocedure use, 60
    superficial chemical peel and, 44–45
    use, after medium-depth chemical peel, 56
Superficial chemical peel(s), 42–46, 48, 48*f*, 69, 81, 81*f*
    agents for, 43
    anatomical considerations in, 43
    complications of, 45–46
    depth of penetration with, 45
    documentation for, 44
    enhanced, 42, 44–45
    erythema with, 45–46
    expected results, 45, 46*f*
    frosting associated with, 45
    healing time for, 45
    indications for, 43
    and laser resurfacing, comparison of, 42
    multiple, 44
    patient selection for, 43–44
    pigmentary changes with, 45–46
    postprocedure care for, 45
    pretreatment for, 42–44
    scientific principles of, 42–43
    sequential application, 44–45
    technical aspects of, 44–45

Superficial musculoaponeurotic system (SMAS), 285, 287*f*
    age-related changes in, 4, 4*f*
    midface, 248
Superior orbital fissure, 31
Supraorbital nerve
    anatomy, 31*f*, 32, 32*f*
    block
        area of anesthesia with, 33
        technical aspects of, 33
Supratrochlear nerve
    anatomy, 31*f*, 33
    block
        area of anesthesia with, 33
        technical aspects of, 33
Surfactant(s), in skin cleansers, 9
Syncope, with local anesthetic injection, 40
Syringoma, chemical peel for, 47, 48*t*

T
Tachyphylaxis, to local anesthetics, 40
Tape, allergic reaction to, 214
Tarsal plate, 234, 234*f*
Tartaric acid, 14
Tazorac, for acne, in Fitzpatrick types IV–VI, 85*t*, 86
TCA. *See* Trichloroacetic acid
Tear trough, anatomy, 249, 249*f*
Tear-trough deformity, 247, 249, 249*f*, 250*t*
    filler for, 150, 168, 169*f*
Telangiectasia
    after rhinoplasty, 210, 211*f*
    intense pulsed light therapy for, 94
    laser treatment of, 110, 114
    spider, laser treatment of, 114
    subtypes of, 114
Telogen effluvium, 315–316, 318
Temporal fat pads, augmentation, dermal filler for, 150,
    150*f*, 230
Temporal hollow, 178*f*
    autologous fat transfer to, 179, 181*f*
    filler for, 230
Temporoparietal flap, 326
Temporoparietal occipital flap, 326
Tetracaine, 22*t*, 23, 29, 30*t*
    ophthalmic, 31
TEWL. *See* Transepidermal water loss
Thiopental, for seizures from local anesthetic toxicity, 39
Tinea versicolor, treatment of, 11
Tissue expander
    in scalp, 327, 327*f*
    and scar revision, 143, 144*f*
Titanium dioxide, 14
Toppik hair-building fibers, 319
TP flap. *See* Temporoparietal flap
TPO flap. *See* Temporoparietal occipital flap
Transderm Scop. *See* Scopolamine
Transepidermal water loss, 9
    inhibition of, 9–10
Tretinoin, 15
    for acne, in Fitzpatrick types IV–VI, 85*t*, 86
    for photodamage, 13
    pretreatment

for Hetter chemical peel, 60–61
for superficial chemical peel, 44
Triamcinolone
  injections
    for scar management, 230
    for supratip problems after rhinoplasty, 209, 210*f*
  for scar revision, 145
Trichloroacetic acid
  for medium-depth chemical peel, 49
  peel, 42–43, 47, 81, 81*f*
    mechanism of action of, 81
    technical aspects of, 84
  for superficial chemical peel, 44–45
Trichophytic incision, 322, 323*f*
Trichotillomania, 316
Trigeminal nerve, sensory distributions of, 31, 31*f*
Tropisetron, 26*t*
Turmeric, 11
  photoprotective effects of, 14
Tyndall effect, 150, 155, 155*f*, 173
Tyrosinase inhibitors, 11–12

U
Ultiva. *See* Remifentanil
Ultraviolet radiation
  and aging of skin, 2
  exposure to, over lifetime, 2
  inflammation caused by, 11
  UVA, 14
  UVB, 14
Urea, 10

V
Valacyclovir hydrochloride
  prophylactic administration, 51
  therapy with, in patients with positive history of HSV, 61
Valium. *See* Diazepam
Valtrex. *See* Valacyclovir hydrochloride
Vancouver scar scale, 130, 130*t*
Vaniqa. *See* Eflornithine hydrochloride cream
Varilite laser, 110
Vascular lesions
  classification of, 108
  historical perspective on, 107
  intense pulsed light therapy for, 94, 95*f*
  laser treatment of, 107–116
    complications of, 115
    results, 114–115
  maternal impression and, 107
  treatment of, options for, 108
Vascular malformation(s), 108
  capillary, laser treatment of, 112–113
  laser treatment of, 110–111
  pathophysiology of, 108
  venous, laser treatment of, 113, 114*f*

Vasovagal response, with local anesthetic injection, 40
Versed. *See* Midazolam
Viafill System, 177
Vision loss, dermal filler embolization in ophthalmic
    artery and, 156
Vitamin C
  photoprotective effects of, 14
  topical, for postlaser erythema, 15
Vitamin E, photoprotective effects of, 14
Volume, facial
  addition, 300–301
  age-related changes in, 3, 300–301
  removal, 300–301
  repositioning, 300–301

W
Walnut oil, 10
Water, as cutaneous chromophore, 125
Wound repair, stages of, 125, 138
W-plasty, for scar revision, 141, 143*f*
Wrinkling. *See also* Rhytids
  age-related factors and, 2–3
  forehead, 3
  of lips, 4–5, 6*f*
  periorbital, 3–4
  ultraviolet radiation exposure and, 2

X
Xanthelasma, chemical peel for, 47, 48*t*
Xeomin, 189, 255. *See also* Botulinum neuromodulator(s)
Xylocaine. *See* Lidocaine

Z
Zinc oxide, 14
Zofran. *See* Ondansetron
Zovirax. *See* Acyclovir
Z-plasty(ies)
  multiple, for scar revision, 141, 142*f*
  for scar revision, 140–141, 141*f*
Zyderm, 166, 228
Zygomatic ligament, 3, 3*f*
Zygomaticofacial nerve
  anatomy, 31*f*, 34, 35*f*
  block
    area of anesthesia with, 34
    technical aspects of, 34
Zygomaticotemporal foramen, 34, 35*f*
Zygomaticotemporal nerve
  anatomy, 31*f*, 34, 35*f*
  block
    area of anesthesia with, 34
    technical aspects of, 34
Zygomaticus major muscle, 190*f*, 192
Zygomaticus minor muscle, 190*f*
Zyplast, 166